STRENGTH AND CONDITIONING

CONDITIONING

A Biomechanical Approach

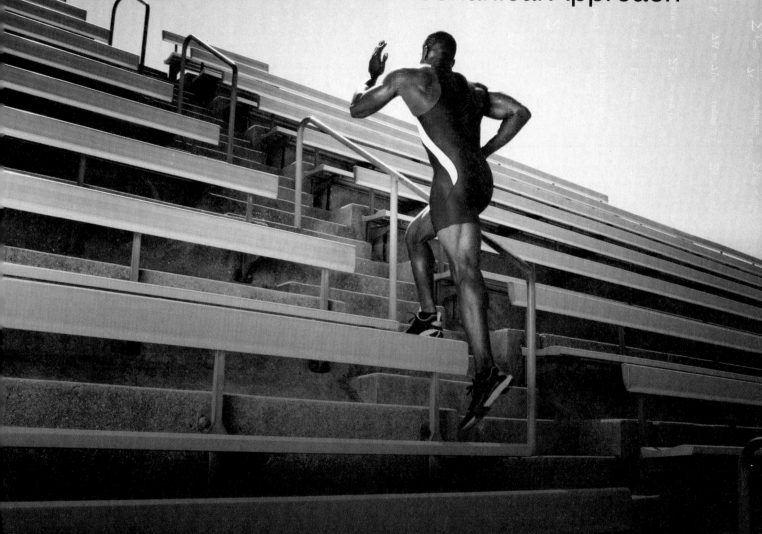

STRENGTH AND CONDITIONING

A Biomechanical Approach

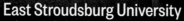

Gavin L. Moir, PhD

Associate Professor
Exercise Science Department
East Stroudsburg University

JONES & BARTLETT
LEARNING

World Headquarters
Jones & Bartlett Learning
5 Wall Street
Burlington, MA 01803
978-443-5000
info@jblearning.com
www.jblearning.com

Jones & Bartlett Learning books and products are available through most bookstores and online booksellers. To contact Jones & Bartlett Learning directly, call 800-832-0034, fax 978-443-8000, or visit our website, www.jblearning.com.

02212-4

Production Credits

Chief Executive Officer: Ty Field
President: James Homer
Chief Product Officer: Eduardo Moura
VP, Executive Publisher: David D. Cella
Publisher: Cathy L. Esperti
Associate Acquisitions Editor: Kayla Dos Santos
Editorial Assistant: Sara J. Peterson
Associate Director of Production: Julie C. Bolduc
Production Assistant: Brooke Appe
Senior Marketing Manager: Andrea DeFronzo

VP, Manufacturing and Inventory Control: Therese Connell
Composition: Cenveo Publisher Services
Cover Design: Kristin Parker
Rights and Media Manager: Joanna Lundeen
Media Development Assistant: Shannon Sheehan
Photo Research and Permissions Coordinator: Amy Rathburn
Cover Image: © Jupiterimages/Stockbyte/Thinkstock
Printing and Binding: Courier Companies
Cover Printing: Courier Companies

Library of Congress Cataloging-in-Publication Data

Moir, Gavin, author.
  Strength and conditioning: a biomechanical approach / by Gavin Moir.
    p. ; cm.
  Includes bibliographical references and index.
  ISBN 978-1-284-03484-4 (pbk. : alk. paper)
  I. Title.
  [DNLM: 1. Biomechanical Phenomena. 2. Physical Conditioning, Human–physiology. 3. Athletic Performance–physiology. 4. Movement–physiology. 5. Muscle Strength–physiology. QT 256]
  QP303
  612.7'6–dc23
                    2014037491
6048

Printed in the United States of America
19 18 17 16 15   10 9 8 7 6 5 4 3 2 1

Brief Contents

Table of Contents

Preface

Physical training is a process through which genetic potential is realized (Tucker & Collins, 2012), and strength and conditioning practitioners are tasked with implementing physical training to optimize the performance of their athletes. It is difficult to quantify the importance of strength and conditioning in the preparation of athletes, but the strength and conditioning coach is now a common element in the training process. The field of strength and conditioning is becoming more professionalized, as highlighted by the founding of organizations such as the Australian Strength and Conditioning Association, the National Strength and Conditioning Association, and the U.K. Strength and Conditioning Association. The academic preparation of strength and conditioning professionals is a high priority of each of these organizations.

Biomechanics is formally defined as the application of mechanics to biological organisms, where the action of forces on the organism is studied within a framework of Newtonian mechanics. The application of biomechanics to strength and conditioning is not well represented in existing texts, yet biomechanics informs our understanding of both the adaptations to exercise and the principles underlying sporting movements. Beyond the formal definition of the subject, Bartlett (2007) defines the focus of biomechanics as being the assessment of movement patterns of athletes, a description that holds great significance for a practitioner. The regrettable lack of emphasis on biomechanics in the study of strength and conditioning may stem from the difficulties associated with the counterintuitive concepts with which the student must grapple (Heishe & Knudson, 2008). Eschewing this subject, however, is unfortunate given the insight the practitioner can gain from an understanding of biomechanical principles.

While biomechanics is underrepresented in strength and conditioning texts, skill acquisition is rarely mentioned at all. This is an enormous oversight for a field in which the practitioners are implicitly concerned with how athletes are able to coordinate their movements in a given situation. When reading the coverage afforded to skill acquisition in extant literature related to strength and conditioning, one may easily infer that the role of the practitioner is to specify which movements the athlete should employ in their given sports. These movements can then be trained for, it would seem, through the administration of specific drills that are repeated until the coach deems that the movement has been learned. This repetitious, drill-based approach to motor skill acquisition is necessarily predicated on the assumption there is a single, optimal model for a given movement task. An obvious corollary to such an approach is that the strength and conditioning coach is aware of such optimal models. This scenario would require the practitioner to demonstrate a clear understanding of biomechanical principles, something that is unlikely to be garnered from existing strength and conditioning texts. Moreover, the "cookie-cutter" approach to skill acquisition contained within the literature ignores the individual constraints that act upon each athlete that must preclude the existence of "optimal" models for specific movements. Indeed, some authors refer to this optimal model approach to coaching simply as *lazy* (Bartlett, 2007). This texts applies a constraints-led approach to skill acquisition (Davids, 2010). Within this framework, strength and conditioning practitioners are encouraged to develop training sessions and practices that allow athletes to explore the movements that are appropriate for them to achieve the goals of a specific task rather than prescribe specific movement patterns.

Another premise of this text is that the practices adopted by strength and conditioning practitioners should be guided by evidence. Evidence-based practice was developed in the medical fields in response to the perceived need to base practice upon evidence accrued from a number of often disparate sources. The call for an evidence-based approach to practice has been proposed in strength and conditioning specifically (English, Amonette, Graham, & Spiering, 2012) due to the misleading and often bogus information that abounds in this field. Before practitioners change their training practices to incorporate new devices or methods, they should have sufficient evidence of their efficacy. This text presents the latest evidence to support the claims made within each chapter.

Content Overview

Chapters 1 through 5 cover aspects of biomechanics pertinent to strength and conditioning. Topics discussed include Newtonian mechanics; the mechanics of biologic tissue, including muscle and tendon; bioenergetics; and the different indices of muscular strength and their importance for specific sports. Chapters 6 through 8 focus on some programming aspects of strength and conditioning, covering training methods to develop muscular strength and power, flexibility, and the development of effective warm-up regimens. Chapter 9 introduces performance analysis techniques in sport that enable the determination of the physiological, mechanical, and technical demands of specific sports in addition to the assessment of the techniques used in the execution of sport-specific skills. The constraints-led approach to skill acquisition is introduced in Chapter 10. Chapters 11 through 13 apply the concepts introduced in the previous chapters to the fundamental movements involved in jumping, landing, and sprint running.

Audience

This text is aimed at higher-level undergraduate students and graduate students studying strength and conditioning. However, it also provides a valuable resource for professionals in the strength and conditioning field. Due to the nature of the material contained within the text, it is expected that the reader has an understanding of basic anatomy and physiology and has completed an introductory class in biomechanics.

Pedagogy

The text contains the following pedagogical elements:

- *Objectives* are presented at the beginning of each chapter.

- *Worked Example* boxes employ real-world scenarios to give sample calculations of the mathematic principles discussed in the chapter.

- *Applied Research* boxes emphasize the research related to the chapter's topic.

- *Concept* boxes within each chapter highlight issues relevant to the chapter's topic.

- Each chapter closes with a *Chapter Summary* and *Review Questions and Projects.*

- An extensive glossary covers terms important to understanding the biomechanics of strength and conditioning.

- Appendices expand on some of the more complex mathematical techniques required to perform biomechanical analyses and offer useful resources to aid the student in locating and evaluating scientific evidence.

About the Author

Gavin Moir works in the Exercise Science Department at East Stroudsburg University where he teaches undergraduate and graduate classes in biomechanics, skill acquisition, and strength and conditioning. Dr. Moir is the Program Director for the MS Exercise Science degree at East Stroudsburg University and has published over 30 research articles and book chapters in the fields of biomechanics and strength and conditioning.

References

Bartlett, R. (2007). *Introduction to biomechanics: Analysing human movement patterns.* Oxford, UK: Routledge.

Davids, K. (2010). The constraints-based approach to motor learning: Implications for a non-linear pedagogy in sport and physical education. In I. Renshaw, K. Davids, & G. J. P. Savelsbergh (Eds.), *Motor learning in practice: A constraints-led approach* (pp. 3–16). Oxfordshire, UK: Routledge.

English, K. L., Amonette, W. E., Graham, M., & Spiering, B. A. (2012). What is "evidence-based" strength and conditioning? *Strength and Conditioning Journal, 34,* 19–25.

Heishe, C., & Knudson, D. (2008). Student factors related to learning in biomechanics. *Sports Biomechanics, 7,* 398–402.

Tucker, R., & Collins, M. (2012). What makes a champion? A review of the relative contribution of genes and training to sporting success. *British Journal of Sports Medicine, 46,* 555–561.

Reviewers

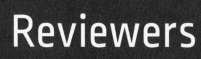

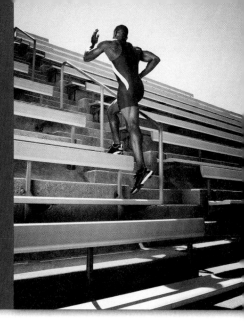

Erin R. Beckwith, MEd, ATC, CSCS
Instructor
The College of Mount St. Joseph
Cincinnati, OH

Greg Ehlers EdD, ATC, CSCS
Associate Professor
Concordia University Wisconsin
Mequon, WI

Rebecca Kudrna, MS, CSCS
Faculty
DeSales University
Center Valley, PA

Kim Puopolo-Larcom
Adjunct Professor
Movement Arts, Health Promotion
Bridgewater State University
Bridgewater, Massachusetts

Hal Strough, PhD, ATR, ATC
Chair
Department of Athletic Training
The College of St. Scholastica
Duluth, MN

Amasay Tal, PhD, CSCS, HFS
Assistant Professor, Physical Education & Coaching Program Coordinator
School of Human Performance & Leisure Sciences
Barry University
Miami Shores, FL

Green T. Waggener, PhD, MPH
Assistant Professor, Exercise Science
Department of Health, Leisure, & Exercise Science
University of West Florida
Pensacola, FL

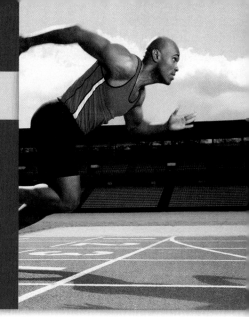

CHAPTER 1

Basic Mechanics: Kinematic Variables

Chapter Objectives

At the end of this chapter, you will be able to:

- Describe the three-dimensional reference frame used to analyze human movements
- Explain the importance of the center of mass of a body
- Describe different types of motion
- Explain the relationships between the kinematic variables of position, velocity, and acceleration
- Use the equations of motion to determine the outcome of movement tasks
- Describe the different technologies that can be used to record linear and angular kinematic variables and the relative merits of each

Key Terms

Acceleration

Angular displacement

Central difference formulae

Equations of motion

First central difference
method

General motion

Kinematic variables

Linear displacement

Position

Radial acceleration

Rotation

Second central difference
method

Translation

Velocity

Chapter Overview

Mechanics is the study of the forces that act on a body and the changes in motion arising from these forces. This chapter will focus on the **kinematic variables** associated with a biomechanical analysis of human movements. Kinematic variables allow the description of the motion of a body without reference to variables that act to change the motion of the body. (The variables that act to change the motion of a body, kinetic variables, will be covered elsewhere.) An appreciation of the kinematic variables associated with an athlete's movements will allow the strength and conditioning practitioner to use specific technologies to assess an athlete's performance in a variety of movement tasks.

This chapter is not intended to be an exhaustive review of mechanical concepts. Rather, the mechanical variables that are pertinent to the fundamental movements covered in subsequent chapters will be addressed. This chapter should therefore be regarded as a reference for the later chapters as well as an introduction to mechanics. Readers should familiarize themselves with the SI units, vectors and scalars, vector analysis, and anatomic terminology before beginning this chapter. We begin our coverage of basic mechanics by defining the three-dimensional reference frame in which all movements take place.

The Mechanical Reference Frame

In any mechanical analysis of human movements, an appropriate reference frame is required that allows the description of the position of the body under analysis. A typical three-dimensional Cartesian coordinate system that is often used in biomechanical analyses is shown in Figure 1.1. In this reference frame, the y-axis corresponds to the principal horizontal direction of movement, while the z-axis corresponds to the vertical direction of movement. Note that this is not the coordinate system adopted by the International Society of Biomechanics, whose convention specifies the principal horizontal direction of movement along the x-axis, with the vertical axis being y. The designation of the orthogonal axes used to define the reference frame really has little effect on the subsequent analysis; what is important is that the reference frame is clearly defined. The convention shown in Figure 1.1, which will be used throughout this text, is that adopted by many technologies that the practitioner will encounter during mechanical analyses of human movements (e.g., motion-analysis systems, force plates).

The use of an appropriate reference frame allows the position of the system under analysis to be described at any point in time through reference to the position along a specific axis relative to the origin of the reference frame. For example, imagine an athlete during a 100-m sprint. If we set our reference frame such that the origin is at the start line and the athlete runs along the y-axis (the principal horizontal direction of motion), then at any point in time during the race we would be able to identify the position of the athlete in one-dimensional space. The selection of an appropriate reference frame during a biomechanical analysis provides meaning to the terms "at rest" and "in motion." Specifically, a body that is at rest will not change its position within the predefined reference frame, while one in motion will be changing its position along one, two, or three of the axes. Clearly, the body's state can be determined only if the body in question is being analyzed within an appropriate reference frame. Furthermore, the

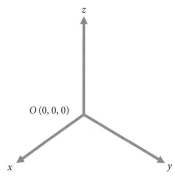

Figure 1.1 A three-dimensional reference frame typical of that used in biomechanical analyses of movements. The y-axis corresponds to the principal horizontal direction of movement. It is assumed that this reference frame does not move during any analysis.

Note: O is the origin of the reference frame.

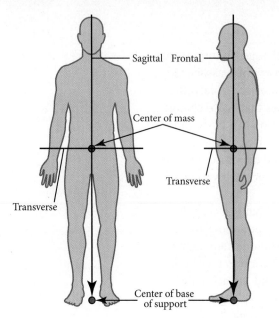

Figure 1.2 When the athlete is in the anatomic position, the center of mass is located close to the navel. The center of mass is located at the intersection of the frontal, sagittal, and transverse planes.

declaration of the reference frame in which the analysis is taking place provides meaning to the direction associated with the vector quantities that are used within a mechanical analysis of movement.

The Center of Mass

In a biomechanical analysis, the human body is often reduced to a point known as the center of mass (CM) when describing whole-body motion. Mass is the quantity of matter contained within a body (measured in kilograms), a quantity that will not be affected by the location in which the individual is being measured. The mass of a body is the same on the moon as it is on the Earth; it is the weight of the body that is dependent upon the magnitude of the gravitational force, and therefore measurement location (see Mechanical Concept 1.1). The CM is then defined as the virtual point about which the mass of the body is evenly distributed. The human body can be reduced to a point-mass system in many biomechanical analyses, with the CM becoming the reference for motion and the action of forces external to the body.

When stood in the anatomical position, the CM is located approximately around the navel (Figure 1.2), although by moving the body segments the location of the CM can move. For example, raising the arms above the head causes the CM to rise within the body. Similarly, when manipulating external masses, such as when performing resistance-training exercises, the location of the CM of the system (mass of athlete + external mass) can be modified considerably. For example, holding a loaded barbell above the head in an overhead squat increases the height of the CM above the ground considerably. As well as being the reference point for the motion of the body and the action of external forces, the CM represents the point through which an axis of rotation passes when the body is free to rotate in space. It should also be recognized that each individual segment that comprises the human body has a CM, while any implement that the athlete is manipulating will also have its own CM.

Mechanical Concept 1.1

Center of mass and center of gravity

The center of mass is the virtual point about which the mass of the body is evenly distributed. The center of gravity is the virtual point at which the gravitational force acts on a body and is the point where the weight force can be said to be acting. We can assume that the center of mass and the center of gravity coincide as humans operate within a constant gravitational field when on the Earth. However, in space, where the influence of gravity has been removed, the center of gravity no longer exists, while the center of mass remains. The term center of mass will be used throughout this text.

Describing Motion with Kinematic Variables

With the identification of a mechanical reference frame and the knowledge of the CM, we now have the beginnings of the mechanical description of motion. Kinematic variables can be used to describe the state of rest or motion of a body, and these variables include the position, velocity, and acceleration of the body under investigation.

Position

We have already introduced the idea that in order to be in motion, a body must be changing its **position** within an appropriate reference frame. Let's use the example of the 100 m sprinter again, where we are expressing the location of the athlete's CM along the principal horizontal direction of movement (y-axis). At time t_0 let's assume that the athlete's CM is located at the origin of the reference frame (0 m along the axis). At time t_1 we record the athlete's CM at 8 m from the origin along the axis. Given this information, we can now record the athlete's change in position as the final position minus the initial position along the y-axis to provide a variable known as the **linear displacement** (s) of the athlete during the time of analysis. In this particular example, the linear displacement of the athlete during the time of analysis is 8 m. It is this linear displacement undergone by the athlete within the reference frame that we use to establish a change in the athlete's linear position. Figure 1.3 provides an example of linear displacement associated with an athlete performing a standing long jump. It can be determined from this illustration that the position of the CM is at 0 m along the y-axis at t_0. At time $t_{1.87}$ the CM is recorded at 2.19 m along the y-axis. The linear displacement undergone by the CM during the time of analysis along the y-axis is therefore 2.19 m. The positive displacement value gives meaning to the direction of motion within the reference frame used. If the athlete had jumped in the opposite direction, the linear displacement undergone would have been – 2.19 m. Recognize

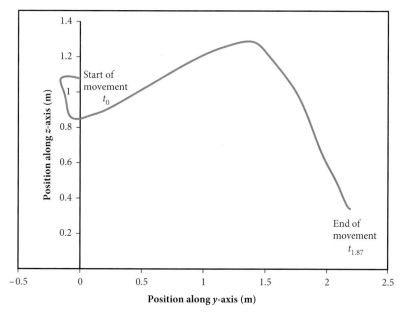

Figure 1.3 A graph showing the two-dimensional position of an athlete's center of mass viewed in the sagittal plane during a standing long jump.

that we have calculated the linear displacement of the CM during the time of the analysis. This is likely to be different from the distance between the feet from takeoff to landing that would typically be recorded during such a movement task. Finally, notice that the position of the CM has changed concomitantly along the z-axis during the time of analysis but that the axes are treated independently during the analysis.

The same methods can be applied to analyze the change in position of a body that is constrained to rotate about a fixed axis. Imagine an athlete performing a biceps curl with the object of the analysis being the motion of the dumbbell held in the hand. During the movement, the dumbbell rotates about an axis defined by the location of the elbow joint. Let the position of the dumbbell at time t_0 be 0° relative to the origin (the athlete is stood in the anatomical position with the elbow joint fully extended). At time t_1 the dumbbell is now 45° relative to the origin (the elbow joint has undergone flexion), so we can calculate the **angular displacement** (θ) by subtracting the initial angular position from the final angular position during the time of analysis. In this example, the angular displacement undergone by the dumbbell is 45° (or 0.79 rad). The positive value assigned to the angular displacement value indicates that the rotation occurred in a counterclockwise direction, which is defined as positive in the analysis of rotational movements.

So here we have two forms of motion both defined by the body under analysis changing position within a reference frame. In the first example, the linear displacement undergone by the athlete during the 100-m sprint resulted in **translation** of the sprinter's CM, while in the example of the biceps curl, the angular displacement moved through resulted in the **rotation** of the dumbbell. These two types of motion are used in all movements performed by athletes (see Mechanical Concept 1.2).

Mechanical Concept 1.2

Translational and rotational motion

Translational motion occurs when a body changes its position within a reference frame, without changing its orientation. Rotational motion occurs around an axis of rotation and requires the body to change its orientation with respect to the reference frame, which is assumed to be stationary. During a 100-m sprint, the CM of the athlete is translated without being rotated (the CM, being a point, cannot change its orientation within the reference frame). However, viewing the body of the sprinter during the race, we notice that the sprinter does change his or her orientation; the sprinter has a distinct forward lean during the early phases of the race and a more upright posture during the later phases. Indeed, during the stance phase of a running stride, the athlete's body may change its orientation as it is rotated about the stance foot. The CM can be translated only during this time. What is important to note, however, is that any translational motion associated with human movement only results from rotational motion as the segments of the body are constrained to rotate about axes defined by the anatomical joints. Using a specific example, the translational motion of a barbell during a back squat occurs as a result of the rotation of the body segments (trunk, thighs, legs, and feet). This combination of translational and rotational motion to achieve the goal of the task is referred to as **general motion**.

Velocity

While the change of position of a system within the reference frame provides information about the state of rest or motion of the system, it is the **velocity** of the system, defined as the rate of change of position during a time interval (Δt), that provides a more formal description of linear motion:

$$\bar{v} = \frac{\Delta s}{\Delta t}$$
Eq. (1.1)

where $\bar{v}$ is the average linear velocity of the body during the time of analysis, Δs is the change in linear displacement over the time of analysis, and Δt is the time taken to undergo the change in linear displacement. (In the strict mechanical sense, the motion of a body is defined by its momentum, the product of mass and velocity. However, given that the mass of the bodies under investigation in a mechanical analysis of sporting movements remains constant, we can use velocity to describe motion.) The angular equivalent is as follows:

$$\bar{\omega} = \frac{\Delta \theta}{\Delta t}$$
Eq. (1.2)

where $\bar{\omega}$ is the average angular velocity of the body during the time of analysis, $\Delta \theta$ is the change in angular displacement over the time of analysis, and Δt is the time taken to undergo the change in angular displacement. Although the average velocity of a body is informative, rarely will an athlete, or an object that is impelled by an athlete, experience a constant velocity. More likely, velocity will be changing either in magnitude or direction (see **Worked Example 1.1**). Therefore, instantaneous values of velocity are often calculated. In differential calculus, the instantaneous velocity can be calculated as the change as time approaches zero:

$$v = \frac{ds}{dt}$$
Eq. (1.3)

where v is the instantaneous linear velocity, ds is an infinitesimal change in linear displacement, and dt is an infinitesimal change in time. In practical terms, the instantaneous velocity can be estimated using the **first central difference method** (see **Worked Example 1.2**).

Worked Example 1.1
Calculating average linear velocity during sprint running

Athlete A completes a 100-m sprint in 9.71 s, while Athlete B completes the race in a time of 9.84 s. Calculate their average linear velocities.

i. Use Equation (1.1)	$v = \Delta s / \Delta t$
ii. Athlete A	$v = 100/9.71$
iii. Athlete B	$v = 100/9.84$
iv. Answers	$A = 10.30$ m/s, $B = 10.16$ m/s

The values represent the average rate of change of linear position of the athlete over the duration of the race. By themselves, these velocity values provide little information to a strength and conditioning coach (other than informing them that both athletes

(continues)

(continued)

under analysis are very fast, with Athlete A being faster than Athlete B). Observing the athletes during the race, we could assume their velocities were not constant throughout, so how much meaning can we attach to the average values that we have just calculated? Furthermore, the average values tell the strength and conditioning coach little about the phases of the race where the athlete could improve and where the coach can potentially direct the focus of training.

Tables 1.1 and 1.2 contain the time taken for the athletes to complete each of the 20-m phases of the race. We have used Equation (1.1) to calculate the athlete's average velocity during each of these phases.

Table 1.1
The Time Taken for Athlete A to Cover Each 20-m Phase of the 100-m Sprint and the Associated Linear Velocity

Displacement (m)	0–20	20–40	40–60	60–80	80–100
Time (s)	2.92	1.78	1.69	1.63	1.69
Velocity (m/s)	6.85	11.24	11.83	12.27	11.83

Table 1.2
The Time Taken for Athlete B to Cover Each 20-m Phase of the 100-m Sprint and the Associated Linear Velocity

Displacement (m)	0–20	20–40	40–60	60–80	80–100
Time (s)	2.91	1.80	1.71	1.68	1.74
Velocity (m/s)	6.87	11.11	11.70	11.90	11.49

Notice how in both cases the average velocity changes as the athlete progresses through the race. Also notice that rarely do the velocity values come close to the average values of 10.30 m/s and 10.16 m/s that were calculated for athletes A and B, respectively, across the duration of the entire race. From the average values calculated over the 20-m phases, the strength and conditioning coach can identify that Athlete B achieves maximal velocity during the same phase as Athlete A, but that the value is 3% lower than that achieved by Athlete A. The mechanical demands of sprint running during the maximal velocity phase of a sprint are distinct from those associated with the acceleration phase. As such, there are specific methods that can be used to improve maximal velocity sprinting. Notice that this information could not be determined from our original analysis using average velocity calculated over the duration of the entire race.

Worked Example 1.2
Calculating instantaneous linear velocity and acceleration

Instantaneous velocities and accelerations can be estimated from displacement data using **central difference formulae**. Instantaneous velocity can be estimated using the **first central difference method** as follows:

$$v_i = \frac{s_{i+1} - s_{i-1}}{2\Delta t}$$

Eq. (1.4)

where v_i is the instantaneous linear velocity of the data point of interest (s_i), s_{i+1} is the displacement data point one time interval after s_i, s_{i-1} is the displacement data point one time interval before s_i, and Δt is the time interval between consecutive data points.

Instantaneous acceleration can be estimated using the **second central difference method** as follows:

$$a_i = \frac{s_{i+1} - 2s_i + s_{i-1}}{\Delta t^2}$$

Eq. (1.5)

where a_i is the instantaneous linear acceleration of the data point of interest (s_i), s_{i+1} is the displacement data point one time interval after s_i, s_i is the displacement data point of interest, s_{i-1} is the displacement data point one time interval before s_i, and Δt is the time interval between consecutive data points.

Table 1.3 shows a small number of data points associated with the vertical position of an athlete's CM during a vertical jump as the athlete ascends from takeoff, measured using a motion-analysis system. Note that the values presented in the table have been rounded. We have calculated the instantaneous values for linear velocity and acceleration of the data points at times 0.005 s through 0.025 s using the first and second central difference formulae.

Table 1.3
The Vertical Position of an Athlete's Center of Mass as It Rises Toward the Apex of Flight During a Vertical Jump and the Instantaneous Vertical Velocity and Acceleration Values

Time (s)	Position (m)	v (m/s)	a (m/s^2)
0.000	1.486428	–	–
0.005	1.489400	(1.492128 – 1.486429)/ (2 × 0.005) = 0.57	(1.492127 – 2 × 1.489400 + 1.486429)/(0.005^2) = –9.80
0.010	1.492127	(1.494608 – 1.489400)/ (2 × 0.005) = 0.52	(1.494608 – 2 × 1.492127 + 1.489400)/(0.005^2) = –9.84
0.015	1.494608	(1.496844 – 1.492127)/ (2 × 0.005) = 0.47	(1.496844 – 2 × 1.494608 + 1.492127)/(0.005^2) = –9.80
0.020	1.496844	(1.498834 – 1.494608)/ (2 × 0.005) = 0.42	(1.498834 – 2 × 1.496844 + 1.494608)/(0.005^2) = –9.84
0.025	1.498834	(1.500578 – 1.496844)/ (2 × 0.005) = 0.37	(1.500578 – 2 × 1.498834 + 1.496844)/(0.005^2) = –9.84
0.030	1.500578	–	–

Note: The first and last data points for velocity and acceleration are not calculated, as the first and second central differences require the data point prior to and following the data point of interest. There are mathematical techniques that can be implemented to calculate these missing data points, but usually in a biomechanical analysis more data are collected to account for these missing values.

From Table 1.3, notice that instantaneous velocity produces a series of positive values. This can be interpreted as the CM moving up in the reference frame used to analyze the athlete, producing a positive velocity vector. Also notice that the magnitudes of the positive values of velocity are decreasing as time progresses. Indeed, the rate at which the positive velocities are decreasing is reflected in the instantaneous accelerations of the CM. Notice that the acceleration values remain almost constant with the change in time (error associated with the

(continues)

(continued)

data collection process and rounding the values precludes the attainment of constant values). We can interpret this as the system experiencing a constant negative acceleration—exactly what would be expected, as gravity is the only force that is acting on the CM following takeoff.

Table 1.4 shows a small number of data points associated with the vertical position of an athlete's CM during a vertical jump as the athlete descends from the apex of flight (the highest vertical position achieved). Notice again that the values presented in the table have been rounded. We have calculated the instantaneous values for linear velocity and acceleration of the data points at times 0.005 s through 0.025 s using the first and second central difference formulae.

Table 1.4
The Vertical Position of an Athlete's Center of Mass as It Descends from the Apex of Flight During a Vertical Jump and the Instantaneous Vertical Velocity and Acceleration Values

Time (s)	Position (m)	v (m/s)	a (m/s^2)
0.000	1.500578	–	–
0.005	1.498834	(1.496844 – 1.500578)/ (2 × 0.005) = –0.37	(1.496844 – 2 × 1.498834 + 1.500578)/(0.005^2) = –9.84
0.010	1.496844	(1.494608 – 1.498834)/ (2 × 0.005) = –0.42	(1.494608 – 2 × 1.496844 + 1.498834)/(0.005^2) = –9.84
0.015	1.494608	(1.492127 – 1.496844)/ (2 × 0.005) = –0.47	(1.492127 – 2 × 1.494608 + 1.496844)/(0.005^2) = –9.80
0.020	1.492127	(1.489400 – 1.494608)/ (2 × 0.005) = –0.52	(1.489400 – 2 × 1.492127 + 1.494608)/(0.005^2) = –9.84
0.025	1.489400	(1.486428 – 1.492127)/ (2 × 0.005) = –0.57	(1.486428 – 2 × 1.489400 + 1.492127)/(0.005^2) = –9.80
0.030	1.486428	–	–

Note: The first and last data points for velocity and acceleration are not calculated, as the first and second central differences require the data point prior to and following the data point of interest. There are mathematical techniques that can be implemented to calculate these missing data points, but usually in a biomechanical analysis more data are collected to account for these missing values.

Notice that instantaneous velocity values are now negative; the CM is now moving down in the reference frame, resulting in a negative velocity vector. Also notice that the magnitudes of the negative values of velocity are increasing as time progresses. The rate at which the negative velocities are increasing remains almost constant with the change in time. This change in velocity, which is the same as that calculated for the data points as the CM was rising after takeoff, is due to the action of gravity on the CM. The acceleration associated with the gravitational force is –9.81 m/s^2. While the example here used linear values, the central difference formulae can be used with angular displacement data as the input.

Acceleration

The rate of change of linear velocity is known as **acceleration**, with average acceleration being calculated as follows:

$$\bar{a} = \frac{\Delta v}{\Delta t}$$

Eq. (1.6)

where $\bar{a}$ is the average linear acceleration of the body during the time of analysis, Δv is the change in linear velocity over the time of analysis, and Δt is the time taken to undergo the change in linear velocity. The angular equivalent is as follows:

$$\bar{\alpha} = \frac{\Delta\omega}{\Delta t} \qquad \text{Eq. (1.7)}$$

where $\bar{\alpha}$ is the average angular acceleration of the body during the time of analysis, $\Delta\omega$ is the change in angular velocity over the time of analysis, and Δt is the time taken to undergo the change in angular velocity. In differential calculus, the instantaneous acceleration can be calculated as the change in time approaches zero:

$$a = \frac{d^2 s}{dt^2} \qquad \text{Eq. (1.8)}$$

where a is the instantaneous velocity, ds is an infinitesimal change in linear displacement, and dt is an infinitesimal change in time. In practical terms, the instantaneous acceleration can be estimated using the second central difference method (see Worked Example 1.2). Table 1.5 shows the values of linear velocity and acceleration achieved during different movement tasks.

Table 1.5
Values of Linear Velocity and Acceleration Achieved During Different Movement Tasks

Movement	Velocity (m/s)	Acceleration (m/s^2)
Baseball struck by bat	41.7[h]	30,000[b]
Typical release of a javelin	30[b]	
Kicking a soccer ball	30[b]	3,000[b]
Cheetah sprinting	29[a]	
Ostrich sprinting	17[a]	
Shot put release	14.1[f]	
Human sprinting	12.4[c]	3.5[d]
Vertical projection of CM during high jump	4.64[e]	26.4[e]
Snatch lift with maximal load	1.65[g]	

Note: CM is center of mass.
[a]Data from Alexander, R. M. (2003). *Principles of Animal Locomotion*. Princeton, NJ: Princeton University Press.
[b]White, C. (2011). *Projectile Dynamics in Sport*. Oxon, UK: Routledge.
[c]Data from http://www.sportscientists.com.
[d]Blazevich, A. (2007). *Sports Biomechanics. The Basics: Optimising Human Performance*. London, UK: A & C Black Publishers.
[e]Ae, M., Nagahara, R., Ohshima, Y., Koyama, H., Takamoto, M., & Shibayama, K. (2008). Biomechanical analysis of the top three male high jumpers at the 2007 World Championships in Athletics. *New Studies in Athletics, 23*, 45–52.
[f]Gutiérrez-Davila, M. (2009). Biomechanical analysis of shot put at the 12th IAAF World Indoor Championships. *New Studies in Athletics, 24*, 45–61.
[g]Hoover, D. L., Carlson, K. M., Christensen, B. K., & Zebas, C. J. (2006). Biomechanical analysis of woman weightlifters during the snatch. *Journal of Strength and Conditioning Research, 20*, 627–633.
[h]Crisco, J. J., Greenwald, R. M., Blume, J. D., & Penna, L. H. (2002). Batting performances of wood and metal baseball bats. *Medicine and Science in Sports and Exercise, 34*, 1675–1684.

Relationships between kinematic variables

The definitions of displacement, velocity, and acceleration allow the relationships between these kinematic variables to be expressed in a series of equations, known as the **equations of motion**:

$$v_f = v_i + at \qquad \qquad \text{Eq. (1.9)}$$

$$s = v_i t + \frac{1}{2}at^2 \qquad \qquad \text{Eq. (1.10)}$$

$$v_f^2 = v_i^2 + 2as \qquad \qquad \text{Eq. (1.11)}$$

where v_f is the linear velocity of the body at the end of the period of analysis, v_i is the linear velocity of the body at the beginning of the period of analysis, a is the linear acceleration experienced by the body, t is the period of time over which the analysis occurs, and s is the linear displacement that the body undergoes during the period of analysis. These equations become very useful in determining the outcome of human movements given the knowledge of certain kinematic variables associated with the movement (see **Worked Example 1.3**).

Worked Example 1.3
Using the equations of motion

1. An athlete performs a vertical jump where the vertical velocity of her CM is 3.25 m/s at takeoff. Calculate the time of flight.
    i. Use Equation (1.9) $\qquad\qquad\qquad v_f = v_i + at$
    ii. Solve for t $\qquad\qquad\qquad\qquad\quad t = (v_f - v_i)/a$
    iii. Input the known variables $\qquad\; t = (0 - 3.25)/-9.81$

    In this instance, v_f represents the vertical velocity at the apex of flight, a known value of 0 m/s. Therefore, the time calculated is the time taken for the CM to reach the apex. a is the acceleration associated with gravity, which needs to be included because the CM is moving along the vertical axis of our reference frame.

    iv. Double the time calculated $\qquad t = 0.33129 \times 2$
    v. Answer $\qquad\qquad\qquad\qquad\qquad t = 0.66258$

    The CM is assumed to follow a parabola during the time of flight such that the time taken to reach the apex of flight will be the same as that taken to descend from the apex. Therefore, the time of flight in this example is 0.66 s.

2. Given the time of flight calculated in Question 1, determine the athlete's jump height.
    i. Use Equation (1.10) $\qquad\qquad\qquad s = v_i t + \frac{1}{2}at^2$

    Given that we are going to calculate jump height (s) from flight time alone, we will have $v_i = 0$ m/s, a value that is achieved when the CM is at the apex of flight. Therefore, what we will actually calculate is the displacement undergone by the CM as it falls from the apex. Assuming the CM follows a parabola during flight, the displacement up to the apex will equal the displacement down from the apex. As we will be analyzing only half of the flight phase, we will require only half of the total flight time ($t = 0.33129$ s).

    ii. Input the known variables $\qquad\; s = (0 \times 0.33129) + (-4.905 \times 0.33129^2)$
    iii. Answer $\qquad\qquad\qquad\qquad\qquad s = -0.54$

    The displacement is calculated as -0.54 m. Remember, this is the displacement undergone by the CM as it descends from the apex of flight. Assuming a parabola during flight, the displacement undergone as the CM rises to the apex, and therefore the jump height, is the same as during its descent. Because the direction of motion is different, however, we remove the negative sign from our answer to get a jump height of 0.54 m.

Note that the CM will only follow a parabola during flight if the posture at takeoff is the same as that upon landing. This is unlikely to be the case, with the athlete more extended at takeoff compared to landing. This will be reflected in the CM undergoing a greater displacement as it descends from the apex compared to its rise to the apex. Therefore, calculating jump height from the time of flight such as when using a contact mat may result in an overestimation of jump height (Moir, 2008).

3. Given the takeoff velocity for the athlete in Question 1, calculate her jump height.

    i. Use Equation (1.11) $v_f^2 = v_i^2 + 2as$
    ii. Solve for s $s = (v_f^2 - v_i^2)/2a$
    iii. Input the known variables $s = (0^2 - 3.25^2)/(2 \times -9.81)$
    iv. Answer $s = 0.54$ m

Notice that the value calculated is positive. In our reference frame, this means that the CM has undergone an upward displacement from takeoff to the apex of flight (compare this to the negative value calculated in Question 2, which calculated the displacement during the descent of the CM from the apex of flight).

In the examples used here, the body was treated as a point-mass system where the behavior of the CM becomes the focus of the analyses. Furthermore, drag forces associated with the movement of the body through the air (air resistance) are ignored. This assumption is valid for a slow-moving body such as a human performing a jump, but is invalid when the body begins to move faster (indeed, the retarding effects of drag increase with v^2 for humans moving through air). A value of $v \geq 5$ m/s is generally used for the inclusion of drag forces in a mechanical analysis (Grimshaw, Lees, Fowler, & Burden, 2006).

We can combine the equations of motion to determine the horizontal range traveled by a body during flight:

$$s = \frac{v^2 \sin\theta \cos\theta + v\cos\theta \sqrt{v^2 \sin^2\theta + 2gh}}{g}$$

Eq. (1.12)

where s is the horizontal range traveled by the body, v is the velocity at release, θ is the angle of release defined by the angle of the velocity vector (determined by the magnitude of the horizontal and vertical components of the release velocity), g is gravitational acceleration, and h is the difference in height between release and landing. The body can be an implement thrown by an athlete (e.g., javelin, discus), a ball that is kicked or thrown, or even the athlete himself or herself, such as during a long-jump event where the body is defined as the CM of the athlete. Although this Equation (1.12) fails to account for the fluid-dynamic forces of drag and lift, which could have substantial effects on the range of the body, it is very informative for the practitioner because it tells us that the linear velocity of the body at release exerts the greatest influence on the range traveled by the body during flight.

Acceleration experienced by a rotating body

Consider a point on a body that is rotating, such as the head of a golf club during a golf swing. If the instantaneous linear velocity of the point of interest is shown at various times during the movement, the direction of the velocity vector will be

Worked Example 1.4
Radial acceleration when running around a bend

Athletes A and B perform a 200-m sprint. Both athletes attempt to achieve the same linear velocity of 10 m/s, but Athlete A runs the bend in lane 1 (radius of 37.4 m) while Athlete B runs the bend in lane 8 (radius of 43.7 m). Calculate the radial acceleration required for both athletes.

i. Use Equation (1.13) $a_R = v^2/r$

ii. Input the known variables for Athlete A $a_R = 10^2/37.4$

iii. Input the known variables for Athlete B $a_R = 10^2/43.7$

iv. Answers $A = 2.67 \text{ m/s}^2, B = 2.29 \text{ m/s}^2$

Notice that the athlete in lane 1 has to produce a greater radial acceleration in order to continue along the curved path compared to the athlete in lane 8, despite the same linear velocity. Of greater concern is the origin of this acceleration. The required acceleration can be generated only when the athlete is in contact with the ground (stance phase), and it comes from a frictional force. Assuming the athletes are of the same mass, our analysis shows that Athlete A has to supply a frictional force that is 17% greater than that supplied by Athlete B. This potentially means less vertical force production for Athlete A, which would have substantial effects on Athlete A's sprinting velocity. An alternative to mitigate the problem, as per Equation (1.13), is, of course, to reduce the linear velocity around the bend—not a satisfactory solution. This is the reason that no athletes are placed in lane 1 in the 200-m race at athletic championships and that the bends are banked on indoor running tracks that have reduced radii.

continually changing in the specified reference frame, even if the magnitude of the vector remains constant. Given that velocity is a vector variable, a change in its direction constitutes a change in velocity, and therefore the rotating body experiences an acceleration. This **radial acceleration** acts toward the axis of rotation and can be calculated as follows:

$$a_R = \frac{v^2}{r}$$

Eq. (1.13)

where a_R is the radial acceleration experienced at the rotating body, v is the instantaneous linear velocity of the rotating point, and r is the radius of the rotating point. It is the radial acceleration that keeps a body moving along a curved path during the movement. Equation (1.13) tells us that the requisite radial acceleration to ensure the continuation of the curved path of the body increases with the square of linear velocity, but is reduced with increases in the associated radius. This has implications for running around a bend (see **Worked Example 1.4**).

Technology to Record Kinematic Variables

There are various technologies available to the strength and conditioning practitioner to assess the kinematic variables associated with the performance of his or her athletes during running, jumping, and resistance training exercises. These technologies include timing gates, contact mats, Global Position System devices, position transducers, accelerometers, and motion-analysis systems. Kinematic data associated with the motion of an athlete's CM can also be gathered from force data collected from a force plate, a technology that is discussed elsewhere.

Timing gates

Timing gates use photocells to record the timing of events (see Mechanical Concept 1.3). For example, timing gates that are positioned at known distances along the path of motion of a body can be used to calculate the speed of the body under investigation (Figure 1.4). (Because the specific axes of motion cannot be identified using this method, the scalar of speed is calculated rather than the vector of velocity.) Timing gates are typically used in the assessment of running performance where the path of motion taken by the body must be known in advance and consideration to the type of timing gate (number of photocells), the height of the timing gates, and the distance between consecutive pairs of timing gates is required (Yeadon, Kato, & Kerwin, 1999; see Applied Research 1.1). It should be recognized that the data recorded from timing gates will only provide the average speed over a known distance. Running speeds recorded from timing gates have been shown to be reliable (Moir, Shastri, & Connaboy, 2004).

Mechanical Concept 1.3

Photocell technology in timing gates

A photocell is a sensor that exhibits photoconductivity, changing its electrical resistance in response to alterations in a light source. In the case of timing gates, the light source is an infrared beam that is reflected back from a reflector placed a short distance from an emitter. An interruption in the beam caused by the motion of a body through the beam causes a change in the resistance of the photocell, resulting in an increase in the voltage output. The time-history of voltage changes can be recorded to provide information about the temporal characteristics of the interruptions of the beam. If emitter–reflector pairs of timing gates are positioned at known distances along the path of the body under investigation, then the average speed can be calculated based upon the time histories of successive beam interruptions.

Some timing gates used for the analysis of running speed have single photocells, while others have multiple photocells (either two or three) located vertically. Timing gates containing multiple photocells produce an increase in the output voltage only when the beams to each of the photocells are interrupted simultaneously. Such an arrangement guards against the occurrence of false signals associated with single photocell timing gates caused by the beam being broken by the outstretched arm or leg of an athlete running through the timing gates. Timing gates comprising multiple photocells are likely to record the times associated with the torso of the athlete breaking the beams, allowing an approximation of the speed of the athlete's CM to be obtained, and are therefore likely to be more accurate than single photocell timing gates for measuring sprint times (Earp & Newton, 2012; Yeadon et al., 1999).

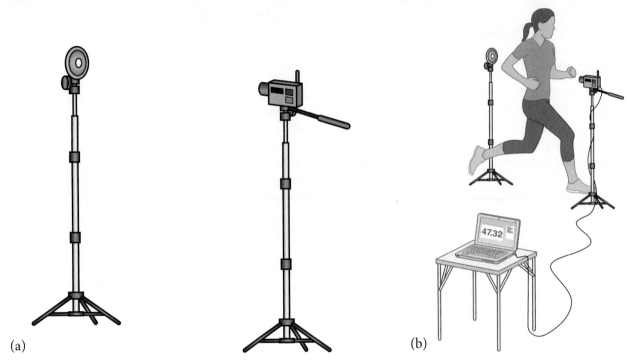

(a)   (b)

Figure 1.4 Timing gates used to record running speed. (a) An emitter–reflector pair. An infrared beam from the emitter (foreground) is reflected back from the reflector placed directly opposite. The interruption of the beams associated with timing gates set at known distances along the path of motion allows the determination of speed. (b) The use of photocells to record the sprinting speed of an athlete.

Applied Research 1.1
Recording sprinting speed using timing gates

The authors assessed the errors in running speeds when using different types of timing gates (single and double photocell) and when setting the gates at different distances along the path of motion. One participant ran at five nominal speeds (5–9 m/s) along a straight running track. Pairs of timing gates were placed along the runway with distances ranging from 1.6 to 2.4 m between consecutive emitter–reflector pairs in the direction of motion. The times obtained from gates using single photocell were compared to those obtained from gates with double photocells. The gates were set at a height such that the lowest photocell was 1.05 m from the ground, corresponding to approximately the height of the participant's hips. A video-based motion-analysis system was used to obtain the actual speed of the participant's CM during each trial, and the speeds from the timing gates were compared to those obtained from the motion-analysis system. The authors reported that the errors in running speed obtained from the timing gates were smaller when the distance between consecutive gates along the path of motion was increased, while the smaller errors in running speed were associated with double photocell gates compared to the single photocell gates. The error in running speeds obtained from single photocell timing gates placed at approximately hip height was 0.1 m/s when the distance between the gates in the direction of motion approximated the stride length of the runner. The authors concluded that timing gates with double photocells should be used when possible and that the distance between the gates in the direction of motion should be set to multiples of the running stride.

Yeadon, M. R., Kato, T., & Kerwin, D. G. (1999). Measuring running speed using photocells. *Journal of Sports Sciences, 17*, 249–257.

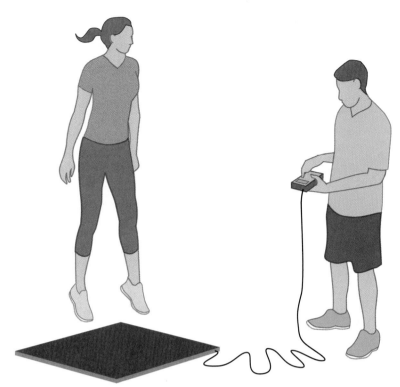

Figure 1.5 A contact mat used to record the time in the air for an athlete during a vertical jump. The pressure exerted by the athlete when stepping on the mat activates microswitches contained within the mat. The pressure is removed when the athlete leaves the mat at takeoff, deactivating the switches and beginning the timing unit. The microswitches are activated upon landing, stopping the timing unit to provide the time in the air.

Contact mats

Contact mats contain microswitches that are activated in response to pressure exerted on the mat, being deactivated once the pressure is removed (Figure 1.5). By connecting the microswitches to a timing unit, a contact mat can be used to provide the time elapsed between consecutive activations caused by the pressure exerted by an athlete's foot contact, allowing contact mats to be used to calculate vertical jump height with the data provided upon completion of the movement. However, the validity of the jump height recorded from a contact mat has been questioned (Buckthorpe, Morris, & Folland, 2012; see Applied Research 1.2), although jump height recorded from a contact mat has been shown to have acceptable reliability (Moir, Shastri, & Connaboy, 2008).

Global Positioning System-based technology

The Global Positioning System (GPS) allows the coordinates of an appropriate receiver to be determined, providing positional information of the receiver in real time (see Mechanical Concept 1.4). GPS receivers can be worn by athletes during practices or competitions (if permitted) to record the distances covered and the speeds achieved (Figure 1.6). Unlike timing gates, the path of motion of the athlete does not have to be determined in advance, allowing the athlete to move freely within the environment, so GPS-based technology can be used to determine kinematic variables associated with player motion in field and court sports. Moreover, the information is gathered online, with no requirements for further calculations, and the high sampling frequency associated with the GPS units allows instantaneous speeds to be approximated. The running speeds obtained from GPS-based technologies are reliable, although the values tend to be lower compared to the speeds obtained from timing gates (Waldron, Worsfold, Twist, & Lamb, 2011; see Applied Research 1.3).

Applied Research 1.2
Recording vertical jump height using a contact mat

The authors compared the height achieved during countermovement vertical jumps performed with an arm swing in a group of 40 participants. Jump height was recorded from a contact mat, a jump-and-reach device (Vertec), and a force plate. The jump height recorded from the force plate served as the criterion measure to which the values from the contact mat and the jump-and-reach device were compared. The vertical force trace derived from the force plate was converted to acceleration by subtracting body mass, and the acceleration was double-integrated to return the vertical displacement of the center of mass (CM) throughout the jump. Jump height was determined as the difference between the height of the CM when the participant was standing before the jump and the maximal vertical displacement achieved during the flight phase of the jump. The time in the air for each jump derived from the contact mat was entered in to an equation of motion to determine the vertical displacement of the CM. The jump-and-reach device comprised a series of plastic swivel vanes arranged in half-inch increments along a telescopic metal pole. The metal pole was adjusted such that the lowest vane was at a height equivalent to the maximal displacement achieved by the participant's dominant hand reaching overhead. Jump height was calculated from the highest vane displaced by an overhead swinging arm motion at the apex of each participant's jump. The authors reported that both the contact mat and the jump-and-reach device returned jump heights that were significantly below that associated with the criterion measure. These differences arose due to the inability of the contact mat and the jump-and-reach devices to account for the rise of the CM prior to takeoff (takeoff height). When this displacement was taken into account, the jump height returned by the contact mat was then greater than that derived from the criterion measure. The authors propose that neither the contact mat nor the jump-and-reach device provide valid measurements of vertical jump height.

Buckthorpe, M., Morris, J., & Folland, J. P. (2012). Validity of vertical jump measurement devices. *Journal of Sports Sciences, 30*, 63–69.

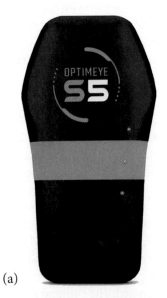

(a)

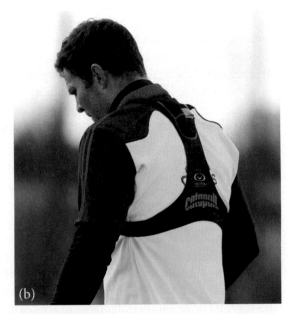

(b)

Figure 1.6 (a) A GPS receiver used to track player motion. (b) The receiver is housed in a vest worn by the player.

Photos courtesy of Catapult Sports.

Mechanical Concept 1.4

GPS-based player tracking technology

The Global Positioning System (GPS) is a U.S.-owned utility that uses 24 satellites orbiting the Earth at a height of approximately 20,200 km to provide accurate positioning and timing information. Each satellite orbits the Earth twice daily, and the constellation of satellites ensures that at least four satellites are within view from almost any area on the planet. GPS devices use radio waves from the orbiting satellites to determine the receiver's geocentric coordinates—that is, the coordinates of the receiver relative to the Earth's center—allowing the positional information of the receiver to be obtained in real time. The calculation of these coordinates is dependent upon accurate measurements of time, which are derived from atomic clock readings. Although largely unaffected by weather, the accuracy of GPS readings can be affected by other atmospheric conditions (e.g., space weather events [Rama Rao et al., 2009]). GPS readings can be affected by obstructions within the environment that interfere with the acquisition of the satellites (e.g., buildings, trees, landscape), which precludes the use of traditional GPS devices in an indoor environment. Even when the GPS units are used in an open-air court setting (e.g., tennis) where multiple satellites are acquired, the reliability of the data have been shown to be compromised (Duffield, Reid, Baker, & Spratford, 2010). However, recent advances in technology have permitted the use of portable "satellites" to be placed within sporting stadia, mitigating the problems associated with satellite reception when using GPS-based systems and allowing the collection of kinematic data during indoor sports.

Applied Research 1.3
Comparing the linear kinematics of athletes recorded from timing gates and GPS devices

Running velocity is an important variable in many sports, so methods to measure it are important in the mechanical analyses of athletes. Typically, an athlete's linear velocity will be recorded using timing gates. However, this method requires that the athlete must follow a specific path during the time of analysis. Global Positioning System (GPS) allows the determination of running velocities as the athlete moves freely within the environment. The authors compared the velocity values recorded from both timing gates and GPS devices for a group of young rugby players over distances ranging from 10 to 30 m. The authors reported that both systems produced reliable velocity values, although the reliability of the values obtained from the timing gates was slightly better. Furthermore, the GPS devices systematically underestimated the magnitude of the athletes' velocities compared to the timing gates. Despite these issues, the authors concluded that GPS devices are able to quantify small, yet practically meaningful, changes in sprint performance.

Waldron, M., Worsfold, P., Twist, C., & Lamb, K. (2011). Concurrent validity and test-retest reliability of a global positioning system (GPS) and timing gates to assess sprint performance variables. *Journal of Sports Sciences, 29*, 1613–1620.

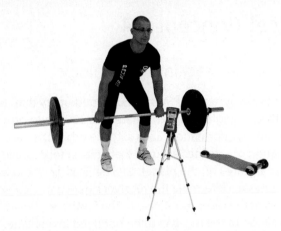

Figure 1.7 A linear position transducer attached to a barbell via a cable is used to record the velocity of the barbell during a snatch movement.

Photo courtesy of Tendo Sport Machines.

Position transducers

A position transducer allows the determination of the displacement of a body in motion (see Mechanical Concept 1.5). Linear position transducers (LPTs) can be used to determine the velocity of the athlete during jumping and running movements, as well as to determine the velocity of the barbell during resistance exercises (Harris, Cronin, Taylor, Boris, & Sheppard, 2010; Figure 1.7). The data obtained from an LPT

Mechanical Concept 1.5

Position transducer technology

A position transducer is a device that converts the change in position of a cable attached to the body under investigation into a voltage. The position transducers typically used in strength and conditioning contain photocells that change their electrical resistance in response to alterations in a light source. The cable of the device rotates a slotted disk when the body under investigation is moved, causing the light source for the photocell to be repeatedly blocked and revealed, which causes a pulse in the voltage signal that is proportional to the rotation of the slotted disk. The time history of the voltage change can then be calibrated to allow the determination of the change in position of the body under investigation. This signal can be differentiated to calculate the velocity and acceleration of the body.

An issue with the use of position transducers for analyzing movements is that the output does not allow for the calculation of the kinematic variables along the specific axes of motion. For example, it is not apparent how much the horizontal motion of the barbell contributes to the output obtained during weightlifting movements. Some commercially available position transducers do record the angle of the cable during the movement, allowing for the determination of the motion along the different axes (Harris et al., 2010), while the use of multiple position transducers will also allow for the calculation of extraneous motion during the movement (Cormie, Deane, & McBride, 2007).

Applied Research 1.4
The use of multiple LPTs increases the accuracy of kinematic data obtained during resistance movements

The authors recorded kinematic and kinetic data during jump squats performed with loads equivalent to 30% and 90% of each participant's one-repetition maximum back squat. The jump squats were performed with different combinations of linear position transducers (LPTs) attached to the barbell, with a single LPT attached to the barbell, or with two LPTs arranged in a triangular formation with the barbell. The use of two LPTs allowed the vertical motion of the barbell to be separated from the horizontal motion during the movement. The authors reported that the peak vertical velocity obtained from the double-LPT arrangement tended to be lower than that obtained from the single LPT during both jumping conditions. This finding was due to the horizontal motion during the movement being unaccounted for with the single-LPT arrangement. The authors concluded that the use of a single LPT is more convenient, although the practitioner should be aware of the overestimation in the kinematic variables obtained during movements that may involve significant horizontal motion.

Cormie, P., Deane, R., & McBride, J. M. (2007). Methodological concerns for determining power output in the jump squat. *Journal of Strength and Conditioning Research, 21*, 424–430.

are provided upon completion of the movement with no need for further calculations. The high sampling frequencies associated with the devices makes them useful for the analysis of kinematic variables during fast movements (e.g., vertical jumps, resistance exercises), and the kinematic data obtained have been shown to be reliable (Hori et al., 2007). However, extraneous movements during the execution of the exercise being performed can compromise the validity of the data obtained, necessitating the use of multiple LPTs for accurate measurements (Cormie et al., 2007; see Applied Research 1.4).

Accelerometers

Accelerometers are devices that are able to detect the acceleration of a body under investigation (see Mechanical Concept 1.6). Accelerometers are small devices that can be attached to an athlete or to an object being manipulated by an athlete (e.g., a barbell)

Mechanical Concept 1.6

Accelerometer technology

An accelerometer is a device that converts a mechanical signal (an acceleration) into an electrical signal (a voltage). This electromechanical effect is achieved by either piezoelectric or capacitance sensors within the device. Piezoelectric accelerometers contain crystal structures (quartz or ceramics) that are deformed as the result of an acceleration, creating a voltage that is recorded. The magnitude of the voltage provides information about the magnitude of the acceleration, while the orientation of the crystal structures allows the direction of the acceleration to be determined. Capacitance accelerometers rely on the change in capacitance of a sensing element (typically silicon) that is converted to a voltage to determine the applied acceleration. Integration of the acceleration data allow the determination of the velocity and displacement of the body under investigation.

(continues)

(continued)

Commercially available accelerometers are calibrated to different axes, with uni-, bi-, or triaxial devices available. However, these axes are orientated to the casing of the device to provide a frame of reference, necessitating the correct orientation of the accelerometer when attaching it to the body under investigation. The inclusion of gyroscopes and magnetometers allow accelerometers to be fixed within a global reference frame, easing the interpretation of the data obtained. Furthermore, the high acceleration amplitudes and sampling frequencies associated with the latest commercially available accelerometers enhance the event detection capabilities of these devices.

without interfering with the movement (Figure 1.8). The high sampling frequencies associated with commercially available devices allow instantaneous acceleration to be estimated, and the signal can be integrated to provide velocity and position data for the movement. Furthermore, accelerometers are portable and the data obtained from accelerometers have been shown to be both valid and reliable (Requena et al., 2012; see Applied Research 1.5).

Motion-analysis systems

Motion-analysis systems use images collected from either video or opto-reflective cameras to provide kinematic data of movements (see Mechanical Concept 1.7). The images are then digitized either manually or automatically to provide the position of the body under analysis within the field of view. Two-dimensional (planar) kinematics are obtained when a single camera is used, while three-dimensional data require the use of a minimum of two cameras. The video-based motion-analysis systems are typically limited to two-dimensional analyses, requiring consideration of the plane in

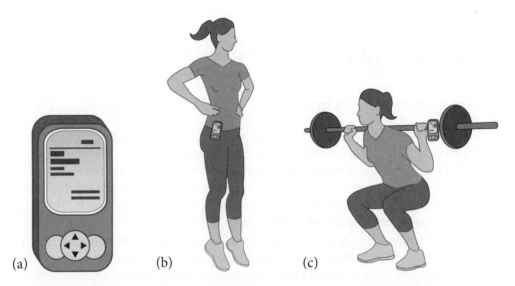

(a)   (b)   (c)

Figure 1.8 (a) An accelerometer used to assess movements. (b) An accelerometer attached to an athlete during a vertical jump test. (c) An accelerometer attached to the barbell during a resistance exercise.

Applied Research 1.5
Recording the kinematics of a vertical jump with an accelerometer

The authors assessed the validity of the data obtained from an accelerometer during a vertical jump by comparing it with that obtained from a high-speed video camera and a linear position transducer. A triaxial accelerometer containing gyroscopes and a magnetometer was placed on the lumbar region of each participant's back during a series of vertical jumps to approximate the location of the center of mass. The acceleration data were sampled at 1,000 Hz and was integrated to provide the vertical velocity of the participant during each jump. The flight time was determined from the acceleration trace at the time when the vertical acceleration was equal to or less than the gravitational acceleration. Each jump was simultaneously videoed with a high-speed digital camera (1,000 frames/s) to provide flight time data, and the cable of a position transducer was attached to a belt worn by the participants to provide velocity data. The authors reported no difference in the flight time obtained from the accelerometer compared to that obtained from the high-speed camera, while the takeoff velocity obtained from the accelerometer was comparable to that obtained from the position transducer. The kinematic data derived from the accelerometer were also found to have acceptable reliability. The authors concluded that an accelerometer attached to the lumbar region of an athlete can be used to obtain valid and reliable kinematic data during a vertical jump.

Requena, B., Requena, F., Garcia, I., Saez-Saez de Villareal, E., & Pääsuke, M. (2012). Reliability and validity of a wireless microelectromechanical-based system (Keimove™) for measuring vertical jumping performance. *Journal of Sports Science and Medicine, 11*, 115–122.

which to view the movement, while the accuracy of the data obtained from the analysis can be limited by the sampling frequency of the video cameras used (Figure 1.9). Both the linear and angular position of the body under analysis can be obtained from motion analysis data, while differentiating the signal allows other kinematic variables

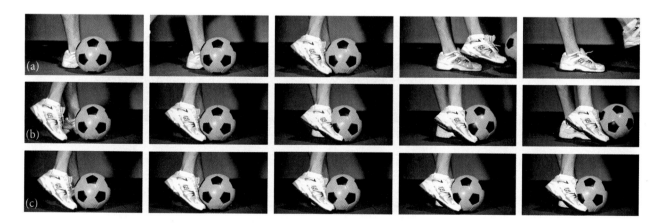

Figure 1.9 The effects of different sampling frequencies in the motion analysis of a soccer kick using a two-dimensional video-based motion analysis system. (a) At a sampling frequency of 50 Hz, foot–ball contact can be observed in only one frame. (b) At a sampling frequency of 250 Hz, foot–ball contact is observed in four frames. (c) At a sampling frequency of 1000 Hz, foot–ball contact is observed in many frames.

Reproduced from Payton, C. J. (2008). Motion analysis using video. In C. J. Payton & R. M. Bartlett (Eds.), *Biomechanical Evaluation of Movement in Sport and Exercise. The British Association of Sport and Exercise Sciences Guidelines* (pp. 8–32). New York, NY: Routledge.

Mechanical Concept 1.7

Opto-reflective motion-analysis systems

Opto-reflective motion-analysis systems provide optical representation of the body under investigation, which is identified via the placement of reflective markers on the body (Figure 1.10). The markers reflect infrared radiation emitted by LED arrays mounted on each camera. The cameras are then able to

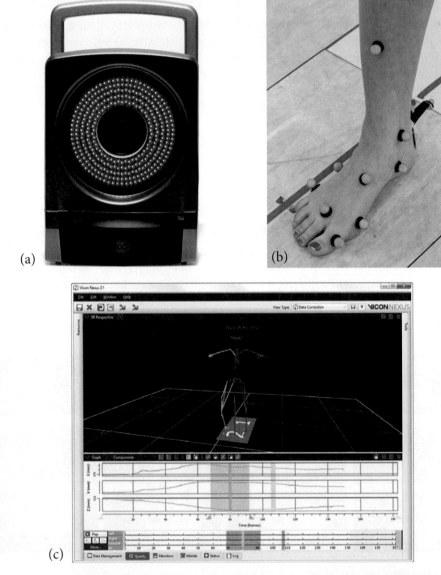

(a)

(b)

(c)

Figure 1.10 (a) An opto-reflective camera with an LED array. (b) Reflective markers placed on anatomical landmarks to allow the body segments to be located within three-dimensional space. (c) The digital output obtained from a three-dimensional opto-reflective motion analysis system.

Photos courtesy of Vicon Motion Systems Ltd.

locate the reflective markers within their field of view, allowing the position of the body under investigation to be determined in two- or three-dimensional space.

The number of reflective markers used depends upon the analysis being performed, but a full-body analysis can require more than 40 markers, increasing the preparation time when these systems are used. Each reflective marker should be viewed by a minimum of two cameras to allow the position within three-dimensional space to be obtained, requiring the use of multiple cameras to reconstruct the marker sets associated with the motion of body segments during most movements. Typically, opto-reflective motion-analysis systems use six to eight cameras placed around the calibrated volume in which the movements will be performed (Milner, 2008). High sampling frequencies can be achieved with opto-reflective motion-analysis systems, with frequencies as high as 10,000 Hz for commercially available systems. However, the spatial resolution of the cameras is severely reduced at these high frequencies.

to be calculated. However, the higher derivatives (e.g., velocity) obtained from commercially available, video-based motion-analysis systems are less reliable than those obtained from opto-reflective systems due to the limited signal processing capabilities of the software (Melton, Mullineaux, Mattacola, Mair, & Uhl, 2011). Furthermore, the errors associated with kinematic data obtained from video-based motion-analysis systems tend to be greater than those obtained from opto-reflective systems (Elliott, Alderson, & Denver, 2007; see Applied Research 1.6).

Applied Research 1.6
Recording angular kinematics of athletes

Motion-analysis systems are used in mechanical analyses to determine the kinematics of a specific movement. There are two broad categories of motion-analysis systems. Video-based systems use video footage of the movement recorded from a digital video camera. The video data are then digitized to determine the relative position of the body segments. Opto-reflective systems use infrared light reflected back by reflective markers that are placed on specific anatomical landmarks to automatically determine the relative position of the body segments. These authors compared the accuracy of a video-based system with an opto-reflective system in determining joint angles during specific movements made by a mechanical arm. The use of a mechanical arm allowed the determination of the actual joint angles to which those derived from the motion-analysis systems were compared. It was found that the opto-reflective system produced the lowest error in the measured joint angle (0.6°), although the error associated with the video-based system was relatively small (2.3°). The authors concluded that motion-analysis systems can be used to accurately record the angular kinematics associated with movements.

Elliott, B. C., Alderson, J. A., & Denver, E. R. (2007). System and modeling errors in motion analysis: implications for the measurement of elbow angle in cricket bowling. *Journal of Biomechanics, 40,* 2679–2686.

Chapter Summary

Any mechanical analysis of human movement requires the selection of an appropriate reference frame to allow the description of the position of the body under investigation; the specific reference frame should be identified prior to any biomechanical analysis. The body being analyzed is often reduced to its CM, defined as the virtual point about which all of the mass of the body is evenly distributed. There are two forms of motion, with linear motion referring to that along a straight or curved path and angular motion referring to the rotation of the body about a fixed axis. All human movements involve both types of motion. The kinematic variables of position, velocity, and acceleration allow the motion of the body to be described. The position of the body defines its location within the specified reference frame; the velocity of the body describes the rate at which the body is changing position; acceleration describes the rate at which the body is changing velocity. The equations of motion define the relationships between these kinematic variables, allowing the practitioner to determine the outcome of movements given knowledge of the initial kinematic conditions of the body. There are different technologies available to the strength and conditioning practitioner that allow them to record both linear and angular kinematic variables, including photocells, GPS, LPTs, accelerometers, and motion-analysis systems. Each of these technologies has benefits and costs associated with its use.

Review Questions and Projects

1. Describe the three-dimensional reference frame used to describe linear motion of a system under analysis, and explain the importance of the different axes when analyzing movements.

2. An athlete runs a 40-yard sprint in 5.05 s. Calculate the average velocity (speed) during the event.

3. Explain why the average speed calculated in Question 2 has limited value for the strength and conditioning practitioner when attempting to develop an effective training program.

4. Explain how you would modify the measurement of the time during the 40-yard sprint to provide more useful information for the strength and conditioning practitioner.

5. What mathematical method allows the estimation of instantaneous velocity from position–time data?

6. A strength and conditioning coach uses video footage to assess an athlete during a vertical jump and determines that the athlete's flight time was 0.58 s. Calculate the jump height for the athlete.

7. Explain why calculating jump height based upon the time in the air tends to overestimate jump height.

8. An athlete performs a vertical jump and produces a vertical velocity of 3.56 m/s at takeoff. Calculate the time taken for the athlete's center of mass to reach the apex of flight.

9. Calculate the vertical jump height for the athlete in Question 8.

10. Discuss the technology that the strength and conditioning practitioner can use to record takeoff velocity during a vertical jump.

11. An athlete performs a running long jump and has a velocity of 9 m/s at takeoff and a takeoff angle of 20°. Calculate the horizontal range traveled by the CM of the athlete during flight assuming that the height of landing is equal to the height of takeoff.

12. Discuss the technology that the strength and conditioning practitioner can use to record the takeoff velocity and the takeoff angle of the long jump athlete.

13. An athlete steps from a 0.30-m box during the performance of a drop jump. Calculate the athlete's vertical velocity upon landing.

14. The contact time associated with the performance of a drop jump provides information about the muscular strength of the athlete beyond the height attained during the jump. Discuss the technology that the strength and conditioning practitioner can use to record this kinematic variable.

15. An athlete performs a bench-throw resistance exercise and projects the barbell 0.45 m vertically from the point of release. Calculate the vertical velocity of the barbell at release.

16. Given the definition of CM and the kinematic factors affecting the horizontal range traveled by the CM during flight, explain how the posture adopted by an athlete at takeoff during a long-jump event influences his or her performance.

17. Explain why the fastest athletes are placed in lanes 4–6 during 200-m sprint events at track and field championships.

18. A strength and conditioning coach wishes to assess the kinematics associated with the athletes' performances during a soccer workout (e.g., distances covered, running velocities). Discuss the relative merits of the different technologies, including timing gates, GPS, and motion-analysis systems.

19. A strength and conditioning coach wishes to measure the vertical jump heights of a group of athletes. The coach has a contact mat, a linear position transducer, an accelerometer, and a motion-analysis system available. Discuss the relative merits of each of these technologies.

20. A strength and conditioning coach is interested in analyzing the angular displacement at the shoulder and elbow joints for an athlete during a bench press. Discuss the limitations associated with a two-dimensional video analysis for the movement.

References

Buckthorpe, M., Morris, J., & Folland, J. P. (2012). Validity of vertical jump measurement devices. *Journal of Sports Sciences, 30,* 63–69.

Cormie, P., Deane, R., & McBride, J. M. (2007). Methodological concerns for determining power output in the jump squat. *Journal of Strength and Conditioning Research, 21,* 424–430.

Duffield, R., Reid, M., Baker, J., & Spratford, W. (2010). Accuracy and reliability of GPS devices for measurement of movement patterns in confined spaces for court-based sports. *Journal of Science and Medicine in Sport, 13*, 523–525.

Earp, J. E., & Newton, R. U. (2012). Considerations for selecting an appropriate timing system. *Journal of Strength and Conditioning Research, 26*, 1245–1248.

Elliott, B. C., Alderson, J. A., & Denver, E. R. (2007). System and modeling errors in motion analysis: implications for the measurement of elbow angle in cricket bowling. *Journal of Biomechanics, 40*, 2679–2686.

Grimshaw, P., Lees, A., Fowler, N., & Burden, A. (2006). *Sport and Exercise Biomechanics*. New York, NY: Taylor and Francis.

Harris, N. K., Cronin, J., Taylor, K. L., Boris, J., & Sheppard, J. (2010). Understanding position transducer technology for strength and conditioning practitioners. *Strength and Conditioning Journal, 32*, 66–79.

Hori, N., Newton, R. U., Andrews, W., Kawamori, N., McGuigan, M., & Nosaka, K. (2007). Comparison of four different methods to measure power output during the hang power clean and the weighted jump squat. *Journal of Strength and Conditioning Research, 21*, 314–320.

Melton, C., Mullineaux, D. R., Mattacola, C. G., Mair, S. D., & Uhl, T. L. (2011). Reliability of video motion-analysis systems to measure amplitude and velocity of shoulder elevation. *Journal of Sport Rehabilitation, 20*, 393–405.

Milner, C. E. (2008). Motion analysis using on-line systems. In C. J. Payton & R. M. Bartlett (Eds.) *Biomechanical Evaluation of Movement in Sport and Exercise. The British Association of Sport and Exercise Sciences Guidelines*. New York, NY: Routledge, pp. 33–52.

Moir, G. L. (2008). Three different methods of calculating vertical jump height from force platform data in men and women. *Measurement in Physical Education & Exercise Science, 12*, 207–218.

Moir, G., Button, C., Glaister, M., & Stone, M. H. (2004). Influence of familiarization on the reliability of vertical jump and acceleration sprinting performance in physically active men. *Journal of Strength and Conditioning Research, 18*, 276–280.

Moir, G., Shastri, P., & Connaboy, C. (2008). Intersession reliability of vertical jump height in women and men. *Journal of Strength and Conditioning Research, 22*, 1779–1784.

Rama Rao, P. V. S., Gopi Krishna, S., Vara Prasad, J., Prasad, S. N. V. S., Prasad, D. S. V. V. D., & Niranjan, K. (2009). Geomagnetic storms effects on GPS based navigation. *Annals of Geophysics, 27*, 2101–2110.

Requena, B., Requena, F., Garcia, I., Saez-Saez de Villareal, E., & Pääsuke, M. (2012). Reliability and validity of a wireless microelectromechanicals based system (Keimove™) for measuring vertical jumping performance. *Journal of Sports Science and Medicine, 11*, 115–122.

Waldron, M., Worsfold, P., Twist, C., & Lamb, K. (2011). Concurrent validity and test-retest reliability of a global positioning system (GPS) and timing gates to assess sprint performance variables. *Journal of Sports Sciences, 29*, 1613–1620.

Yeadon, M. R., Kato, T., & Kerwin, D. G. (1999). Measuring running speed using photocells. *Journal of Sports Sciences, 17*, 249–257.

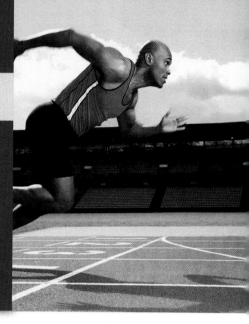

CHAPTER 2

Basic Mechanics: Kinetic Variables

Chapter Objectives

At the end of this chapter, you will be able to:

- Describe the effect of forces on kinematic variables
- Apply Newton's laws of motion to specific movement tasks
- Describe the components of the ground reaction force (GRF) and their importance during movement tasks
- Use the impulse–momentum relationship to determine the outcome of specific movement tasks
- Use the work–energy theorem to determine the outcome of specific movement tasks
- Describe the different forms of mechanical energy and the importance of energy exchanges in specific movement tasks
- Explain the effects of a moment of force applied to a body
- Describe the different technologies that can be used to record kinetic variables and the relative merits of each

Key Terms

Body weight

Center of pressure

Centripetal force

Compressive action

Conservation laws

Elastic collision

Energy

External forces

Free-body diagrams

Frictional component

Gravitational potential energy

Impulse–momentum relationship

Inelastic collision

Inertia

Internal forces

Inverse dynamics

Kinetic energy

Kinetic variables

Moment arm

Moment of force

Momentum

Normal component

Normal force

Potential energy

Power

Principle of conservation of mechanical energy

Static equilibrium

Strain potential energy

Support moment

Tensile action

Work–energy theorem

Chapter Overview

Kinematic variables associated with a biomechanical analysis allow the description of the motion of a body. For a complete mechanical analysis, however, we need to explore the variables that are responsible for changing the motion of a body. It is to these **kinetic variables** that we now turn our attention. The current chapter is not intended to be an exhaustive review of kinetic variables, serving instead to introduce the pertinent kinetic variables that will provide a foundation to support the biomechanical analyses and explanations used in this discipline. We begin our exploration of kinetic variables with the concept of forces.

Forces

A force is an agent that changes or tends to change the motion of a body. We have already proposed that the motion of a body is determined by its velocity. As velocity is a vector variable, a force can be considered to act to change either the magnitude or direction of motion of a body, and therefore produce an acceleration. The qualification of *tends to change motion* is included in the definition of force because the magnitude of a force may not always be sufficient to actually change the motion of the body that it acts upon. Thus, an absence of acceleration observed in an analysis does not necessarily mean that there are no forces acting upon the body; the acceleration of a body is therefore the result of unbalanced forces acting on the body.

Forces are vector quantities that can be broadly categorized as inducing a pull on a body, where we refer to the **tensile action** of the force, or the force can invoke a push on a body, where we refer to the **compressive action** of the force. For example, during a muscular contraction, the muscle develops tension and pulls on a body segment to induce a change in the motion of that segment (muscle tension is covered in more depth elsewhere), whereas the tibia of the leg experiences a compressive force during upright stance as a result of the body weight and the ground reaction force acting upon the bone.

In a biomechanical analysis of human movements, it is often useful to consider **internal forces**, such as those associated with muscular contractions, and **external forces**, such as gravity and the ground reaction force. The **ground reaction force (GRF)** is an external force that is imposed on a body when it is in contact with a supporting surface. While internal muscular forces are able to displace body segmental masses with respect to one another, it is external forces such as the GRF that act to change the motion of the center of mass (CM) of the body. Some forces that act on a body are constant, whereas others are nonconstant. For example, the force of gravity (see Mechanical Concept 2.1) is a constant force, whereas the GRF represents a nonconstant force acting on the body during many movement tasks. The nonconstant GRF is crucial in establishing changes in motion of the human body. The action of forces acting on a body can be determined from the construction of **free-body diagrams** that are often used in mechanical analyses (see Mechanical Concept 2.2).

Newton's Laws of Motion

Forces and their actions are central tenets in a mechanical analysis of movements and the relationships between forces and the motion of bodies upon which they act are highlighted in Newton's three laws of motion.

Mechanical Concept 2.1

Gravitational acceleration

Newton's law of universal gravitation states that every particle in the universe is attracted to every other particle with a force that is proportional to the product of their masses and inversely proportional to the square of the distance between them. This can be expressed mathematically as follows:

$$F_g = G\frac{m_1 m_2}{r^2}$$

Eq. (2.1)

where F_g is the force of attraction, G is the universal gravitational constant of 6.67×10^{-11} N (m/kg)^2, m_1 and m_2 are the masses of the bodies involved, and r is the distance between the center of the bodies. We can use this equation to determine the strength of the attractive force between an athlete of mass 75 kg and the Earth. Taking the mass of the Earth as 5.98×10^{24} kg, and the radius of the Earth as 6.38×10^6 m, we calculate the attractive force between the two bodies as 735 N. Because the Earth is the most massive body in our locale, this force represents the force with which the athlete is attracted toward the center of the Earth; this attractive force represents the athlete's body weight.

When analyzing sporting movements where the body or an implement is projected into the air, thereby moving its mass farther from the center of the Earth, we can ignore this projection because it is negligible compared to the Earth's radius. The attractive force can therefore be considered constant in our analyses, a consideration known as the "flat Earth assumption." We can rearrange Equation (2.1) to determine the magnitude of the acceleration associated with the gravitational force:

$$g = G\frac{m_e}{r_e^2}$$

Eq. (2.2)

where g is the acceleration due to gravity, G is the universal gravitational constant, m_e is the mass of the Earth, and r_e is the radius of the Earth. Equation (2.2) provides an acceleration of 9.81 m/s^2, which is constant close to the Earth's surface (indeed, moving 100 km from the surface of the Earth reduces g by approximately 3%). Returning to our athlete, whose body weight we calculated as 735 N, if we divide this force of attraction by the acceleration due to gravity, we arrive back at the athlete's mass of 75 kg. Because the gravitational force acts toward the center of the Earth, which has a downward direction in our reference frame, the acceleration due to the gravitational force is -9.81 m/s^2.

Newton's law of inertia

A body at rest will remain at rest, while a body in motion will remain in uniform motion unless acted upon by unbalanced external forces.

The first of Newton's laws of motion tells us that a change in motion of a body occurs when there is an imbalance of forces acting on it. Referring to the barbell shown in Mechanical Concept 2.2, the forces of weight and the normal component

Mechanical Concept 2.2

Free-body diagrams

A free-body diagram is used in mechanical analyses to determine the effects of external forces acting on the body of interest. The use of a free-body diagram provides a generalization of the forces acting on the body that simplifies but informs our mechanical analyses of human movements by providing a visual representation of the forces. Through the construction of a free-body diagram, the resultant motion of the body can be determined.

In order to construct a free-body diagram, we first identify the reference frame in which the body is being analyzed. We then draw a minimalist representation of the body free from the surrounding environment, identifying the location of the CM of the body, and place arrows to represent the vectors associated with the external forces acting on the body. Figure 2.1 shows a free-body diagram of a loaded barbell that is at rest on a lifting platform.

Notice that although the gravitational force (weight force, F_w) will act upon all of the particles associated with the barbell and the disks, this force is represented as acting at the CM. Furthermore, the GRF is drawn as acting at the CM in opposition to the weight force of the barbell. The GRF is an external force that is exerted on a body by virtue of its contact with a supporting surface and will therefore act on all of the particles of the body that are in contact with the supporting surface. Placing the resultant GRF at the CM is mechanically equivalent. The resultant GRF in this example acts perpendicular to the supporting surface, and we can therefore refer to it as the **normal component** of the GRF (N). From this free-body diagram, we can determine that the barbell will remain in its present state of rest; the forces acting on the body are equal in magnitude but opposite in direction, so the net force is zero. This interpretation comes from Newton's first law of motion.

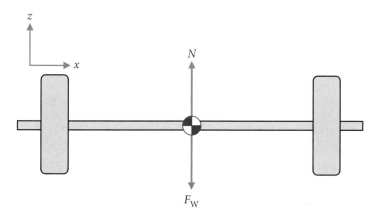

Figure 2.1 A free-body diagram of a loaded barbell at rest on a lifting platform. Notice the center of mass, the force vectors, and the reference frame, which shows the x and z axes because the barbell is viewed in the frontal plane.

Note: N is the normal reaction force; F_w is the weight of the barbell.

(continues)

(continued)

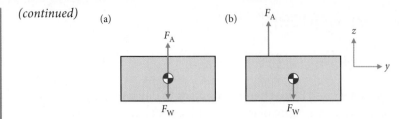

Figure 2.2 Two bodies of equal mass that have an external force applied to them. The magnitude and direction of the applied force is the same in each diagram. The external force exceeds the weight of the body in both examples. Because the external force in (a) has a line of action that passes through the CM, the body will experience translation. Because the external force in (b) has a line of action that does not pass through the CM, the body will experience both translation and rotation about an axis passing through the CM.

Note: F_W is the weight force; F_A is external force.

In Figure 2.2, there are two free-body diagrams that show bodies of equal mass that have an external force applied to them (F_A). This external force has the same magnitude and direction in each of the diagrams. However, its line of action, determined by its point of application on the body, differs.

Both bodies will experience a change in motion as a result of the unbalanced forces acting on them. What will differ between the two bodies is the form taken by the resultant motion. In the Figure 2.2a, the external force has a line of action that acts through the CM, whereas in Figure 2.2b, the line of action does not pass through the CM. As noted elsewhere, the CM represents the point through which an axis passes in a body that is free to rotate in space. From these free-body diagrams, we can determine that the first body will experience linear translation, commensurate with Newton's first and second laws of motion. In the second example, however, the body will be rotated as well as being linearly translated. In this second example, the external force that was applied to the body acted at a distance from the axis of rotation (CM), which produced a **moment of force**.

of the GRF are balanced (they are equal in magnitude but opposite in direction), so the barbell will not experience a change in motion (an acceleration), remaining in its present state of rest. It can therefore be describes as being in a state of **static equilibrium** because the forces acting on it sum to zero. If an athlete applies an upward force to the barbell that exceeds the weight force, such as during a clean movement, the barbell will experience an acceleration and will begin to rise. In this instance, there is a net upward force acting on the barbell. The concept of **inertia** tells us something about the difficulty associated with attempting to change the motion of a body, and we use the mass of the body as an indication of its inertia. Experience shows us that it is more difficult to change the motion of a heavily laden barbell than it is to change the motion of a lightly laden barbell because of their different masses; a greater force needs to be applied to the more massive barbell to change its motion.

Newton's law of acceleration

The change in motion of a body is proportional to and acts in the same direction as the net force acting on the body.

To fully establish the basis of this law, we must introduce a new mechanical variable: that of **momentum**. The momentum of a body describes the quantity of motion possessed by the body and is the product of mass and velocity:

$$p = mv \qquad\qquad \text{Eq. (2.3)}$$

where p is linear momentum, m is the mass of the body, and v is the linear velocity of the body. Momentum becomes a very important variable when bodies collide, and the conservation law associated with the variable allows the outcome of a collision to be determined (see Mechanical Concept 2.8). Newton's second law of motion tells us that the rate of change in momentum is proportional to the net force applied to the body:

$$F = \frac{\Delta p}{\Delta t} \qquad\qquad \text{Eq. (2.4)}$$

As the mass of the body remains constant, we can rewrite Equation (2.4) as:

$$F = \frac{m\Delta v}{\Delta t} \qquad\qquad \text{Eq. (2.5)}$$

Given that the rate of change in velocity is an acceleration, we can rewrite Equation (2.5) as:

$$F = ma \qquad\qquad \text{Eq. (2.6)}$$

where F is force, m is the mass of the body, and a is the linear acceleration. This equation provides a direct means of measuring the force being applied to a body. Equation (2.6) also tells us that **body weight** is a force equal to the product of the mass of a body being accelerated by gravity (see Mechanical Concept 2.3). **Worked Example 2.1** provides a practical example of using the relationship between force and momentum.

Mechanical Concept 2.3

Body mass versus body weight

Body mass refers to the quantity of matter contained within a body. It is a scalar quantity that has the units of kilogram. Body weight, on the other hand, is a force associated with the mass of the body being accelerated by the attractive force of gravity, as per Newton's second law of motion. Body weight is therefore a vector quantity and has the unit of the newton (N). It is a distributed force with the net effect acting at the CM.

The two variables of mass and weight are often thought of as interchangeable, probably due to their proportionality; the weight of a body is proportional to its mass multiplied by the constant of gravitational acceleration. However, the consequences of erroneously interchanging these variables are significant in

(continues)

(continued)

biomechanical analyses, as will become apparent when we integrate the vertical GRF during a jump to calculate jump height. Vogel (2003) provides an example to illustrate the difference between mass and weight. Imagine an astronaut locomoting on the Earth and the moon. While a constant gravitational force acts on the surface of both the Earth and the moon, gravity on the moon is about one-sixth of that on the Earth. An astronaut with a mass of 70 kg on the Earth will have exactly that mass on the moon, as mass is unaffected by the acceleration associated with gravity. Body weight, on the other hand, will be very different in these two locations: –687 N on the Earth and –114 N on the moon. Vogel (2003) noted that this difference has a profound effect on the movements used by the astronaut. Hopping upward works well on the moon and also on the Earth, as an equivalent muscular force acting on the same mass results in a greater vertical acceleration in the face of the reduced gravitational force. Hopping forward is also successful on the moon, but here the astronaut must lean forward considerably in order to initiate the movement. This is because the astronaut's forward motion is generated by a frictional force in response to his or her backward push on the lunar surface; this frictional force is dependent upon the magnitude of the normal force, which is itself dependent upon the weight force (see Equation 2.23). Obviously, the weight force is reduced due to the reduced gravitational force. Recognize that the mass of the astronaut has not changed. Weight is certainly proportional to mass, but the two are distinct variables.

Worked Example 2.1
Calculating momentum and force

An athlete with a mass of 70 kg performs a countermovement vertical jump. At the beginning of the propulsion phase, the athlete's vertical velocity is 0 m/s; at takeoff, the vertical velocity is 3 m/s. Calculate the change in momentum during the propulsive phase of the jump.

i. Use Equation (2.3)	$p = mv$
ii. At the beginning of propulsion	$p_1 = 70 \times 0$
iii. At the beginning of propulsion	$p_1 = 0$ kg m/s
iv. At takeoff	$p_2 = 70 \times 3$
v. At takeoff	$p_2 = 210$ kg m/s
vi. Change in momentum	$\Delta p = p_2 - p_1$
vii. Answer	$\Delta p = 210$ kg m/s

If the duration of the propulsive phase was 0.72 s, calculate the average vertical force acting on the athlete.

i. Use Equation (2.4)	$F = \Delta p / \Delta t$
ii. Input the known variables	$F = 210/0.72$
iii. Answer	$F = 292$ N

The force applied here represents the average net force acting on the athlete during the propulsive phase—that is, the average force acting on the athlete once body weight has been removed from the analysis. Remember that the body weight force of –687 N is acting on the athlete at all times. Analyzing the instantaneous force, we would notice that the vertical force was changing continuously during the propulsive phase of the jump.

Newton's law of reaction

When one body exerts a force upon another body, the force of the first body is counteracted by a force exerted by the second body back onto the first that is equal in magnitude but opposite in direction.

The GRF is a consequence of Newton's third law of motion (**Figure 2.3**). Consider an athlete who is at rest and in contact with the ground. The athlete's body weight is a downward force due to the attractive force of gravity, and it is applied to the ground. The ground reacts to this force by applying an upward force back to the athlete. These two forces are equal in magnitude but opposite in direction, and therefore the athlete remains in a state of rest. However, it was noted previously that the force of gravity is constant, whereas the GRF can be altered. The athlete is able to alter the magnitude of the GRF through internal muscular forces (see **Mechanical Concepts 2.4** and 2.12). In most sporting events, it is the GRF that the athlete should be exploiting in order to improve performance. The GRF can provide an indication of total muscular effort in a given movement (Zatsiorsky, 2002), so strength and conditioning practitioners should be interested in this force. The GRF can be measured directly from a force plate or pressure insoles and also from kinematic variables associated with the motion of the body under analysis (see the Technology to Record Kinetic Variables section later in the chapter).

The importance of Newton's laws in determining the change in motion observed during a given task is highlighted in **Mechanical Concept 2.5.**

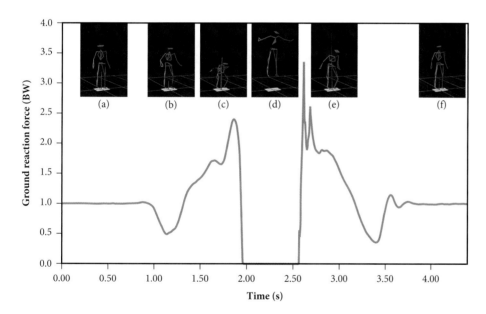

Figure 2.3 The vertical component of the ground reaction force (GRF) during a countermovement jump. The units are multiples of body weight. The images are from an opto-reflective motion analysis system recording the movement of the athlete performing the jump on a force plate. The GRF is shown as a red arrow. (a) The GRF is equal to body weight, and the athlete remains stationary. (b) The GRF is less than body weight, causing the center of mass to descend. (c) The GRF exceeds bodyweight, arresting the athlete's descent and beginning ascent. (d) The athlete is airborne, so there is no GRF recorded. (e) Upon landing, the GRF greatly exceeds body weight to arrest the downward motion of the center of mass. (f) The GRF is equal to body weight, and the athlete remains stationary once again.

Mechanical Concept 2.4

The ground reaction force (GRF)

The GRF represents the force provided by the support surface on which the athlete is moving, and it is a consequence of Newton's third law. Although the GRF is distributed across the entire body part that is in contact with the supporting surface, we can determine the resultant GRF as acting at a virtual point on the supporting surface known as the **center of pressure**.

The resultant GRF can be resolved into three orthogonal components: the anteroposterior, the mediolateral, and the normal component. A **normal force** is that which acts perpendicular to the surface supporting the body; the normal component of the GRFs acts vertically along the z-axis. The anteroposterior and mediolateral components act along the y- and x-axes, respectively. These horizontal components are shear or **frictional components**. These three components represent the reaction provided by the support surface to the actions of the athlete that are transmitted to the surface. Each of the components acts to accelerate the CM of the athlete in the respective directions, so the performance in many sports is affected by the magnitude of these components.

The GRF can be considered the reaction to the accelerations of the body's segmental masses during a given movement task. If an athlete is stationary, then the force applied to the supporting surface is simply the product of the mass of the entire body being accelerated by gravity. The force provided by the surface is simply a reaction to this body weight force and will only have a normal component (that along the z-axis) given that there are no other accelerations being experienced by the athlete. If the athlete then pushes backwards against the ground, this action will establish a horizontal reaction force acting to propel the athlete forward. It should be recognized that the internal muscular forces exerted by the athlete are what accelerate the athlete's segmental masses and cause the forward motion of the CM. No change in motion of the CM would be possible without the external GRF acting on the athlete; however, the causes of the GRF are body weight and the internal muscular forces.

Figure 2.4 shows the component of the GRF along the y-axis (solid line) and that along the z-axis (dashed line) as an athlete runs across a force platform. Notice that the frictional component along the y-axis not only changes magnitude during the stance phase, but it also changes from being negative during the first half of stance to positive during the second half. The initial negative value for the force is caused by the athlete's foot being in front of the CM when it contacts the ground: The motion of the foot is forward relative to the ground, and the reaction to this is a force acting back onto the athlete, which constitutes a negative force in our reference frame. The positive force during the second half of stance results from the body being rotated over the stance foot such that the CM is located in front of the stance foot, and the foot now applies a backward force to the ground. The reaction to this is a forward-directed force acting on the athlete. The GRF acting along the y-axis determines the CM acceleration

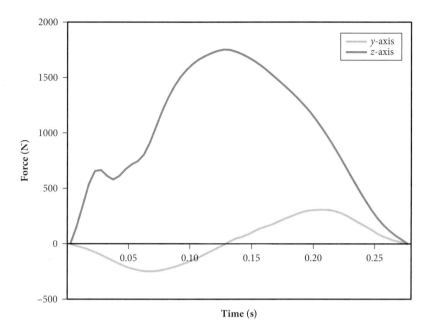

Figure 2.4 The horizontal components of the GRF along the *y*-axis (anteroposterior) and those along the *z*-axis (vertical) as an athlete runs across a force plate.

in this direction and will be influenced by the orientation of the athlete's leg at touchdown, the acceleration of the segmental masses during stance, and the coefficient of friction associated with the materials in contact.

Mechanical Concept 2.5

Applying Newton's laws of motion to the vertical jump

Figure 2.5a shows the normal component of the GRF (*z*-axis) for an athlete performing a vertical jump from a stationary starting position. This force acts to accelerate the CM vertically during the movement. The graphs of vertical acceleration, velocity, and displacement of the CM are also shown.

The following descriptions relate to the regions highlighted in each of the graphs shown in Figure 2.5a–d.

Region 1

The GRF is a consequence of Newton's third law of motion and represents a reaction to the forces applied by the athlete to the supporting surface. In Figure 2.5, the initial force represents the reaction to the athlete's body weight. These two forces, the GRF and body weight, are equal in magnitude but opposite in direction. These balanced forces result in a net zero vertical force acting on the athlete, and by Newton's first law of motion, there will be no acceleration of the athlete's CM.

(continues)

(continued)

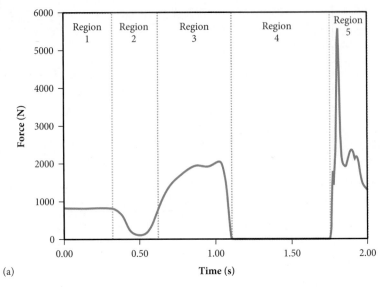

(a)

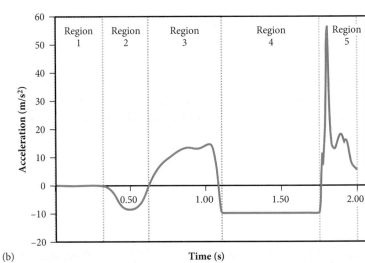

(b)

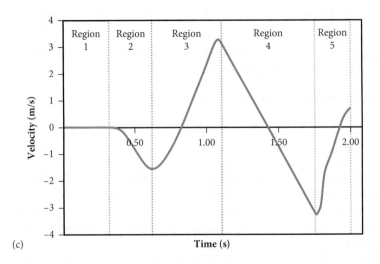

(c)

(continues)

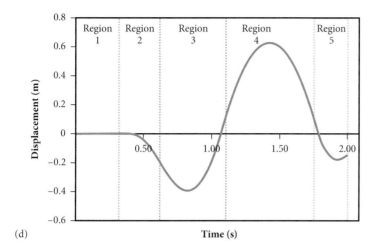

(d)

Figure 2.5 (a) The vertical GRF recorded from a force plate for an athlete performing a countermovement vertical jump. The acceleration (b), velocity (c), and displacement (d) of the center of mass of an athlete during the countermovement vertical jump.

Region 2

At the beginning of the propulsion phase, the athlete flexes the hip, knee, and ankle joints. This downward acceleration of the associated segmental masses results in the GRF falling below body weight. At this time, the net negative force acting on the CM results in the acceleration of the CM, as per Newton's first law of motion. Newton's second law of motion informs us that the acceleration experienced by a body is proportional to and acts in the same direction as the net force acting on the body. Therefore, the athlete's CM undergoes a negative acceleration and begins to move down at this time. This is referred to as a countermovement or unloading phase of the jump.

Region 3

As the CM descends during the countermovement, the athlete begins to activate the extensor muscles of the hip, knee, and ankle joints. This muscle activity results in the acceleration of the trunk segment. Newton's second law of motion informs us that a force is the product of a mass and an acceleration. The reaction to this upward force acting on the trunk is a downward force that is transmitted to the surface via the feet, resulting in an increase in the magnitude of the GRF acting on the athlete (Newton's third law of motion). At this time, the GRF exceeds the force of body weight, and the CM experiences a net positive force, and therefore a positive acceleration (Newton's second law of motion). This positive acceleration of the CM first manifests as a decrease in its negative vertical velocity until the CM achieves its lowest vertical position, and then as an increase in the positive vertical velocity of the CM. Notice that the greatest magnitude of the GRF is seen at a time when the athlete is close to the lowest position during the countermovement. At this time, the musculature crossing the joints of the lower body is able to exert large forces to accelerate the body segments. This illustrates the dependence of the GRF on muscular forces.

(continues)

(continued)

Region 4

After the athlete has achieved the lowest position during the countermovement, the CM begins to increase its positive vertical velocity by virtue of the GRF exceeding the body weight force. As the lower-body joints extend and increase their angular velocity during the propulsive phase, the forces necessary to accelerate the segmental masses to continue to produce a GRF in excess of the body weight force become greater than the forces the musculature can generate. When this occurs, the net negative force results in a negative acceleration (Newton's first and second laws of motion), and the positive velocity of the athlete's CM is decreased slightly before takeoff. However, the CM possesses sufficient vertical motion that it will continue to move upward.

Region 5

Eventually, the rate and magnitude of the extension of the joints of the lower body prevent the athlete's feet from maintaining contact with the supporting surface given the vertical motion of the CM. The feet are therefore pulled from the floor at the point of takeoff. Once this occurs, the action of the GRF is removed from the CM, and the only force acting on the athlete will be that of gravity; due to Newton's first law of motion, the CM will experience an acceleration. This acceleration will be negative, from Newton's second law of motion, and the vertical velocity of the CM will be reduced, being 0 m/s at its highest vertical position. Following this, the gravitational force will increase the negative vertical velocity of the CM until the athlete lands back on the supporting surface and has the GRF applied once again.

One final issue requires explanation. If the athlete applies a force to the supporting surface that reacts with a force back to the athlete that is equal in magnitude, why does the athlete's CM experience an acceleration? This situation produces balanced forces, and therefore there should be no acceleration, as per Newton's first law of motion. However, the masses of the bodies involved in the analysis should to be included. The athlete possesses considerably less mass than that of the Earth. Newton's second law of motion informs us that the acceleration experienced by a body will be proportional to the force applied, but inversely proportion to the mass. The Earth will experience a negligible acceleration compared to the athlete during the movement by the virtue of its much greater mass. In any analysis of the motion of a body, the mass of the body is important.

The Impulse of a Force and Momentum

Forces take time to act on bodies, as can be seen from the example shown in Mechanical Concept 2.5. Therefore we should be concerned with both the magnitude of the applied force and the time over which the force acts. The product of the force and the time over which it acts is the impulse of the force:

$$J = Ft \qquad \text{Eq. (2.7)}$$

where J is the impulse of the applied force measured in newton-seconds, F is the average force applied, and t is the time over which the force is applied (see **Worked Example 2.2**).

Worked Example 2.2
Calculating the impulse of a force

Figure 2.6 shows the vertical GRF during a countermovement vertical jump performed from a stationary starting position by an athlete. The propulsive phase of the jump is shown by the shaded area on the graph.

The mass of the athlete was 79.4 kg, the time of propulsion was 1.23 s, and the average net force acting on the athlete during propulsion was 188.25 N. Calculate the net impulse of the applied force.

i. Use Equation (2.7) $J = Ft$

ii. Input the known variables $J = 188.25 \times 1.23$

iii. Answer $J = 231.55 \text{ Ns}$

The impulse calculated represents the net vertical impulse acting on the athlete during the propulsive phase of the jump. This impulse informs us of the change in momentum experienced by the athlete during the time of force application; this is the basis of the impulse–momentum relationship. We know that the athlete did not possess any momentum at the beginning of the propulsive phase, as the athlete was not moving. This allows us to determine that the impulse of the force is equal to the vertical momentum at the end of the propulsive phase (takeoff). From this, we can determine the athlete's vertical velocity at takeoff.

i. Use Equation (2.10) $J = m\Delta v$

ii. Input the known variables $231.55 = 79.4 \times (v_f - 0)$

iii. Solve for v_f $v_f = 231.55/79.4$

iv. Answer $v_f = 2.92 \text{ m/s}$

The takeoff velocity can then be inserted into the following kinematic equation, described elsewhere, to determine the jump height:

$$v_f^2 = v_i^2 + 2as \qquad \text{Eq. (2.8)}$$

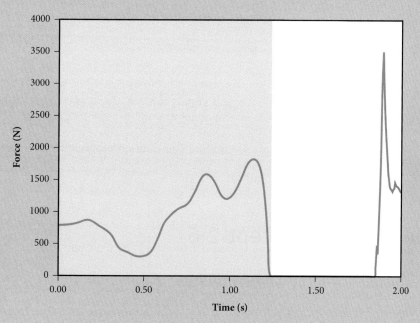

Figure 2.6 The vertical GRF during a countermovement vertical jump performed by an athlete.

(continues)

(continued)

A more accurate method of calculating the impulse of the force would be to integrate the force trace using the trapezoid method. This provides an impulse of 234.32 N, leading to a takeoff velocity of 2.95 m/s, which produces a jump height of 0.44 m.

The importance of the impulse of a force becomes clear when it is related to the linear momentum of the body to which the force is being applied. Newton's second law of motion shows that the rate of change in momentum is proportional to the net force applied to the body. Summing Equation (2.7) over a time interval for a body of constant mass, we can get:

$$\int F \mathrm{d}t = m \int \mathrm{d}v$$

Eq. (2.9)

where F is the net external force acting on the body during the time interval, t is the time interval over which the force acts, m is the mass of the body, and v is the linear velocity of the body. The symbol $\int$ refers to the integral, while d refers to an infinitesimal change. Remember that the impulse of an applied force is the product of force and time, while linear momentum is the product of mass and velocity. Equation (2.9) therefore shows that the impulse of the force is equal to the change in linear momentum produced, and the equation summarizes the **impulse–momentum relationship**:

$$J = m\Delta v$$

Eq. (2.10)

where J is the impulse of the applied force, and $m\Delta v$ is the change in momentum of a body of constant mass. Notice that this relationship can be derived from the following equation:

$$v_f = v_i + at$$

This simple relationship becomes very important in the mechanical analyses of human movements. We use momentum to quantify the motion possessed by a body, and every sport requires the change in momentum of a body, whether it is the increase in momentum of the athlete during running (see Mechanical Concept 2.6) or the increase in momentum of a projectile such as a javelin, baseball, or soccer ball. It may be that the situation requires momentum to be reduced, such as during landing tasks or intercepting a projectile, or the situation simply demands a change in direction of momentum, such as during an agility movement performed by an athlete. All of these examples require that the momentum of a body is changed; all of the examples therefore require the application of an impulse. One could make the argument that, from a mechanical perspective, success in the majority of sports is determined by the ability to generate impulse.

An appreciation of the impulse of a force is also important because in most sports the athletes are limited in the time they have to apply a force, and therefore the impulse of force may be more informative than the maximal force that the athlete is able to apply in an unrestricted time. The importance of the impulse–momentum relationship is demonstrated in Worked Examples 2.3 and 2.4.

Mechanical Concept 2.6

The impulse–momentum relationship

Figure 2.7 shows the GRF along the y-axis as an athlete runs across a force plate under three different conditions: acceleration (solid line), constant velocity (dashed line), and deceleration (broken line). The data have been time-normalized to the duration of each stance phase for the purposes of

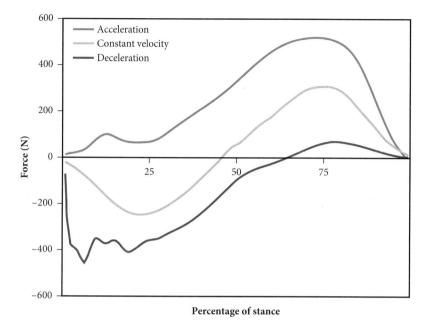

Figure 2.7 The GRF along the *y*-axis as an athlete runs across a force plate under three different conditions.

the comparison. Recall that the horizontal components of the GRF represent frictional forces.

Graphically, the impulse of a force is the area under the force–time curve. Numerically we obtain the impulse through integration of the force–time trace. In all the examples shown here, the athlete is moving along the *y*-axis so the linear momentum of the CM is always positive. In the graph associated with the acceleration trial (green line), the athlete experiences a positive impulse during the entire stance phase. The net impulse was calculated as 58.4 N. This impulse will act to increase the positive linear momentum of the CM and its velocity will be increased across the duration of stance; the athlete is getting faster.

In the graph associated with the constant velocity trial (yellow line), we can see that the athlete first experiences a negative impulse followed by a positive impulse. The two areas appear equal, implying that the net change in momentum of the CM should be 0 kg m/s during the stance phase, resulting in a constant velocity across stance. In fact, the net impulse was calculated as 7.3 N, a very small positive impulse, which would produce a very small increase in momentum, and therefore velocity, during the stance phase. However, the athlete would slow down during the subsequent aerial phase of the running step due to the retarding effect of air resistance.

Finally, in the deceleration trial (red line), we can see that the area of negative impulse is greater than that of the positive impulse. The net impulse was calculated as −71.0 N during the stance phase. This negative impulse acts to reduce the positive linear momentum of the CM such that the athlete's positive velocity will be reduced during the stance phase. Here, the athlete is slowing down.

Worked Example 2.3
Using the impulse–momentum relationship

An athlete with a mass of 80 kg performs a countermovement vertical jump. Figure 2.8 shows the vertical GRF during the time of propulsion associated with the jump recorded from a force plate.

Once body weight has been removed from the force–time curve, we can calculate the area under the curve using integration. This area represents the net impulse acting on the athlete during the time of propulsion (the sum of the positive and negative areas). We find that the net impulse acting on the athlete is 224.5 N. Given this information, calculate the takeoff velocity of the athlete.

i. Use Equation (2.10) $\qquad$ $J = m\Delta v$

ii. Input the known variables $\qquad$ $224.5 = 80 \times (v_f - v_i)$

iii. As the athlete was initially stationary $\qquad$ $224.5 = 80 \times (v_f - 0)$

iv. Rearrange to get v_f $\qquad$ $v_f = 224.5/80$

v. Answer $\qquad$ $v_f = 2.81$ m/s

The net impulse represents the change in the momentum of the athlete's CM over the time of analysis. Given that the initial momentum was 0 kg m/s (the athlete began the propulsive phase in a state of rest), this change in momentum represents the momentum at the end of propulsion—that is, the point of takeoff. Given that momentum is mv (Equation 2.3), by dividing the momentum at takeoff by the body mass of the athlete, we have the vertical velocity at takeoff. We can then calculate the athlete's jump height.

i. Use Equation (2.8) $\qquad$ $v_f^2 = v_i^2 + 2as$

ii. Input the known variables $\qquad$ $0^2 = 2.81^2 + 2 \times -9.81 \times s$

iii. Rearrange for s $\qquad$ $s = (0^2 - 2.81^2)/(2 \times -9.81)$

iv. Answer $\qquad$ $s = 0.40$ m

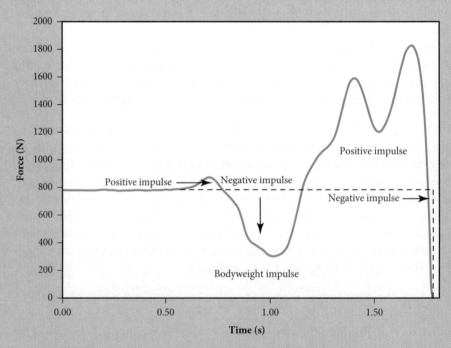

Figure 2.8 The vertical component of the GRF recorded during a countermovement vertical jump.

Worked Example 2.4
Using the impulse–momentum relationship

An athlete with a mass of 80 kg drops from a 0.30-m box and lands on a force plate on two occasions. During the first trial, the athlete prevents the hip, knee, and ankle joints from flexing excessively during landing (stiff-leg trial) and the vertical GRF and displacement of the CM is shown in **Figure 2.9a**. For the second trial, the athlete flexes the lower-limb joints during landing (bent-leg trial) with the vertical GRF and CM displacement shown in **Figure 2.9b**. The displacement of the CM was collected from a motion-analysis system and is used to define the absorption phase of the landing. Absorption is defined as the event between initial contact with the ground and the lowest vertical position of the CM, shown by the colored area on the figures.

From the graphs, we can determine the time of absorption for each of the trials. For the stiff-leg trial, the time of absorption was 0.075 s, while for the bent-leg trial the time of absorption was 0.545 s. Calculate the average force acting on the athlete during both trials.

i. Use Equation (2.8) to determine v upon landing $\qquad v_f^2 = v_i^2 + 2as$

ii. Input known variables $\qquad v_f^2 = 0^2 + 2 \times -9.81 \times -0.30$

iii. Velocity upon landing $\qquad v_f = -2.43$ m/s

iv. Use Equation (2.3) to determine initial momentum $\qquad p = mv$

v. Initial momentum $\qquad p = -194.4$ kg m/s

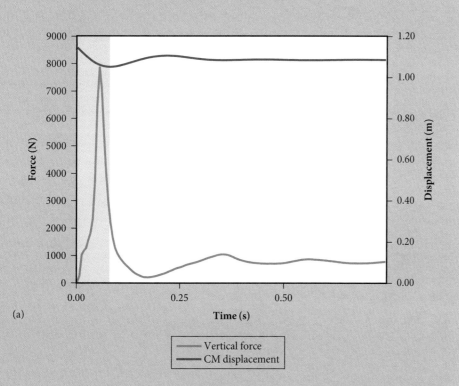

(a)

Vertical force
CM displacement

Figure 2.9 (a) The vertical GRF and the displacement of the center of mass of an athlete who lands and keeps the joints stiff after having stepped from a 0.30-m box. (*continues*)

(continues)

(continued)

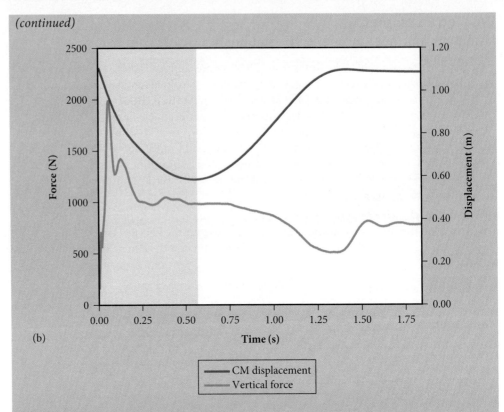

(b)

Figure 2.9 (b) The same athlete landing after having stepped from the same box, but flexing the joints of the lower body. *(continued)*

This becomes the initial vertical momentum of the athlete in both trials. During landing the GRF will act to change the initial momentum to 0 kg m/s (the CM will have a momentum of 0 kg m/s when it is at its lowest point during the landing). The difference between the two trials is the time taken by the GRF to achieve this. First we will calculate the average force during the stiff-leg trial.

i. Use Equation (2.10) $J = m\Delta v$

ii. Input known variables $F \times 0.075 = (0 - -194.4)$

iii. Rearrange for F $F = 194.4/0.075$

iv. Answer $F = 2592$ N

Now repeat the calculations for the bent-leg trial.

i. Use Equation (2.10) $J = m\Delta v$

ii. Input known variables $F \times 0.545 = (0 - -194.4)$

iii. Rearrange for F $F = 194.4/0.545$

iv. Answer $F = 357$ N

These forces represent the average forces acting on the athlete during absorption once body weight has been removed from the analysis. We can see that by increasing the time of absorption during the landing the athlete is able to reduce the average force acting on him or her during the time of landing. This is likely to have significant consequences for injury prevention.

The Work Done by a Force and Mechanical Energy

It is often informative to consider the displacement undergone by a body as a result of a force being applied. Whenever a force applied to a body results in a displacement of the body in the direction that the force acts, the force has done work on the body. Mathematically we can write this as:

$$W = Fs$$ Eq. (2.11)

where W is the work done by the force measured in joules, F is the average force applied, and s is the displacement undergone by the body in the same direction as the force acts (see Worked Example 2.5).

Worked Example 2.5
Calculating the work done by a force

Calculate the work done by the forces shown in the following free-body diagrams:

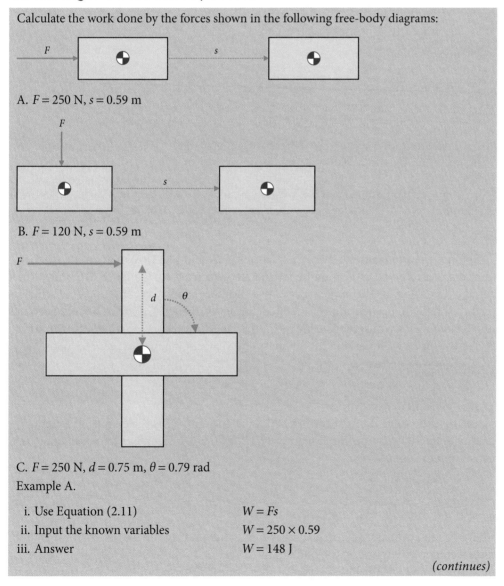

A. $F = 250$ N, $s = 0.59$ m

B. $F = 120$ N, $s = 0.59$ m

C. $F = 250$ N, $d = 0.75$ m, $\theta = 0.79$ rad

Example A.

  i. Use Equation (2.11) $W = Fs$

  ii. Input the known variables $W = 250 \times 0.59$

  iii. Answer $W = 148$ J

(continues)

(continued)

Example B.

i. Use Equation (2.11)	$W = Fs$
ii. Input the known variables	$W = 120 \times 0$
iii. Answer	$W = 0 \text{ J}$

Notice here that the body did not undergo a displacement in the direction that the applied force acts. Remember, there is a qualification provided in the calculation of work that the displacement of the body must correspond to the direction that the force is applied to the body for the force to do work. Therefore, $W = F\Delta s \cos \theta$, where θ refers to the angle between the force and displacement vectors. This is the dot product of the vector variables of force and displacement, which returns the scalar of work. If the vectors of force and displacement act in the same direction, then the work done by the force is maximized because of the cosine involved in the calculation; if the vectors are orthogonal to one another, then no work is performed by the force.

Example C.

This example requires the calculation of the work done in rotating the body.

i. Use Equation (2.26) to calculate the moment of force	$M = Fd$
ii. Input the known variables	$M = 250 \times 0.75$
iii. Answer	$M = 187.5 \text{ Nm}$
iv. Use the angular equivalent of Equation (2.11)	$W = M\theta$
v. Input the known variables	$W = 187.5 \times 0.79$
vi. Answer	$W = 148 \text{ J}$

Notice that the work done by the force of 250 N in rotation here is the same as that done by the same magnitude of force in translation in Example A. This is because the points of force application have undergone equivalent linear displacements in both situations; the force acting at 0.75 m from an axis of rotation has undergone a curvilinear displacement of 0.59 m when it rotates through an angular displacement of 0.79 rad ($0.75 \times 0.79 = 0.59$).

Notice the similarities between Equations (2.7) and (2.11). Work is done when a force displaces a body, while impulse is generated when a force is applied to a body over a defined time interval. The importance of the impulse of a force became apparent when its relationship with momentum was defined. Similarly, the work done by a force becomes important when we observe the effects on the mechanical energy of a body. By multiplying the terms in Equation (2.8) by mass and rearranging, we can get the following:

$$Fs = \frac{\Delta mv^2}{2}$$

Eq. (2.12)

where Fs is the work done by the applied force and $\Delta mv^2/2$ is the change in kinetic energy of the body. Summing Equation (2.12) over a displacement for a body of constant mass, we can get:

$$\int Fds = \frac{m \int dv^2}{2}$$

Eq. (2.13)

where F is the net external force acting on the body during the displacement, s is the displacement undergone by the body in the direction of the applied force, m is the mass of the body, and v is the linear velocity of the body. The symbol $\int$ refers to the integral, while d refers to an infinitesimal change. Equation (2.13) shows that the work done by the force is equal to the change in translational kinetic energy produced, and the equation summarizes the **work–energy theorem**:

$$W = \frac{\Delta m v^2}{2}$$

Eq. (2.14)

where W is the work done by the applied force and $\Delta mv^2/2$ is the change in translational kinetic energy. **Kinetic energy** is the energy possessed by a body due to its motion, so Equation (2.14) tells us that we can change the kinetic energy of the body only by performing work on the body. The work–energy theorem becomes important when we want to determine the effects of a force acting on a body (see Worked Example 2.6).

Worked Example 2.6
Using the work–energy theorem

Returning to the example shown in Worked Example 2.4, an athlete with a mass of 80 kg drops from a 0.30-m box and lands on a force plate on two occasions. During the first trial, the athlete prevents the hip, knee, and ankle joints from flexing excessively during landing (stiff-leg trial); during the second trial, the athlete flexes the lower-limb joints during landing (bent-leg trial).

The vertical displacement undergone by the CM during each of the trials can be determined from a motion analysis system. For the stiff-leg trial, the displacement of the CM was 0.091 m, while for the bent-leg trial, the displacement was 0.652 m. Calculate the average force acting on the athlete during both trials.

i. Velocity upon landing	$v_f = -2.43$ m/s
ii. Determine initial kinetic energy	$E_K = mv^2/2$
iii. Initial kinetic energy	$E_K = 236.2$ J

This becomes the initial kinetic energy of the athlete in both trials. During the landing, the forces acting on the CM will change the kinetic energy to 0 J, which will be achieved when the CM is at its lowest point. The difference between the two trials is the displacement gone through by the CM to achieve this. First, we will calculate the average force during the stiff-leg trial.

i. Use Equation (2.12)	$Fs = \Delta mv^2/2$
ii. Input known variables	$F \times 0.091 = (0 - 236.2)$
iii. Rearrange for F	$F = 236.2/0.091$
iv. Answer	$F = 2596$ N

Now repeat the calculations for the bent-leg trial.

i. Use Equation (2.12)	$Fs = \Delta mv^2/2$
ii. Input known variables	$F \times 0.652 = (0 - 236.2)$
iii. Rearrange for F	$F = 236.2/0.652$
iv. Answer	$F = 362$ N

These forces represent the average forces acting on the athlete during absorption once body weight has been removed from the analysis. We can see that by increasing the displacement

(continues)

(continued)

undergone by the CM during the landing, the athlete is able to reduce the average force acting on the body. This is likely to have significant consequences for injury prevention. Comparing the average force values with those calculated in Worked Example 2.4, we observe differences of less than 2% when using the impulse–momentum and work–energy theorem in these specific examples.

A final note is warranted here. While it may be convenient to consider the vertical component of the GRF as performing work on the athlete to change the kinetic energy in this example, strictly speaking, the vertical component of the GRF does no work on the athlete by virtue of the point of application of the force not undergoing a displacement. It is the internal forces that have done the work to reduce the kinetic energy of the body, the muscles having displaced the body segments during the absorption phase in this example. However, the GRF can be used to indicate the total muscular effort during a movement task.

From the work–energy theorem we can view *work* as the amount of energy transferred by a force to a body, while *energy* can be defined as the capacity to do work. Energy, like momentum, obeys a conservation law (see Mechanical Concept 2.7). Earlier, it was noted that performance in the majority of sports is determined by the ability to generate impulse given the requirement to change momentum of a body that accompanies success in most sports. The work–energy theorem provides us with a slightly different, but related, mechanical perspective. We could argue that every sport requires the change in kinetic energy of a body—the increase in the kinetic energy of the athlete during a sprint, of the projectile during javelin, baseball, or soccer; or the decrease in kinetic energy during landing tasks or intercepting a projectile. Like the impulse–momentum relationship, the work–energy theorem provides us with a mechanical means to analyze many sporting tasks (see Mechanical Concept 2.8).

Mechanical Concept 2.7

Conserved variables in biomechanical analyses

There exist a number of variables pertinent to mechanical analyses of human movements that obey **conservation laws**. What this means is that there are certain variables that remain unchanged over the period of analysis under certain mechanical conditions (mainly, the removal of nonconstant external forces such as friction, air resistance, etc.). The momentum possessed by a body follows a conservation law, and this provides a powerful tool when analyzing the aftermath of a collision between two or more bodies. If the momentum of the bodies is known prior to the collision, then the conservation of momentum informs us that the total momentum of the bodies must remain conserved during the collision; therefore, the momentum of the bodies following the collision can be calculated.

Energy also obeys a conservation law, a fact that forms the focus of the first law of thermodynamics. Using an example of a collision between bodies of equal mass traveling in opposite directions, kinetic energy is conserved such that each body may continue in motion following the collision (although the direction of motion may have changed), denoting an **elastic collision**. Furthermore, energy remains conserved during the collision even if the two bodies adhere to one another and their kinetic energy (energy due to motion) is dissipated. In this example of an **inelastic collision**, the energy is transformed from that due to the motion of the bodies to other forms (e.g., heat energy, sound energy), but total energy remains conserved. The conservation of mechanical energy also informs us that there will be energy exchanges between the different forms of mechanical energy during the flight phase of a vertical jump (see Worked Example 2.8).

Other variables associated with biomechanical analyses do not obey a conservation law. Force is not conserved. The motor system exploits this by using bones as levers with appropriate moment arms, allowing muscular forces to be amplified through these anatomical structures. Power (the rate of change of energy) also does not obey a conservation law. The existence of tendons and ligaments allows the strain potential energy accumulated during the performance of negative work associated with the countermovement of a vertical jump to be returned rapidly such that power is amplified toward the time of takeoff, enhancing jump height. Again, the motor system exploits this nonconserved variable through appropriate anatomical structures.

Mechanical Concept 2.8

Comparing the impulse–momentum relationship to the work–energy theorem

Notice the similarities between Equation (2.10) and Equation (2.14). The work–energy theorem can be derived from the impulse–momentum relationship. Given $Ft = m(v_f - v_i)$, we can assume that the change in v increases proportionally with t during the application of a constant force, and therefore the average velocity during the time of analysis can be calculated as $(v_f - v_i)/2$. The average velocity can also be determined from the ratio of displacement undergone during the time of analysis, such that $s/t = (v_f - v_i)/2$. Multiplying $Ft = m(v_f - v_i)$ by $s/t = (v_f - v_i)/2$ we get $Fs = (mv_f^2 - mv_i^2)/2$, which, of course, is the work–energy theorem. These variables have the same dimensions.

It appears, then, that we have two mechanical relationships that tell us the same thing, just using slightly different variables. This apparent mechanical redundancy can actually be helpful. In sports, we are attempting to change the motion of some body—our own, or that of an opponent, a projectile, or an implement. The momentum and kinetic energy of a body informs us of the motion. Sometimes it is useful to think about the time over which a force has been applied to a body to change its motion; here, we invoke the impulse–momentum relationship for our analysis. On other occasions, however, it might be more informative to consider the displacement undergone by the force as it changes the motion of the body. In this case, we would use the work–energy theorem for our analysis.

Forms of Mechanical Energy

As well as the kinetic energy that a body possesses due to motion ($E_{TK} = mv^2/2$), there are other forms of mechanical energy that are important in biomechanical analyses. The work–energy theorem states that the work done by a force is equal to the change of kinetic energy produced. The change in the kinetic energy of the body results in it undergoing a displacement. If the change in displacement is opposed by another force that does not change direction, then the body will possess energy that can be used when the displacement-causing force is removed (Enoka, 2008). This form of energy is known as **potential energy**, of which there are two forms pertinent to biomechanical analyses: **gravitational potential energy** and **strain potential energy**.

Gravitational potential energy is that possessed by the body due to its position in a gravitational field and is expressed as follows:

$$E_{GP} = mgh \qquad\qquad \text{Eq. (2.15)}$$

where E_{GP} is the gravitational potential energy possessed by the body measured in joules, m is the mass of the body, g is gravitational acceleration, and h is the height of the body in the reference frame (above the ground). In order to raise the body within the gravitational field, we must do work against the constant force of gravity; the more work we do, the higher we raise the body, and the more gravitational potential energy the body has (see **Worked Example 2.7**).

Worked Example 2.7
Calculating work using the change in gravitational potential energy

An athlete performs a clean movement with an 85-kg barbell. When the barbell is initially resting on the lifting platform, it is 0.22 m above the ground. The athlete catches the barbell at a height of 1.52 m above the ground at the end of the movement. Calculate the work done on the barbell during the clean.

i. Use Equation (2.15) to calculate the initial E_{GP}	$E_{GPi} = mgh$
ii. Input known variables	$E_{GPi} = 85 \times 9.81 \times 0.22$
iii. Answer	$E_{GPi} = 183.4 \text{ J}$
iv. Use Equation (2.15) to calculate the final E_{GP}	$E_{GPf} = mgh$
v. Input known variables	$E_{GPf} = 85 \times 9.81 \times 1.52$
vi. Answer	$E_{GPf} = 1267.5 \text{ J}$
vii. Calculate the change in E_{GP}	$\Delta E_{GP} = E_{GPf} - E_{GPi}$
viii. Input known variables	$\Delta E_{GP} = 1267.5 - 183.4$
ix. Answer	$\Delta E_{GP} = 1084.1 \text{ J}$

The work–energy theorem informs us that the work done on a body is equal to the change in energy produced. In Equation (2.14), we introduced this as relating to E_{TK}, allowing us to calculate the work done in changing E_{TK} in Worked Example 2.6. In the example presented here, however, the initial and final E_{TK} would be 0 J. We do know that the barbell has been raised within the gravitational field, and therefore a force has been applied to the barbell that has resulted in its displacement. This allows us to use E_{GP} to calculate that the athlete has done 1084.1 J of work on the barbell to raise it. Notice that more work would be required to raise the barbell to a greater height or to raise a more massive barbell to the same height.

We can show that the sum of mechanical energies, in the forms of kinetic and gravitational potential, are conserved under appropriate circumstances. The work–energy theorem states that the work done by a force is equal to the change of kinetic energy produced. The work done by a force can be considered to act against both constant and nonconstant forces (Enoka, 2008). Therefore:

$$\Delta E_{TK} = W_C + W_{NC} \qquad\qquad \text{Eq. (2.16)}$$

where ΔE_{TK} is the change in translational kinetic energy produced by the work, W_C is the work done against a constant force, and W_{NC} is the work done against a nonconstant force. Given that W_C results in the acquisition of potential energy, we can rewrite Equation (2.16) as follows:

$$\Delta E_{TK} = \Delta E_{GP} + W_{NC} \qquad\qquad \text{Eq. (2.17)}$$

where ΔE_{TK} is the change in translational kinetic energy produced by the work, ΔE_{GP} is the change in gravitational potential energy, and W_{NC} is the work done against a nonconstant force. When the only forces acting on the body are constant, we can rewrite Equation (2.17) as follows:

$$\Delta E_{TK} + \Delta E_{GP} = \text{constant} \qquad\qquad \text{Eq. (2.18)}$$

This is the **principle of conservation of mechanical energy**. Given that the only constant force that acts on the body in a biomechanical analysis is likely to be gravity, this principle applies to situations when the body is in flight and we consider its vertical motion (see **Worked Example 2.8**).

Worked Example 2.8
Calculating mechanical energy exchanges during the flight phase of a vertical jump

The total mechanical energy of a body (the sum of E_{TK} and E_{GP}) is conserved when the only force acting on the body is that of gravity. Consider an athlete with a mass of 80 kg during a vertical jump. **Figure 2.10** shows the vertical displacement and velocity of the CM during the jump, and the flight phase is shown by the colored area. The data were recorded from an opto-reflective motion-analysis system.

As the CM rises, its E_{GP} (mgh) increases, while its E_{TK} ($mv^2/2$) decreases. As the CM descends following the apex of flight, the E_{GP} decreases while E_{TK} increases. **Table 2.1** shows instantaneous vertical displacement and velocity of the CM during its ascent to the apex of flight recorded from a motion-analysis system, and **Table 2.2** shows its descent from the apex.

Notice in Table 2.1 that as the CM rises, the E_{GP} increases at the same time as E_{TK} is decreasing. The rate of change in these variables must be equivalent, as the sum of the two, E_{TOTAL}, remains practically constant during the time of analysis. In Table 2.2, the changes in E_{GP} and E_{TK} are reversed, but E_{TOTAL} remains constant. This demonstrates that E_{GP} and E_{TK} of the CM are exchanged, and E_{TOTAL} is conserved during the flight phase of the vertical jump when the constant force of gravity is the only force acting on the body. We can ignore the fluid dynamic force of drag here because the body is not moving with sufficient velocity.

(continues)

(continued)

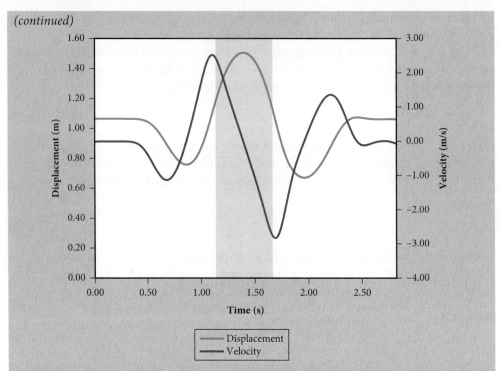

Figure 2.10 The vertical displacement and the vertical velocity of the center of mass of an athlete performing a countermovement vertical jump from a stationary starting position.

Table 2.1
The Vertical Displacement, Vertical Velocity, and Mechanical Energy of an Athlete's Center of Mass as It Rises to the Apex of Flight During a Vertical Jump

Time (s)	s (mm)	v (m/s)	E_{GP} (J)	E_{TK} (J)	E_{TOTAL} (J)
0.000	1501.89	0.27	$(80 \times 9.81 \times 1.50189)$ $= 1178.68$	$(80 \times 0.27^2/2)$ $= 2.92$	1181.60
0.005	1503.11	0.22	$(80 \times 9.81 \times 1.50311)$ $= 1179.64$	$(80 \times 0.22^2/2)$ $= 1.94$	1181.58
0.010	1504.10	0.17	$(80 \times 9.81 \times 1.50410)$ $= 1180.42$	$(80 \times 0.17^2/2)$ $= 1.16$	1181.58
0.015	1504.85	0.13	$(80 \times 9.81 \times 1.50485)$ $= 1181.00$	$(80 \times 0.13^2/2)$ $= 0.68$	1181.68
0.020	1505.35	0.08	$(80 \times 9.81 \times 1.50535)$ $= 1181.40$	$(80 \times 0.08^2/2)$ $= 0.26$	1181.66
0.025	1505.62	0.03	$(80 \times 9.81 \times 1.50562)$ $= 1181.61$	$(80 \times 0.03^2/2)$ $= 0.04$	1181.65
0.030	1505.65	−0.02	$(80 \times 9.81 \times 1.50565)$ $= 1181.63$	$(80 \times -0.02^2/2)$ $= 0.02$	1181.65

Note: s is the vertical position of the CM within the reference frame; v is the vertical velocity of the CM; E_{GP} is the gravitational potential energy of the CM; E_{TK} is the translational kinetic energy of the CM; E_{TOTAL} is the total mechanical energy of the CM.

Table 2.2
The Vertical Displacement, Vertical Velocity, and Mechanical Energy of an Athlete's Center of Mass as It Falls from the Apex of Flight During a Vertical Jump

Time (s)	s (mm)	v (m/s)	E_{GP} (J)	E_{TK} (J)	E_{TOTAL} (J)
0.000	1505.65	−0.02	$(80 \times 9.81 \times 1.50565)$ $= 1181.63$	$(80 \times -0.02^2/2)$ $= 0.02$	1181.65
0.005	1505.43	−0.07	$(80 \times 9.81 \times 1.50543)$ $= 1181.46$	$(80 \times -0.07^2/2)$ $= 0.20$	1181.66
0.010	1504.97	−0.12	$(80 \times 9.81 \times 1.50497)$ $= 1181.10$	$(80 \times -0.12^2/2)$ $= 0.58$	1181.68
0.015	1504.27	−0.16	$(80 \times 9.81 \times 1.50427)$ $= 1180.56$	$(80 \times -0.16^2/2)$ $= 1.02$	1181.57
0.020	1503.33	−0.21	$(80 \times 9.81 \times 1.50333)$ $= 1179.82$	$(80 \times -0.21^2/2)$ $= 1.76$	1181.57
0.025	1502.15	−0.26	$(80 \times 9.81 \times 1.50215)$ $= 1178.89$	$(80 \times -0.26^2/2)$ $= 2.70$	1181.59
0.030	1500.72	−0.31	$(80 \times 9.81 \times 1.50072)$ $= 1177.77$	$(80 \times -0.31^2/2)$ $= 3.84$	1181.61

Note: s is the vertical position of the CM within the reference frame; v is the vertical velocity of the CM; E_{GP} is the gravitational potential energy of the CM; E_{TK} is the translational kinetic energy of the CM; E_{TOTAL} is the total mechanical energy of the CM.

Strain potential energy is the energy that a body possesses due to the deformation induced by the work done by a force, expressed as:

$$E_{SP} = \frac{kx^2}{2}$$

(Eq. 2.19)

where E_{SP} is strain potential energy measured in joules, k is the stiffness of the material being deformed, and x is the displacement over which the material is deformed. There are many materials, both naturally occurring and manmade, that athletes use in sport to take advantage of E_{SP} to enhance performance. Tendons and ligaments are elastic tissues by virtue of the protein bundles comprising them. The elasticity is exploited by the motor system, which employs the associated storage of E_{SP} in these tissues when they are deformed to minimize metabolic energy costs and enhance performance (see Mechanical Concept 2.9). Other materials able to store E_{SP} that are used to

Mechanical Concept 2.9

Potential energy as stored work

The foot is placed ahead of the CM at the beginning of each stance phase when walking, inducing a frictional force that acts to slow the forward velocity of the CM during the first half of stance. However, the leg remains relatively stiff during

(continues)

(continued)

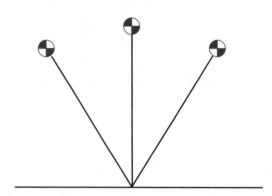

Figure 2.11 The human body modeled as an inverted pendulum during the stance phase of walking. At the beginning of stance the foot contacts the ground ahead of the center of mass, inducing a frictional force to reduce the translational kinetic energy possessed by the center of mass. The leg remains relatively stiff, causing the center of mass to rise over the first half of stance, increasing the gravitational potential energy of the center of mass. The center of mass falls over the second half of stance such that the gravitational potential energy of the center of mass is reduced with a concomitant increase in the translational kinetic energy.

the stance phase and the CM rises over the first half of stance, falling during the second half. The stiff stance leg and the concomitant rise and fall of the CM means that the body acts like an inverted pendulum during the stance phases of walking gait (Farley & Ferris, 1998; Figure 2.11).

If we graph the E_{TK} and E_{GP} of the CM during the stance phase of walking, we get the data shown in Figure 2.12. Notice that over the first half of stance E_{TK} is reduced, while E_{GP} is increased, as per an inverted pendulum. E_{TK} is being transformed to E_{GP} over the first half of stance due to the frictional force acting on the participant and the relatively stiff leg. The CM then uses the E_{GP} to do work to increase E_{TK} over the second half of stance. This exchange of energy reduces the requirement for metabolic energy expenditure during the stance phase of walking by minimizing the requirement for muscular work to maintain the motion of the CM.

The greater forward velocities achieved when running preclude the use of the inverted pendulum and the body is modeled as a mass-spring system where the leg acts like a spring, being compressed over the first half of stance and returning to its original configuration over the second half of stance, as shown in Figure 2.13 (Farley & Ferris, 1998).

This spring-like action of the stance leg is necessary to reduce the magnitude of the impact forces that would be incurred during running gait if the leg were to remain stiff as per the inverted pendulum model. The spring-like action of the leg means that E_{TK} and E_{GP} possessed by the CM are now in-phase during stance, falling and rising in synchrony; these forms of mechanical energy can no longer

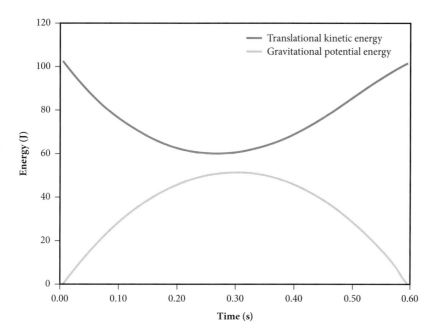

Figure 2.12 A graph showing the translational kinetic and gravitational potential energy of the center of mass during the stance phase of walking. Notice that the two forms of mechanical energy have an antiphase relationship meaning that they are exchanged during the stance phase of walking.

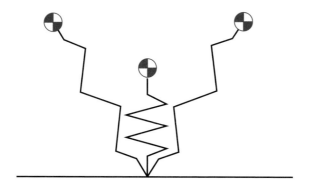

Figure 2.13 The human body modeled as a mass-spring system during the stance phase of running. At the beginning of stance the foot contacts the ground ahead of the center of mass, inducing a frictional force to reduce the translational kinetic energy possessed by the center of mass. The shorter stance durations associated with the greater speeds achieved during running gait mean that the leg acts like a spring to reduce the impact forces experienced. The compression of the leg over the first half of stance allows the leg spring to accumulate strain potential energy as the elastic tissues associated with the tendons and ligaments are deformed. Strain potential energy is then returned during the second half of stance to allow the leg spring to do work on the center of mass to increase translational kinetic energy.

(continues)

(continued)

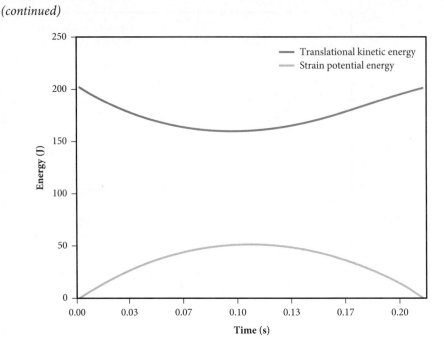

Figure 2.14 This graph shows the translational kinetic energy of the CM and the strain potential energy of the leg spring during the stance phase of running. Notice that the two forms of mechanical energy have an antiphase relationship, meaning that they are exchanged during the stance phase of running.

be exchanged. However, the compression of the leg over the first half of stance allows the leg spring to accumulate E_{SP} as the elastic tissues associated with the tendons and ligaments are deformed. E_{SP} is then returned during the second half of stance to allow the leg spring to do work on the CM to increase E_{TK} (Figure 2.14). Again, metabolic energy expenditure is reduced by this energy exchange. Essentially, both forms of potential energy, E_{GP} and E_{SP}, act as mechanisms to store work from E_{TK} during the first half of stance that can be used to increase E_{TK} over the second half of stance. Metabolic energy is therefore saved during both walking and running gait by exchanging mechanical energy.

enhance sports performance include golf clubs and balls, soccer balls, running tracks, and poles used in the pole vault (see **Mechanical Concept 2.10**). Elastic bands are also used to alter the mechanical response when performing resistance-training exercises (see Chapter 6).

Power

Power is defined as the rate of doing work. Much like the variable of the impulse of force, power is likely to have a significant effect in sports where the athletes are limited by time; their performance is limited not by the maximal amount of work that they

Mechanical Concept 2.10

Energy exchanges during the pole vault

The poles used in the pole vault event in track and field are made of a carbon-composite material that is able to store and return strain potential energy. Consider an athlete holding the pole while sprinting down the runway. At this point, the system (athlete + pole) possesses energy due to its velocity (E_{TK}). This energy can be used to do work on the pole once it is planted in the box. The work done on the pole acts to deform it, so it stores energy (E_{SP}). This energy is then returned and the pole does work to raise the CM of the athlete (increasing E_{GP}). Although there are obviously mechanical energy losses during the movement, this simple analysis of the energy exchanges is very helpful. It tells us that in order to be successful, that athlete must possess large E_{GP} before attempting to negotiate the bar, but this energy is due in large part to the initial E_{TK} possessed by the system. Therefore, a good pole vaulter needs to be a good sprinter (Schade, Arampatzis, Brüggeman, & Komi, 2004).

Essentially, both forms of potential energy, E_{GP} and E_{SP}, act as mechanisms to store work from E_{TK} during the first half of stance that can be used to increase E_{TK} over the second half of stance. Metabolic energy is therefore saved during both walking and running gaits by exchanging mechanical energy.

---

are able to perform, but rather the rate at which they are able to perform work. For this reason, power is considered to be a very important mechanical variable in determining success in sports.

Average power can be expressed as follows:

$$\bar{P} = \frac{W}{\Delta t}$$

Eq. (2.20)

where $\bar{P}$ is average power measured in watts, W is the work done by the applied force, and Δt is the change in time (see **Worked Example 2.9**). Given that $W = Fs$, Equation (2.20) can be rewritten in terms of velocity as:

$$P = Fv$$

Eq. (2.21)

where P is power, F is the applied force, and v is the linear velocity of the body (see **Worked Example 2.10**). Given the work–energy theorem, we can also express power as the rate of change in mechanical energy:

$$P = \frac{\Delta E_{TOTAL}}{\Delta t}$$

Eq. (2.22)

where P is the net power, ΔE_{TOTAL} is the change in mechanical energy (sum of E_{TK}, E_{GP}, and E_{SP}), and Δt is the change in time.

Worked Example 2.9
Calculating average power output from kinematic data

An athlete performs a power clean from the floor with an 87.5-kg barbell. Figure 2.15 shows the vertical displacement and velocity of the barbell CM recorded from an opto-reflective motion-analysis system.

At the start of the movement ($t = 0$ s) the vertical position of the CM is 0.22 m, while at the highest point ($t = 1.70$ s), the vertical position of the CM is 1.49 m. Calculate the average power output from the start of the clean to the highest position of the barbell.

i. Calculate the energy at $t = 0$ s using Equation (2.15)	$E_{GP} = mgh$
ii. Input known variables at the start	$E_{GPi} = 87.5 \times 9.81 \times 0.22$
iii. Answer	$E_{GPi} = 188.8$ J
iv. Calculate the energy at $t = 1.70$ s using Equation (2.15)	$E_{GPf} = 87.5 \times 9.81 \times 1.49$
v. Answer	$E_{GPf} = 1279.0$ J
vi. Calculate the change in E_{GP}	$\Delta E_{GP} = 1090.2$ J
vii. Use Equation (2.20)	$P = W/\Delta t$
viii. Input known variables	$P = 1090.2/(1.70 - 0)$
ix. Answer	$P = 641.3$ W

The value of 641.3 W represents the average rate at which work was done by the athlete on the barbell when raising it to its highest position. We could also calculate instantaneous

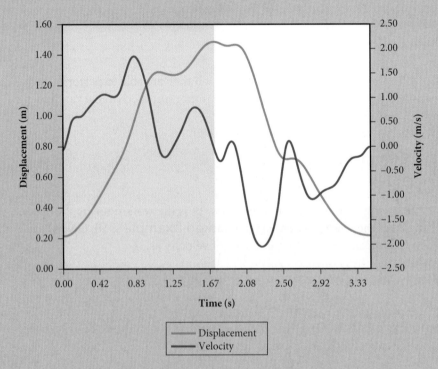

Figure 2.15 The vertical displacement and velocity of the center of mass of a barbell during a power clean from the floor. The shaded area highlights the event from the start of the lift to the time when the athlete stands up with the barbell, having caught it.

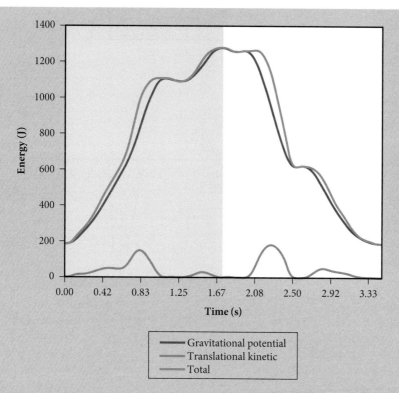

Figure 2.16 The graphs of gravitational potential, translational kinetic, and total mechanical energy of the barbell during the power clean. The shaded area highlights the event from the start of the lift to the time when the athlete stands up with the barbell, having caught it.

power output during the lift by using the work–energy theorem. Remember, this theorem informs us that the work done on a body is equal to the change in energy produced. Power is the rate of performing work; therefore, power is the rate at which energy is changed. By calculating the instantaneous values for E_{GP} and E_{TK}, we can calculate the total mechanical energy of the barbell ($E_{GP} + E_{TK}$). The instantaneous mechanical energy graphs are shown in Figure 2.16.

We can calculate the instantaneous rate of change in energy by calculating the first derivative of the total mechanical energy. This variable is the instantaneous power output, as shown in Figure 2.17.

If we average the instantaneous power output shown in Figure 2.17 from the start of the movement to the time of highest vertical displacement, we arrive at a value of 640.3 W, a value that is almost identical to that calculated from the average rate of change of gravitational potential energy. Furthermore, from Figure 2.15, we are able to determine a peak power output of over 2000 W that occurs during the second pull of the movement. If we integrate the area under the power output curve between $t = 0$ and $t = 1.70$, we get a value of 1090.9 J, representing the work done in raising the barbell. Notice how close this value is to the change in gravitational potential energy calculated earlier. A change in energy reflects the work done on a body; power is the time-derivative of work, so work is the time-integral of power.

(continues)

(continued)

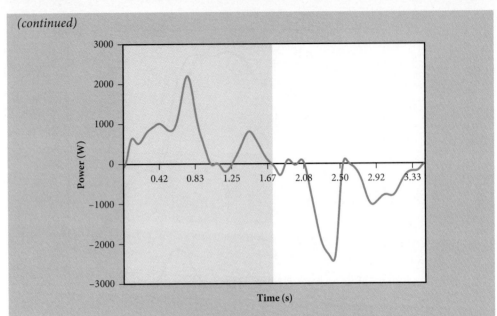

Figure 2.17 The graph of instantaneous power output of the barbell during the power clean. The shaded area highlights the event from the start of the lift to the time when the athlete stands up with the barbell, having caught it.

Worked Example 2.10
Calculating peak power output from kinetic data

An athlete performs a countermovement vertical jump. Figure 2.18 shows the vertical force measured from a force plate during the jump along with the vertical velocity of

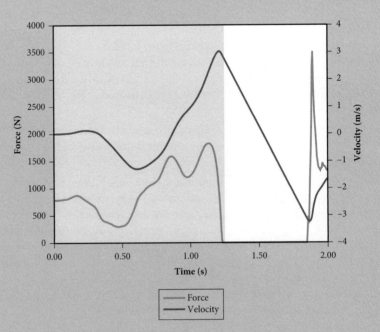

Figure 2.18 The vertical GRF and vertical velocity during a countermovement vertical jump from a stationary starting position.

the CM calculated through integration of the force trace. The shaded area represents the propulsive phase of the jump.

Calculate the peak power output of the CM during the jump.

  i. Use Equation (2.21) $\qquad\qquad\qquad\qquad$ $P = Fv$

Figure 2.19 shows the instantaneous power output calculated from this method. The peak power output can then be determined.

  ii. Answer $\qquad\qquad\qquad\qquad\qquad$ $P = 4613 \text{ W}$

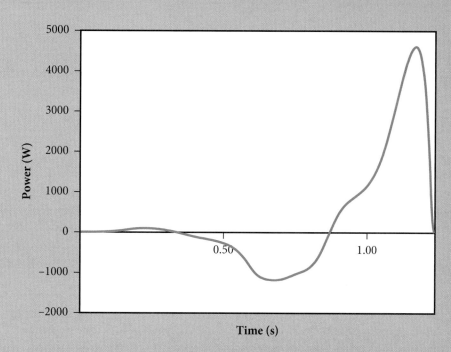

Figure 2.19 The instantaneous power output of the CM during the propulsive phase of a countermovement vertical jump calculated from the product of the vertical GRF and the vertical velocity of the CM.

Friction and the Coefficient of Friction

When decomposing the GRF into the components that act along the three axes, it was noted that the component along the z-axis was the normal force, while those along the x- and y-axes were frictional forces (see Mechanical Concept 2.4). Friction is induced whenever two bodies in contact move or tend to move relative to one another. The frictional force resists the motion or intended motion of the bodies and can be expressed as follows:

$$F_F = \mu N \qquad\qquad\qquad\qquad \textbf{Eq. (2.23)}$$

where F_F is the frictional force measured in newtons, μ is the coefficient of friction, and N is the force normal to the surface. The normal force acting on the body is equal to the weight of the body when the surface is level, but the athlete can increase the normal force through muscular forces (see Mechanical Concept 2.10). The coefficient of friction is a dimensionless number that is determined by the characteristics of the surfaces of the two bodies in contact, including the relative roughness, hardness, temperature, lubricating material interposed between the surfaces, and relative velocity of the bodies. The effect of relative velocity gives rise to two types of friction coefficient. The coefficient of static friction (μ_s) applies to situations when there is no movement of the bodies in contact. The static frictional force can then be expressed:

$$F_{Fs} \leq \mu_s N \qquad\qquad \text{Eq. (2.24)}$$

where F_{Fs} is the static frictional force, μ_s is the coefficient of static friction, and N is the force normal to the surface. The inequality symbol in Equation (2.24) indicates that the frictional force is evident even when it exceeds the force being applied to the body and the body is not moving. In situations when there is movement of the bodies in contact, the coefficient of kinetic friction (μ_k) applies. The kinetic frictional force is then expressed as follows:

$$F_{Fk} = \mu_k N \qquad\qquad \text{Eq. (2.25)}$$

where F_{Fk} is the kinetic frictional force, μ_k is the coefficient of kinetic friction, and N is the force normal to the surface. The coefficient of kinetic friction remains relatively constant up to velocities of approximately 10 m/s (Bartlett, 2007). It should be noted that the coefficient of static friction is greater than the coefficient of kinetic friction, resulting in greater frictional forces when there is no relative motion between the two surfaces. Although Equations (2.24) and (2.25) are simplifications of real situations (Blau, 2009), they will suffice for most of our mechanical analyses of human movements. Table 2.3 shows coefficients of static and kinetic friction for a variety of materials in contact. The frictional components of the GRF are very important in many sporting movements (see Mechanical Concept 2.11 and Applied Research 2.1).

Table 2.3
Coefficients of Static and Kinetic Friction for a Variety of Materials

Materials	μ_s	μ_k
Finger on mild steel		1.8
Tennis ball on synthetic carpet		0.61
Finger on paper		0.6
Tennis ball on hard court		0.5
Waxed ski on snow (0°C)	0.1	0.05
Ice on ice (melting point)	0.05–0.15	
Teflon on Teflon	0.04–0.08	

Data from Blau, P. J. (2009). *Friction Science and Technology. From Concepts to Applications.* Boca Raton, FL: Taylor and Francis; White, C. (2011). *Projectile Dynamics in Sport.* Oxon, UK: Routledge.

Mechanical Concept 2.11

Manipulating the frictional components of the GRF

The two horizontal components of the GRF (x- and y-axes) represent the friction between the athlete and the supporting surface. The frictional force is very important in determining an athlete's ability to accelerate in a horizontal plane. Equation (2.23) summarizes the relationship between the coefficient of friction and the normal component of the ground reaction, which determines the frictional force. This equation, $F_F = \mu N$, provides two basic solutions available to the athlete in order to increase or decrease the frictional force: either change the coefficient of friction or change the normal component of the GRF. The coefficient of friction is determined by the characteristics of the materials comprising the surfaces in contact and is difficult for the athlete to change in the short term, with the exception of changing footwear. What the athlete is able to affect, however, is the magnitude of the normal component of the GRF. A reduction of the normal component can be achieved by flexing the lower-body joints to induce a negative acceleration of the CM, such as occurs during the unweighting at the beginning of a countermovement jump. Conversely, by forcefully extending the lower-body joints, the normal component can be increased. An athlete may use this flexion and extension of the lower-body joints when performing a change-of-direction maneuver involving rotation about the stance foot. Initially the athlete flexes, producing an unweighting that reduces the normal component, and therefore the frictional force at the foot. This allows the body to be rotated about the ground foot. The athlete then extends the joints, thereby increasing the normal component and increasing the frictional force while accelerating away from the turn.

Applied Research 2.1
The effects of friction on change-of-direction performance and injury potential

The horizontal components of the GRF have a significant effect on the ability of the athlete to change direction rapidly. Therefore, increasing frictional forces at the shoe–ground interface are likely to improve change-of-direction performance, although concomitant increases in the lower-body joint kinetics are likely, which would have implications for injuries. The authors compared lower-body joint kinetics during the performance of a change-of-direction movement when wearing a shoe with a tread versus a shoe with a smooth sole. The coefficients of friction were significantly different between the tread and smooth shoes (1.00 vs. 0.87, respectively). While performance of the change-of-direction task was not different between the two conditions, the peak joint moments were significantly greater when the movement was performed with the high-friction, tread shoe. This implies an upper threshold for frictional forces above which performance improvements are not realized, but the potential for musculoskeletal injury is increased.

Wannop, J. W., Worobets, J. T., & Stefanyshyn, D. J. (2010). Footwear traction and lower extremity joint loading. *American Journal of Sports Medicine, 38*, 1221–1228.

The Moment of a Force

It was noted that forces are vector quantities so their magnitude and direction of application are important in determining the changes of motion of the body to which the forces are applied. A third variable associated with a force is required to allow a full description of its effect on a body, and that is the line of action of the force. So far we have considered the effects of forces on the linear motion of bodies, yet consideration of the line of action of the force allows us to determine their effects on rotational motion. Rotational motion is defined as that taking place around an axis. If a net force is applied to a rigid body such that the line of action of the force passes through the axis of rotation, then the body will undergo translation. However, if the line of action of the net force does not pass through the axis, then the body will undergo both translation and rotation. The perpendicular distance between the line of action of the force and the axis of rotation is known as the **moment arm** of the force and can be used to calculate the moment of force:

$$M = Fd \hspace{6cm} \textbf{Eq. (2.26)}$$

where M is the moment of force measured in newton-meters, F is the force applied to the body, and d is the moment arm of the force measured in meters. Both F and d are vectors, and the moment of force is calculated as the cross-product of the two vectors. The moment of force informs us of the rotational effect of the applied force. Examples that are pertinent to the analysis of sporting movements include moments of force acting at joints (joint moments; see Mechanical Concept 2.12) and moments of force acting on an athlete associated with the GRF (see Mechanical Concept 2.13).

Mechanical Concept 2.12

Calculating joint moments

Forces that act on body segments are responsible for the rotations of the segments relative to one another such as those observed during movements. The forces acting on the body segments include the following (Winter, 2009):

1. Gravitational force: This force acts at the CM of each segment and is equal to the product of the segmental mass and gravitational acceleration (-9.81 m/s^2).

2. Ground reaction or external forces: External forces are exerted on the body when it is in contact with another body, which will be the ground in most of our analyses. The GRF can be represented as a single vector acting at the center of pressure.

3. Joint structural forces: The many internal forces acting across a joint that are exerted on the body segment under analysis include those from muscles, ligaments, the joint capsule, and even the skin. Of these forces, those exerted by muscular contractions are considered to present the greatest contribution.

4. Joint reaction forces: The body segments on either side of a joint exert equal and opposite forces on one another in accordance with Newton's third law of motion.

5. Articulating forces: The forces associated with the joint structures produce not only a rotational force but also compressive and shear forces. These compressive and shear forces are exerted across the articulating surfaces of the joint.

By considering the forces acting on a segment, we are able to calculate the net moment acting at a joint using a segmental analysis. In such an analysis, the body segments are considered rigid bodies that do not deform and therefore have constant inertial properties (i.e., mass, CM, distribution of mass). Furthermore, frictional forces that may be induced by the motion of the body segments acting at the joint are neglected. Consider the free-body diagram of the foot segment shown in Figure 2.20.

The segment is considered free to rotate in space about an axis that passes through the CM. Figure 2.21 shows the free-body diagram with the variables of linear and angular accelerations of the segment as well as the moment arms associated with the forces acting on the segment.

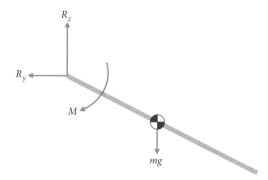

Figure 2.20 A free-body diagram of the foot segment during a mechanical analysis as viewed in the sagittal plane. The ankle joint is placed at the left side of the segment.

Note: mg is the weight of foot segment; R_y is the joint reaction force along the y-axis; R_z is the joint reaction force acting along the z-axis; M is the net joint moment.

The joint reaction forces can be calculated from Newton's equation of motion (Equation 2.6) applied to the forces along the y- and z-axes:

$$\Sigma F_y = ma, \text{ therefore } R_y = m \times a_y \qquad\qquad \text{Eq. (2.27)}$$

$$\Sigma F_z = ma, \text{ therefore } R_z = m \times a_z - mg \qquad\qquad \text{Eq. (2.28)}$$

where ΣF_y is the sum of the forces acting on the segment along the y-axis, ΣF_z is the sum of the forces acting on the segment along the z-axis, m is the mass of the segment, a is the linear acceleration of the CM of the segment, and g is gravitational acceleration. The mass of a body segment can be obtained from various sources (e.g., Dempster, 1955), while the linear acceleration of the segment CM can be measured using a motion-analysis system. The joint reaction forces R_y and R_z are responsible for the acceleration of the segment CM we measure from

(continues)

(continued)

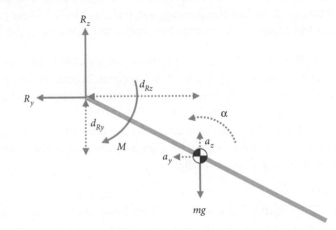

Figure 2.21 The free-body diagram of the foot segment during a mechanical analysis showing the linear and angular accelerations of the segment and the moment arms of the forces.

Note: mg is the weight of foot segment; R_y is the joint reaction force along the y-axis; R_z is the joint reaction force acting along the z-axis; M is the net joint moment; a_y is the acceleration of the CM along the y-axis; a_z is the acceleration of the CM along the z-axis; α is the angular acceleration of the segment; d_{Ry} is the moment arm of R_y; d_{Rz} is the moment arm of R_z.

our motion-analysis system. Given the knowledge of R_y and R_z, we can calculate the net moment acting on the segment by using Euler's equation of motion:

$$\sum M = I\alpha \qquad \text{Eq.(2.29)}$$

where ΣM is the sum of the moments of force acting on the segment, I is the mass moment of inertia of the segment defining the resistance that the body provides to an angular acceleration, and a is the angular acceleration of the segment. Essentially, Equation (2.5) is the angular equivalent of Newton's equation of motion. The mass moment of inertia of the segment about an axis of rotation can again be obtained from various sources (e.g., Dempster, 1955), while the angular acceleration of the CM can again be measured using a motion-analysis system. Given that the forces R_y and R_z represent moments of force that act to rotate the segment about the CM, we can rewrite Equation (2.5) as:

$$M + (R_y \times d_{Ry}) - (R_z \times d_{Rz}) = I\alpha \qquad \text{Eq. (2.30)}$$

Note that the addition of the term $(R_y \times d_{Ry})$ and the subtraction of the term $(R_z \times d_{Rz})$ in Equation (2.30) simply denote the direction of rotation induced by these forces (counterclockwise is positive, clockwise is negative). The moment arms d_{Ry} and d_{Rz} can be measured from our motion-analysis system, leaving the only unknown in Equation (2.30) as M, the net moment of force acting at the ankle joint about the mediolateral axis. This net moment of force does not represent the actual muscle force exerted on the segment during the analysis; other structures such as the ligaments that cross the joint and the associated joint capsules also contribute to this moment of force (Winter, 2009). Muscular forces are certainly considered to represent the major contributors to the observed joint moment. However, it should be recognized that the activity of antagonistic muscles will have a considerable effect on the net joint moment of force during a given movement.

Notice that the foot was not in contact with a supporting surface in our analysis, and therefore there was no GRF exerted on the segment. The GRF represents a boundary condition that would need to be included in our previous analysis if the athlete was in contact with a supporting surface. The GRF can be measured from a force plate and would act on the segment at a point defined by the center of pressure. The effects of the GRF can be determined by data recorded from force plate that have been synchronized with a motion-analysis system, allowing the calculation of joint moments using the **inverse dynamics** approach (Winter, 2009).

Joint moments of force hold considerable interest in the mechanical analysis of movements because of the effect the joint moments have on the GRF acting on the athlete. Figure 2.22 shows the moment of force summed across the hip, knee, and ankle joints of both legs for an athlete performing a vertical jump. The joint moments were those calculated about the *x*-axis representing flexion–extension at each of the joints (positive values reflect a net extensor moment at the joints). The sum of these moments is known as the **support moment** (Winter, 2009). Also shown in Figure 2.22 is the vertical GRF during the movement. The relationship between the combined joint moments and the resulting GRF is obvious. In this way the GRF can provide an indication of total muscular effort in a given movement (see Applied Research 2.2).

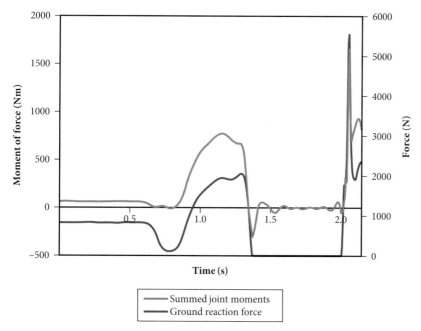

Figure 2.22 The net moment of force summed across the hip, knee, and ankle joints of both legs and the vertical GRF during a countermovement vertical jump. Note that a positive value represents an extensor moment at the joints.

Applied Research 2.2

The effects of barbell load on the lower-body joint moments during the back squat exercise

The joint moments of the lower-body joints contribute substantially to the GRF recorded during movements such that the GRF should change in proportion to the changes in the support moment (the sum of the hip, knee, and ankle joint moments). These authors recorded the GRF and lower-body joint moments during back squats performed with loads equivalent to 25%, 50%, 75%, and 100% of each participant's three-repetition maximum. It was reported that the average GRF increased with the load on the barbell and the increases were proportional to the increases in the average support moment. However, while the magnitude of the moments at the hip, knee, and ankle joints increased with external load, their individual contributions to the support moment were not consistent across the loading conditions. This suggests that the control of force output during multi-segment movements is complex.

Flanagan, S. P., & Salem, G. J. (2008). Lower extremity joint kinetic responses to external resistance variations. *Journal of Applied Biomechanics, 24,* 58–68.

Mechanical Concept 2.13

Moments of force when running around a curve

Consider an athlete running around a curve such as during a 200-m sprint. If we plotted the velocity vector of the CM in the transverse plane, we would observe it changing direction at each time instant. Even if the magnitude of the velocity vector remained constant throughout the task, the change in direction of the velocity vector constitutes an acceleration, which must be caused by a force acting on the CM (as per Newton's first law of motion). This force is the **centripetal force**, the magnitude of which is given by $F_c = m(v^2/r)$. This equation informs us that the centripetal force required to keep the direction of the velocity vector changing—and therefore the athlete running around the curve—will increase as running velocity increases or as the radius of the curve decreases. The source of the centripetal force for the sprinter is the friction exerted between the athlete's foot and the running surface; the athlete's foot is placed laterally with respect to the CM when viewed in the frontal plane, inducing a frictional force acting toward the center of the curve, as shown in Figure 2.23a.

Notice in Figure 2.23a that the frictional force acts at a distance from the CM. This will induce a moment of force acting to rotate the athlete in the counter-clockwise direction. Clearly, this outward rotation will impede the forward progression of the athlete. In Figure 2.23b, the athlete leans into the curve while running. By adopting this posture, the force associated with body weight acts a distance from the foot, producing a moment to rotate the athlete in the clockwise direction. This moment counters that caused by the frictional force.

This inward lean of the athlete, which is required to counter the moment induced by friction, reduces the athlete's ability to exert vertical force, and therefore interferes with running velocity. Indeed, it has been shown that

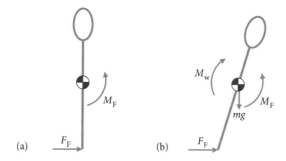

Figure 2.23 (a) A free-body diagram showing the frontal view of an athlete running around a bend in an upright posture. (b) A free-body diagram showing the frontal view of an athlete running around a bend while leaning into the bend.

Note: F_F is the frictional force, M_F is the moment of force due to friction; mg is the weight force; M_w is the moment of force due to weight.

athletes run faster on a straight track when compared to running around a flat curve (Jain, 1980). However, running tracks have curves. When the radius of the curve is reduced, such as on an indoor track, the curves are banked, and the requirement for the frictional force to act as a centripetal force is reduced. The influence of the biomechanics associated with speed when running around a flat curve are different than those of a straight track.

Technology to Record Kinetic Variables

There are various technologies available to the strength and conditioning practitioner to assess the kinetic variables associated with the performance of athletes during jumping and running tasks, as well as resistance-training exercises. These technologies include position transducers, motion-analysis systems, and accelerometers whereby Newton's equation of motion (second law of motion) can be used to calculate kinetic variables, including force and power output. Other technologies, including pressure insoles and force plates, allow the direct measurement of the GRF during movements.

Position transducers

Position transducer technology allows the linear position of a body to be determined and can be very useful when recording the kinematic variables associated with jumping and resistance exercises. The position data recorded by a position transducer can be double differentiated to return the acceleration of the body, which can then be entered into Equation (2.6), along with the mass of the body, to determine the force acting on the body. Differentiating the position data derived from a position transducer to return the velocity of the body can allow the power output of the body to be determined by using Equation (2.21). This approach has been used to calculate the force and power output during resistance exercises, including bench throws and squat jumps (Comstock, Solomon-Hill, Flanagan, 2011; Crewther et al., 2011). While the kinetic data derived from a position transducer have been shown to have acceptable reliability, the validity of the kinetic variables derived from kinematic data recorded from position transducers has been questioned (Cormie, McBride, & McCaulley, 2007; see Applied Research 2.3).

Applied Research 2.3
Measuring kinetic variables directly versus calculating them from kinematic data

Kinetic variables such as force and power during resistance-training exercises can be calculated from the instantaneous position of the barbell recorded from linear position transducers (LPTs) by using Newton's equation of motion ($F = ma$). Alternatively, the forces acting on the system can be measured directly from force-plate data, which can be integrated to provide kinematic variables as well. Finally, force plate data can be combined with that from LPTs to allow the calculation of power output. These authors compared the difference in force, velocity, and power output recorded during jump squats, squats, and power cleans calculated from different combinations of kinematic and kinetic data recorded from an LPT and a force plate. The authors found that the force calculated from LPT data was overestimated compared to the force recorded directly from the force plate. This resulted in an overestimation of power output. Conversely, the velocity calculated from the force plate data tended to be below that recorded from the LPT, resulting in an underestimation of power output. The authors reported that calculation methods that rely solely on kinematic or kinetic data have limitations that preclude their use in mechanical analyses, so kinematic data should be combined with kinetic data for accurate measurement of power output. These findings have significant implications for determining the specific load during resistance training exercises that maximize the kinetic variables of force and power.

Cormie, P., McBride, J. M., & McCaulley, G. O. (2007). Validation of power measurement techniques in dynamic lower body resistance exercises. *Journal of Applied Biomechanics, 23*, 103–118.

Accelerometers

Accelerometers are devices that record the acceleration of a body to which they are attached. Given knowledge of the mass of the body, the acceleration data can be used with Equation (2.6) to provide the force acting on the body. Integrating the acceleration data allows the velocity of the body to be calculated, which can be combined with the force data to return the power output, as per Equation (2.21). This approach has been used to calculate force and power output from accelerometers attached to the barbell during resistance exercises including bench throws and squat jumps (Comstock et al., 2011; Crewther et al., 2011; see Applied Research 2.4), and the kinetic data calculated have been shown to be reliable (Choukou, Laffaye, & Taiar, 2014). Furthermore, the peak GRF during walking and running can be predicted from the acceleration data collected from an accelerometer placed on the hip of the participant (Neugebauer, Hawkins, & Beckett, 2012). The use of this device allows the athlete to move freely within the environment rather than the individual's movements being confined to a laboratory, although event detection becomes an issue.

Pressure insoles

Pressure insoles are composed of thin pressure sensors that can be inserted into athletic shoes in order to record the plantar pressure during locomotor tasks including walking and running (see Mechanical Concept 2.14). The use of

Applied Research 2.4

Using accelerometers to calculate force and power output during resistance exercises

The authors investigated the validity of force and power output calculated from a linear position transducer (LPT) and an accelerometer during loaded jump squats by comparing the values to those derived from a force plate. Resistance-trained men completed jump squats with loads of 20, 40, 60, and 80 kg while standing on a force plate with an LPT and an accelerometer attached to the barbell. Power output was calculated from the force-plate data by multiplying the instantaneous vertical force with instantaneous vertical velocity returned by integrating the force trace. The instantaneous vertical position of the barbell from the LPT was double differentiated to return the instantaneous vertical acceleration, which was then multiplied by the mass of the barbell and the athlete to provide the vertical force. This was multiplied by the barbell velocity, which was calculated by differentiating the vertical position data to return the power output during each jump. The vertical acceleration data collected from the accelerometer were multiplied by the mass of the athlete and the barbell to return the vertical force during each jump, which was then multiplied by the vertical velocity, calculated by integrating the acceleration data, to return the power output. The authors reported that the kinetic variables of force and power output calculated from the LPT and the accelerometer were not significantly different from the values calculated from the force plate. However, the force values calculated from the kinematic data tended to be greater than the values recorded directly from the force plate, particularly at the lower loads. Power output calculated from the LPT tended to be greater than that calculated from the force-plate data, while the values derived from the accelerometer were greater than the force-plate data under the lowest and highest load conditions, being lower than the force plate values with the 40- and 60-kg loads. The authors suggested that the differences were likely caused by the lower sampling frequencies associated with the LPT and accelerometer, and the inability of the LPT and accelerometer to accurately account for horizontal motion of the barbell.

Crewther, B. T., Kilduff, L. P., Cunningham, D. J., Cook, C., Owen, N., & Yang, G.-Z. (2011). Validating two systems for estimating force and power. *International Journal of Sports Medicine, 32,* 254–258.

pressure insoles allows the normal (vertical) component of the GRF to be recorded while the athlete moves freely about the environment, and pressure insoles have been shown to produce reliable force traces, although the magnitude of the force tends to be lower than that recorded from a force plate (Low & Dixon, 2010; see Applied Research 2.5). Unlike force plates, however, pressure insoles allow the distribution of the applied force over the contact surface to be determined.

Force plates

Force plates allow the practitioner to record the GRF acting on the athlete through either piezoelectric or strain-gauge transducers (see Mechanical Concept 2.15). Force plates allow the determination of the GRF along each of the three axes associated with the three-dimensional reference frame. As the GRF reflects the motion of the CM during a given movement task, the kinematic variables of the CM (e.g., position, velocity) are calculated using numerical integration of the force trace. A force plate is therefore a very useful device that can provide valid and reliable kinetic and

Mechanical Concept 2.14

Pressure sensor technology

The pressure sensors in pressure insoles are typically either capacitance or conductance type (Lees & Lake, 2008). A capacitance pressure sensor is composed of two layers of conductive electrically charged material separated by a thin layer of a nonconducting, dielectric elastic material. A pressure exerted on the sensor deforms the dielectric elastic layer, which reduces the distance between the two electrically charged layers, producing a voltage change that is proportional to the applied pressure (Razak, Zayegh, Begg, & Wahab, 2012). A conductance sensor has a conductive polymer separating two layers of conductive material. When a pressure is exerted on the sensor, the resistance of the conductive polymer decreases in proportion to the magnitude of the applied pressure, resulting in a change in voltage that can be recorded (Razak et al., 2012).

Pressure insoles contain an array of sensors that allow the plantar pressure exerted during foot–ground contact to be recorded, with the resolution of the plantar pressure being influenced by the number of sensors within the insole. However, the sensors are only responsive to the normal (vertical) loading during contact, precluding the magnitude of the horizontal forces from being recorded. Another important issue concerning the use of pressure insoles is that the sensors are sensitive to changes in temperature. The temperature of the midsole of the foot can increase by 15°C when running, potentially reducing the accuracy of the data recorded from a pressure insole (Lees & Lake, 2008). Finally, the insole should be securely fitted within the shoe, as any slippage can affect the accuracy of the recording (Razak et al., 2012).

Applied Research 2.5
The ground reaction force (GRF) during running measured from a force plate compared to pressure insoles

The criterion measure for the GRF is that recorded from a force plate. However, such analyses are constrained by the number of plates used and their location within the laboratory. Furthermore, the participant being analyzed is required to contact the plate in an appropriate manner, which often requires the participant to aim for the plate, thereby altering his or her movements. Such issues are likely to be circumvented through the use of pressure insoles worn by the participant during the analysis. The authors compared the GRFs recorded from pressure insoles to those recorded from a force plate with participants running at a speed of 3.8 m/s ($\pm$5%). While both instruments produced reliable forces, those recorded from the pressure insoles were significantly lower than those recorded from the force plate.

Low, D. C., & Dixon, S. J. (2010). Footscan pressure insoles: accuracy and reliability of force and pressure measurements in running. *Gait and Posture, 32*, 664–667.

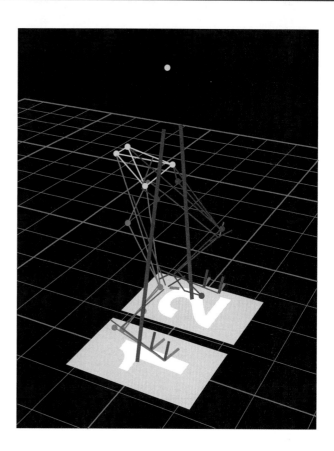

Figure 2.24 The output from an opto-reflective motion analysis system synchronized with two piezoelectric force plates during a biomechanical analysis of an athlete performing a squat jump with a loaded barbell held on the back. The position of the lower-body segments are determined from the 16 reflective markers placed at specific anatomical landmarks. A further reflective marker placed on the center of the barbell is visible toward the top of the image. The GRFs recorded from both force plates are visible as red arrows. The virtual point where each of these vectors acts on the surface of the force plate represents the center of pressure of the contact force. The knowledge of the location of the center of pressure and the magnitude and direction of the ground reaction forces with respect to the lower-body segments allows the determination of the three-dimensional joint moments using inverse dynamic methods.

kinematic variables when used appropriately (Hunter, Marshall, & McNair, 2004; Moir, Garcia, & Dwyer, 2009; Street, McMillan, Board, Rasmussen, & Heneghan, 2001; see Applied Research 2.6). However, a potential issue arises from the need of the athletes to "aim" for the force plate during locomotor tasks, potentially resulting in the athletes modifying their movements to accommodate the necessary contact with the plate. Force plates are often used in conjunction with motion-analysis systems to provide both kinetic and kinematic data (Figure 2.24). The combination of the GRF recorded from force plates and the kinematic data from a motion-analysis system allows the determination of joint moments during movement tasks (see Mechanical Concept 2.12).

Mechanical Concept 2.15

Piezoelectric and strain gauge transducers in force plates

A force plate comprises a rigid top plate that is supported at each corner by transducers that convert the applied force into a voltage that can be recorded and calibrated to allow the measurement of the applied forces (Figure 2.25). The transducers used in commercially available force plates are usually

(continues)

(continued)

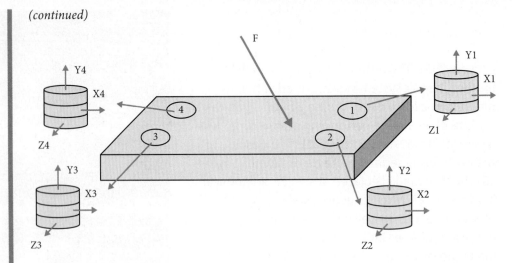

Figure 2.25 The general construction of a force plate. The rigid top plate is supported at each corner by a transducer. Each transducer comprises elements that are sensitive to forces applied along each of the three orthogonal axes. Notice that the axes shown in this image conform to the system recommended by the International Society of Biomechanics. Typically the manufacturers of force plates denote the vertical axis as *z*, the anteroposterior axis as *y* (along the length of the plate), and the mediolateral axis as *x* (along the width of the plate).

Note: *F* is the external force applied to the top plate.
Reproduced from Lees, A., & Lake, M. (2008). Force and pressure measurement. In C. J. Payton & R. M. Bartlett (Eds.), *Biomechanical Evaluation of Movement in Sport and Exercise. The British Association of Sport and Exercise Sciences Guidelines.* (pp. 53–76). New York, NY: Routledge.

piezoelectric or strain gauges. Piezoelectric force transducers contain crystal structures (quartz or ceramics) that are deformed as the result of an applied force, creating a voltage that is recorded. Strain-gauge force transducers comprise foil strips that are deformed in response to an applied force, with the deformation resulting in a change in voltage that is proportional to the magnitude of the applied force. The change in the voltage provides information about the magnitude of the applied force, while the orientation of the transducers allows the determination of the magnitude of the applied force along three orthogonal axes. The voltage output from multiple transducers allows the location of the center of pressure of the applied force to be determined. The center of pressure represents the virtual point on the contact surface where the GRF vector acts and becomes very important when calculating the moment of force acting at joints during movements.

Generally, piezoelectric force plates have greater sensitivity to dynamic loading conditions compared to strain gauge plates, rendering them better suited to the analysis of fast movements such as running and jumping. However, the voltage from piezoelectric force transducers tends to drift during long recording times such that the recording time should be as short as possible. Strain gauge transducers do not suffer from this issue.

Applied Research 2.6
Sources of errors when using force plates to calculate jump height

The authors investigated the errors in vertical jump height caused by the selection of sampling frequency, the selection of force threshold to identify takeoff, and filtering the data. Participants performed a countermovement vertical jump for maximal height on a strain-gauge force plate. The vertical force was sampled at frequencies ranging from 180 to 2,700 Hz, and the force signal was numerically integrated using the trapezoid method to return the net vertical impulse during the propulsive phase of the jump. This was used to establish the vertical velocity of the CM at takeoff as per the impulse–momentum relationship. The authors reported that the selection of a sampling frequency below 1,000 Hz resulted in an underestimation of jump height, while filtering the force signal prior to numerical integration also resulted in an underestimation of jump height. Identifying takeoff using a force threshold of >2 N was found to overestimate jump height. These errors arose due to the failure to accurately identify the point of takeoff in the jump. The authors concluded that the accuracy of jump height can be ensured when the data collection and signal processing are appropriate.

Street, G., McMillan, S., Board, W., Rasmussen, M., & Heneghan, J. M. (2001). Sources of error in determining countermovement jump height with the impulse method. *Journal of Applied Biomechanics, 17,* 43–54.

Chapter Summary

A force is an agent that changes or tends to change the motion of a body. Types of forces are internal forces (e.g., muscular forces) and external forces (e.g., GRF, gravitational force). Muscular forces exert moments of force acting at joints to change the motion of the body segments to which the muscles attach. The GRF acts on the athlete when in contact with a supporting surface, comprising vertical (normal) and horizontal components. The horizontal components of the GRF represent frictional forces. The magnitude of the GRF is dependent upon body weight and the muscular forces exerted by the athlete during a given movement, and the GRF reflects the motion of the CM when the athlete is in contact with a supporting surface given that it is a nonconstant force. Newton's three laws of motion inform us of the action of forces on bodies and provide a mechanical framework in which to analyze the motion of bodies. Because forces take time to exert their influence on bodies, the impulse of force is an informative kinetic variable given the relationship between the impulse of a force and the resulting change in momentum of the body. This mathematical dependence is captured in the impulse–momentum relationship, which can be used to calculate the kinematic and kinetic variables during specific movement tasks. The application of a force that displaces a body results in mechanical work being done. This work acts to change the mechanical energy of the body and is characterized by the work–energy theorem. This theorem can also be used to determine the kinematic and kinetic variables associated with a specific movement task. There are different forms of mechanical energy, and both manmade and anatomical structures can be used to exchange the different forms of mechanical energy during sporting tasks, thereby enhancing performance. Different technologies can be used by the strength and conditioning practitioner to record kinetic variables, including force plates, pressure insoles, accelerometers, and LPT and motion analysis systems, each with associated benefits and costs.

Review Questions and Projects

1. Construct a free-body diagram for each of the images in Figure 2.3 showing an athlete performing a vertical jump. Include the GRF and body weight.

2. Construct a free-body diagram of an athlete during the stance phase of sprint running. Include the GRF, body weight, and air resistance.

3. Apply Newton's laws of motion to an athlete performing a back squat beginning from the starting position through the descent and ascent phases.

4. An athlete with a mass of 72 kg steps from a 0.50-m box during the performance of a depth jump. Calculate the athlete's momentum upon landing.

5. If the absorption phase of the landing for the athlete in Question 3 lasts 0.25 s, calculate the average vertical GRF acting on the athlete.

6. Explain what the athlete can do to reduce the magnitude of the average vertical force during the landing task.

7. An athlete generates a net vertical impulse of force of 234 N/s during the propulsive phase of a countermovement vertical jump. If the mass of the athlete is 78 kg, what is the jump height?

8. An athlete with a mass of 70 kg is sprinting at maximal velocity. At the beginning of the stance phase the vertical velocity of the CM is –0.50 m/s while at the end of the stance phase the vertical velocity is 0.50 m/s. If the duration of the stance phase is 0.10 s, calculate the vertical impulse of the GRF (ensure that the impulse to support body weight is included in your calculation).

9. What is the average vertical GRF for the athlete in Question 8?

10. Explain why the curves are banked on indoor running tracks.

11. Explain how the normal component of the GRF influences the frictional force exerted by an athlete during a change-of-direction task.

12. An athlete raises a barbell 1.03 m during the ascent of a bench press exercise. If the barbell has a mass of 105 kg, what is the mechanical work done on the barbell by the athlete?

13. Assuming the duration of the barbell ascent in Question 12 is 0.83 s, calculate the average mechanical power output during the exercise.

14. Explain the exchanges of mechanical energy during the propulsive and flight phases of a countermovement vertical jump.

15. Discuss some of the sporting equipment used by athletes to enhance performance through exchanges of mechanical energy.

16. Explain how increasing muscle force through resistance training methods may increase the magnitude of the GRF during a given movement task.

17. A strength and conditioning practitioner wants to assess the GRF during a drop jump. Explain the different technologies that he or she could use.

18. What technology could the practitioner in Question 17 utilize to calculate the lower-body joint moments during the drop jump task?

19. Discuss the relative merits of force plates and pressure insoles for the determination of GRFs during running tasks.

20. What mathematical procedure should a practitioner use to calculate the kinematic variables associated with the CM from force-plate data?

References

Bartlett, R. (2007). *Introduction to Sports Biomechanics. Analysing Human Movement Patterns.* Oxon, UK: Routledge.

Blau, P.J. (2009). *Friction Science and Technology. From Concepts to Applications.* Boca Raton, FL: Taylor and Francis.

Choukou, M.-A., Laffaye, G., & Taiar, R. (2014). Reliability and validity of an accelerometric system for assessing vertical jumping performance. *Biology of Sport, 31,* 55–62.

Comstock, B.A., Solomon-Hill, G., Flanagan, S.D., Earp, J. E., Luk, H. W., Dobbins, K. A., . . . Kraever, W. J. (2011). Validity of the Myotest® in measuring force and power production in the squat and bench press. *Journal of Strength and Conditioning Research, 25,* 2293–2297.

Cormie, P., McBride, J.M., & McCaulley, G.O. (2007). Validation of power measurement techniques in dynamic lower body resistance exercises. *Journal of Applied Biomechanics, 23,* 103–118.

Crewther, B.T., Kilduff, L.P., Cunningham, D.J., Cook, C., Owen, N., & Yang, G.-Z. (2011). Validating two systems for estimating force and power. *International Journal of Sports Medicine, 32,* 254–258.

Dempster, W.T. (1955). *Space Requirements for the Seated Operator.* WADC-TR-55-159, Wright Patterson Air Force Base.

Enoka, R.M. (2008). *Neuromechanics of Human Movement.* Champaign, IL: Human Kinetic Publishers.

Hunter, J.P., Marshall, R.N., & McNair, P. (2004). Reliability of biomechanical variables of sprint running. *Medicine and Science in Sports and Exercise, 36,* 850–861.

Jain, P.C. (1980). On a discrepancy in track race. *Research Quarterly in Exercise and Sport, 51,* 432–436.

Lees, A., & Lake, M. (2008). Force and pressure measurement. In C.J. Payton & R.M. Bartlett (Eds.), *Biomechanical Evaluation of Movement in Sport and Exercise. The British Association of Sport and Exercise Sciences Guidelines* (pp. 53–76). New York, NY: Routledge.

Low, D.C., & Dixon, S.J. (2010). Footscan pressure insoles: accuracy and reliability of force and pressure measurements in running. *Gait and Posture, 32,* 664–667.

Moir, G.L., Garcia, A., & Dwyer, G.B. (2009). Intersession reliability of kinematic and kinetic variables during vertical jumps in men and women. *International Journal of Sports Physiology and Performance, 4,* 317–330.

Neugebauer, J.M., Hawkins, D.A., & Beckett, L. (2012). Estimating youth locomotion ground reaction forces using an accelerometer-based activity monitor. *PLoS One, 7,* e48182.

Razak, A.H.A., Zayegh, A., Begg, R.K., & Wahab, Y. (2012). Foot plantar pressure measurement system: a review. *Sensors, 12,* 9884–9912.

Schade, F., Arampatzis, A., Brüggeman, G.-P., & Komi, P.V. (2004). Comparison of the men's and the women's pole vault at the 2000 Sydney Olympic Games. *Journal of Sports Sciences, 22,* 835–842.

Street, G., McMillan, S., Board, W., Rasmussen, M., & Heneghan, J.M. (2001). Sources of error in determining countermovement jump height with the impulse method. *Journal of Applied Biomechanics, 17,* 43–54.

Vogel, S. (2003). *Comparative Biomechanics. Life's Physical World.* Princeton, NJ: Princeton University Press.

Winter, D.A. (2009). *Biomechanics and Motor Control of Human Movement.* Hoboken, NJ: John Wiley and Sons, Inc.

Zatsiorsky, V.M. (2002). *Kinetics of Human Motion.* Champaign, IL: Human Kinetic Publishers.

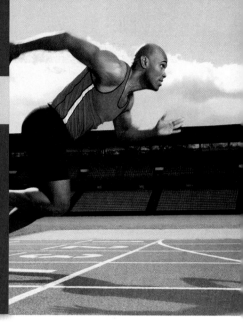

CHAPTER 3

Structure and Mechanical Function of Skeletal Muscle and Tendon

Chapter Objectives

At the end of this chapter, you will be able to:

- Explain the mechanical characteristics associated with different types of skeletal muscle actions
- Explain the specific arrangements of the skeleton and muscles that produce force and distance advantages
- Describe the macro- and microstructure of skeletal muscle
- Explain the processes underlying the sliding-filament theory of generating muscular tension
- Describe the processes involved in the excitation–contraction coupling that lead to the development of muscular tension
- Understand the physiological and mechanical factors that affect the development of muscular tension
- Understand the factors affecting the energetic cost of different muscle actions
- Describe the macro- and microstructure of tendon
- Describe the mechanical characteristics of tendon
- Explain the integration of skeletal muscle and tendon during multijoint movements

Key Terms

α-motoneuron

Acetylcholine

Actin

Action potential

Adenosine-5'-triphosphate (ATP)

Afferent

Agonist

Amplitude

Anatomical cross-sectional area

Antagonist

Atrophy

Basal lamina

Central fatigue

Coactivation

Concentric action

Crossbridge

Depolarized

Dihydropyridine receptors

Discharge doublets

Distance advantage

Eccentric action

Effective mechanical advantage

Efferent

Elastin

Electromechanical delay

Electromyographic analysis

Endomysium

Endotenon

End-plate potential

Enthesis

Epimysium

Epitenon

Equilibrium potential

Extrafusal fibers

Fascicles

Fatigue

Force advantage

Frequency

Functional physiological cross-sectional area

Fusiform

γ-motoneurons

Golgi tendon organs

Hyperplasia

Hypertrophy

Innervation ratio

Interneurons

Intrafusal fibers

Isokinetic

Isometric action

Lateral sacs

Mechanical advantage

Mitochondria

Moment of force

Motoneuron

Motor unit

Muscle fiber

Muscle fiber action potential

Muscle spindles

Myofibrils

Myofilaments

Myonuclear domain

Myosin

Myosin heavy chain (MHC)

Myotendinous junction

Nebulin

Neuromuscular junction

Normalized tendon length

Nuclear bag fibers

Nuclear chain fibers

Nuclei

Paratenon

Pennate

Pennation angle

Perimysium

Peripheral fatigue

Postactivation potentiation

Primary endings

Rate coding

Repolarized

Resting membrane potential

Ryanodine receptors

Sarcolemma

Sarcomeres

Sarcopenia

Sarcoplasm

Sarcoplasmic reticulum

Satellite cells

Secondary endings

Size principle

Sliding-filament theory

Somatosensory receptors

Specific tension

Strain

Stretch reflex

Stretch–shortening cycle

Task agonist

Task antagonist

Terminal cisternae

Titin

Transverse tubules

Tropomyosin

Troponin

Viscoelastic

Young's module

Z-discs

Chapter Overview

The volitional motion of the athlete within the environment demands that the motor system generate the necessary forces, so the biologic tissue comprising the motor system, which is responsible for these forces, should be of concern to the strength and conditioning practitioner. The main biologic tissue with which we are concerned is skeletal muscle, the biologic motors that power human movements. While the function of skeletal muscle and the factors that affect the generation of force are indeed central to understanding how athletes move, it is the interaction between skeletal muscle and tendon that gives rise to the movements of the athletes that are observed during specific tasks, as well as the source of energetic costs associated with performing the tasks. The structure and mechanical behavior of these biologic tissues will be discussed in the present chapter. An understanding of the interaction between skeletal muscle and tendon will allow strength and conditioning practitioners to develop training programs to enhance the athletic performance of their athletes.

This chapter is not intended to be an exhaustive review of the mechanical behavior of skeletal muscle and tendon; rather, it presumes a base knowledge of mechanics and physiology, while introducing new mechanical and physiological concepts to allow further understanding. The present chapter will therefore provide a reference for readers that will aid their understanding of how anatomical structures operate, allowing them to develop training regimens to improve athletic performance.

Skeletal Muscle

Skeletal muscle comprises approximately 30–40% of total body mass in humans (Janssen, Heymsfield, Wang, & Ross, 2000) and accounts for approximately 23% of total resting energy expenditure (Gallagher et al., 1998). Skeletal muscle also represents the biologic motors that power the volitional movements of athletes by producing mechanical work to accelerate the segments of the body. However, beyond this obvious function, the role of skeletal muscle in thermoregulation of the body and the contribution of receptors within the muscles to somatosensory feedback during movements should not be overlooked. The human body contains over 600 skeletal muscles, and Figure 3.1 shows many of the superficial muscles.

When a muscle is activated, it exerts a tensile force. An active muscle can exert tension under three conditions: while maintaining a constant length, which we refer to as an **isometric action**; while it is shortening, resulting in a **concentric action**; or while it is lengthening, producing an **eccentric action**. The active muscle exerts a force during all of these actions, but given the mechanical definition of work, not all muscle actions will result in mechanical work being performed. Specifically, during an isometric action no mechanical work is performed by the muscle, as it does not change length. During a concentric action the muscle performs mechanical work as it shortens, while during an eccentric action the muscle will absorb mechanical work as it lengthens. Such issues have significant implications for the energetic cost of the muscle action, as will be highlighted later in this chapter.

A fourth type of muscle action, **isokinetic**, is often mentioned in the literature. The definition of an isokinetic action is a dynamic muscle action where the velocity of shortening or lengthening of the muscle remains constant throughout the action. However, recent evidence gathered from ultrasonographic analyses has shown that muscle fiber velocities do not remain constant during joint motions recorded *in vitro*

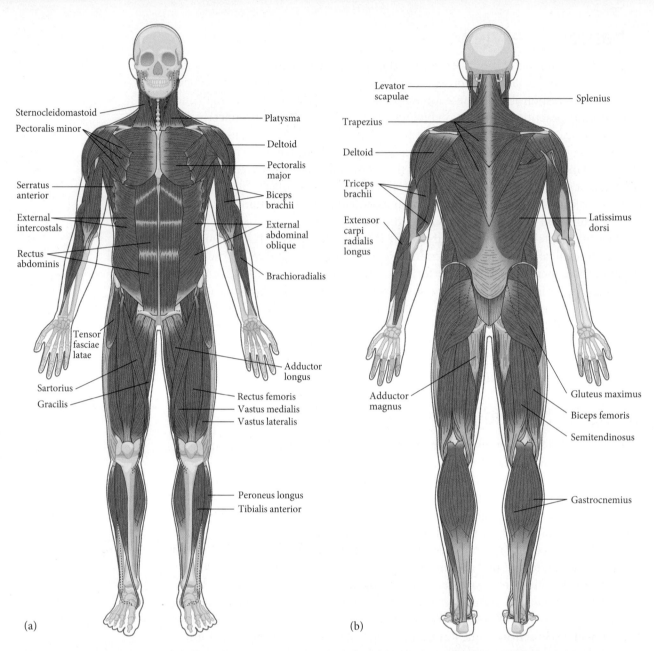

Figure 3.1 Anterior and posterior views of the human body showing the superficial muscles.

(Ichinose, Kawakami, Ito, Kanehisa, & Fukunaga, 2000; see Applied Research 3.1). This brings in to question the validity of the physiological assumptions underlying isokinetic muscle actions. Therefore, the term isokinetic should be reserved for the description of dynamometers used to test and train muscular strength rather than a description of a muscle action.

The tension developed by an active muscle is transmitted to the skeleton, to which it attaches via elastic tissues (tendons and aponeuroses) that are in series with the muscle (Figure 3.2). The effect of the muscular tension transmitted to the skeleton results in an acceleration of the specific body segment about an anatomical axis of rotation, depending upon the magnitude of the opposing force. A muscle that, when

Applied Research 3.1
Muscle shortening velocity during isokinetic actions

The authors used ultrasonic measurements of fascicles during dynamic knee-extension exercise performed in an isokinetic dynamometer. The dynamometer allowed the joint angular velocity to be held constant at two different speeds during the movement (30°/s and 150°/s), allowing the authors to determine the differences in fascicle-shortening velocity and joint angular velocity. It was found that the fascicle-shortening velocity did not remain constant during the movement, tending to follow a parabolic relationship with knee joint angle reaching peak shortening velocity at a joint angle of 71° and 57° in the 30°/s and 150°/s conditions, respectively. The differences were explained in terms of the effects of changes in moment arm lengths, pennation angle, the influence of the series elastic components, and activation dynamics associated with the changing joint angles. This study highlights the difference between joint angular velocity and the underlying fiber shortening velocities of the active musculature.

Ichinose, Y., Kawakami, Y., Ito, M., Kanehisa, H., & Fukunaga, T. (2000). In vivo estimation of contraction velocity of human vastus lateralis muscle during "isokinetic" action. *Journal of Applied Physiology, 88*, 851–856.

activated, produces a specific motion observed at a joint is known as an **agonist**, while a muscle that opposes the action of the agonist is known as an **antagonist**. Antagonistic pairings about joints allow the muscles to produce a wide variety of movements in the face of the limitation of muscle only being capable of exerting tensile forces. For example, biceps brachii and triceps brachii constitute an antagonistic pairing for

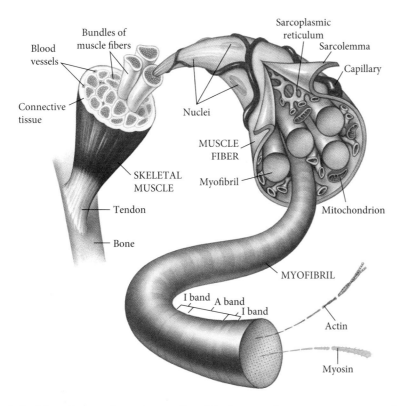

Figure 3.2 Muscle tension transmitted to bone via aponeuroses and tendinous structures.

flexion and extension of the elbow joint, with the biceps brachii being the agonist for flexion and the triceps brachii being the agonist for extension.

The nomenclature of agonist and antagonist is based upon the anatomical location of the muscle relative to a joint. However, it is rare for a muscle to be aligned such that the tensile force exerted results in a rotation about a single axis; thus, the contributions of a specific muscle to a given movement must be considered relative to the task being performed. For example, biceps brachii acts to accelerate both the elbow joint into flexion and the radioulnar joint into supination, so the muscle can be described as a **task agonist** for elbow flexion and a **task antagonist** for pronation during the biceps curl exercise. Furthermore, the interconnection between the segments of the human motor system results in muscle forces being distributed between body segments such that muscles can affect the motion of segments to which they do not attach (Zajac, Neptune, & Kautz, 2002). Such matters complicate the analysis of even simple movements. What is presented here is a simplified introduction to the behavior of skeletal muscle that will allow us to develop some basic principles that can be applied to fundamental movements.

Muscular and Skeletal Couplings to Produce Movement

As previously stated, a muscle is only capable of exerting a tensile force, and force is not a conserved variable. Therefore, the force exerted by a muscle can be amplified or attenuated simply through the muscle's mechanical arrangement with the skeleton to which it attaches. The arrangement of a muscle and the skeleton can be simplified to a lever system comprising a rigid beam (bone) that rotates about a fulcrum (anatomical joint) due to the action of forces (muscular forces and those associated with gravity and external loads). The forces acting on the beam will tend to induce rotations of the beam given their application at a distance from the fulcrum. We are therefore interested in the **moment of force** associated with the muscle force and that associated with the external load. A moment of force can be calculated as follows:

$$M = Fd \qquad \text{Eq. (3.1)}$$

where M is the moment of force measured in newton-meters, F is the magnitude of the applied force, and d is the moment arm of the force. The moment arm of the force is the perpendicular distance between the line of action of the force and the fulcrum. Figure 3.3 shows a schematic representation of a lever system within the human body, displaying the moments of force associated with a muscle ($F_M \times M_M$) and a load held in the hand ($F_R \times M_R$).

The effectiveness of a given lever system can be evaluated by calculating the **mechanical advantage** (MA) of the system:

$$MA = \frac{M_M}{M_R} \qquad \text{Eq. (3.2)}$$

where MA is the mechanical advantage of the lever system, M_M is the moment arm of the muscle force, and M_R is the moment arm

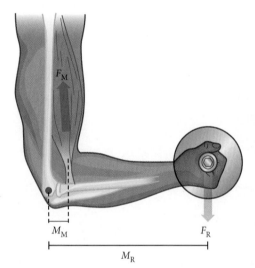

Figure 3.3 Schematic representation of the moments of force associated with a muscle crossing the elbow joint and an external load held in the hand.

Note: F_M is the muscular force; F_R is the force associated with the load; M_M is the moment arm of the muscular force; M_R is the moment arm of the force associated with the load.

of the external force. Three functional categories of lever system can be defined based upon the mechanical advantage:

- *MA* > 1. Muscular force is amplified with this arrangement such that a large external load can be overcome through the application of a lesser muscular force. This type of lever system has a **force advantage** (Vogel, 2003). An example of this category of lever system is shown in Figure 3.4b.
- *MA* < 1. The linear distance moved through by the point of application of the external force is amplified in this arrangement. This type of lever system therefore has a **distance advantage**, calculated as the reciprocal of *MA* (Vogel, 2003). Figures 3.4a and c show lever systems with *MA* < 1.

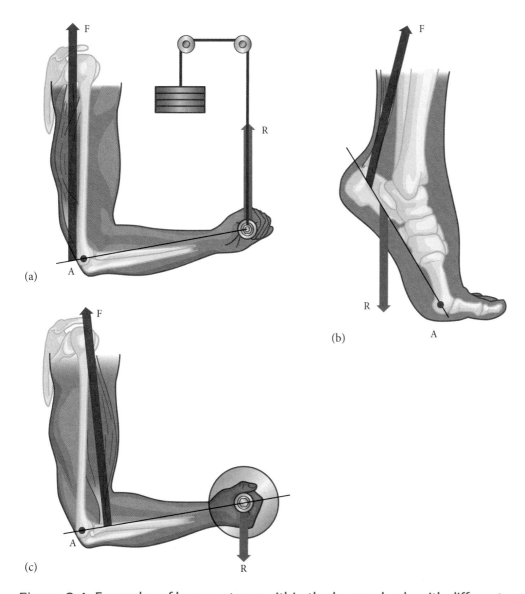

Figure 3.4 Examples of lever systems within the human body with different functional arrangements. The lever system in (b) has a force advantage, while those in (a) and (c) have distance advantages.

Note: F is the muscular force; A is the fulcrum; R is the resistance force.

- $MA = 1$. This type of lever system amplifies neither force nor distance, being employed to redirect the direction that the muscular force acts. The patellar can be considered to function as a beam within a lever system with an MA of 1.

Most of the lever systems in the human body have $MA < 1$ (Table 3.1), a fact that initially seems counterintuitive given the attenuation of muscular force associated with such arrangements. Skeletal muscle, while being well suited at developing force, is unable to shorten over large distances, and therefore lever systems with distance advantages appear to be appropriate. Furthermore, the distance advantage also confers a speed advantage. If the beam of the lever system is considered to be completely rigid, then it can be assumed that the point of application of external force will also be moving with greater speed than the point of application of muscular force, as it will cover a greater distance in the same amount of time. When the lever system has a $MA < 1$, both distance and speed are amplified at the distal end of the lever.

From Equation (3.1), it is obvious that the moment of force associated with a muscle action is dependent not only upon the magnitude of the force exerted, but also on the moment arm of the applied force. Both the force exerted by a muscle and its moment arm will change as the joint is accelerated through a range of motion, which will affect the moment of force associated with a given muscle action (Figure 3.5). In this situation, of course, there will be a concomitant change in the moment arm associated with the external load.

The moment of force associated with an external force acting at a joint (e.g., the force associated with an external load or the ground-reaction force) must be balanced by the moment of force associated with muscular forces. We can express this algebraically as follows:

$$F_M \times M_M = F_R \times M_R \qquad \text{Eq. (3.3)}$$

where F_M is the muscular force at the joint of interest, M_M is the moment arm of the muscular force, F_R is the external force acting on the joint, and M_R is the moment arm associated with the external force. Rearranging Equation (3.3), we get:

$$\frac{M_M}{M_R} = \frac{F_R}{F_M} \qquad \text{Eq. (3.4)}$$

Table 3.1
Mechanical and Distance Advantages for Specific Skeletal Muscles

Muscle	Mechanical Advantage	Distance Advantage
Biceps brachii	0.18	5.45
Triceps brachii	0.05	22.0
Quadriceps femoris	0.06	2.30

Note: The mechanical advantage is calculated as the ratio of the moment arm of the muscular force to the moment arm of the external force. The distance advantage is the reciprocal of the mechanical advantage.

Data from Vogel, S. (2003). *Comparative Biomechanics. Life's Physical World*. Princeton, NJ: Princeton University Press.

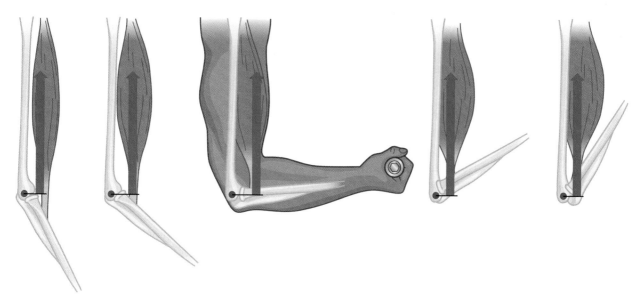

Figure 3.5 Changes in the muscle moment arm as the joint is accelerated through a range of motion.

The ratio of F_R to F_M is known as the **effective mechanical advantage** (EMA), which can be altered by changing the segment positions during a given movement (Biewener, 2003). For example, knee flexion increases when transitioning from walking to running in order to absorb the greater impact forces experienced during each stance phase. This causes a substantial decrease in the EMA at the joint (i.e., the moment arm of the ground-reaction force greatly exceeds that of the knee extensor musculature). This change in the EMA necessitates greater muscular forces be exerted during running compared to walking. It is possible that the change in EMA also contributes to the sticking region associated with many resistance-training exercises (see Skeletal Muscle Concept 3.1).

Skeletal Muscle Concept 3.1

The sticking region in the bench press

The sticking region during a resistance-training exercise such as a back squat or the bench press is defined as a period of decreasing vertical velocity during the ascent of the barbell and is evident when performing lifts with near maximal loads (Elliott, Wilson, & Kerr, 1989; Newton et al., 1997). The region has been associated with failed lifts, although not all authors report failure during this region (Van den Tillaar & Ettema, 2009). The sticking region begins between approximately 0.20 and 0.30 s after the initial upward movement of the barbell and lasts for approximately 25% of the time of ascent (Elliott, Wilson, & Kerr, 1989; Van den Tillaar & Ettema, 2010). The mechanical explanation for the sticking region is straightforward: It represents a phase of the lift when the force exerted by the athlete on the barbell is less than the weight of the barbell,

(continues)

(continued)

resulting in deceleration. However, the biomechanical reasons underpinning *why* the force exerted by the athlete is attenuated during this phase are more complex.

Some researchers proposed that the sticking region in the bench press occurs due to changes in the moment arms associated with the barbell and the agonist muscles crossing the shoulder and elbow joints (Madsen & McLaughlin, 1984). However, Elliott, Wilson, & Kerr (1989) reported that the change in moment arms associated with the barbell and muscular forces was not solely responsible. Furthermore, there was no change in muscle activation during the sticking region. These authors concluded that the sticking region occurs at a time when the strain potential energy that was stored in the musculotendinous unit during the descent of the barbell dissipates, reducing the work that can be done on the barbell at that time. The sticking region therefore represents a transition phase during the lift between the strain potential energy-assisted acceleration phase and the phase where the active muscles are able to generate maximal force.

Van den Tillaar and Ettema (2010) reported that the activation of the agonist muscles tended to increase after the sticking region had been negotiated. The authors suggested that this increase in activity was in response to the sticking region and represented a delayed neural reaction that followed a diminution of the potentiation of the active muscles resulting from the eccentric action during barbell descent prior to the ascent of the barbell. However, Van den Tillaar, Sæterbakken, and Ettema (2012) recently compared the mechanics and muscle activation during dynamic bench press movements with those of isometric bench press. They reported that both dynamic and isometric performance of the movement was associated with regions of diminished force and with similar muscle activation patterns, suggesting that the sticking region may in fact coincide with a mechanically poor position resulting from changes in the moment arm at the elbow joint, rather than a reduction of potentiation of the active muscles.

Macrostructure of Skeletal Muscle

Figure 3.2 shows the macrostructure of skeletal muscle. As can be seen from this figure, skeletal muscle consists of groups of **fascicles** surrounded by a sheath of connective tissue known as the **epimysium**. A fascicle is a bundle of muscle fibers, and each fascicle is contained within another connective tissue sheath, the **perimysium**. The perimysial connective tissue contributes significantly to passive stiffness of muscle (Purslow, 1989), a factor that may have significant implications for measures of flexibility. Each **muscle fiber** within a fascicle has a cellular membrane, the **sarcolemma**, that is further surrounded by yet another connective tissue sheath, the **endomysium**. The sarcolemma is an excitable membrane across which a potential difference in electrical charge exists due to the location of different charged particles (ions). The **basal lamina** connects the endomysium to the sarcolemma of a muscle fiber. Located in the basal lamina of adult muscle fibers are myogenic progenitor cells, known as **satellite cells**. These cells lie quiescent until the muscle fiber is injured, at which time the satellite cells are activated, proliferate, and then migrate to the site of the injury to repair or replace damaged muscle fibers (Adams, 2006). Satellite cells also appear to play a very important role in the processes involved in muscle hypertrophy (Kadi et al., 2004; see Skeletal Muscle Concept 3.8).

Enclosed by the sarcolemma is a fluid known as the **sarcoplasm**. Within the sarcoplasm, there are fuel sources (e.g., lipid droplets, glycogen granules) as well as organelles, including the **mitochondria** and the **nuclei**. Muscle fibers are multinucleated cells, and it is believed that each nucleus serves a finite volume of the sarcoplasm (**myonuclear domain**), controlling protein synthesis and potentially providing a limit to the size of the fiber (Kadi et al., 2004). Within the sarcoplasm, there is also a membranous system that runs parallel to the myofibrils within each fiber. This system includes the **sarcoplasmic reticulum**, the **transverse tubules**, **terminal cisternae**, and **lateral sacs** (Figure 3.6), all of which are involved in the activation of the muscle fiber.

Muscles differ in their fiber arrangements (Figure 3.7). The fiber arrangement has consequences for the force developed by the muscle. Specifically, **pennate** muscles with their oblique fiber arrangement tend to generate large forces, while **fusiform** muscles with their parallel fiber arrangement tend to generate lesser forces but shorten over long ranges. The number of muscle fibers also differs substantially between muscles within the body, with a greater number of fibers contained within muscles that function to develop large forces (Figure 3.8).

It is unlikely that the muscle fibers run the entire length of a given muscle, meaning that the tension developed by a muscle fiber must be transmitted laterally to adjacent fibers. The length of a muscle fiber with a given muscle has a functional significance, with muscles that have high fiber length:muscle length ratios being able to accomplish large excursions with high velocities of shortening (Table 3.2). This is due to the proportionality of maximal muscle excursion and shortening velocity to fiber length (Zatsiorsky & Prilutsky, 2012). Within each muscle fiber, there are

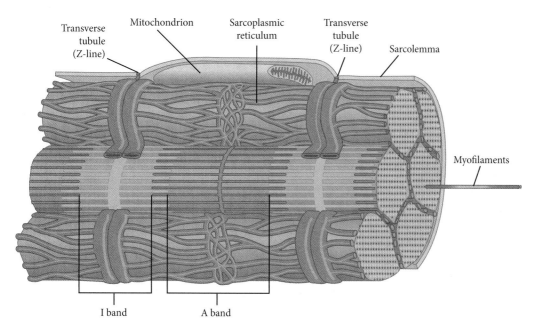

Figure 3.6 The structures within a single muscle fiber.

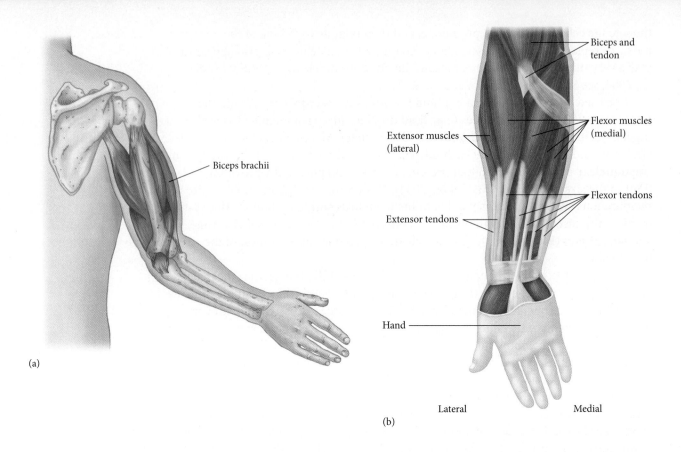

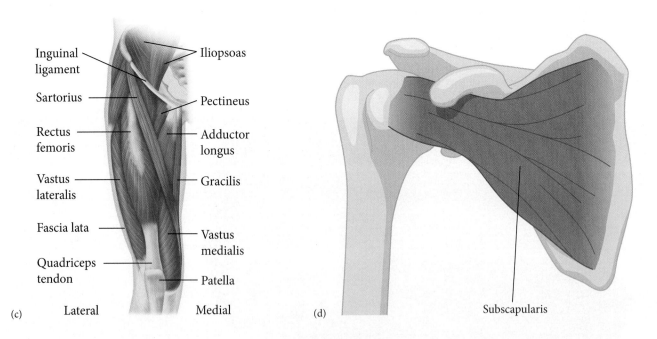

Figure 3.7. Muscles with different fiber arrangements. (a) Biceps brachii is a fusiform muscle, (b) flexor pollicis longus is a unipennate muscle, (c) rectus femoris is a bipennate muscle, and (d) subscapularis is a multipennate muscle. The arrangements shown here reflect the fascicles, which can be used to determine the orientation of the muscle fibers.

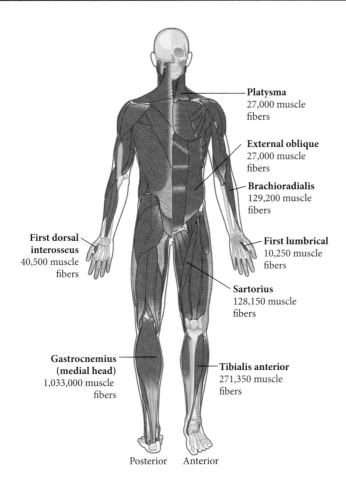

Platysma
27,000 muscle
fibers

External oblique
27,000 muscle
fibers

Brachioradialis
129,200 muscle
fibers

First lumbrical
10,250 muscle
fibers

Sartorius
128,150 muscle
fibers

**First dorsal
interosseus**
40,500 muscle
fibers

Tibialis anterior
271,350 muscle
fibers

**Gastrocnemius
(medial head)**
1,033,000 muscle
fibers

Posterior   Anterior

Figure 3.8 The number of muscle fibers within selected muscles.

Data from MacIntosh, B. R., Gardiner, P. F., & McComas, A. J. (2006). *Skeletal Muscle. Form and Function*.
Champaign, IL: Human Kinetic Publishers.

Table 3.2
Architectural Properties for Selected Lower-Body Muscles

Muscle	Muscle Length (mm)	Fiber Length (mm)	Sarcomere Length (µm)	Pennation Angle (°)	PCSA (mm²)	I_f/I_M ratio
Psoas	242.5 ± 47.5	116.9 ± 16.6	3.11 ± 0.28	10.6 ± 3.2	77 ± 23	0.50 ± 0.14
Gluteus maximus	269.5 ± 64.2	156.9 ± 25.7	2.60 ± 0.36	21.9 ± 26.2	334 ± 88	0.62 ± 0.22
Sartorius	448.1 ± 41.9	403.0 ± 46.3	3.11 ± 0.19	1.3 ± 1.8	19 ± 7	0.90 ± 0.04
Rectus femoris	362.8 ± 47.3	75.9 ± 12.8	2.42 ± 0.30	13.9 ± 3.5	135 ± 50	0.21 ± 0.03
Vastus lateralis	273.4 ± 4.62	99.4 ± 17.6	2.14 ± 0.29	18.4 ± 6.8	351 ± 161	0.38 ± 0.11
Vastus intermedius	412.0 ± 81.7	99.3 ± 20.3	2.17 ± 0.42	4.5 ± 4.5	167 ± 69	0.24 ± 0.04
Vastus medialis	439.0 ± 98.5	96.8 ± 23.0	2.24 ± 0.46	29.6 ± 6.9	206 ± 72	0.22 ± 0.04
Soleus	405.4 ± 83.2	44.0 ± 9.9	2.12 ± 0.24	28.3 ± 10.1	518 ± 149	0.11 ± 0.02
Medial gastrocnemius	269.4 ± 46.5	51.0 ± 9.8	2.59 ± 0.26	9.9 ± 4.4	211 ± 57	0.19 ± 0.03
Lateral gastrocnemius	223.5 ± 37.0	58.8 ± 9.5	2.71 ± 0.24	12.0 ± 3.1	97 ± 33	0.27 ± 0.03

Modified from Ward, S. R., Eng, C. M., Smallwood, L. H., & Lieber, R. L. (2009). Are current measurements of lower extremity muscle architecture accurate? *Clinical Orthopedics Related Research, 467*, 1074–1082, with kind permission from Springer Science and Business Media.

myofibrils, which are composed of **sarcomeres**. A sarcomere represents the smallest functional unit of the muscle and contains the contractile proteins (**myofilaments**) that are responsible for developing tension during muscle actions.

Microstructure of Skeletal Muscle

Within each myofibril there are serially connected sarcomeres that are separated from one another by **Z-discs** and that contain a number of proteins that serve different functions, such as supporting structures and contractile elements (Figure 3.9).

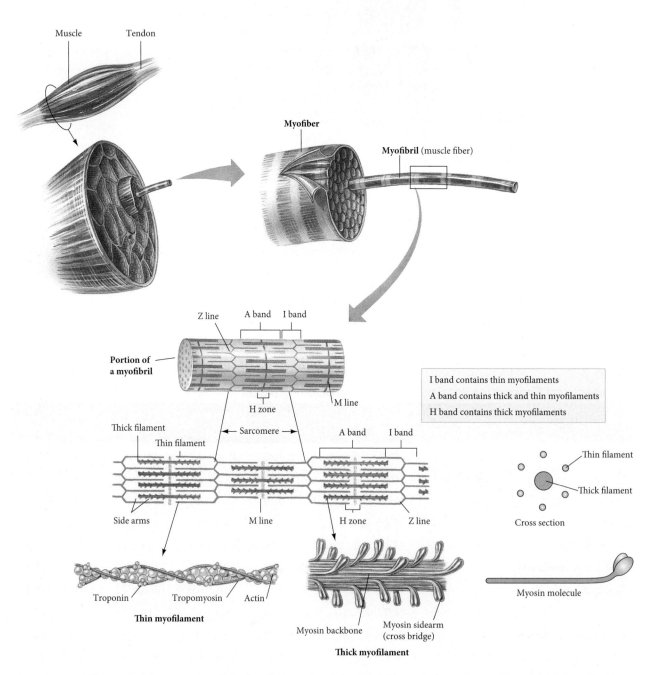

I band contains thin myofilaments
A band contains thick and thin myofilaments
H band contains thick myofilaments

Figure 3.9 The microstructure of skeletal muscle showing the contractile and structural proteins.

Most of these proteins exist in many isoforms, which has important consequences for the function of the muscle fiber. (An isoform is a different form of the same protein; one that has a slightly different structure when compared to other forms of that protein but performs the same task.) The number of sarcomeres arranged in series will determine the maximum displacements and shortening velocities of the muscle fibers (Zatsiorsky & Prilutsky, 2012), while the number of sarcomeres arranged in parallel will determine the overall tension developed by the fiber (Close, 1972; see Skeletal Muscle Concept 3.2). Different types of exercises have been shown to have differential effects on the number of serial and parallel sarcomeres (see Applied Research 3.2).

There are three main myofilaments within each sarcomere: **actin**, **myosin**, and **titin**. The interaction between the crossbridge of the thick myofilament of myosin and the thin myofilament of actin is responsible for the tension developed within each sarcomere. Specifically, the crossbridges attach to the actin molecule and rotate, pulling the thin myofilament and the Z-disc toward the center of the sarcomere. This is the basis of the **sliding-filament theory** of muscle action. For this reason, myosin and actin molecules are known as the contractile proteins within the sarcomere. However, titin has recently been proposed to modulate the tension developed within

Skeletal Muscle Concept 3.2

Sarcomeres arranged in series and parallel

A sarcomere is the smallest functional unit of a muscle fiber, and it contains the contractile proteins associated with tension development according to the **crossbridge** theory (the thick and thin myofilaments). The arrangement of sarcomeres within a muscle fiber can have a substantial effect on the mechanical output of the fiber, with a greater number of sarcomeres arranged in parallel corresponding to greater tension, while a greater number of sarcomeres arranged in series corresponds to greater shortening velocity of the fiber.

Consider a single myofibril with a serial arrangement of sarcomeres in which tension during activation is transmitted to an external load. Not all of the crossbridges within the myofibril will pull directly on the external load during activation; the tension generated by the crossbridges will be transmitted to neighboring sarcomeres, pulling on them as opposed to exerting a force directly on the load. However, the velocity of shortening will be additive across the sarcomeres because of this serial arrangement such that the more sarcomeres in series, the greater the overall shortening velocity of the myofibril. Conversely, if we arrange a number of myofibrils side by side such that the same number of sarcomeres that were arranged serially in the original myofibril now appear in parallel, the tension developed will be proportional to the number of sarcomeres in parallel. In this situation, the crossbridges acting in parallel would exert a tensile force directly to the external load, but the velocity of shortening of the myofibrils would be reduced.

Applied Research 3.2
Differential effects of resistance training on serial and parallel sarcomere number

The authors compared the effects of 14 weeks of resistance training in older adults using only eccentric actions with a regimen employing combined concentric and eccentric actions on strength and muscle architecture in older adults. While the increases in maximal isometric strength were similar between the groups (~8%), the eccentric-only training induced a greater increase in fascicle length, whereas increases in pennation angle were greater following the combined concentric–eccentric mode of training. Increases in fascicle length were proposed to reflect increases in serial sarcomere numbers in the muscle fibers, while the increases in pennation angle reflected increases in parallel sarcomere number. These findings suggest that there are different mechanisms underpinning adaptations in sarcomeres in series and in parallel in response to resistance training.

Reeves, N. D., Maganaris, C. N., Longo, S., & Narici, M. V. (2009). Differential adaptations to eccentric *versus* conventional resistance training in older humans. *Experimental Physiology*, *94*, 825–833.

a sarcomere during muscle activation as a muscle is stretched (see Skeletal Muscle Concept 3.3).

Composition of thin and thick myofilaments

The thin myofilament comprises actin molecules arranged around the protein **nebulin**; the inextensibility of nebulin renders the thin myofilament inelastic (Zatsiorsky & Prilutsky, 2012). The actin molecule does not have isoforms within

Skeletal Muscle Concept 3.3

The role of titin in regulating force

In addition to the myofilaments of actin and myosin, titin has been proposed to modulate the tension developed by a muscle fiber, particularly following muscle stretch (Herzog, Duvall, & Leonard, 2012). The titin myofilament spans each half-sarcomere from the M line to the Z-disc, crossing through the A and I bands of the sarcomere (Figure 3.10).

Titin is fixed to the thick myofilament within the A band of the sarcomere but is free in the I band, where its extensibility has been proposed to be primarily responsible for the passive elasticity observed when myofibrils are stretched (Herzog, Leonard, Joumaa, & Mehta, 2008). However, the stiffness of the titin myofilament can be increased through Ca^{2+} binding, enhancing the tension development during muscle activation during stretch (Rassier, 2012). Furthermore, titin has been shown to bind to actin in the region of the I band, which decreases the length of titin in this region, producing a corresponding increase in its stiffness (Leonard & Herzog, 2010). Therefore, tension development

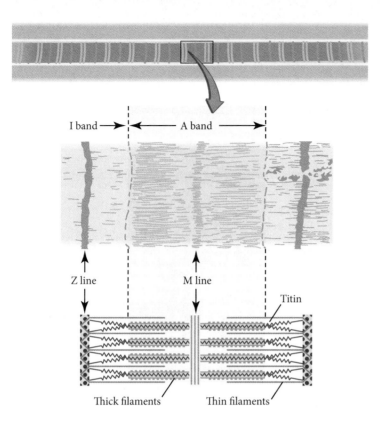

I band   A band

Z line   M line

Titin

Thick filaments   Thin filaments

Figure 3.10 The location of the thick, thin, and titin myofilaments within a sarcomere. The titin myofilament attaches the thick myofilament to the Z-disc and spans the A and I bands. The region of titin that spans the I band is proposed to be responsible for the passive elasticity of the sarcomere.

when the muscle fiber is stretched is regulated not only by the actin–myosin interaction but also by the titin myofilament.

Although the functional role of titin in athletic performance has yet to be determined, there is evidence of a differential expression of titin isoforms between athletes involved in strength and power sports compared to nonathletic subjects (McBride, Triplett-McBride, Davie, Abernethy, & Newton, 2003). Future research may reveal the importance of titin for athletic performance as well as the adaptations in this molecule in response to different training regimens.

human skeletal muscle (Pette, 1998; Schiaffino & Reggiani, 1994). Wrapped around the thin myofilament is the protein **tropomyosin**, which has the **troponin** protein attached to it (Figure 3.11). The tropomyosin–troponin complex plays an important role in the excitation–contraction coupling by regulating the exposure of the active binding sites on the actin molecule.

The thick myofilament is composed of heavy and light chains. While both the heavy and light chains regulate the tension developed by the sarcomere, it is the **myosin heavy chain (MHC)** that endows the fiber with its main functional characteristics, the

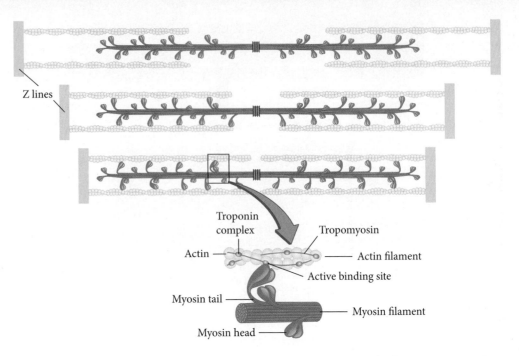

Figure 3.11 The thin myofilaments, comprising actin with the tropomyosin–troponin complex wrapped around them, and the thick myofilaments, comprising myosin within a sarcomere.

most important of which is its shortening velocity. There are three isoforms of MHC present in human skeletal muscle fibers: types Iβ, IIa, and IIx (note the lowercase letters used to represent the specific MHC isoform). The specific MHC content is used to differentiate the fiber types within skeletal muscle (see Skeletal Muscle Concept 3.4).

Crossbridge cycling

There are multiple crossbridges located along each thick myofilament that can bind to actin molecule located on the thin myofilament. Close to the actin binding site located on the crossbridges, there is a binding site for **adenosine-5′-triphosphate**

Skeletal Muscle Concept 3.4

Determining fiber types within skeletal muscle

Schiaffino (2010) provides the following historical perspective of determining the different types of muscle fibers within skeletal muscle. Early investigations into the composition of skeletal muscle led researchers to promote the view that there were two types of muscles and corresponding muscle fibers: "fast" white fibers and "slow" red fibers. This distinction was based upon the enzymatic and metabolic characteristics of the fibers, with the white fibers characterized by low myoglobin content and mitochondria, relying on glycolytic energy pathways, while the red fibers favored oxidative metabolism and were rich in myoglobin and mitochondria.

The development of histochemical staining procedures allowed investigators to differentiate fibers based upon their ATPase activity, leading to the classification of type I, IIA, and IIB fibers. Using this classification system, it was found that human type IIB fibers had higher glycolytic enzyme capacity than type IIA, with the IIA fibers having higher glycolytic capacity than type I fibers. This confirmed the classification of fast glycolytic, fast oxidative glycolytic, and slow oxidative fibers corresponding to types IIB, IIA, and I, respectively, that had been developed in animals.

Finally, the advent of monoclonal antibody-generation techniques and electrophoretic separation techniques allowed investigators to classify muscle fibers based upon their myosin heavy chain (MHC) isoform, leading to the categories of types I, IIA, IIX, and IIB in rodent muscle. Furthermore, it was reported that rodent muscle contained hybrid fibers with preferential combinations of MHC according to the sequence:

$$I \leftrightarrow I - IIA \leftrightarrow IIA \leftrightarrow IIA - IIX \leftrightarrow IIX \leftrightarrow IIX - IIB \leftrightarrow IIB.$$

It was found that the human fiber type IIB, as identified through ATPase staining techniques, contained the genetic equivalent of the rat IIX MHC, and that human muscle fibers tended not to express IIB MHC (although it is expressed in human extraocular and laryngeal muscles). Therefore, only three fiber types were identified within human skeletal muscle based upon MHC isoforms: types I, IIA, and IIX. The more restricted MHC repertoire of human MHC isoforms in comparison with rodent muscle, together with different relative proportions (human skeletal muscle tends to have a greater proportion of types I and IIA fibers, with rodent muscle composed mainly of types IIB and IIX) and metabolic properties, mean that one should interpret the research relating to muscle fiber types taken from the rodent model with caution when attempting to relate the findings to humans.

(ATP). The ATPase enzyme that is responsible for hydrolyzing the ATP molecule and energizing the crossbridge, an important step in excitation–contraction coupling, is located here. The specific isozyme of ATPase that exists on the crossbridge determines the rate of ATP hydrolysis, and therefore the rate of crossbridge cycling during muscle activation.

The proposed steps involved in the cycling of crossbridges during a shortening action in an activated muscle fiber are shown in Figure 3.12. In a resting muscle, the crossbridges are in an energized state due to the hydrolysis of ATP; however, the actomyosin interaction is prevented by the position of the regulatory troponin–tropomyosin complex blocking the active binding sites on the actin molecules. Following an increase in the sarcoplasmic concentration of Ca^{2+}, the active binding sites on actin are exposed; the crossbridges attach, and adenosine diphosphate (ADP) and inorganic phosphate (P_i) are released from the myosin head. The crossbridge undergoes a power stroke, pulling the thin myofilament toward the center of the

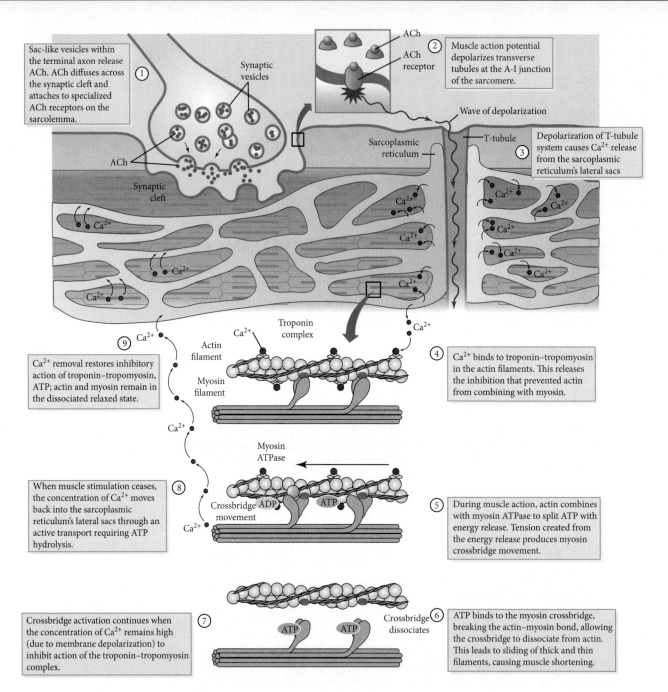

Sac-like vesicles within the terminal axon release ACh. ACh diffuses across the synaptic cleft and attaches to specialized ACh receptors on the sarcolemma.

Muscle action potential depolarizes transverse tubules at the A-I junction of the sarcomere.

Depolarization of T-tubule system causes Ca^{2+} release from the sarcoplasmic reticulum's lateral sacs

Ca^{2+} binds to troponin–tropomyosin in the actin filaments. This releases the inhibition that prevented actin from combining with myosin.

During muscle action, actin combines with myosin ATPase to split ATP with energy release. Tension created from the energy release produces myosin crossbridge movement.

ATP binds to the myosin crossbridge, breaking the actin–myosin bond, allowing the crossbridge to dissociate from actin. This leads to sliding of thick and thin filaments, causing muscle shortening.

Crossbridge activation continues when the concentration of Ca^{2+} remains high (due to membrane depolarization) to inhibit action of the troponin–tropomyosin complex.

When muscle stimulation ceases, the concentration of Ca^{2+} moves back into the sarcoplasmic reticulum's lateral sacs through an active transport requiring ATP hydrolysis.

Ca^{2+} removal restores inhibitory action of troponin–tropomyosin, ATP; actin and myosin remain in the dissociated relaxed state.

Figure 3.12 The proposed steps associated with crossbridge cycling in an activated muscle.

sarcomere, thereby developing tension. The detachment of the crossbridge requires an ATP molecule to attach to the ATP binding site of the myosin head. The detachment of the myosin molecule in conjunction with the hydrolysis of the ATP molecule energizes the crossbridge in readiness for the next cycle. It should be noted that there is turnover of crossbridges even under isometric conditions where the muscle fiber develops tension while maintaining constant length (Edman, 2003). Table 3.3 provides some measurements associated with the microstructural elements of skeletal muscle.

Table 3.3
Measurements of the Microstructural Elements of Skeletal Muscle

Element	Measurement
Actin filament thickness	50–60 Å
Actin filament length	2.0 μm
Myosin filament thickness	110 Å
Myosin filament length	1.65 μm
Force exerted by single crossbridge	5.3 pN
Number of crossbridges at each end of myosin filament	≈100
Sarcomeres in tibialis muscle	8,000–15,000
Sarcomeres in soleus muscle	14,000
Sarcomeres in gastrocnemius, medial head	15,000–16,000

Note: Å = angstroms (10^{-10} m)

Data from Zatsiorsky, V. M., & Prilutsky, B. I. (2012). *Biomechanics of Skeletal Muscles.* Champaign, IL: Human Kinetics.

Excitation–Contraction Coupling

In order to develop force, a muscle must be activated by the central nervous system. The stimulus responsible for this activation is an **action potential**. An action potential is transmitted by a **motoneuron** (an **α-motoneuron**), a nerve cell that originates in the ventral horn of the spinal cord, to the muscle fibers within a given muscle. A single motoneuron and the muscle fibers that it innervates are known as a **motor unit** and form the functional unit used by the central nervous system during the activation of a muscle.

An action potential transmitted down the axon of a motoneuron arrives at the **neuromuscular junction**, where the neurotransmitter **acetylcholine** is released into the synaptic cleft. Acetylcholine diffuses across the synaptic cleft and attaches to receptors located on the sarcolemma, which open Na^+-K^+ channels. There then follows an influx of Na^+ into the muscle fiber and an efflux of K^+ from the muscle fiber, resulting in the development of an **end-plate potential** that generates a muscle fiber action potential. The electrical activity associated with the activation of a muscle can be recorded in an electromyographic analysis (see Skeletal Muscle Concept 3.5).

Skeletal Muscle Concept 3.5

Recording the electrical activity of muscle

In a resting muscle fiber, there is a difference in electrical charge across the sarcolemma such that the interior of the cell is more negatively charged than the outside of the cell. This difference in charge results from the different concentration of ions, mainly sodium (Na^+) and potassium (K^+), across the

(continues)

(continued)

sarcolemma. In a resting muscle cell, the concentration of Na⁺ is greater on the outside of the cell, while K⁺ is found in greater concentrations on the interior of the cell, resulting in a difference in charge across the sarcolemma (an electrical potential) of approximately −90 mV. This value represents the **resting membrane potential** of a muscle fiber.

Each of the ions in a muscle fiber has an associated **equilibrium potential** that can be calculated from the Nernst equation (see Equation 3.5). For both Na⁺ and K⁺, the equation can be simplified to the following (MacIntosh, Gardiner, & McComas, 2006):

$$E_x = 61.5\,mV\ log_{10}\frac{[X]_o}{[X]_i} \qquad \text{Eq. (3.5)}$$

where E_x is the equilibrium potential of the specific ion in mV, $[X]_o$ is the concentration of the ion on the outside of the cell in mM, and $[X]_i$ is the concentration of the ion on the inside of the cell. The first term on the right-hand side of Equation (3.5) represents the electrical force (opposite charges attract) while the second term represents the chemical force (concentration gradient), both of which drive the diffusion of the ions across the sarcolemma. The equilibrium potential represents the resting membrane potential required to maintain the concentrations of ions on either side of the sarcolemma if the membrane were freely permeable to the specific ion. The equilibrium potential for Na⁺ is 71 mV, while that for K⁺ is −95 mV. The equilibrium potential occurs when the electrical and chemical forces are equal and there is no movement of the specific ion across the membrane. Notice that the resting membrane potential is very close to the equilibrium potential for K⁺, reflecting the fact that the resting membrane potential is mainly due to K⁺ concentrations across the sarcolemma at rest (MacIntosh, Gardiner, & McComas, 2006).

The value of the membrane potential at any time is related to the permeability of the membrane to specific ions (membrane conductance) and the equilibrium potentials of the specific ions. The membrane potential can be calculated from the Goldman-Hodgkin-Katz equation (MacIntosh, Gardiner, & McComas, 2006):

$$E_m = 61.5\,mV\ log_{10}\frac{P_K[K]_o + P_{Na}[Na]_o + P_{Cl}[Cl]_o}{P_K[K]_i + P_{Na}[Na]_i + P_{Cl}[Cl]_i} \qquad \text{Eq. (3.6)}$$

where E_m is the membrane potential and P is the permeability of the membrane for a specific ion. The sarcolemma has a much greater permeability to K⁺ compared to Na⁺ due to the concentration gradient of this ion across the membrane and the greater number of K⁺-specific channels in the membrane. Changing the concentration of the specific ions will tend to alter the difference in charge from inside to outside the cell, such that the membrane potential approximates the equilibrium potential of the specific ion. When a muscle fiber is activated by stimulation from a motoneuron, Na$^+$ channels on the sarcolemma are opened by acetylcholine binding to post-synaptic receptors. This increases the permeability of the sarcolemma to Na$^+$, allowing it to move down its concentration gradient and into the interior of the cell. This change in concentration of Na$^+$ will have the effect of moving the membrane potential toward the equilibrium potential of Na$^+$ (71 mV); the membrane potential becomes less negative, and therefore the membrane has been **depolarized**. The increased permeability of the membrane to Na$^+$ is very short-lived and the channels are rapidly inactivated. At the same time, the permeability of the membrane to K$^+$ is increased, causing efflux of the ion down its concentration gradient, returning the membrane potential back to a negative value; the membrane has been **repolarized**. This transient change in the membrane potential as a result of the movement of Na$^+$ and K$^+$ across the membrane characterizes a **muscle fiber action potential** (Figure 3.13).

A change occurs in the concentrations of Na$^+$ and K$^+$ across the sarcolemma in response to a muscle fiber action potential, but the quantities are so small that a muscle fiber is capable of conducting several thousand action potentials (MacIntosh, Gardiner, & McComas, 2006). Furthermore, during voluntary muscle actions there will be conduction of multiple action potentials associated with

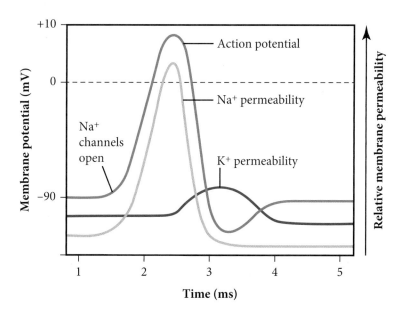

Figure 3.13 The changes in the membrane potential associated with an action potential caused by the movement of sodium and potassium ions across the sarcolemma.

Reproduced, with permission, from Kamen, G., & Gabriel, D. A. (2010). *Essentials of Electromyography*. Champaign, IL: Human Kinetics.

(continues)

(continued)

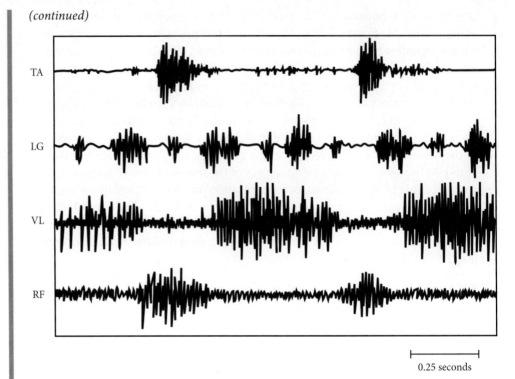

0.25 seconds

Figure 3.14 The electromyographic signals from four lower-body muscles during a movement task.

Note: TA is tibialis anterior; LG is the long head of the gastrocnemius; VL is vastus lateralis; RF is rectus femoris.

all of the muscle fibers that have been activated in response to the activation of multiple motor units. The motor unit action potentials can be recorded in an **electromyographic (EMG) analysis** (Figure 3.14).

As with other biomechanical signals, important information can be gleaned from the **amplitude** and the **frequency** of the EMG signal. The amplitude of the EMG signal can be determined using various methods (e.g., peak-to-peak amplitude, average rectified amplitude, root mean squared amplitude [Kamen, 2004]). The amplitude of the EMG signal reflects the average conduction velocity of the muscle fibers, the number of active motor units, the synchronization of active motor units, and the size of the active motor units (Enoka, 2008; MacIntosh, Gardiner, & McComas, 2006). There is some evidence that EMG amplitude increases linearly with muscle force during isometric actions, while reductions in EMG amplitude occur during fatigue associated with maximal isometric actions (Kamen & Gabriel, 2010).

The frequency content of the EMG signal is largely influenced by the average conductance velocity of the muscle fibers (Enoka, 2008). It is known that fast fibers have a greater conduction velocity than slow fibers (Kamen & Gabriel, 2010), so researchers have investigated the relationship between muscle force and the frequency content of the EMG signal, although the findings are inconsistent (Enoka, 2008). A clearer relationship exists between the frequency content of the EMG signal and muscular fatigue, certainly during isometric actions, where the median frequency of the EMG signal declines with fatigue (Kamen & Gabriel, 2010). This may reflect the reduced activation of fast fibers during such activities, as these fibers are unable to resist fatigue.

Despite the physiologic conclusions that can be drawn from the amplitude and frequency of the EMG signal, there are a number of other variables that can influence the signal. These include the thickness of subcutaneous tissue; number and distribution of muscle fibers; muscle fiber length; pennation angles; movement of the muscle relative to the electrodes; and the size, shape, and placement of the electrodes (Enoka, 2008). These factors need to be considered when interpreting the EMG signal.

Propagation of action potentials

The muscle fiber action potential is propagated along the sarcolemma at a velocity of between 2 and 6 m/s, being higher in fast-muscle fibers (Kamen & Gabriel, 2010). When the action potential reaches the transverse tubules (T-tubules), it is propagated into the interior of the muscle fiber. This T-tubule action potential activates the **dihydropyridine receptors**, which then transmit the signal to the **ryanodine receptors** in the sarcoplasmic reticulum, which results in the movement of Ca^{2+} down its concentration gradient from the terminal cisternae into the sarcoplasm. An increase in the concentration of Ca^{2+} in the sarcoplasm causes the ion to bind to the regulatory protein troponin associated with the thin myofilament, whereby tropomyosin undergoes a structural change and exposes the active binding sites on the actin molecule. At this time, the myosin crossbridge, which is in an energized state due to the hydrolysis of ATP, binds to the actin molecule and undergoes a power stroke, moving the thin myofilament toward the center of the sarcomere. A reuptake of Ca^{2+} occurs via the Ca^{2+} pump (an active process that requires ATP), which returns the Ca^{2+} concentrations in the sarcoplasm to resting levels, and it is the reuptake of Ca^{2+} into the sarcoplasmic reticulum that determines the rate of relaxation of the muscle. The main events associated with the excitation–contraction coupling are summarized in Figure 3.15. Three of the steps require ATP and therefore consume metabolic energy:

- The actomyosin interaction during crossbridge cycling
- The Na^+-K^+ pump to establish the concentration of these ions on either side of the sarcolemma to their resting values
- Ca^{2+} pump required to reuptake this ion back into the sarcoplasmic reticulum

These steps have important implications for the energetics associated with muscle actions.

There is a short delay (between 25 and 100 ms) following the activation of a muscle until the force is detected that is known as **electromechanical delay** (Zatsiorsky & Prilutsky, 2012). The source of this delay likely resides in an initial stretch of the connective tissue following crossbridge cycling. The electromechanical delay is shorter for eccentric actions where the connective tissue is pre-stretched compared to concentric actions and decreases with the increase of lengthening velocity (Zatsiorsky & Prilutsky, 2012). This highlights the importance of performing initial eccentric muscle actions during activities that require high rates of force development.

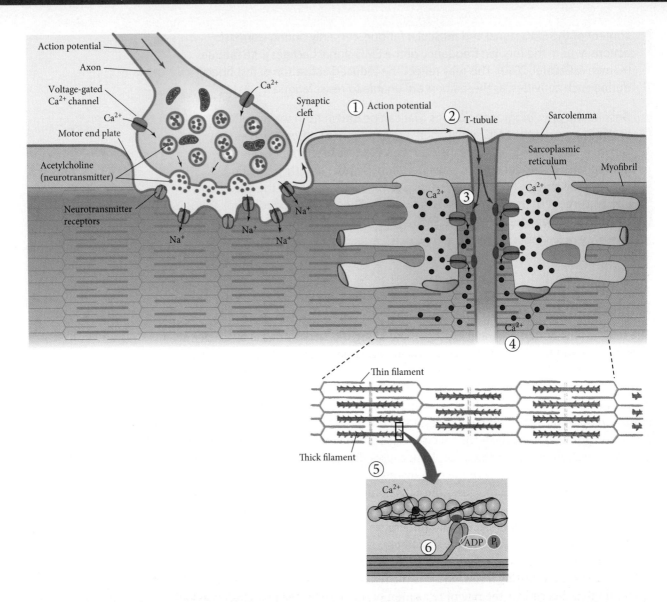

Figure 3.15 The steps involved in the excitation–contraction coupling: (1) propagation of an action potential along the sarcolemma; (2) propagation of the action potential down the T-tubule; (3) activation of the dihydropyridine and ryanodine receptors of the sarcoplasmic reticulum; (4) movement of Ca^{2+} into the sarcoplasm; (5) binding of Ca^{2+} to troponin; (6) binding of myosin crossbridge to the actin molecule.

Factors Affecting the Mechanical Output of Skeletal Muscle

There are a number of factors that determine the force generated by a muscle, as well as the work and power. These include the length of the muscle, the velocity of dynamic muscle actions, muscle fiber type, cross-sectional area, architecture, activation dynamics, spinal reflexes, and contractile history.

Length of the muscle

When a muscle operates isometrically, the maximal tension that it can develop is dependent upon the length of the muscle (Edman, 2003). This length-dependence of tension has been demonstrated from experiments performed on sarcomeres of uniform length, producing the curve shown in **Figure 3.16**.

The length–tension relationship shown in Figure 3.16 occurs due to the variation in the overlap between the thick and thin myofilaments, whereby the reduced overlap at longer sarcomere lengths reduces the maximal developed tension, while at short sarcomere lengths double filament overlap and the abutment of the thick myofilament against the Z-discs reduce the maximal tension developed. This functional relationship highlights the proportionality between active force development within the sarcomeres and the overlap between the thick and thin myofilaments, while also highlighting the optimal length of sarcomeres to develop maximal tension.

The active length–tension relationship shown for sarcomeres does not reflect the relationship for whole muscle. Skeletal muscle contains passive elastic elements (e.g., connective tissue such as tendon and aponeuroses), so the tension developed at a given muscle length is the sum of the passive and active components (**Figure 3.17**).

In Figure 3.17, the overall length–tension properties are shown for two muscles: One has fibers arranged at an angle to the line of action of the muscle (pennation angle), while the other has a parallel arrangement of fibers. Muscles that have pennate fibers tend to contain considerable connective tissue, and thus have a larger passive

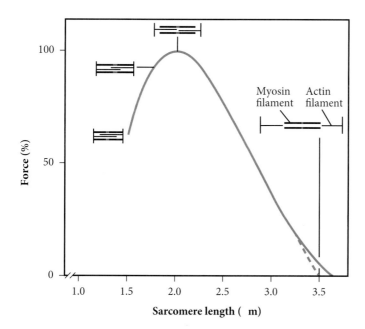

Figure 3.16 The length–tension relationship of skeletal muscle. The graph shows the variation in maximal tension associated with changes in the length of sarcomeres.

Reproduced from Edman, K. A. P. (2003). Contractile performance of skeletal muscle fibers. In P. V. Komi (Ed.), *Strength and Power in Sport*. Oxford, UK: Blackwell Publishing.

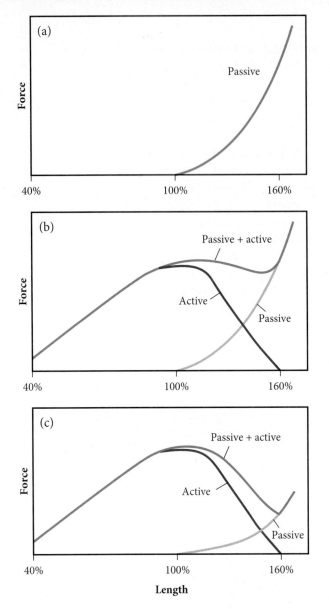

Figure 3.17 The contribution of passive and active components to tension within a whole muscle. (a) The passive length–tension curve for a muscle showing that the resistance to stretch increases as the muscle is lengthened. The resistance comes from passive elastic elements including the tendon and aponeurosis. (b) The contribution of passive and active components to the length–tension curve for a typical pennate muscle, which has considerable connective tissue. Notice that high tension is developed at long muscle lengths. (c) The contribution of passive and active components to the length–tension curve for a typical fusiform muscle, which has little connective tissue. Notice that there is a reduction in tension at long muscle lengths.

Reproduced from Biewener, A. A. (2003). *Animal Locomotion*. Oxford, UK: Oxford University Press.

component (Biewener, 2003). This arrangement allows the development of higher tensions at longer lengths in comparison to muscles with a parallel arrangement of fibers. The practical significance of the length–tension relationship for the strength and conditioning practitioner is that joint angle will determine the length of a muscle, which will therefore influence the isometric force developed (see Applied Research 3.3). Furthermore, serial sarcomere addition resulting from changes in contractile activity of the activated fibers is likely to change the muscle length associated with maximal tension development (Butterfield & Herzog, 2006).

The length–tension relationship is determined experimentally during isometric actions performed under predetermined muscle and sarcomere lengths. It does not accurately reflect the instantaneous length–tension relationship that would be elicited during natural movements, because the manner in which the muscle arrived at the

Applied Research 3.3
The joint-specific effects of isometric training are affected by muscle length

The authors investigated the effects of 12 weeks of isometric knee extension training on isometric knee extension torque. Each subject trained one leg at a knee angle of 50° (short muscle length), with the knee of the contralateral leg at 100° (long muscle length). Isometric torque was measured at eight knee angles between 40° and 110° for both legs after the training period. It was reported that training at the short muscle length resulted in increases in extension torque close to the trained angle (40° to 80°), while training at the longer length produced increases in isometric torque across all test angles. The authors attributed the greater range of improvements accompanying the 100° knee angle condition as resulting from the increased tendon stiffness. As the moment arm associated with the knee extensors was greater at the shorter muscle length (50° knee angle), the muscular force was greater at the longer muscle length for the same absolute joint torque. This implies that the tension developed by the musculotendinous unit is important for adaptations in tendinous structures.

Kubo, K., Ohgo, K., Takeishi, R., Yoshinaga, K., Tsunoda, N., Kanehisa, H., & Fukunaga, T. (2006). Effects of isometric training at different knee angles on the muscle-tendon complex *in vivo*. *Scandinavian Journal of Medicine Science Sports, 16,* 159–167.

length is ignored (i.e., the contractile history is neglected) and the velocity of the movement is also neglected. It is to this issue that we turn our attention.

Velocity of dynamic muscle actions

The velocity at which a muscle is shortening or lengthening can have a considerable effect on the observed tension developed. Figure 3.18 shows the force–velocity relationship of an active skeletal muscle fiber.

The reduction in force development with increasing shortening velocity can be explained in terms of chemical reaction rates associated with the ATPase enzyme associated with actomyosin cycling, as described by the crossbridge theory of muscle

Figure 3.18 The force–velocity relationship of a single muscle fiber. The graph shows that the velocity of shortening increases (positive values on the y-axis) as the magnitude of the external load, and therefore the force exerted by the fiber, is decreased. Conversely, the velocity of lengthening increases (negative values on the y-axis) as the magnitude of the external load, and therefore the force exerted by the fiber, is increased.

Note: v_{max} is the maximal velocity or shortening; P_o is the maximal isometric tension.

Reproduced from Edman, K. A. P. (2003). Contractile performance of skeletal muscle fibers. In P. V. Komi (Ed.), *Strength and Power in Sport.* Oxford, UK: Blackwell Publishing.

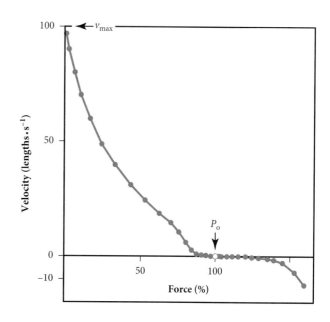

contraction (Lieber, 2002). However, the rise in force as the muscle is lengthened while developing tension cannot readily be explained by the original crossbridge theory. During eccentric muscle actions, the crossbridges are forcibly detached as a result of the external force applied to the muscle exceeding muscular tension. Crossbridges that are detached in this manner have been shown to reattach at much higher rates, so that the number of crossbridges attached even during rapid muscle lengthening remains high (Lombardi & Piazzesi, 1990). This allows the tension developed during eccentric actions to remain greater than that associated with concentric and even isometric actions, a finding shown *in vitro* as well as *in vivo* (Drury, Stuempfle, Mason, & Girman, 2006; Harry, Ward, Heglund, Morgan, & McMahon, 1990). This aspect has important implications for the mechanical behavior of skeletal muscle during natural movements, with eccentric actions allowing the absorption of large amounts of work and being important in landing movements.

The ability to develop high power outputs has been identified as the most important factor in determining sporting success (Wilson, Newton, Murphy, & Humphries, 1993). Power is the rate of performing work, which can be calculated as the product of force and velocity. We can therefore determine the power output of muscle fibers from their force–velocity curves. The shortening velocities of type II fibers have been reported to be twice that of the type I fibers (Lionikas, Li, & Larsson, 2006). This, combined with greater force-generating capabilities of the fast fibers (Linari et al., 2003), confers much greater power outputs in the fast fibers compared to the slow fibers (Bottinelli, Pellegrino, Canepari, Rossi, & Reggiani, 1999). It is therefore no surprise that those athletes competing in sports requiring high power outputs tend to have a greater proportion of fast-muscle fiber types (Andersen, Klitgaard, & Saltin, 1994). There is some evidence that different training regimens may increase the power output of skeletal muscle fibers through different mechanisms (see Skeletal Muscle Concept 3.6). For example, resistance training appears to increase power output through hypertrophy of the muscle fibers (Shoepe, Stelzer, Garner, & Widrick, 2003), while there is evidence that endurance training may increase fiber power output through increases in shortening velocity (Harber & Trappe, 2008).

Skeletal Muscle Concept 3.6

Comparing single fiber power output with whole-body power output

The force–velocity relationship shown in Figure 3.18 was generated from a series of experiments where the muscle fiber was allowed to shorten against various constant loads. It is therefore strictly the load–velocity relationship. Calculating power output during shortening of the fiber shown in Figure 3.18 produces a parabolic curve with maximal power occurring at approximately 0.4 v_{max} (Biewener, 2003).

When power output is calculated in this manner for the whole body using multijoint movements such as vertical jumps performed under different loaded conditions, the derived power output plot is linear, with power output maximized at the highest movement velocities, decreasing with movement velocity. The difference in the plots of power output for an isolated muscle fiber and for multijoint movements likely reflects different levels of muscle activation, reflexive input, and the combined output of many muscles of differing fiber type and architectural characteristics operating with continually changing moment arms during multijoint movements. Furthermore, the shape of the relationship in multijoint activities is influenced by the specific movement used (e.g., squat jump versus back squat [Cormie, McCaulley, Triplett, & McBride, 2007]) and the training background of the athlete (e.g., strength trained versus power trained [Samozino, Rejc, Di Prampero, Belli, & Morin, 2012]). The power–load relationship measured during multijoint movements has been shown to be modifiable through specific training regimens (Cormie, McCaulley, & McBride, 2007).

Fiber type

Skeletal muscles are composed of fibers that possess different structural and molecular components that result in different functional properties. Human skeletal muscle contains type I, IIA, and IIX fibers in varying degrees. This nomenclature comes from the isoform of the myosin molecule, specifically the heavy chain of the myosin molecule (Baldwin & Haddad, 2001), as this protein endows the fiber with specific functional characteristics. Table 3.4 shows the physiological and mechanical characteristics of the different fiber types based upon their MHC content.

Type I fibers extracted from the vastus lateralis have been shown to develop less isometric tension than type IIA fibers, which developed less tension than hybrid type IIA/IIX fibers (Linari et al., 2003). Furthermore, greater specific tension has been reported for type IIX fibers compared to MHC type I (Stienen, Kiers, Bottinelli, & Reggiani, 1996). These findings are substantiated *in vivo*, with positive correlations between the percentage of fast fibers within a muscle and measures of strength

Table 3.4
Physiological and Mechanical Characteristics of the Different Fiber Types

Characteristics	Type I	Type IIA	Type IIX
Specific tension	Low	Intermediate	High
Velocity of shortening	Slow	Moderate to fast	Fast
Rate of force development	Low	Intermediate	High
Myosin ATPase activity	Low	High	High
CS and SDH activity	High	Intermediate	Low
Myoglobin content	High	High	Low
Glycogen granules	Sparse	Intermediate	Many
Mitochondria and capillaries	Many	Intermediate	Few
Resistance to fatigue	High	Intermediate	Low

Note: CS is citrate synthase; SDH is succinate dehydrogenase.

Reproduced from Biewener, A. A. (2003). *Animal Locomotion*. Oxford, UK: Oxford University Press.

(Aagaard & Andersen 1998). There are unlikely to be fiber type transformations beyond those associated with type IIA ↔ IIX, although there is likely to be an increase in hybrid muscle fibers following different modes of training (see **Skeletal Muscle Concept 3.7** and Applied Research 3.4).

Cross-sectional area

The maximal tension developed by a muscle is determined by the number of sarcomeres in parallel (Close, 1972), so one would expect the force-generating capacity of muscle to be related to its cross-sectional area (CSA). It has been demonstrated that the force generated by a muscle follows a linear relation with the CSA of the muscle such that the greater the cross-section, the greater the force developed (Jones, Rutherford, & Parker, 1989; see Applied Research 3.5).

Skeletal Muscle Concept 3.7

Can muscle fiber type be changed through physical training?

Given that the classification of muscle fiber types is based upon their MHC isoform content, this question is better expressed as whether the MHC isoforms are responsive to physical training. Evidence from animal models has shown that a fast muscle can be transformed to a slow muscle by chronic low-frequency (10-Hz) electrical stimulation (Pette, Smith, Staudte, & Vrbová, 1973). Similarly, cross-innervation of a muscle, whereby the motoneurons of fast and slow muscles are switched, results in the reversal of their characteristic contractile velocities such that the fast muscle becomes slow, the slow muscle becoming fast (Buller, Eccles, & Eccles, 1960). It was later confirmed that these findings were due to changes in the specific MHC isoforms within the muscle fibers (Pette, 2001). In humans, spinal cord injury resulting in paralysis leads to the affected muscles expressing fast MHC isoforms exclusively (Andersen, Mohr, Biering-Sørensen, Galbo, & Kjær, 1996). What these studies show is that a complete transformation between MHC isoforms is possible. However, the situations in which the transformations were induced do not relate to the mechanical and metabolic changes associated with a period of physical training.

Different regimens of physical training (e.g., endurance training, resistance training, sprint training) tend to induce a fast-to-slow transformation of MHC isoforms, with type IIX fibers transitioning to IIA (Andersen & Aagaard, 2010; Kraemer et al., 1995; Ross & Leveritt, 2001). Conversely, a period of detraining has been shown to induce a slow-to-fast transition (Pette & Staron, 1997). Hybrid fibers are classified as those fibers that coexpress two or more MHC isoforms; therefore, there exists a continuum from the "pure" type I fibers to the "pure" type IIX fibers (Pette, 1998). The appearance of fibers coexpressing MHC isoforms has been observed in fibers undergoing molecular and functional transformations (Pette, Peuker, & Staron, 1999; Stephenson, 2001). Thus, while complete fiber transformations between the fast and slow pure muscle fiber types are unlikely in response to physical training, there is likely to be an increase in hybrid muscle fibers in response to the altered contractile activity that accompanies an increase or decrease in an exercise stimulus.

The effects of physical training on MHC transformations has been shown to be influenced by the MHC isoforms present in the muscle prior to training (Gehlert et al., 2012), and there is evidence that fiber types within human skeletal muscle have a significant genetic component (Ahmetov, Vinogradova, & Williams, 2012). There also is evidence that mechanical characteristics such as v_{max} can be significantly increased in all fiber types following a regimen of plyometric training despite a concomitant transformation of type IIX to IIA (Malisoux, Francaux, Nielens, & Theisen, 2006). Furthermore, single muscle fibers with apparently identical MHC isoforms can vary considerably in their metabolic capacities (Pette, Peuker, & Staron, 1999). While these findings complicate the matter of the characteristics of the different fiber types, it should be remembered that these adaptations represent one in a number of factors that will contribute to performance improvements following a period of physical training. Indeed, some have argued that other adaptations within a muscle fiber that accompany a regimen of physical training (e.g., cross-sectional area and architectural changes) are more important in affecting performance than fiber type transformations (Lieber, 2002).

Applied Research 3.4
Muscle fiber types of different athletes

The authors compared the muscle fiber characteristics of the vastus lateralis of 72 athletes from various sports. Fiber types were determined using ATPase staining techniques. Long-distance runners were found to have the greatest percentage of type I fibers, with athletes involved in explosive sports (karate and triple jump) possessing the smallest percentage of these fibers. Sprint athletes (100–400 m) had a low percentage of type I fibers and a high percentage of type II fiber (~ 40% and 60%, respectively), comparable to the sedentary controls in the investigation. However, the diameter of these fibers was much greater in the sprint athletes than in the controls. Whether these differences reflect a genetic predisposition or a training effect could not be ascertained from the data.

Ricoy, J. R., Encinas, A. R., Cabello, A., Madero, S., & Arenas, J. (1998). Histochemical study of the vastus lateralis muscle fibre types of athletes. *Journal of Physiology and Biochemistry, 54*, 41–47.

Applied Research 3.5
Comparison of muscle fiber characteristics between resistance-trained and sedentary individuals

The authors compared the mechanical characteristics of muscle fibers in a group of men who had been regularly resistance training for an average of 7.6 years with a group of sedentary individuals. Biopsies were obtained from the vastus lateralis muscle and tested for maximal isometric tension, unloaded shortening velocity, and power output. The CSA of the fibers was also recorded. The authors reported that the resistance-trained group had fibers with significantly greater CSA across all fiber types (I, IIA, and IIX); however, there were no differences in the unloaded shortening velocities between the two groups. Absolute power output was significantly greater for all fiber types in the resistance-trained group compared to the sedentary group. The authors concluded that muscle fiber hypertrophy resulting from long-term resistance training produces greater power outputs.

Shoepe, T. C., Stelzer, J. E., Garner, D. P., & Widrick, J. J. (2003). Functional adaptability of muscle fibers to long-term resistance exercise. *Medicine and Science in Sports and Exercise, 35*, 944–951.

The area of the section of muscle that reflects the circumference of the muscle is known as the **anatomical cross-sectional area** (ACSA) of the muscle. The irregular shape of many skeletal muscles and the orientation of the fibers preclude the use of circumferential measurements to reflect the intrinsic force capabilities of the muscle. In order to ensure that the CSA reflects a section orthogonal (perpendicular) to the direction of muscle fibers within the muscle, the **functional physiological cross-sectional area** (PCSA) can be calculated (Zatsiorsky & Prilutsky, 2012):

$$PCSA = \frac{m \times cos\theta}{\rho \times l_f}$$

Eq. (3.7)

where *PCSA* is the functional physiological cross-sectional area of the muscle, m is the mass of the muscle in grams, θ is the pennation angle of the fibers, ρ is the density of muscle (1.056 g/cm^3), l_f is the length of the fibers within the muscle in millimeters. The PCSA is equal to the ACSA in parallel-fibered muscles, while in those muscles with pennate arrangements of the fibers, the PCSA can be considerably larger than the ACSA (Fukunaga et al., 1992). The CSA of the muscle fibers is sensitive to the changing mechanical demands associated with an increased or decreased use (see Skeletal Muscle Concept 3.8).

Skeletal Muscle Concept 3.8

Hypertrophy and atrophy of skeletal muscle fibers

Hypertrophy is defined as an increase in the CSA of muscle fibers as a result of an increase in the number and area of the myofibrils contained within (MacDougall, 2003). This is in contrast with **hyperplasia**, which is an increase in the number of fibers within a muscle (MacDougall, 2003). Despite evidence for hyperplasia in animal models (Kelley, 1996), it is unlikely to contribute to the increase in muscle CSA observed in humans (MacDougall, 2003). The increase in the number and area of myofibrils is induced as a result of the increase in muscle protein synthesis and/or a decrease in the breakdown of proteins in response to an increased contractile activity (Kumar, Atherton, Smith, & Rennie, 2009; Sandri, 2008). Because of the increase in size of the muscle fibers, there is a concomitant increase in the myonuclear domain (i.e., the sarcoplasmic volume that is controlled by each nucleus [Kadi et al., 2004]). The myonuclear domain limits the increase in fiber size by controlling the accretion of protein within the sarcoplasm; a myonuclear domain ceiling of approximately 25% hypertrophy of the original fiber CSA has been suggested (Kadi et al., 2004). At this point, the satellite cells that are located at the periphery of the muscle fibers (basal lamina) donate their nuclei to allow the process to continue (Adams, 2006; Kadi et al., 2004; Petrella, Kim, Mayhew, Cross, & Bamman, 2008). Although all fiber types can undergo hypertrophy, fast fibers demonstrate the greatest increases, certainly in response to a resistance-training regimen (Kosek, Kim, Petrella, Cross, & Bamman, 2006), possibly due to greater damage induced by the greater forces generated by these fibers and structural differences (Schoenfeld, 2010).

It should be noted that the CSA of whole muscle can be affected by the pennation angle of the fibers, with significant positive correlations reported between muscle thickness and pennation angles (Ichinose, Kanehisa, Ito, Kawakami, & Fukunaga, 1998; Kawakami, Abe, & Fukunaga, 1993). This suggests that increases in pennation angle may contribute to the increases in muscle CSA observed following a period of resistance training in addition to fiber hypertrophy.

In contrast to hypertrophy, **atrophy** is a decrease in the CSA of muscle fibers as a result of protein breakdown exceeding protein synthesis, which can accompany a decrease in contractile activity (Sandri, 2008). Various mechanisms have been forwarded to explain this disuse atrophy, including activation of proteolytic pathways (Sandri, 2008). It is important to note that the signaling pathways activated during hypertrophy and atrophy of the muscle are distinct, despite the apparent reversal in morphology that accompanies each state (Coffey & Hawley, 2007). While all fibers are affected by a reduction in contractile activity resulting from disuse, there is evidence that slow fibers accrue greater atrophy than the fast fibers (Baldwin & Haddad, 2001; di Prampero & Narici, 2003). **Sarcopenia** is a loss of muscle mass usually associated with aging muscle. This condition is distinct from disuse atrophy due to the loss of muscle fibers (hypoplasia) that accompanies fiber atrophy, which is believed to be caused by the activation of proteolytic processes and apoptosis within the affected muscle fibers (Dirks & Leeuwenburgh, 2005).

Specific tension

Specific tension refers to the force capacity of a muscle fiber relative to the CSA of the fiber; it is a functional measure of the number of myofibrils per unit of CSA (Enoka, 2008), reflecting the myofilament packing density. It has been shown that the specific tension differs between muscle fiber types, with fast fibers demonstrating greater specific tension than the slow fibers (Bottinelli et al., 1996; D'Antona et al., 2006; see Applied Research 3.6).

Applied Research 3.6
Changes in specific tension of the quadriceps following resistance training

The authors investigated the effects of nine weeks of high-intensity resistance training on the strength of the quadriceps femoris muscle and the concomitant changes in architecture, volume, and PCSA of the muscle group. A 31% increase in the force exerted during a maximal voluntary isometric action was accompanied by a 6% increase in muscle volume and a 5% increase in fascicle pennation angle (only observed in the vastus lateralis muscle), while there was no change in fascicle length. Muscle activation assessed through EMG increased by only 3%. The structural changes in the muscle resulted in a 6% increase in the PCSA of the quadriceps. Given the change in PCSA, specific tension of the quadriceps was increased by 20% as a result of the resistance-training regimen. The increase in specific tension may have arisen from increases in the myofilament packing density, changes in muscle fiber type, or increases in lateral force transmission within the activated muscles. Increases in specific tension could possibly explain the disproportionate changes in muscular strength and size following resistance training.

Erskine, R. M., Jones, D. A., Williams, A. G., Stewart, C. E., & Degens, H. (2010). Resistance training increases *in vivo* quadriceps femoris muscle specific tension in young men. *Acta Physiologica, 199*, 83–89.

Architecture

The length of the fibers within a muscle is dependent upon the number of sarcomeres arranged serially. This architectural feature of the muscle will influence the length, and therefore joint angle, at which the greatest force is developed. Furthermore, the length of a fiber will influence the rate of shortening, and the fastest sprinters have been shown to have the longest fascicles (Abe, Fukashiro, Harada, & Kawamoto, 2001; Kumagai et al., 2000). Figure 3.19 shows the number of serial sarcomeres within the fibers of different muscles.

The architectural characteristic that has the greatest effect on the tension developed by skeletal muscle is the **pennation angle** of the muscle fibers. The pennation angle is defined as the angle between the direction of the muscle fibers and the line of action of force associated with the muscle (Zatsiorsky & Prilutsky, 2012). Because of the inherent difficulties in assessing the orientation of the muscle fibers directly, researchers use the orientation of the fascicles within the muscle. Because more fibers are contained within a given volume of a pennate muscle when compared to a fusiform muscle, pennate

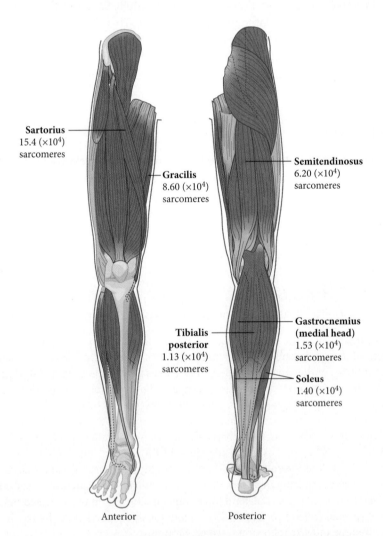

Sartorius
15.4 (×10^4)
sarcomeres

Gracilis
8.60 (×10^4)
sarcomeres

Semitendinosus
6.20 (×10^4)
sarcomeres

**Tibialis
posterior**
1.13 (×10^4)
sarcomeres

**Gastrocnemius
(medial head)**
1.53 (×10^4)
sarcomeres

Soleus
1.40 (×10^4)
sarcomeres

Anterior   Posterior

Figure 3.19 The number of serial sarcomeres in fibers from different muscles.

Data from MacIntosh, B. R., Gardiner, P. F., & McComas, A. J. (2006). *Skeletal Muscle. Form and Function*. Champaign, IL: Human Kinetic Publishers.

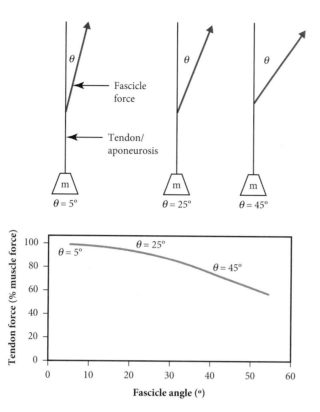

Figure 3.20 The influence of pennation angle on tendon force. Notice that the proportion of muscle-fiber force directed along the tendon decreases as the pennation angle increases, with a concomitant decrease in tendon force. However, the decrease in tendon force is small with typical anatomical pennation angles (≤30°).

Reproduced from Blazevich, A. J. (2006). Effects of physical training and detraining, immobilization, growth and aging on human fascicle geometry. *Sports Medicine, 36*, 1003–1017, with kind permission from Springer Science and Business Media.

muscles are able to generate greater force (Zatsiorsky & Prilutsky, 2012). Pennation angles typically range between 0° and 30° in human skeletal muscle (Figure 3.20), and greater angles are associated with greater force capabilities (Ichinose, Kanehisa, Ito, Kawakami, & Fukunaga, 1998).

Because of the oblique angle of the muscle fibers in pennate muscles, only a component of the fiber tension contributes to the tension produced by the whole muscle, with the contribution of each fiber to the overall force being proportional to the cosine of the pennation angle. However, some authors suggest that the increase in fibers in a given volume of these muscles offsets this reduced contribution (Biewener, 2003), while the reduction in tension within the range of pennation angles observed *in vivo* is limited (Figure 3.20). There is some evidence that the pennation angle changes with joint angle (Kawakami et al., 2000), which will affect the joint angle at which maximal force is generated, while the pennation angle has been shown to increase in response to resistance-training regimens (Blazevich, Gill, Bronks, & Newton, 2003; see Applied Research 3.7).

Although pennate muscles generate greater tension, they tend to have shorter fibers, limiting both the excursion of the muscle during shortening and the maximal

Applied Research 3.7
Changes in pennation angles and fiber length following resistance training

The authors investigated the effects of five weeks of resistance training on athletic performance and muscle architecture changes. Participants performed either (1) back-squat training combined with sprint and jump training, (2) forward hack-squat training combined with sprint and jump training, or (3) sprint and jump training only. It was reported that the groups did not differ in their changes in the measures of athletic performance (accelerative sprint time, vertical jump height, isometric and isokinetic measures of strength). However, pennation angle in the vastus lateralis muscle increased in the squat training groups, while decreasing in the combined sprint and jump training group. The sprint and jump training group demonstrated an increase in fascicle length in the vastus lateralis muscle, with no changes reported for the two squat training groups. The authors concluded that the differential responses in pennation angle and fascicle length likely reflect the different force and velocity characteristics of the training exercises.

Blazevich, A. J., Gill, N. D., Bronks, R., & Newton, R. U. (2003). Training-specific muscle architecture adaptations after 5-wk training in athletes. *Medicine and Science in Sports and Exercise, 35*, 2013–2022.

shortening velocity (Zatsiorsky & Prilutsky, 2012). It has been shown that the fibers of pennate muscles actually rotate during shortening of the muscle such that the pennation angle increases (Azizi, Brainerd, & Roberts, 2008), allowing the fibers to contribute to the shortening velocity of the muscle. However, the increase in pennation angle as a result of the rotations decreases the contribution of the fibers to overall muscle force, so the rotations tend to be limited to situations where the external load is low.

Activation dynamics

The activation dynamics of skeletal muscle refer to the recruitment of motor units, rate coding, and the timing and coordination of activation.

Motor-unit recruitment

The functional unit used by the central nervous system to control muscular tension is the motor unit, a motoneuron and the muscle fibers that it innervates. The **innervation ratio** reflects the number of muscle fibers per motor unit and informs us of the force-generating capacity of the motor unit, with large innervation ratios reflecting large force capacity. Skeletal muscles differ in the number of motor units that they contain as well as their respective innervation ratios. For example, the external rectus muscle of the eye has 2,970 motor units and an innervation ratio of 9; the tibialis anterior muscle has 445 motor units and an innervation ratio of 562; and the medial head of the gastrocnemius has 579 motor units and an innervation ratio of 1,934 (MacIntosh, Gardiner, & McComas, 2006). The tension developed within a muscle can be modulated simply by increasing the number of motor units recruited at any time (Duchateau, Semmler, & Enoka, 2006), with large forces requiring the recruitment of more motor units.

The motoneuron associated with a specific motor unit can be characterized by its size. Various morphological features of the motoneuron have been used as a marker of size including the diameter of the neuron cell body, surface area, the number of dendrites, and the responses of the membrane to stimulation (Enoka, 2008). Such measures allow the grouping of motoneurons, and therefore motor units, based upon size. This grouping is important because the recruitment of motor units during a given muscle action follows a specific order beginning with the small motor units and progressing to large motor units in accordance with the **size principle** (Henneman, Somjen, & Carpenter, 1965). The small motor units have a lower threshold for excitation (MacIntosh, Gardiner, & McComas, 2006) and are therefore more likely to respond to a given level of excitatory input from the motor cortex, resulting in their initial recruitment during the activation of a muscle. The size principle of motor-unit recruitment appears to be set for both isometric and dynamic muscle actions as well as during the stretch reflex (Chalmers, 2008; Duchateau, Semmler, & Enoka, 2006). However, it is possible to reverse the recruitment order of motor units during evoked actions using transcutaneous stimulation (Bickel, Gregory, & Dean, 2011).

There is a relationship between the size of the motoneuron cell body and the muscle fibers innervated by the neuron such that the small motor units innervate type I fibers, with the larger motor units innervating the faster fibers (MacIntosh, Gardiner, & McComas, 2006). This means that the recruitment of small motor units corresponds to low tension generated by the muscle and provides a mechanism for the central nervous system to control tension during the activation of a muscle.

There is evidence that motor units are activated earlier during rapid muscle actions in movements characterized by high rates of force development when compared to tasks in which force levels increase slowly (Duchateau, Semmler, & Enoka, 2006). Furthermore, more motor units are recruited to produce a given level of force during a rapid muscle action than during slow actions (Duchateau, Semmler, & Enoka, 2006). Finally, motor unit activation is affected by the orientation of the body segments during the task and the direction of force application in a given task (Brown, Kautz, & Dairaghi, 1996; ter Haar Romeny, van der Gon, & Gielen, 1984). This highlights the mechanical specificity associated with the movement task that influences motor-unit recruitment.

Rate coding

The rate at which a motoneuron discharges action potentials is known as **rate coding**. The average value of rate coding for a muscle during a voluntary contraction is between 30 and 50 Hz, although the values vary among muscles, with those composed of predominantly slow fibers generally having lower values (Duchateau, Semmler, & Enoka, 2006). As the rate of action-potential discharge increases, the tension developed by the muscle increases, although the relationship is sigmoidal, implying an upper limit on rate coding (Duchateau, Semmler, & Enoka, 2006). However, an increase in rate coding represents a mechanism, along with motor-unit recruitment, that the central nervous system can employ to increase muscular tension, with motor-unit recruitment allowing an approximate 100-fold increase in tension, whereas an increase in rate coding produces an approximate 10-fold increase in muscle tension (MacIntosh, Gardiner, & McComas, 2006). Indeed, muscles differ in the relative contribution of motor-unit recruitment and rate coding to develop maximal tension (Moritz, Barry, Pascoe, & Enoka, 2005; Oya, Riek, & Cresswell, 2009), with an apparent general rule that smaller muscles tend to rely on rate coding to achieve maximal tension (MacIntosh, Gardiner, & McComas, 2006). More subtle gradations in tension are likely to be achieved by modulating rate coding rather than through the activation or deactivation of entire motor units (Kamen & Gabriel, 2010).

The rate coding observed during a maximal voluntary contraction actually reduces as maximal force is achieved. For example, discharge frequency of action potentials at the onset of voluntary contractions can be as high as 100–200 Hz, reducing to 15–35 Hz at the time of maximal force production (Aagaard, 2003). The high rate coding values early during a voluntary contraction are likely to contribute to high rates of force development. Furthermore, **discharge doublets** (consecutive action potentials with an interspike interval < 10 ms) are often observed during the periods of high rate coding at the onset of voluntary contraction (Aagaard, 2003). It is likely that these discharge doublets are also responsible for achieving high rates of force development.

Timing and coordination of activation

During cyclical movements involving the repeated lengthening and shortening of a muscle, such as would occur during many sporting movements, the length at which the muscle is activated will affect force generation and the work done by the active muscle. Therefore, the timing of muscle activation as well as the duration of the period of activation should be considered. The muscle fibers of the lower-limb muscles have been reported to move through multiple lengths at various times during the gait cycle (Arnold & Delp, 2011), covering most of the associated length–tension relationship for the fibers. However, it was noted that the fibers were only actually active over a much more restricted range corresponding to the plateau or descending limb of the length–tension relationship. Therefore, in natural movements it would appear that muscles are activated at a length whereby their mechanical output is optimized.

Figure 3.21 shows examples of the timing of the activation of muscles during cyclical lengthening and shortening. In Figure 3.21a, the activation of the muscle occurs prior to shortening and continues into the shortening phase. In this situation, both muscular tension and the amount of mechanical work during shortening are likely to be maximized due to the muscle being initially activated while it is being lengthened, a situation similar to that which occurs during the **stretch–shortening cycle**, where it has been established that the mechanical output of the muscle is enhanced during the subsequent shortening phase (Komi, 2003). Conversely, in Figure 3.21b, the muscle is activated later in the cycle at the end of shortening, with the period of activation lasting into the lengthening phase of the cycle. Here, the muscle performs little positive mechanical work but absorbs energy while developing a large amount of tension associated with an eccentric action. This pattern would be observed when a muscle acts to "brake" the body, such as occurs during landing tasks.

In contrast to an isolated muscle, the mechanical output during multijoint movements results from the interaction of the tension developed by groups of muscles. Considering a single joint, the acceleration of a limb segment is produced by the agonist muscle while the antagonist muscle produces an opposite acceleration. The mechanical output of the agonist muscle is therefore dependent upon the activity of its antagonist during a given task such that the mechanical output at a joint will be determined by the degree of **coactivation** between the antagonistic pair of muscles about the joint. Previous researchers have shown that physical training decreases the amount of coactivation between antagonistic pairs during tests of muscular strength, which may partially account for the increases in muscular strength (Amiridis et al., 1996). However, the coactivation of antagonistic pairs can increase the stability of a joint and distributes the load across a greater surface area of the joint structures, thereby limiting the potential for musculoskeletal injury (Aagaard, 2011). Furthermore, coactivation of monoarticular and biarticular muscles can enhance

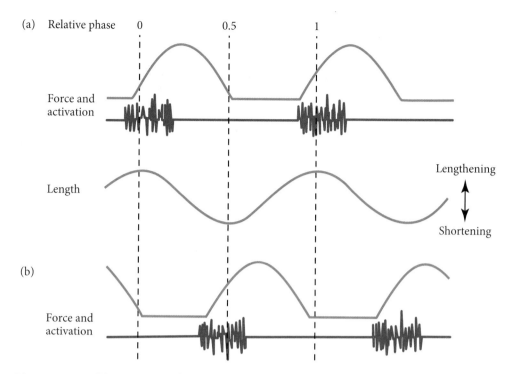

Figure 3.21 The timing of muscle activation during cyclical lengthening and shortening of a muscle. In example (a), the muscle is activated as it is lengthened prior to shortening. In example (b), the muscle is shortening as it is activated.

Reproduced from Biewener, A. A. (2003). *Animal Locomotion.* Oxford, UK: Oxford University Press.

performance by allowing the work performed by the monoarticular muscles to be transferred to other joints by the biarticular muscles (van Ingen Schenau, 1989).

Spinal reflexes

Spinal reflexes are rapid responses that involve the coupling between **afferent** and **efferent** signals within the central nervous system in order to elicit a response in an organ. These reflexes allow the central nervous system to modulate the response of an organ with respect to changes in the environment. An afferent signal refers to an action potential that is propagated by afferent neurons and that conveys sensory information relating to a specific stimulus from the periphery to the central nervous system. An efferent signal refers to an action potential propagated by neurons that transmit information from the central nervous system to a specific organ; the efferent neurons that innervate skeletal muscles are the α-motoneurons. The interaction of the neurons involved in the afferent–efferent coupling is influenced by **interneurons** that can modulate the membrane potentials of neurons, thereby changing the excitability of the neuron (Enoka, 2008). In skeletal muscle there are a number of **somatosensory receptors** that are sensitive to mechanical stimuli (Table 3.5), conveying afferent feedback to the central nervous system, of which the most important are **muscle spindles** and **Golgi tendon organs** (MacIntosh, Gardiner, & McComas, 2006). These sensory receptors can also modulate the tension developed by a muscle.

Table 3.5
Characteristics of Somatosensory Receptors

Receptor	Stimulus	Type of Afferent	Action Potential Conduction Velocity (m/s)
Muscle spindle (primary)	Rate of muscle stretch	Ia	40 to 90
Golgi tendon organ	Muscle force	Ib	30 to 75
Muscle spindle (secondary)	Muscle stretch	II	20 to 45
Joint receptors	Force around joint	II to III	4 to 45
Haptic receptors	Skin movement	I to III	4 to 80

Reproduced, with permission, from Enoka, R. M. (2008). *Neuromechanics of Human Movement*. Champaign, IL: Human Kinetic Publishers.

Muscle spindles

A muscle spindle consists of a series of **intrafusal fibers** enclosed in a connective tissue capsule. An intrafusal fiber has contractile proteins at the polar (end) regions, while the equatorial (central) region of each fiber is innervated by group Ia and II afferent nerve endings. The limited contractile proteins within the intrafusal fibers means that they do not contribute significantly to the tension developed within a muscle, in contrast to the **extrafusal fibers** (skeletal muscle fibers) that surround them (Figure 3.22).

Two types of intrafusal fibers can be identified based upon the arrangement of their nuclei. **Nuclear bag fibers** have their nuclei arranged in a central group, while **nuclear chain fibers** have their nuclei arranged sequentially along their length. The nuclear bag fibers are innervated mainly by group Ia afferents, while the nuclear chain fibers have both group Ia and II afferents (Enoka, 2008). The terminus of the group Ia afferents in an intrafusal fiber are known as **primary endings**, while the terminus of the group II afferents are known as the **secondary endings**. The polar regions of the intrafusal fibers are innervated by **γ-motoneurons**, which are efferent neurons. Activation of the γ-motoneurons results in the shortening of the intrafusal fiber at the polar regions and a concomitant stretch of the equatorial region, thereby altering the responsiveness of the fiber to a given rate and magnitude of stretch. The γ-motoneurons therefore modulate the feedback to the central nervous system in response to an imposed stretch (Enoka, 2008).

When a stretch is imposed on a muscle, the Ia and II afferents associated with the muscle spindles discharge action potentials. The Ia afferents discharge high-frequency action potentials during the stretch (dynamic response), with a steady discharge when the muscle achieves its new length (static response). The group II afferents only have a static response (MacIntosh, Gardiner, & McComas, 2006). The Ia and II afferents enter the spinal cord through the dorsal roots and make monosynaptic excitatory

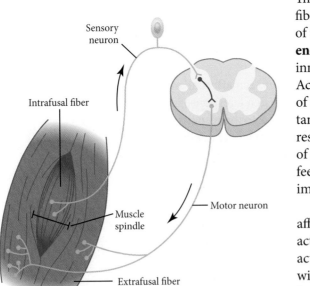

Figure 3.22 The intrafusal fibers located within a muscle.

connections with α-motoneurons that innervate the same (homonymous) muscle (Enoka, 2008). Furthermore, the Ia afferent can inhibit the α-motoneurons that innervate the antagonist muscle via an interneuron. The result is an efferent signal to increase the contractile activity of the stretched muscle and a reduction in the output of the antagonistic muscle. This **stretch reflex** has multiple components, the first of which has a latency of approximately 30 ms with another component having a latency of approximately 60 ms (Enoka, 2008).

Evidence for changes in the stretch reflex as a result of physical training is currently inconclusive. The reflex excitability of power-trained athletes tends to be lower than of endurance-trained counterparts (Kyröläinen & Komi, 1994; Maffiuletti et al., 2001), although these differences may reflect fiber-type distributions in the tested muscles or a genetic predisposition. Following a period of resistance training, Aagaard, Simonsen, Andersen, Magnusson, and Dyhre-Poulsen (2002) found that the H-reflex was increased. The H-reflex provides information regarding the excitability of the motoneuron pool within a muscle as well as the inhibition of Ia afferents. Others have reported that the stretch reflex was unchanged following four weeks of resistance training, while balance training resulted in a depression of the stretch reflex (Gruber et al., 2007). However, differences in both testing as well as training protocols complicate the interpretation of these studies.

Golgi tendon organs

Golgi tendon organs (GTOs) reside in the musculotendinous junction (**Figure 3.23**) and comprise a Ib afferent and a small group (10 to 20) of extrafusal fibers enclosed within a capsule (Enoka, 2008). The Ib afferent contacts collagen strands associated with an aponeurosis. As they are in series with the muscle fibers (extrafusal fibers), GTOs are sensitive to the tension developed in the muscle. The discharge of a Ib afferent may inhibit the α-motoneurons of the homonymous muscle while exciting those of the antagonistic muscle (Enoka, 2008; MacIntosh, Gardiner, & McComas, 2006). Such a response would reduce the contractile activity associated with a given muscle. It was believed that GTOs were mainly sensitive to large forces developed by a muscle and that their activity conferred a protective mechanism to a muscle during periods of high force. However, this view may be too simplistic (Chalmers, 2002; Enoka, 2008; MacIntosh, Gardiner, & McComas, 2006). It is likely that GTOs provide the central nervous system with information concerning muscular tension during movement tasks. Furthermore, while some authors propose a decrease in GTO-mediated inhibition during force generation as a result of resistance training (Zatsiorsky & Kraemer, 2006), evidence for this adaptation is lacking (Chalmers, 2002), although such an adaptation would be conducive to improved performance in many movements requiring the generation of large forces.

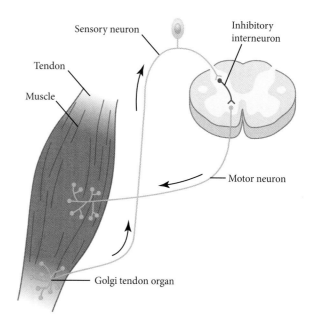

Figure 3.23 The Golgi tendon organ located within a muscle.

Contractile history

The mechanical output of a muscle during shortening can be enhanced when the concentric action is immediately preceded by either an isometric or eccentric action (Finni, Ikegawa, & Komi, 2001; Walshe, Wilson, & Ettema, 1998). Greater enhancement in the mechanical output of the muscle occurs when the concentric action is preceded by an eccentric compared to an isometric action (Walshe, Wilson, & Ettema, 1998). The sequence of muscle actions where a concentric action follows an immediate eccentric action is known as the stretch–shortening cycle (SSC) and is a naturally occurring coupling of muscle actions that can be observed in many movements (Komi, 2003). The proposed mechanisms behind the mechanical improvements that occur as a result of the SSC include strain potential energy contributions, reflex activation, and alterations in the crossbridge dynamics prior to muscle shortening (Bobbert, Gerritsen, Litjens, & Van Soest, 2005; Komi, 2003). The functional consequences of the SSC during movements become apparent when, for example, performing a vertical jump for maximal height. In this situation it has been shown that the performance of an initial countermovement (i.e., an initial downward movement of the center of mass) results in a greater jump height compared to those jumps performed without a preparatory countermovement (Bobbert et al., 1996; Komi & Bosco, 1978; Kubo, Kawakami, & Fukunaga, 1999; see Skeletal Muscle Concept 3.9).

Skeletal Muscle Concept 3.9

The performance benefits of the stretch–shortening cycle

The combination of an eccentric muscle action followed immediately by a concentric action is known as a stretch–shortening cycle (SSC). Most movements in sports incorporate the SSC, including running, jumping, and change of direction, and performance in the movements is likely to be enhanced through the involvement of the SSC. It has long been known that stretching an active muscle before it shortens increases the force and work performed during the subsequent concentric action compared to that achieved in a concentric-only action (Cavagna, Saibene, & Margaria, 1965; Edman, Elzinga, & Noble, 1978). This potentiation of mechanical output during the concentric phase is transient, lasting between 300 and 500 ms after the start of shortening (Ettema & Huijing, 1992; Walshe, Wilson, & Ettema, 1998). A large transitional force is important for enhanced concentric phase mechanics, meaning that the activation of the muscle prior to the shortening phase is important (Komi, 2003).

A functional consequence of utilizing the SSC is that performance in explosive movements is improved. For example, jump height achieved in a countermovement that incorporates the SSC is greater than that achieved in a static vertical jump where the SSC is absent (Bobbert et al., 1996). Furthermore, greater enhancements in jump performance can be accrued when the magnitude and rate of eccentric loading are increased, such as when performing a drop jump (McBride, McCaulley, & Cormie, 2008; McCaulley et al., 2007). The improvements in the concentric phase accrued from the SSC are greater than those when the concentric action is preceded by a maximal isometric action (Walshe, Wilson, & Ettema, 1998).

There are many mechanisms that have been forwarded to explain the performance benefits associated with the SSC:

- **Active state.** The tension developed during an eccentric action is greater than that during both isometric and concentric actions, reflecting a greater proportion of attached crossbridges during an eccentric action. This is known as the active state of the muscle. A greater active state at the commencement of the concentric phase of the SSC as a result of the prior eccentric action allows the muscle to perform more work early during the concentric action (Bobbert, Gerritsen, Litjens, & Van Soest, 2005).

- **Activation of the stretch reflex.** During the eccentric phase of the SSC, the active muscles are stretched. This activates the intrafusal fibers (muscle spindles) in the muscles, which have excitatory connections with the α-motoneurons of the target muscle and inhibitory connections with the antagonist muscle (Enoka, 2008). This results in a greater force being generated during the subsequent concentric action (Komi, 2003).

- **Storage and return of strain potential energy.** During the eccentric phase of the SSC, the series of elastic components of the musculotendinous unit (e.g., crossbridges, aponeurosis, tendon) are stretched, storing strain potential energy. During the subsequent concentric phase of the movement, this mechanical energy can be reused, allowing the musculotendinous unit to perform greater work during shortening compared to that during a concentric-only action (Komi, 2003).

- **Interaction of contractile and elastic elements.** The stretch of the tendinous structures during the eccentric phase of the SSC and their subsequent recoil during the concentric phase limit the amount of lengthening and shortening of the fascicles within the active muscle. Therefore, the fascicles can operate under near-isometric conditions while the musculotendinous unit lengthens and shortens. Such behavior would allow the fascicles to operate closer to their optimal length and generate greater force during the concentric phase than if they were required to shorten (Fukashiro, Hay, & Nagano, 2006).

It is difficult to determine whether the performance benefits of the SSC arise from any one mechanism alone; it may be that a combination of mechanisms contributes to the gains in performance observed when utilizing the SSC.

Another factor that has been highlighted by some authors as influencing the mechanism of the SSC is the mechanics of the movement. For example, van Ingen Schenau, Bobbert, and de Haan (1997) proposed that the speed of the SSC is likely to determine the mechanisms underpinning the performance enhancement. Certainly the SSC is a technique that can be incorporated in many explosive movements that can result in performance improvements. Furthermore, it should be noted that the SSC may be responsible for the greater efficiency of whole-body cyclical movements such as running and hopping compared to the efficiency of isolated skeletal muscle (Cavagna, Saibene, & Margaria, 1964; Dean & Kuo, 2011). Finally, the ability to utilize the SSC has been shown to be improved following a period of resistance training (Cormie, McCaulley, & McBride, 2007; McBride, Triplett-McBride, Davie, & Newton, 2002).

As well as the immediate effects of the coupling of specific muscle actions on subsequent mechanical output of the activated muscle, enhancements can be accrued when maximal or near-maximal muscle actions are performed and a rest interval is interposed prior to the performance movement of interest. This phenomenon is known as **post-activation potentiation** (PAP) (Hodgson, Docherty, & Robbins, 2005). The mechanisms proposed as responsible for PAP include the phosphorylation of the myosin light chains that render the crossbridges more sensitive to Ca^{2+} and an increase in the excitability of the motoneurons, both of which would result in an increased mechanical response of the activated muscles, particularly the rate of force development (Hodgson, Docherty, & Robbins, 2005; Sale, 2002). The PAP effect can be exploited by including maximal or near-maximal muscle actions in exercises performed during a warm-up, while long-term use of PAP may result in increases in power output beyond those observed following traditional training methods (Robbins, 2005).

While an enhancement of the mechanical output of the muscle can be induced by the completion of prior contractile activity in the PAP response, if the rest between the potentiating activity and the performance activity is insufficient, then the mechanical output is likely to be compromised as the muscle will be in a state of **fatigue**. Fatigue can be defined as a reversible decline in the mechanical output associated with contractile activity that is marked by a progressive reduction in the contractile response of the active muscle (Allen, Lamb, & Westerblad, 2008). The reduction in force associated with fatigue may not be as pronounced during submaximal contractions compared to situations requiring maximal contractions, in which case fatigue manifests itself as an inability to maintain the activity at the required intensity (Allen, Lamb, & Westerblad, 2008). Furthermore, while a reduction in force can be easily identified during isometric tasks, it is more difficult to determine during dynamic muscle actions. Therefore, rather than force, contractile response including shortening, velocity of shortening, work, and power are used to assess fatigue during dynamic actions (MacIntosh, Gardiner, & McComas, 2006).

The mechanisms behind fatigue are complex, with almost any step from the descending motor pathways to those involved in the excitation–contraction coupling representing a potential site for fatigue (MacIntosh, Gardiner, & McComas, 2006). In general, the mechanisms of fatigue can be categorized as those associated with the central nervous system (**central fatigue**) and those associated directly with the motor units themselves (**peripheral fatigue**). The mechanisms implicated in fatigue are shown in Table 3.6. It is important to note that fatigue is not just an acute phenomenon that occurs immediately following muscular contractions. Under certain circumstances, the depression in the expected contractile response following muscular contractions could last days, especially when the movements involve the SSC (Nicol, Avela, & Komi, 2006; Stewart, Duhamel, Rich, Tupling, & Green, 2008). The strength and conditioning practitioner therefore needs to manage fatigue in order to optimize the performance of his or her athletes.

It is clear that the mechanical behavior of skeletal muscle is determined by the complex interaction of multiple factors that are summarized in Figure 3.24. The factors highlighted in this figure should be considered when attempting to assess the mechanical capacity in athletes. Furthermore, the plasticity of skeletal muscle in response to different regimens of physical training means that modifications to all of the factors highlighted in Figure 3.24 are possible (see Skeletal Muscle Concept 3.10).

Table 3.6
The Mechanisms Associated with Fatigue

Mechanism	Explanation
Cerebral cortex	Function of the neurons in the cerebral cortex impeded through a disturbance in neurotransmitters (e.g., serotonin, dopamine, norepinephrine), hyperthermia, hypoglycemia, and hyperammonemia
Descending drive	A reduction in the excitation delivery from supraspinal centers (motor cortex) to motoneurons manifest in an increased perceived effort and a reduction in voluntary activation
Spinal activation	A reduction in rate coding
Afferent feedback	Depressed discharge from the muscle spindle and Golgi tendon organ afferents
Neuromuscular propagation	Reduction in ability of axonal action potential mobilize vesicles in the presynaptic terminal
	Depletion of neurotransmitter
Activation failure	Decrease in the sensitivity of myofibrils to Ca^{2+}
	Reduction in the release of Ca^{2+} from sarcoplasmic reticulum
Metabolite accumulation	Accumulation of P_i impairing crossbridge functioning and reducing maximal isometric tension (*myofibrillar fatigue*)
	Accumulation of Mg-ADP impairing crossbridge functioning and reducing maximal speed of shortening
	H^+ competing with Ca^{2+} for troponin C
	Reactive oxygen species/reactive nitrogen species reducing Ca^{2+} sensitivity
Metabolic substrates	Glycogen depletion limiting ATP resynthesis
Blood flow	Increased intramuscular pressure associated with muscle actions compressing blood vessels and limiting the delivery of substrate, removal of metabolites, and the dissipation of heat

Note: Ca^{2+} = calcium; P_i = inorganic phosphate; Mg = magnesium; ADP = adenosine diphosphate; H^+ = hydrogen ions; ATP = adenosine triphosphate

Data from Allen, D. G., Lamb, G. D., & Westerblad, H. (2008). Skeletal muscle fatigue: cellular mechanisms. *Physiological Review, 88*, 287–332; Enoka, R. M. (2008). *Neuromechanics of Human Movement*. Champaign, IL: Human Kinetics Publishers.

Energetics of Muscular Actions

It was noted in the discussion of the excitation–contraction coupling that ATP is required during the cycling of crossbridges associated with the activation of a muscle. Although there is some evidence to the contrary, it is generally believed that one ATP

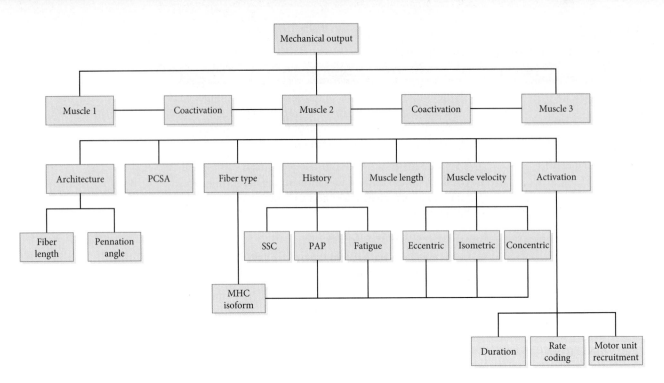

Figure 3.24 The interacting factors that affect the mechanical output of skeletal muscle.

Note: PSCA is physiological cross-sectional area; SSC is stretch shortening cycle; PAP is post-activity potentiation; MHC is myosin heavy chain.

Reproduced, with permission, from Moir, G. L. (2012). Muscular strength. In T. Miller (Ed.), *NSCA's Guide to Tests and Assessments* (pp. 147–191). Champaign, IL: Human Kinetics.

Skeletal Muscle Concept 3.10

What are the signals causing skeletal muscle adaptations?

Skeletal muscle is a remarkably plastic tissue, able to alter its structure and function in response to the physical demands imposed upon it. The adaptations observed in skeletal muscle following a period of physical training correspond to the changes in proteins that comprise the tissue. It has long been known that concurrent resistance and endurance training results in less adaptation of skeletal muscle than training for either separately (Hickson, 1980). If we characterize resistance training as an exercise mode involving high intensities and short durations and endurance training as involving low intensities and long durations, we can generalize the muscular adaptations to both modes of exercise. Resistance training tends to produce an increase in muscle fiber size (hypertrophy), while increases in oxidative metabolism (e.g., increased mitochondrial and capillary density, oxidative enzymes) follow a period of endurance training. These adaptations reflect alterations in the types and amounts of specific proteins within the activated muscle fibers. The functional consequences of the protein changes are largely determined by the mode of physical training, as well as the intensity, frequency, and duration of the training.

Adaptations in the proteins following a period of physical training involve specific signaling mechanisms that initiate the replication of DNA genetic sequences that result in the translation of the genetic code into a series of amino acids. These amino acids form the basis for the specific proteins. Resistance training typically influences the contractile proteins while endurance training influences mitochondrial and metabolic proteins within the muscle cell. Recently, the specific molecular pathways that are activated by different modes of physical training, specifically resistance training and endurance training, have been elucidated (Coffey & Hawley, 2007). These signaling pathways are initiated by the primary processes associated with the contractile activity that accompanies a specific exercise stimulus (Figure 3.25).

Mechanical stretch of the sarcolemma

The generation of muscular forces induces considerable stretch of the sarcolemma, which mediates signaling cascades within the muscle fiber. The mechanical stretch of the sarcolemma induced by a regimen of resistance training is likely to be much greater than that in response to endurance training.

Intracellular Ca²⁺ flux

During muscular actions, Ca^{2+} is released from the sarcoplasmic reticulum into the sarcoplasm in response to an action potential. The Ca^{2+} is resequestered back into the sarcoplasmic reticulum following the action potential. The Ca^{2+}

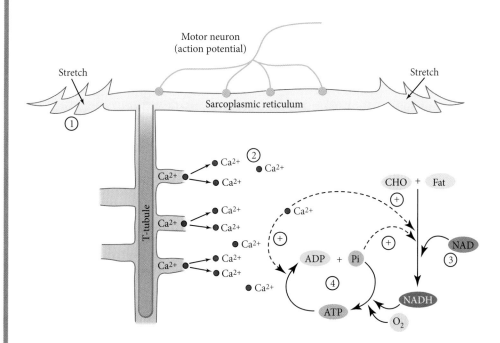

Figure 3.25 The primary processes associated with contractile activity that accompany an exercise stimulus. (1) Mechanical stretch of the sarcolemma; (2) intracellular Ca^{2+} flux; (3) redox potential; (4) phosphorylation potential.

(continues)

(continued)

flux is likely to be very different during a resistance-training workout compared to a bout of endurance exercise. Specifically, resistance training will induce short periods of high intracellular Ca^{2+}, while an endurance workout will induce prolonged periods of elevated intracellular Ca^{2+} concentrations.

Redox potential

The energy demands associated with exercise influence the nucleotide pool in the mitochondria, specifically nicotinamide adenine dinucleotide (NAD) and NADH (the reduced form of NAD). The ratio of NAD to NADH is known as the redox potential of the cell, the maintenance of which produces reactive oxygen species (ROS). Due to the greater demands for oxygen and the increased activity of the metabolic pathways, a bout of endurance exercise is likely to generate higher levels of ROS compared to resistance training.

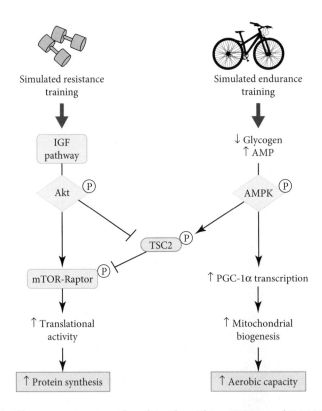

Figure 3.26 The proteins involved in the Akt-mTOR and AMPK pathways associated with a bout of resistance training and endurance training, respectively.

Note: IGF is insulin-like growth factor; Akt is protein kinase B; mTOR is mammalian target of rapamycin; AMP is adenosine monophosphate; AMPK is adenosine monophosphate kinase; PGC-1α is peroxisome proliferator activated receptor γ co-activator-1α; TSC2 is tuberous sclerosis complex 2; P is phosphorylation.

Reproduced from Coffey, V. G., & Hawley, J. A. (2007). The molecular bases of training adaptations. *Sports Medicine, 37,* 737–763, with kind permission from Springer Science and Business Media.

Phosphorylation potential

The resynthesis of ATP to provide energy to sustain muscular actions results in the accumulation within the muscle fiber of metabolites such as adenosine diphosphate (ADP) and inorganic phosphate (P_i). The ratio of intracellular ATP concentrations to the concentrations of ADP and P_i is known as the phosphorylation potential of the cell. There is likely to be a greater change in the phosphorylation potential of the muscle cell in response to a bout of endurance exercise compared to resistance training.

These primary mechanical and metabolic signals associated with an exercise stimulus result in the activation of a series of signaling proteins. There have been two distinct signaling pathways identified, one associated with a bout of resistance training, the other with a bout of endurance training (Coffey & Hawley, 2007; see Figure 3.26).

It has been proposed that the competition between the Akt–mTOR and the AMPK signaling pathways acts as a "switch" to mediate the synthesis of myofibrillar protein and mitochondrial protein (Atherton et al., 2005; Baar, 2006), and it is therefore responsible for the specific adaptations following resistance training and endurance training. It has been demonstrated that these molecular responses to physical training are influenced by the nutritional status of the athlete (e.g., amino acid and carbohydrate ingestion) as well as the athlete's training history (Coffey et al., 2006; Deldicque et al., 2008). Furthermore, the order in which the athlete performs bouts of different exercise modes influences the activation of the specific signaling pathways when diverse exercise modes are undertaken in close proximity (Coffey, Pilegaard, Garnham, O'Brien, & Hawley, 2009).

molecule is hydrolyzed per power stroke of a myosin crossbridge (Huxley, 1998). The requirement for ATP demands metabolic energy be expended during the activation of a muscle. As a rough approximation, it is useful to consider the metabolic energy consumed by a muscle as coming from two sources (Alexander, 1992):

$$E_{Met} = F_{Cost} + W_{Cost}$$

Eq. (3.8)

where E_{Met} is the total metabolic energy cost measured in oxygen consumption, F_{Cost} is the metabolic cost of generating force, and W_{Cost} is the metabolic cost of performing mechanical work. Mechanical work is the product of a force and the displacement undergone by the point of application of the force in the direction in which the force acts.

Although the distinction between the metabolic cost of force and the metabolic cost of work as highlighted in Equation (3.8) is somewhat artificial, given that a muscle is required to generate force when performing mechanical work, it is useful for explanatory purposes. During an isometric action, the muscle develops force, but there is no mechanical work done by the muscle given the absence of a change in its length. There is still crossbridge cycling during an isometric action, and therefore a requirement for ATP with a concomitant increase in metabolic energy consumption. However, because no mechanical work is done during an isometric action, the metabolic cost will be below that of a concentric action, as per Equation (3.8). Indeed, Jones (1993) estimated the metabolic cost of an isometric action at 4.7 mM ATP/s, with the cost for a concentric action estimated at 9.3 mM ATP/s. During an eccentric action, work is done on the muscle and the crossbridges are forcibly detached (Huxley, 1998; Lombardi & Piazzesi, 1990), a process that does not required ATP and therefore reduces the metabolic energy costs associated with this form of dynamic muscle action.

Equation (3.8) also informs us that the larger the force generated by the muscle, the greater the associated metabolic cost. This is due to the requirement to activate more fascicles to contribute to the overall force. Furthermore, the metabolic cost of generating muscular force is affected by the architecture of the muscle (the longer the fascicles, the greater the metabolic cost due to the increased number of associated crossbridges) and the time of the muscle action (a 2-s isometric action will consume twice the energy of a 1-s isometric action in the same muscle). Therefore, the metabolic cost of generating force can be expressed as follows (Alexander, 1992):

$$F_{Cost} = \frac{(F \times l_f \times t_{Action})}{Efficiency} \qquad \text{Eq. (3.9)}$$

where F_{Cost} is the metabolic cost of generating force, F is the magnitude of the developed force, l_f is the length of the fascicles, t_{Action} is the time of the muscle action during which tension is developed, and *Efficiency* of the muscle fibers is the ratio of mechanical work output to the metabolic energy input and is dependent upon the fiber type, with faster fibers having lower economy due to higher crossbridge cycling rates.

Skeletal muscle has been reported to have an efficiency of ~25% when performing positive mechanical work during a concentric action at relatively low velocity of shortening (Margaria, 1968; Margaria, Cerretelli, Aghemo, & Sassi, 1963). This implies a considerable loss of energy associated with this type of muscle action. Despite this, the efficiency of cyclical movements such as hopping and running, which utilize the SSC, has been reported to be as high as 45% (Cavagna, Saibene, & Margaria, 1964; Dean & Kuo, 2011). This increased efficiency of movement associated with the SSC arises due to compliant tendons allowing the fascicles to undergo less displacement during each movement cycle, reducing the amount of mechanical work to be performed by the active muscles (see Skeletal Muscle Concept 3.11).

Tendon

Tendons are dense bands of connective tissues that are integral structures within the human motor system, influencing both the force-generating capacity and the energetics of the system during movements. Tendons are responsible for transmitting force from skeletal muscle to bone, and they therefore must bear very large forces. For example, the force transmitted by the Achilles tendon during running has been reported to be as large as 9000 N, or 12.5 times body weight (Komi, 2003). The tensile strength of skeletal muscle is around 250 kPa, while that of tendon is approximately 50 to 100 MPa (Zatsiorsky & Prilutsky, 2012). Therefore, tendon has a tensile strength approximately 400 times higher than that of skeletal muscle.

When a tendon deforms during a stretch imposed by an external force, it does not consume metabolic energy. Hence, it is referred to as providing passive resistance to the stretch (Figure 3.17). Furthermore, when a tendon is stretched, it stores strain potential energy that can be used at a later time. For example, the elongation of the Achilles

Skeletal Muscle Concept 3.11

Why is walking less energetically costly than running?

Figure 3.27 shows the net energy cost of walking and running in humans.

Running incurs a greater energetic cost compared to walking. Furthermore, there is a sharp increase in cost of transport when changing from walking to running. One reason for this is that the leg position is different during stance when walking compared to running: The knee is more extended during walking and more flexed during running. This change likely reflects the requirement of the athlete to absorb the more forceful impacts that accompany the greater speeds associated with running. However, the increased knee flexion reduces the effective mechanical advantage (EMA) of the knee extensors (Figure 3.28).

Notice in Figure 3.28 how the average EMA calculated during the stance phase remains relatively constant at the hip and ankle joints, while that at the knee decreases substantially at the transition from the walking to the running gait. The reduction in the EMA at the knee joint results in a requirement for greater force to be generated by the quadriceps muscle group. Given Equation (3.8), the greater muscular force will increase the metabolic cost of the running gait compared to walking (Biewener, 2003). Equation (3.8) can also be used to explain why running uphill increases the associated energy costs (Minetti, Ardigò, & Saibene, 1994), as the muscles must shorten to perform mechanical work to raise the center of mass. Similarly, metabolic cost increases when running on a compliant surface such as sand (Lejeune, Willems, & Heglund, 1998) due to the requirement to perform mechanical work to deform the surface.

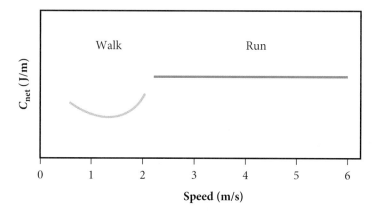

Figure 3.27 The net energy cost of walking and running in humans.

Note: C_{net} is the net cost of locomotion.

Reproduced from Biewener, A. A. (2003). *Animal Locomotion*. Oxford, UK: Oxford University Press.

(continues)

(continued)

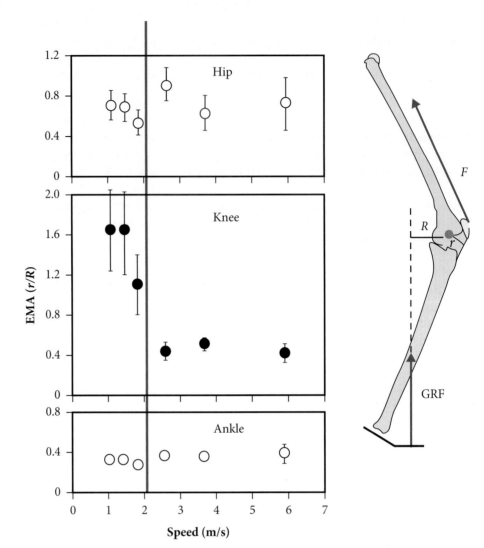

Figure 3.28 The effective mechanical advantage at the hip, knee, and ankle joints during speeds associated with walking and running in humans. Notice the large decrease in the effective mechanical advantage at the knee joint at speeds exceeding 2 m/s. These speeds are typical of those associated with running in humans.

Reproduced from Biewener, A. A. (2003). *Animal Locomotion*. Oxford, UK: Oxford University Press.

Another explanation for the increase in metabolic cost is the associated decrease in stance duration that accompanies the increased speed associated with running compared to walking. The reduced stance duration demands an increase in the rate at which force is developed, a factor that favors the activation of the less energetically efficient fast-muscle fibers as opposed to the slow-muscle fibers (Biewener, 2003).

tendon, measured as **strain** (the ratio of the elongation of the tendon to its initial length), is typically 7% during the stance phase of running (Zatsiorsky & Prilutsky, 2012), allowing the tendon to store strain potential energy. Moreover, the stored energy is able to be reused, reducing the metabolic cost incurred during the task.

Macro- and microstructure of tendon

Tendons are composed of collagens (mainly type I, with small proportions of type III and V collagens), proteoglycans, glycoproteins, water, and cells (Wang, 2006). The structural arrangement of collagen within a tendon is shown in **Figure 3.29**. The tendon is surrounded by a loose connective tissue known as the **paratenon**. Below the paratenon is the **epitenon**, another connective tissue layer. These connective tissue layers serve to reduce friction between the adjacent tissues. Each bundle of collagen fibers is surrounded by the **endotenon**, within which blood vessels and nerves are contained. The junction between the tendon and the bone is known as the **enthesis** whereas the **myotendinous junction** forms the connection between the muscle fibers and the tendon. The tensile forces at the enthesis have been proposed to be four times

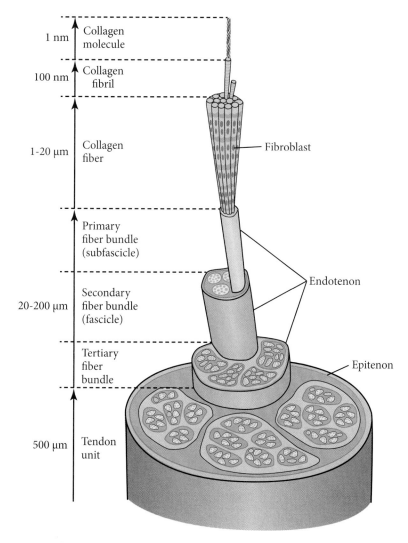

Figure 3.29 The structural arrangement of collagen within a tendon.

Applied Research 3.8
Differences in tendon and aponeurosis strain during muscle stretch

The authors assessed the elongation of the patellar tendon and aponeurosis of the knee extensors during a maximal isometric knee extension task. These data were compared to the elongation of the Achilles tendon and the aponeurosis of the ankle plantar flexors during a maximal isometric plantar flexion task. The elongation of the tendon and aponeuroses were recorded using ultrasonography. The authors reported that the strain of the knee extensor aponeurosis (12.1%) was greater than the strain of the patellar tendon (8.3%). Conversely, the strain of the ankle plantar flexor aponeurosis (2.7%) was less than the strain of the Achilles tendon (5.9%). These results imply that tendons and aponeuroses may serve different mechanical functions about the knee and ankle joints during human movements. Specifically, the compliant aponeurosis of the knee extensors may confer a protective mechanism by attenuating damage during impacts while also storing strain potential energy during loading. The stiff aponeurosis of the ankle plantar flexors may be better suited to transmitting the tensile forces generated by the muscle fibers rapidly to the tendon.

Kubo, K., Kanehisa, H., & Fukunaga, T. (2005). Comparison of elasticity of human tendon and aponeurosis in knee extensors and ankle plantar flexors in vivo. *Journal of Applied Biomechanics*, *21*, 129–142.

greater than those experienced in other regions of the tendon, while the myotendinous junction has been identified as the weakest region of the musculotendinous unit (Wang, 2006).

While all muscles have a tendon, pennate muscles have an extension of the external tendon that runs within the muscle known as the aponeurosis, and it is the aponeurosis that the muscle fibers innervate. Although the external tendon and the internal aponeurosis may be schematically represented as being arranged in series with one another, these structures should not be considered as mechanically serial (Epstein, Wong, & Herzog, 2006; see Applied Research 3.8).

Mechanical characteristics of tendon

The mechanical characteristics of tendon can be described by their stress–strain response and viscoelastic qualities.

Stress–strain characteristics

During unloaded conditions, the collagen fibers within the tendon have a wavy, "crimped" appearance, with the fibers straightening in response to an applied load. These changes in fiber orientation confer the mechanical properties of tendon that are displayed in the stress–strain curve (**Figure 3.30**). Stress is defined as the ratio of force applied to a material to the CSA of the material, while strain is the ratio of the elongation of the material to its initial length. Stiffness can be calculated as the ratio between the force applied to a body and the deformation caused by the force. It should be noted that the stress–strain characteristics of a material are mathematically distinct from the force–deformation characteristics of a material, which define the stiffness of the material. The stress–strain curve of tendon is characterized by three regions: (1) an initial toe region, (2) a linear region, and (3) a failure region.

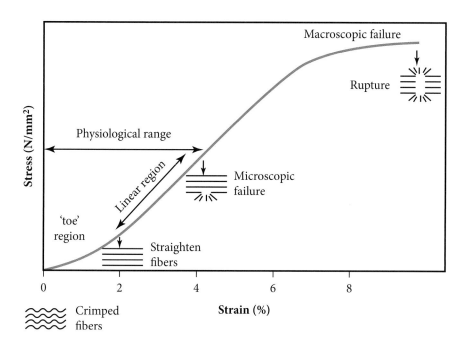

Figure 3.30 The stress–strain curve of a tendon.

Reproduced from Wang, J. H.-C. (2006). Mechanobiology of tendon. *Journal of Biomechanics, 39*, 1563–1582, with permission from Elsevier.

The toe region is associated with an increase of the slope of the stress–strain relationship and occurs at a strain of between 1.5% and 4% for most tendons (Zatsiorsky & Prilutsky, 2012). The collagen fibers begin to straighten in this region, although the collagen bundles (subfascicles and fascicles) are not yet stretched. In the linear region the collagen fibers lose their crimped appearance and the region usually begins with imposed stresses of between 5 and 30 MPa, ending at stresses between 70 and 100 MPa (Zatsiorsky & Prilutsky, 2012). The slope of the linear region of the stress–strain curve provides the **Young's modulus** of the tendon, which provides a measure of the elasticity of the tendon (Table 3.7).

The stiffness of the tendon is likely to influence the rate of force development of the musculotendinous unit, with higher tendon stiffness increasing the rate of force development (Bojsen-Møller, Magnusson, Rasmussen, Kjær, & Aagaard, 2005). The stiffness of tendon has been shown to be affected by gender and age, with greater stiffness reported in men compared to women and in the young compared to the old (Kubo, Kanehisa, & Fukunaga, 2003; Kubo, Kanehisa, Miyatani, Tachi, & Fukunaga, 2003). Furthermore, resistance training has been shown to increase tendon stiffness (Kubo, Kanehisa, & Fukunaga, 2002; Kubo et al., 2009; see Applied Research 3.9), while detraining and disuse decreases tendon stiffness (Kubo et al., 2000; Kubo, Ikebukuro, Yata, Tsunoda, & Kanehisa, 2010). However, stiffness has been shown to be negatively correlated with the ability to utilize the SSC (Kubo, Kanehisa, & Fukunaga, 2005). Furthermore, there appears to be an inverse relationship between tendon stiffness and exercise economy in trained distance runners, with reduced tendon stiffness being related to increased exercise economy (Kubo, Tabata, Ikebukuro, Igarashi, & Tsunoda, 2010).

Table 3.7
The Mechanical Characteristics of Tendons and Aponeuroses Recorded *In Vivo*

Tendon/ Aponeurosis	Activity	Stress (MPa)	Strain (%)	Stiffness (N/mm)	Young's Modulus (GPa)
Patellar tendon (young)	Maximal isometric	30.2 ± 2.2	6.9 ± 0.6	4334 ± 562	1.09 ± 0.12
Patellar tendon (older)	Maximal isometric	40 ± 11	9.9 ± 2.2	2187 ± 713	1.3 ± 0.3
Achilles tendon	Maximal isometric	41.6 ± 3.9	4.4–5.6		1.05–1.47
Achilles tendon	One-leg hopping		8.3	145–231	0.67–1.07

Data from Zatsiorsky, V. M., & Prilutsky, B. I. (2012). *Biomechanics of Skeletal Muscles*. Champaign, IL: Human Kinetics.

Viscoelastic characteristics

Tendons are **viscoelastic** due to the interaction between the collagens, water, and proteoglycans. Viscoelasticity is exemplified by time-dependent mechanical behavior (Zatsiorsky & Prilutsky, 2012; Wang, 2006), including:

- Sensitivity to strain rate
- Stress relaxation
- Creep
- Hysteresis

Sensitivity to strain. Tendons tend to be more deformable under conditions where the rate of strain is low, increasing their stiffness under high strain rates (Wang, 2006). This behavior means that strain potential energy is more likely to be stored in tendon

Applied Research 3.9
Differential effects of resistance training on tendon and aponeurosis stiffness

The authors investigated the effects of 12 weeks of isometric and dynamic (repetitions involving both concentric and eccentric actions) knee extension resistance-training exercises on muscular strength and stiffness of the patellar tendon and aponeurosis of the knee extensors. Each participant trained one leg under each of the conditions four times per week during the study. The resistance training protocols resulted in significant increases in muscle volume, maximal isometric strength, and muscle activation (electromyography) of the knee extensors. While there were no changes in CSA of the patellar tendon, both resistance-training protocols increased the stiffness of the tendon-aponeurosis complex, although the relative changes were greater following the isometric training. However, only the isometric resistance training resulted in a significant increase in the stiffness of the tendon. This finding highlights the different responses in the tendon and aponeuroses following a period of training, exemplifying the mechanical independence of these two structures.

Kubo, K., Ikebukuro, T., Yaeshima, K., Yata, H., Tsunoda, N., & Kanehisa, H. (2009). Effects of static and dynamic training on the stiffness and blood volume of tendon in vivo. *Journal of Applied Physiology, 106,* 412–417.

under low strain rates, while at higher strain rates, the tendon is more suited to transfer muscular tension to bone.

Stress relaxation. When a tendon experiences a constant deformation, the stress reduces over time.

Creep. The strain experienced by a tendon increases over time when a constant load is applied.

Hysteresis. The difference between the stress–strain curve during loading and unloading cycles represents the hysteresis of the tendon. A tendon elongates when a force is applied to it, and the integral of the applied force and the elongation of the tendon represents the mechanical work done on the tendon to deform it. With the removal of the applied force, the tendon will tend to return to its original length due to **elastin** and other microfibrillar proteins. The area under the unloaded curve represents the energy recovered by the tendon due to this elastic recoil. However, the mechanical work during unloading is less than that during loading, the difference representing a loss of energy by the tendon and providing a measure of the hysteresis of the material. The energy loss has been attributed to damping as a result of internal structures, so the hysteresis of the tendon reflects the viscosity of the tissue (Butler, Grood, Noyes, & Zernicke, 1978). A typical value for the hysteresis of tendon is approximately 20% (Kubo et al., 2002).

Tendon hysteresis has been reported to be lower in women than in men (Kubo, Kanehisa, & Fukunaga, 2003) and greater in older subjects (Kubo, Kanehisa, Miyatani, Tachi, et al., 2003), while long-term stretching has been shown to reduce hysteresis without any changes in tendon stiffness or elongation during imposed stretch (Kubo et al., 2002; see Applied Research 3.10). This is important because lower tendon hysteresis has been shown to be related to the ability to utilize the SSC (Kubo, Kanehisa, & Fukunaga, 2005).

Applied Research 3.10
The combination of stretching and resistance training reduces tendon hysteresis

The authors investigated the effects of eight weeks of dynamic resistance training or a combination of resistance training and stretching on the stiffness and hysteresis of the Achilles tendon. Each participant trained one leg under each of the conditions with resistance training being performed four times per week, while stretching was performed twice a week before and after the resistance-training exercises. Stiffness and hysteresis were recorded using ultrasonography during a maximal isometric plantar flexion task. It was found that both training protocols increased maximal isometric force and the volume of the triceps surae with no changes in muscle activation (EMG). Tendon stiffness was increased following both training protocols in the absence of any changes in tendon CSA. However, only the combination of resistance training and stretching reduced tendon hysteresis. The reduction in tendon hysteresis might increase the capacity of the tendon to store and reuse strain potential energy, which has implications for performance during movements involving the stretch–shortening cycle.

Kubo, K., Kanehisa, H., & Fukunaga, T. (2002). Effects of resistance and stretching training programmes on the viscoelastic properties of human tendon structures *in vivo*. *Journal of Physiology*, *538*, 219–226.

Muscle–Tendon Integration During Movements

It was noted earlier that the efficiency of cyclical movements such as hopping and running were greater than the efficiency of isolated skeletal muscle (Cavagna, Saibene, & Margaria, 1964; Dean & Kuo, 2011). The increased efficiency in these movements was attributed to the utilization of the SSC, whereby the displacement of the fascicles was limited during each cycle by the compliant tendons. Voigt, Bojsen-Møller, Simonsen, and Dyhre-Poulsen (1995) reported that the tendons were responsible for between 52% and 60% of the mechanical work performed on the center of mass during repetitive jumping, where the efficiency of the movement was almost 70%. These authors also reported that the efficiency of the movement was shown to be sensitive to changes in the Young's modulus of the tendon.

A reasonable estimate for strain potential energy recovery of tendon is (Biewener, 2003):

$$E_{\mathrm{SP}} = 0.465\,F\Delta l \qquad\qquad \textbf{Eq. (3.10)}$$

where E_{SP} is the magnitude of the strain potential energy recovered from the tendon, F is the maximum force transmitted by the tendon, and Δl is the total change in length experienced by the tendon. Furthermore, an indication of the ability of the musculotendinous unit to store and return strain potential energy is provided by the **normalized tendon length** (Zatsiorsky & Prilutsky, 2012):

$$\text{Normalized } l_{\mathrm{t}} = \frac{l_{\mathrm{t\,Slack}}}{l_{\mathrm{o}}} \qquad\qquad \textbf{Eq. (3.11)}$$

where $l_{\mathrm{t\,Slack}}$ is the tendon slack length (threshold length at which a stretched tendon develops force) and l_{o} is optimal fiber length (length at which active fibers develop maximum force). Equation (3.11) informs us that the larger the normalized tendon length, the longer the tendon and the shorter the muscle fibers. Therefore, the higher the ratio the greater the ability of the musculotendinous unit to store and reuse strain potential energy. Figure 3.31 shows the normalized tendon length for selected muscles in the body.

What is noticeable from Figure 3.31 is that the normalized tendon length decreases from the distal to proximal musculature of the leg. During walking the interaction between the horizontal and vertical components of the ground-reaction force during stance tends to produce a resultant force that is directed toward the hip joint, while the excursion of the force from the ankle joint increases during stance. This results in lower joint moments at the hip compared to the ankle joint (Biewener, Farley, Roberts, & Temaner, 2004). However, the metabolic costs of the task are likely to be reduced, given the greater ability of the distal musculotendinous units to store and reuse strain potential energy during each stance phase (see Skeletal Muscle Concept 3.12). The integration of skeletal muscle and tendon also influence the performance of explosive movements by influencing the mechanical power output of the musculotendinous unit. Recall that mechanical power is not a conserved variable, and a tendon can be used to amplify muscular power output (see Skeletal Muscle Concept 3.13).

During typical sporting movements, skeletal muscle and tendons interact to produce the specific movements. Indeed, the integration of skeletal muscle and tendon during movements increases the functional capacity of muscle beyond the constraints imposed by the force–velocity and length–tension relationships. Furthermore, both biologic tissues adapt in response to an exercise stimulus, although the rates of adaptation

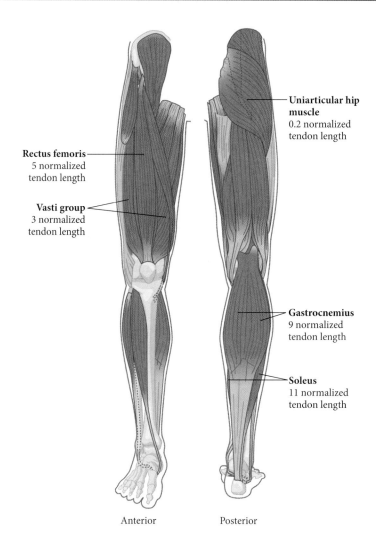

Uniarticular hip
muscle
0.2 normalized
tendon length

Rectus femoris
5 normalized
tendon length

Vasti group
3 normalized
tendon length

Gastrocnemius
9 normalized
tendon length

Soleus
11 normalized
tendon length

Anterior   Posterior

Figure 3.31 Normalized tendon lengths of selected muscles in the human body.

Data from Zatsiorsky, V. M., & Prilutsky, B. I. (2012). *Biomechanics of Skeletal Muscles*. Champaign, IL: Human Kinetics.

Skeletal Muscle Concept 3.12

Muscle–tendon integration reduces the metabolic energy costs of running

Kram (2000) notes that the main metabolic cost during running is the requirement of the active musculature to generate force during each stance phase. Given this information, we can design an efficient muscle that we can activate to generate force during the stance phase of running: a slow muscle (greater efficiency), short fascicles (low numbers of sarcomeres in series), a high pennation angle (larger force generation for a given volume of muscle activated), and

(continues)

(continued)

a short time of contraction. Furthermore, we would probably require our athlete to have a low body weight, minimizing the magnitude of the required force. Given what we know about the force–velocity characteristics of the different fiber types, a slow muscle may not be able to generate sufficient force in a short time of contraction (the rate of force development in type I fibers is low). As such, Kram (2000) noted that a relatively longer stance phase would reduce the metabolic cost of running by allowing the activation of the more economical slow fibers. Finally, we would want our muscle to innervate a long tendon. This would allow the muscle to operate isometrically, minimizing the requirement of performing mechanical work, which has high metabolic costs, while the tendon stores strain potential energy as it lengthens during the first half of stance, returning this energy rapidly (and at no metabolic cost) during the second half of stance when it shortens. This highlights how the integration of skeletal muscle and tendon can reduce the metabolic cost incurred during running.

Skeletal Muscle Concept 3.13

Muscle–tendon integration amplifies power output

The mechanical definition of power is the rate at which mechanical work is performed, with work being the integral of force and the displacement undergone by the point of application of the force. A functional property of skeletal muscle is that the force generated as it shortens decreases as the velocity of shortening increases, exemplified in the force–velocity relationship. This will limit the amount of mechanical work performed and the power output of the muscle under conditions of high shortening velocity, such as might be encountered during the concentric phase of the stretch–shortening cycle. However, the integration of tendon with skeletal muscle allows the musculotendinous unit to maintain a high power output. Specifically, during the eccentric phase of the stretch–shortening cycle the tendon accumulates strain potential energy by virtue of the deformation experienced by the tissue. The strain potential energy can be reused during the subsequent concentric phase. A key in this scheme is the high rate at which the strain potential energy is returned by the tendon. As energy represents the capacity of a body to perform work, the tendon is able to perform work at a high rate during the concentric phase of the stretch–shortening cycle; therefore, the power output (rate of performing work) of the musculotendinous unit remains high at a time when the work performed and the power output of the muscle is constrained by the force–velocity relationship. Furthermore, the energy can be stored in the tendon at a low rate but released at a much higher rate. Power output is amplified in a manner akin to the action of a catapult. Finally, the stretch and subsequent recoil of the tendon allow the muscle fascicles to maximize their force generation by limiting their shortening velocity while the shortening of the musculotendinous unit is high (Finni, Ikegawa, & Komi, 2001). This highlights how the integration of skeletal muscle and tendon can amplify power output during explosive movements.

differ between skeletal muscle and tendon, with muscle increasing its force-generating capacity before any mechanical changes are observed in tendon (Kubo, Ikebukuro, et al., 2010). This may have implications for the potential to damage tendon.

Chapter Summary

Skeletal muscle is the biological motor that powers movement. The mechanical output of skeletal muscle is modified by the arrangement with the skeleton, producing lever systems that have either force or distance advantages. Skeletal muscle contains groups of fascicles that comprise bundles of fibers, while each fiber is made up of myofibrils. Each myofibril contains sarcomeres, the smallest functional unit of the muscle, that house the contractile proteins (myofilaments) that are responsible for developing tension during muscle actions. The number of sarcomeres arranged in series has implications for the shortening velocity of the muscle fiber, while the number of sarcomeres arranged in parallel affects the force generated by the fiber. The myofilaments within each sarcomere are the actin, myosin, and titin proteins that interact to generate tension, while numerous structural proteins also support the contractile machinery. Most of these proteins adapt their structure in response to an exercise stimulus. The excitation–contraction coupling includes the processes from the propagation of an action potential along the sarcolemma to the actomyosin binding associated with the generation of tension commensurate with the sliding-filament theory. A concentric muscle action occurs when the muscle shortens while developing tension, with an eccentric muscle action occurring when the muscle lengthens while developing tension. During an isometric muscle action, tension is developed in the absence of any length change of the muscle. There are many factors that affect the tension developed by an active muscle, including the length of the muscle, the velocity of dynamic muscle actions, fiber type, CSA, activation dynamics, spinal reflexes, and contractile history. These factors can influence any assessment of the mechanical output of skeletal muscle while also driving the selection of specific training regimens to enhance the mechanical output. The energetics of muscle activity can be related to the requirement to generate force and also the requirements associated with performing mechanical work. Concentric muscle actions necessarily include both of these requirements and are therefore more energetically costly than isometric actions, which are themselves more energetically costly than eccentric actions. During human movements, skeletal muscle functions in series with tendons, which are dense bands of connective tissue. The integration of skeletal muscle and tendons minimizes the energetic costs during whole-body movements and amplifies the power output of the musculotendinous units during explosive movements.

Review Questions and Projects

1. Explain the steps that are associated with the excitation–contraction coupling.

2. What are the three myofilaments within skeletal muscle?

3. Most muscles operate with a distance advantage. How is this calculated and what are the mechanical implications?

4. What is the sticking region associated with the bench press exercise, and what are the mechanisms that are proposed to be responsible?

5. List the factors that affect the mechanical output of skeletal muscle.

6. Given the factors that affect the mechanical output of skeletal muscle, discuss the implications for testing muscular strength.

7. Identify the physiological and mechanical differences between type I, IIA, and IIX muscle fibers.

8. Resistance training has been shown to produce a shift from type IIX fibers to IIA. Explain why measures of muscular strength are usually increased following a period of resistance training.

9. Describe the length–tension relationship of skeletal muscle.

10. Explain the differences in the length–tension relationship between a typical pennate skeletal muscle and a typical fusiform muscle.

11. Describe the force–velocity relationship in an isolated muscle fiber and explain the physiological processes underpinning the changes in force that occur when the velocity of shortening and the velocity of lengthening are increased.

12. Why do muscles with greater pennation angles typically produce greater force than fusiform muscles?

13. What is an action potential, and how is it generated?

14. Describe the spinal reflexes that influence muscle tension.

15. List the factors associated with the energetics of different actions in isolated muscle.

16. Rank eccentric, concentric, and isometric actions in the order of their energetic costs.

17. Explain why the efficiency of whole-body movements tends to be greater than the efficiency of isolated skeletal muscle.

18. To what does *hysteresis* refer with regard to tendon?

19. Explain why an athlete jumps higher when executing an initial countermovement compared to when the jump is performed without a countermovement.

20. Design a musculotendinous unit that would optimize performance in endurance activities and another that would optimize performance in explosive activities. Consider fiber type, fiber length, fiber architecture, and tendon characteristics.

References

Aagaard, P. (2003). Training-induced changes in neural function. *Exercise and Sport Sciences Reviews, 31,* 61–67.

Aagaard, P. (2011). Neural adaptations to resistance exercise. In M. Cardinale, R. Newton, & K. Nosaka (Eds.), *Strength and Conditioning. Biological Principles and Practical Applications* (pp. 105–124). West Sussex, UK: Wiley-Blackwell.

Aagaard, P. & Andersen, J.L. (1998). Correlation between contractile strength and myosin heavy chain isoform composition in human skeletal muscle. *Medicine and Science in Sports and Exercise, 30,* 1217–1222.

Aagaard, P., Simonsen, E.B., Andersen, J.L., Magnusson, P., & Dyhre-Poulsen, P. (2002). Neural adaptation to resistance training: changes in evoked V-wave and H-reflex responses. *Journal of Applied Physiology, 92,* 2309–2318.

Abe, T., Fukashiro, S., Harada, Y., & Kawamoto, K. (2001). Relationship between sprints performance and muscle fascicle length in female sprinters. *Journal of Physiological Anthropology and Applied Human Sciences, 20,* 141–147.

Adams, G.R. (2006). Satellite cell proliferation and skeletal muscle hypertrophy. *Applied Physiology, Nutrition, and Metabolism, 31*, 782–790.

Ahmetov, I.I., Vinogradova, O.L., & Williams, A.G. (2012). Gene polymorphisms and fiber-type composition of human skeletal muscle. *International Journal of Sport Nutrition and Exercise Metabolism, 22*, 292–303.

Alexander, R. Mc. (1992). *Exploring Biomechanics. Animals in Motion.* New York, NY: Scientific American Library.

Allen, D.G., Lamb, G.D., & Westerblad, H. (2008). Impaired calcium release during fatigue. *Journal of Applied Physiology, 104*, 296–305.

Amiridis, I.G., Martin, A., Morlon, B., Martin, L., Cometti, G., Pousson, M., & van Hoecke, J. (1996). Coactivation and tension-regulating phenomena during isokinetic knee extension in sedentary and highly skilled humans. *European Journal of Applied Physiology, 73*, 149–156.

Andersen, J.L., & Aagaard, P. (2010). Effects of strength training on muscle fiber types and size; consequences for athletes training for high-intensity sport. *Scandinavian Journal of Medicine and Science in Sports, 20*, S32–S38.

Andersen, J.L., Klitgaard, H., & Saltin, B. (1994). Myosin heavy chain isoforms in single fibres from m. vastus lateralis of sprinters, influence of training. *Acta Physiologica Scandinavica, 151*, 135–142.

Andersen, J.L., Mohr, T., Biering-Sørensen, F., Galbo, H., & Kjær, M. (1996). Myosin heavy chain isoform transformation in single fibres from m. vastus lateralis in spinal cord injured individuals: effects of long-term functional electrical stimulation (FES). *Pflugers Archives, 431*, 513–518.

Arnold, E.M., & Delp, S.L. (2011). Fibre operating lengths of human lower limb muscles during walking. *Philosophical Transactions of the Royal Society, 366*, 1530–1539.

Atherton, P.J., Babraj, J.A., Smith, K., Singh, J., Rennie, M.J., & Wackerhage, H. (2005). Selective activation of AMPK-PGC-1α or PKB-TSC2-mTOR signaling can explain specific adaptive responses to endurance or resistance training-like electrical muscle stimulation. *FASEB Journal, 19*, 786–788.

Azizi, E., Brainerd, E.L., & Roberts, T.J. (2008). Variable gearing in pennate muscles. *Proceedings of the National Academy of Science, 105*, 1745–1750.

Baar, K. (2006). Training for endurance and strength: lessons from cell signaling. *Medicine and Science in Sports and Exercise, 38*, 1939–1944.

Baldwin, K.M., & Haddad, F. (2001). Effects of different activity and inactivity paradigms on myosin heavy chain gene expression in striated muscle. *Journal of Applied Physiology, 90*, 345–357.

Bickel, C.S., Gregory, C.M., & Dean, J.C. (2011). Motor unit recruitment during neuromuscular electrical stimulation: a critical appraisal. *European Journal of Applied Physiology, 111*, 2399–2407.

Biewener, A.A. (2003). *Animal Locomotion.* Oxford, UK: Oxford University Press.

Biewener, A.A., Farley, C.T., Roberts, T.J., & Temaner, M. (2004). Muscle mechanical advantage of human walking and running: implications for energy cost. *Journal of Applied Physiology, 97*, 2266–2274.

Blazevich, A.J., Gill, N.D., Bronks, R., & Newton, R.U. (2003). Training-specific muscle architecture adaptations after 5-wk training in athletes. *Medicine and Science in Sports and Exercise, 35*, 2013–2022.

Bobbert, M.F., & Casius, L.J. (2005). Is the effect of a countermovement on jump height due to active state development? *Medicine and Science in Sports and Exercise, 37*, 440–446.

Bobbert, M.F., Gerritsen, K.G.M., Litjens, M.C.A., & van Soest, A.J. (1996). Why is countermovement jump height greater than squat jump height? *Medicine and Exercise in Sports and Exercise, 28*, 1402–1412.

Bojsen-Møller, J., Magnusson, S.P., Rasmussen, L.R., Kjær, M., & Aagaard, P. (2005). Muscle performance during maximal isometric and dynamic contractions is influenced by the stiffness of the tendinous structures. *Journal of Applied Physiology, 99*, 986–994.

Bottinelli, R., Canepari, M., Pellegrino, C., & Reggiani, C. (1996). Force-velocity properties of human skeletal muscle fibres: myosin heavy chain isoform and temperature dependence. *Journal of Physiology, 495*, 573–586.

Bottinelli, R., Pellegrino, M.A., Canepari, R., Rossi, R., & Reggiani, C. (1999). Specific contributions of various muscle fibre types to human muscle performance: an in vitro study. *Journal of Electromyography and Kinesiology, 9*, 87–95.

Brown, D.A., Kautz, S.A., & Dairaghi, C.A. (1996). Muscle activity patterns altered during pedaling at different body orientations. *Journal of Biomechanics, 29*, 1349–1356.

Buller, A.J., Eccles, J.C., & Eccles, R.M. (1960). Interactions between motoneurones and muscles in respect of the characteristic speeds of their responses. *Journal of Physiology, 150*, 417–439.

Butler, D.L., Grood, E.S., Noyes, F.K., & Zernicke, R.F. (1978). Biomechanics of ligaments and tendons. *Exercise and Sport Science Reviews, 6,* 125–181.

Butterfield, T.A., & Herzog, W. (2006). The magnitude of muscle strain does not influence serial sarcomere number adaptations following eccentric exercise. *Pflugers Archives, 451,* 688–700.

Cavagna, G.A., Saibene, F.P., & Margaria, R. (1964). Mechanical work in running. *Journal of Applied Physiology, 19,* 249–256.

Cavagna, G.A., Saibene, F.P., & Margaria, R. (1965). Effect of negative work on the amount of positive work performed by an isolated muscle. *Journal of Applied Physiology, 20,* 157–158.

Chalmers, G.R. (2002). Do Golgi tendon organs really inhibit muscle activity at high force levels to save muscles from injury, and adapt to strength training? *Sports Biomechanics, 1,* 239–249.

Chalmers, G.R. (2008). Can fast-twitch muscle fibres be selectively recruited during lengthening contractions? Review and applications to sports movements. *Sports Biomechanics, 7,* 137–157.

Close, R.I. (1972). Dynamic properties of mammalian skeletal muscles. *Physiology Reviews, 52,* 129–197.

Coffey, V.G., & Hawley, J.A. (2007). The molecular bases of training adaptations. *Sports Medicine, 37,* 737–763.

Coffey, V.G., Pilegaard, H., Garnham, A.P., O'Brien, B.J., & Hawley, J.A. (2009). Consecutive bouts of diverse contractile activity alter acute responses in human skeletal muscle. *Journal of Applied Physiology, 106,* 1187–1197.

Coffey, V.G., Shield, A., Canny, B.J., Carey, K.A., Smith, D., & Hawley, J.A. (2006). Interaction of contractile activity and training history on mRNA abundance in skeletal muscle from trained athletes. *American Journal of Physiology, 290,* E849–E855.

Cormie, P., McCaulley, G.O., & McBride, J.M. (2007). Power versus strength-power jump squat training: influence on the load-power relationship. *Medicine and Science in Sports and Medicine, 39,* 996–1003.

Cormie, P., McCaulley, G.O., Triplett, N.T., & McBride, J.M. (2007). Optimal loading for maximal power output during lower-body resistance exercises. *Medicine and Science in Sports and Exercise, 39,* 340–349.

D'Antona, G., Lanfranconi, F., Pellegrino, M.A., Brocca, L., Adami, R., Rossi, R., . . . Bottinelli, R. (2006). Skeletal muscle hypertrophy and structure and function of skeletal muscle fibres in male body builders. *Journal of Physiology, 570,* 611–627.

Dean, J.C., & Kuo, A.D. (2011). Energetic costs of producing muscle work and force in a cyclical human bouncing task. *Journal of Applied Physiology, 110,* 873–880.

Deldicque, L., Atherton, P., Patel, R., Theisen, D., Nielens, H., Rennie, M.J., & Francaux, M. (2008). Decrease in Akt/PKB signaling in human skeletal muscle by resistance exercise. *European Journal of Applied Physiology, 104,* 57–65.

di Prampero, P.E., & Narici, M.V. (2003). Muscles in microgravity: from fibres to human motion. *Journal of Biomechanics, 36,* 403–412.

Dirks, A.J., & Leeuwenburgh, C. (2005). The role of apoptosis in age-related skeletal muscle atrophy. *Sports Medicine, 35,* 473–483.

Drury, D.G., Stuempfle, K.J., Mason, C.W., & Girman, J.C. (2006). The effects of isokinetic contraction velocity on concentric and eccentric strength of the biceps brachii. *Journal of Strength and Conditioning Research, 20,* 390–395.

Duchateau, J., Semmler, J.G., & Enoka, R.M. (2006). Training adaptations in the behavior of human motor units. *Journal of Applied Physiology, 101,* 1766–1775.

Edman, K.A.P. (2003). Contractile performance of skeletal muscle fibers. In P.V. Komi (Ed.), *Strength and Power in Sport* (pp. 114–133). Oxford, UK: Blackwell Science Ltd.

Edman, K.A.P., Elzinga, G., & Noble, M.I. (1978). Enhancement of mechanical performance by stretch during tetanic contractions of vertebrate skeletal muscle fibres. *Journal of Physiology, 281,* 139–155.

Elliott, B.C., Wilson, G.J., & Kerr, G.K. (1989). A biomechanical analysis of the sticking region in the bench press. *Medicine and Science in Sports and Exercise, 21,* 450–462.

Enoka, R.M. (2008). *Neuromechanics of Human Movement.* Champaign, IL: Human Kinetics Publishers.

Epstein, M., Wong, M., & Herzog, W. (2006). Should tendon and aponeurosis be considered in series? *Journal of Biomechanics, 39,* 2020–2025.

Ettema, G.J., & Huijing, P.A. (1992). The potentiating effect of prestretch on the contractile performance of rat gastrocnemius medialis muscle during subsequent shortening and isometric contractions. *Journal of Experimental Biology, 165,* 121–136.

Finni, T., Ikegawa, S., & Komi, P.V. (2001). Concentric force enhancement during human movement. *Acta Phyiologica Scandinavica, 173,* 369–377.

Fukashiro, S., Hay, D.C., & Nagano, A. (2006). Biomechanical behavior of muscle-tendon complex during dynamic human movements. *Journal of Applied Biomechanics, 22,* 131–147.

Fukunaga, T., Roy, R.R., Shellock, F.G., Hodgson, J.A., Day, M.K., Lee, P.L., . . . Edgerton, V.R. (1992). Physiological cross-sectional area of human leg muscles based on magnetic resonance imaging. *Journal of Orthopaedic Research, 10,* 928–934.

Gallagher, D., Belmonte, D., Deurenberg, P., Wang, Z., Krasnow, N., Pi-Sunyer, F.X., & Heymsfield, S.B. (1998). Organ-tissue mass measurement allows modeling of REE and metabolically active tissue mass. *American Journal of Physiology, 275,* E249–E258.

Gehlert, S., Weber, S., Weidmann, B., Gutsche, K., Platen, P., Graf, C., . . . Bloch, W. (2012). Cycling exercise-induced myofiber transitions in skeletal muscle depend on basal fiber type distribution. *European Journal of Applied Physiology, 112,* 2393–2403.

Gruber, M., Taube, W., Gollhofer, A., Beck, S., Amtage, F., Schubert, M. (2007). Training-specific adaptations of H- and stretch reflexes in human soleus muscle. *Journal of Motor Behavior, 39,* 68–78.

Harber, M., & Trappe, S. (2008). Single muscle fiber contractile properties of young competitive distance runners. *Journal of Applied Physiology, 105,* 629–636.

Harry, J.D., Ward, A.W., Heglund, N.C., Morgan, D.L., & McMahon, T.A. (1990). Cross-bridge cycling theories cannot explain high-speed lengthening behavior in frog muscle. *Biophysical Journal, 57,* 201–208.

Henneman, E., Somjen, G., & Carpenter, D.O. (1965). Functional significance of cell size in spinal motoneurons. *Journal of Neurophysiology, 28,* 560–580.

Herzog, W., Duvall, M., & Leonard, T.R. (2012). Molecular mechanisms of muscle force regulation: a role for titin? *Exercise and Sports Science Reviews, 40,* 50–57.

Herzog, W., Leonard, T.R., Joumaa, V., & Mehta, A. (2008). Mysteries of muscle contraction. *Journal of Applied Biomechanics, 24,* 1–13.

Hickson, R.C. (1980). Interference of strength development by simultaneously training for strength and endurance. *European Journal of Applied Physiology, 45,* 255–263.

Hodgson, M., Docherty, D., & Robbins, D. (2005). Post-activation potentiation: underlying physiology and implications for motor performance. *Sports Medicine, 35,* 585–595.

Huxley, A.F. (1998). Biological motors: energy storage in myosin molecules. *Current Biology, 8,* 485–488.

Ichinose, Y., Kanehisa, H., Ito, M., Kawakami, Y., & Fukunaga, T. (1998). Relationship between muscle fiber pennation angle and force generation capability in Olympic athletes. *International Journal of Sports Medicine, 19,* 541–546.

Ichinose, Y., Kawakami, Y., Ito, M., Kanehisa, H., & Fukunaga, T. (2000). In vivo estimation of contraction velocity of human vastus lateralis muscle during "isokinetic" action. *Journal of Applied Physiology, 88,* 851–856.

Janssen, I., Heymsfield, S.B., Wang, Z.M., & Ross, R. (2000). Skeletal muscle mass and distribution in 468 men and women aged 18–88 yr. *Journal of Applied Physiology, 89,* 81–88.

Jones, D.A. (1993). How far can experiments in the laboratory explain fatigue of athletes in the field? In A.J. Sargeant & D. Kernell (Eds.), *Neuromuscular Fatigue* (pp. 100–108). Amsterdam: North Holland.

Jones, D.A., Rutherford, O.M., & Parker, D.F. (1989). Physiological changes in skeletal muscle as a result of strength training. *Quarterly Journal of Experimental Physiology, 74,* 233–256.

Kadi, F., Schjerling, P., Andersen, L.L., Charifi, N., Madsen, J.L., Christensen, L.R., & Andersen, J.L. (2004). The effects of heavy resistance training and detraining on satellite cells in human skeletal muscles. *Journal of Physiology, 558,* 1005–1012.

Kamen, G. (2004). Electromyographic kinesiology. In D.G.E. Robertson, J. Hamill, G.E. Caldwell, & G. Kamen (Eds.), *Research Methods in Biomechanics* (pp. 163–181). Champaign, IL: Human Kinetics Publishers.

Kamen, G., & Gabriel, D.A. (2010). *Essentials of Electromyography.* Champaign, IL: Human Kinetics Publishers.

Kawakami, Y., Abe, T., & Fukunaga, T. (1993). Muscle-fiber pennation angles are greater in hypertrophied than in normal muscles. *Journal of Applied Physiology, 74,* 2740–2744.

Kawakami, Y., Ichinose, Y., Kubo, K., Ito, M., Imai, M., & Fukunaga, T. (2000). Architecture of contracting human muscles and its functional significance. *Journal of Applied Biomechanics, 16,* 88–97.

Kelley, G. (1996). Mechanical overload and skeletal muscle fiber hyperplasia: a meta-analysis. *Journal of Applied Physiology, 81*, 1584–1588.

Komi, P.V. (2003). Stretch-shortening cycle. In P.V. Komi (Ed.), *Strength and Power in Sport* (pp. 184–202). Oxford, UK: Blackwell Science Ltd.

Komi, P.V., & Bosco, C. (1978). Utilization of stored elastic energy in leg extensor muscles by men and women. *Medicine and Science in Sports, 10*, 261–265.

Kosek, D.J., Kim, J.S., Petrella, J.K., Cross, J.M., & Bamman, M.M. (2006). Efficacy of 3 days/wk resistance training on myofiber hypertrophy and myogenic mechanisms in young vs. older adults. *Journal of Applied Physiology, 101*, 531–544.

Kraemer, W.J., Patton, J.F., Gordon, S.E., Harman, E.A., Deschenes, M.R., Reynolds, K., . . . Dziados, J.E. (1995). Compatibility of high-intensity strength and endurance training on hormonal and skeletal muscle adaptations. *Journal of Applied Physiology, 78*, 976–989.

Kram, R. (2000). Muscular force or work: what determines the metabolic energy cost of running? *Exercise and Sport Science Reviews, 28*, 138–143.

Kubo, K., Akima, H., Kouzaki, M., Ito, M., Kawakami, Y., Kanehisa, H., & Fukunaga, T. (2000). Changes in the elastic properties of tendon structures following 20 days bed-rest in humans. *European Journal of Applied Physiology, 83*, 463–468.

Kubo, K., Ikebukuro, T., Yaeshima, K., Yata, H., Tsunoda, N., & Kanehisa, H. (2009). Effects of static and dynamic training on the stiffness and blood volume of tendon in vivo. *Journal of Applied Physiology, 106*, 412–417.

Kubo, K., Ikebukuro, T., Yata, H., Tsunoda, N., & Kanehisa, H. (2010). Time course of changes in muscle and tendon properties during strength training and detraining. *Journal of Strength and Conditioning Research, 24*, 322–31.

Kubo, K., Kanehisa, H., & Fukunaga, T. (2002). Effect of stretching training on the viscoelastic properties of human tendon structures in vivo. *Journal of Physiology, 92*, 595–601.

Kubo, K., Kanehisa, H., & Fukunaga, T. (2003). Gender differences in the viscoelastic properties of tendon structures. *European Journal of Applied Physiology, 88*, 520–526.

Kubo, K., Kanehisa, H., & Fukunaga, T. (2005). Effects of viscoelastic properties of tendon structures on stretch-shortening cycle exercise *in vivo*. *Journal of Sports Sciences, 23*, 851–860.

Kubo, K., Kanehisa, H., Miyatani, M., Tachi, M., & Fukunaga, T. (2003). Effect of low-load resistance training on the tendon properties in middle-aged and elderly women. *Acta Physiological Scandinavica, 178*, 25–32.

Kubo, K., Kawakami, Y., & Fukunaga, T. (1999). Influence of elastic properties of tendon structures on jump performance in humans. *Journal of Applied Physiology, 87*, 2090–2096.

Kubo, K., Tabata, T., Ikebukuro, T., Igarashi, K., & Tsunoda, N. (2010). A longitudinal assessment of running economy and tendon properties in long-distance runners. *Journal of Strength and Conditioning Research, 24*, 1724–31.

Kumagai, K., Abe, T., Brechue, W.F., Ryushi, T., Takano, S., & Mizuno, M. (2000). Sprint performance is related to muscle fascicle length in male 100-m sprinters. *Journal of Applied Physiology, 88*, 811–816.

Kumar, V., Atherton, P., Smith, K., & Rennie, M.J. (2009). Human muscle protein synthesis and breakdown during and after exercise. *Journal of Applied Physiology, 106*, 2026–2039.

Kyröläinen, H., & Komi, P.V. (1994). Neuromuscular performance of lower limbs during voluntary and reflex activity in power- and endurance-trained athletes. *European Journal of Applied Physiology, 69*, 233–239.

Lejeune, T.M., Willems, P.A., & Heglund, N.C. (1998). Mechanics and energetics of human locomotion on sand. *Journal of Experimental Biology, 201*, 2071–2080.

Leonard, T.R., & Herzog, W. (2010). Regulation of muscle force in the absence of actin-myosin-based cross-bridge interaction. *American Journal of Cell Physiology, 299*, C14–C20.

Lieber, R.L. (2002). *Skeletal Muscle Structure, Function, and Plasticity.* Baltimore, MD: Lippincott Williams and Wilkins.

Linari, M., Bottinelli, R., Pellegrino, M.A., Reconditi, M., Reggiani, C., & Lombardi, V. (2003). The mechanism of the force response to stretch in human skinned muscle fibres with different myosin isoforms. *Journal of Physiology, 554*, 335–352.

Lionikas, A., Li, M., & Larsson, L. (2006). Human skeletal muscle myosin function at physiological and non-physiological temperatures. *Acta Physiologica, 186*, 151–158.

Lombardi, V., & Piazzesi, G. (1990). The contractile response during steady lengthening of stimulated frog muscle fibers. *Journal of Physiology, 431*, 141–171.

MacDougall, J.D. (2003). Hypertrophy and hyperplasia. In P.V. Komi (Ed.), *Strength and Power in Sport* (pp. 252–264). Oxford, UK: Blackwell Science Ltd.

MacIntosh, B.R., Gardiner, P.F., & McComas, A.J. (2006). *Skeletal Muscle. Form and Function.* Champaign, IL: Human Kinetics Publishers.

Madsen, N., & McLaughlin, T.M. (1984). Kinematic factors influencing performance and injury risk in the bench press exercise. *Medicine and Science in Sports and Exercise, 16,* 376–381.

Maffiuletti, N.A., Martin, A., Babault, N., Pensini, M., Lucas, B., & Schieppati, M. (2001). Electrical and mechanical H(max)-to-M(max) ratio in power- and endurance-trained athletes. *Journal of Applied Physiology, 90,* 3–9.

Malisoux, L., Francaux, M., Nielens, H., & Theisen, D. (2006). Stretch-shortening cycle exercises: an effective training paradigm to enhance power output of human single muscle fibers. *Journal of Applied Physiology, 100,* 771–779.

Margaria, R. (1968). Positive and negative work performances and their efficiencies in human locomotion. *Internationale Zeitschrift für Angewandte Physiologie, 25,* 339–351.

Margaria, R., Cerretelli, P., Aghemo, P., & Sassi, G. (1963). Energy cost of running. *Journal of Applied Physiology, 18,* 367.

McBride, J.M., McCaulley, G.O., & Cormie, P. (2008). Influence of preactivity and eccentric muscle activity on concentric performance during vertical jumping. *Journal of Strength and Conditioning Research, 23,* 750–757.

McBride, J.M., Triplett-McBride, T., Davie, A.J., Abernethy, P.J., & Newton, R.U. (2003). Characteristics of titin in strength and power athletes. *European Journal of Applied Physiology, 88,* 553–557.

McBride, J.M., Triplett-McBride, T., Davie, A., & Newton, R.U. (2002). The effects of heavy- vs. light-load jump squats on the development of strength, power, and speed. *Journal of Strength and Conditioning Research, 16,* 75–82.

McCaulley, G.O., Cormie, P., Cavill, M.J., Nuzzo, J.L., Urbiztondo, Z.G., & McBride, J.M. (2007). Mechanical efficiency during repetitive vertical jumping. *European Journal of Applied Physiology, 101,* 115–123.

Minetti, A.E., Ardigò, L.P., & Saibene, F. (1994). Mechanical determinants of the minimum energy cost of gradient running in humans. *Journal of Experimental Biology, 195,* 211–225.

Moritz, C.T., Barry, B.K., Pascoe, M.A., & Enoka, R.M. (2005). Discharge rate variability influences the variation in force fluctuations across the working range of a hand muscle. *Journal of Neurophysiology, 93,* 2449–2459.

Newton, R., Murphy, A.J., Humphries, B., Wilson, G., Kraemer, W., & Häkkinen, K. (1997). Influence of load and stretch shortening cycle on the kinematics, kinetics and muscle activation that occur during explosive upper body movements. *European Journal of Applied Physiology, 75,* 333–342.

Nicol, C., Avela, J., & Komi, P.V. (2006). The stretch-shortening cycle: a model to study naturally occurring neuromuscular fatigue. *Sports Medicine, 36,* 977–999.

Oya, T., Riek, S., & Cresswell, A.G. (2009). Recruitment and rate coding organization for soleus motor units across entire range of voluntary isometric plantar flexions. *Journal of Physiology, 587,* 4737–4748.

Petrella, J.K., Kim, J.S., Mayhew, D.L., Cross, J.M., & Bamman, M.M. (2008). Potent myofiber hypertrophy during resistance training in humans is associated with satellite cell-mediated myonuclear addition: a cluster analysis. *Journal of Applied Physiology, 104,* 1736–1742.

Pette, D. (1998). Training effects on the contractile apparatus. *Acta Physiologica Scandinavica, 162,* 367–376.

Pette, D. (2001). Historical perspectives: plasticity of mammalian skeletal muscle. *Journal of Applied Physiology, 90,* 1119–1124.

Pette, D., Peuker, H., & Staron, R.S. (1999). The impact of biomechanical methods for single muscle fiber analysis. *Acta Physiologica Scandinavica, 166,* 261–277.

Pette, D., Smith, M.E., Staudte, H.W., & Vrbová, G. (1973). Effects of long-term electrical stimulation on some contractile and metabolic characteristics of fast rabbit muscle. *Pflügers Archives, 338,* 257–272.

Pette, D., & Staron, R.S. (1997). Mammalian skeletal muscle fiber type transitions. *International Review of Cytology, 170,* 143–223.

Purslow, P.P. (1989). Strain-induced reorientation of an intramuscular connective tissue network: implications for passive muscle elasticity. *Journal of Biomechanics, 22,* 21–31.

Rassier, D.E. (2012). The mechanisms of the residual force enhancement after stretch of skeletal muscle: non-uniformity in half-sarcomeres and stiffness of titin. *Proceedings of the Royal Society, 279,* 2705–2713.

Robbins, D.W. (2005). Postactivation potentiation and its practical applicability. *Journal of Strength and Conditioning Research, 19*, 453–458.

Ross, A., & Leveritt, M. (2001). Long-term metabolic and skeletal muscle adaptations to short-sprint training: implications for sprint training and tapering. *Sports Medicine, 31*, 1063–82.

Sale, D.G. (2002). Postactivation potentiation: role in human performance. *Exercise and Sports Science Reviews, 30*, 138–143.

Samozino, P., Rejc, E., Di Prampero, P.E., Belli, A., & Morin, J-B. (2012). Optimal force-velocity profile in ballistic movements—*Altius: Citius* or *Fortius*? *Medicine and Science in Sports and Exercise, 44*, 313–322.

Sandri, M. (2008). Signaling in muscle atrophy and hypertrophy. *Physiology, 23*, 160–170.

Schiaffino, S. (2010). Fibre types in skeletal muscle: a personal account. *Acta Physiologica, 199*, 451–463.

Schiaffino, S., & Reggiani, C. (1994). Myosin isoforms in mammalian skeletal muscle. *Journal of Applied Physiology, 77*, 493–501.

Schoenfeld, B.J. (2010). Does exercise-induced muscle damage play a role in skeletal muscle hypertrophy? *Journal of Strength and Conditioning Research, 26*, 1441–1453.

Shoepe, T.C., Stelzer, J.E., Garner, D.P., & Widrick, J.J. (2003). Functional adaptability of muscle fibers to long-term resistance exercise. *Medicine and Science in Sports and Exercise, 35*, 944–951.

Stephenson, G.M.M. (2001). Hybrid skeletal muscle fibers: a rare or common phenomenon? *Clinical and Experimental Pharmacology and Physiology, 28*, 692–702.

Stewart, R.D., Duhamel, T.A., Rich, S., Tupling, A.R., & Green, H.J. (2008). Effects of consecutive days of exercise and recovery on muscle mechanical function. *Medicine and Science in Sports and Exercise, 40*, 316–325.

Stienen, G.J., Kiers, J.L., Bottinelli, R., & Reggiani, C. (1996). Myofibrillar ATPase activity in skinned human skeletal muscle fibres: fibre type and temperature. *Journal of Physiology, 493*, 299–307.

ter Haar Romeny, B.M., van der Gon, J.J., & Gielen, C.C. (1984). Relation between location of a motor unit in the human biceps brachii and its critical firing levels for different tasks. *Experimental Neurology, 85*, 631–650.

Van den Tillaar, R., & Ettema, G.J. (2009). A comparison of successful and unsuccessful attempts in maximal bench pressing. *Medicine and Science in Sports and Exercise, 41*, 2056–2063.

Van den Tillaar, R., & Ettema, G.J. (2010). The "sticking period" in a maximum bench press. *Journal of Sports Sciences, 28*, 529–535.

Van den Tillaar, R., Sæterbakken, A.H., & Ettema, G.J. (2012). Is the occurrence of the sticking region the result of diminishing potentiation in bench press? *Journal of Sports Sciences, 30*, 591–599.

van Ingen Schenau, G.J. (1989). From rotation to translation: constraints on multi-joint movements and the unique action of biarticular muscles. *Human Movement Sciences, 8*, 301–337.

van Ingen Schenau, G.J., Bobbert, M.F., & de Haan, A. (1997). Mechanics and energetics of the stretch-shortening cycle: a stimulating discussion. *Journal of Applied Biomechanics, 13*, 484–496.

Vogel, S. (2003). *Comparative Biomechanics. Life's Physical World*. Princeton, NJ: Princeton University Press.

Voigt, M., Bojsen-Møller, F., Simonsen, E.B., & Dyhre-Poulsen, P. (1995). The influence of tendon Young's modulus, dimensions and instantaneous moment arms on the efficiency of human movement. *Journal of Biomechanics, 28*, 281–291.

Walshe, A.D., Wilson, G.J., & Ettema, G.J. (1998). Stretch-shorten compared with isometric preload: contributions to enhanced muscular performance. *Journal of Applied Physiology, 84*, 97–106.

Wang, J.-C. (2006). Microbiology of tendon. *Journal of Biomechanics, 39*, 1563–1582.

Wilson, G.J., Newton, R.U., Murphy, A.J., & Humphries, B.J. (1993). The optimal training load for the development of dynamic athletic performance. *Medicine and Science in Sports and Exercise, 25*, 1279–1286.

Zajac, F.E., Neptune, R.R., & Kautz, S.A. (2002). Biomechanics and muscle coordination of human walking. Part I: introduction to concepts, power transfer, dynamics and simulations. *Gait and Posture, 16*, 215–232.

Zatsiorsky, V.M., & Kraemer, W.J. (2006). *Science and Practice of Strength Training*. Champaign, IL: Human Kinetics Publishers.

Zatsiorsky, V.M., & Prilutsky, B.I. (2012). *Biomechanics of Skeletal Muscle*. Champaign, IL: Human Kinetics Publishers.

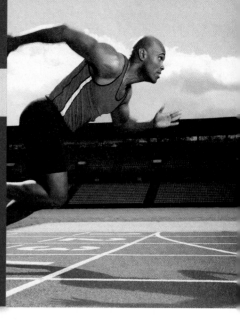

CHAPTER 4

Bioenergetics of Exercise

Chapter Objectives

At the end of this chapter, you will be able to:

- Describe the systems that provide energy to sustain muscle activity during exercise
- Explain the relative contributions of the energy systems to the transition from rest to exercise
- Explain the relative contributions of the energy systems to continuous exercise of differing intensities and durations
- Explain the relative contributions of the energy systems to repeated-sprint activities
- Explain the role of bioenergetics in fatigue

Key Terms

Adenosine-5′-triphosphate (ATP)

Adenylate kinase reaction

Alactic glycolysis

AMP deaminase reaction

β-alanine

Beta-oxidation

Bioenergetics

Citric acid cycle

CK–PCr shuttle

Creatine kinase reaction

Efficiency

Electron transport chain

Gibbs free energy

Glycolysis

Indirect calorimetry

Lactate dehydrogenase

Lactate threshold

Lactic glycolysis

Magnetic resonance spectroscopy

Mitochondrial biogenesis

Monocarboxylate transporters

Muscle biopsies

Muscle-specific hormone sensitive lipase

Oxidative phosphorylation

Oxygen debt

Oxygen deficit

Phosphagen system

Phosphofructokinase

Phosphorylase

Pyruvate dehydrogenase

Respiratory control

Respiratory exchange ratio

Sodium bicarbonate

Sodium citrate

Substrate-level phosphorylation

Teleoanticipatory model

Chapter Overview

Bioenergetics describes the processes involved in the energy transfer associated with the metabolic reactions that sustain the physiological functioning of the human motor system. During exercise, energy expenditure can increase 100-fold above that observed at rest; in the present chapter, we will limit our discussion to the energetic processes involved in the activity of skeletal muscle during exercise. The various reactions that occur within the muscle fiber, either in the cytosol or within the mitochondria, liberate chemical energy that ultimately allows the contractile machinery of the fibers to produce force and perform mechanical work as required. As we will see, these chemical reactions are regulated such that the provision of energy is closely matched to the demand imposed by the intensity of the exercise. An understanding of the bioenergetic processes involved in different exercises is important to the strength and conditioning practitioner because these processes underpin the development of effective training programs for athletes.

Bioenergetics and Exercise Intensity

When an athlete is required to run at maximal speed for different durations, a hyperbolic relationship is evident from the resultant speed–duration graph (**Figure 4.1**). The graph shows that over short durations, sustainable running speeds decrease markedly with small increases in the duration of the sprint; that is, as the duration of each run becomes longer, there is a reduction in the sustainable speed. This relationship becomes apparent when the speeds of world-record performances in track events are scrutinized (**Table 4.1**). Notice that the average speed for the 100-m sprint, which lasts in the region of 10 s, is almost twice the average speed for the 42,195-m distance of the marathon, which lasts around 2 hours. However, the average speed for the 10,000-m distance is only slightly faster than the values associated with the marathon, yet the event lasts less than a quarter of the time. The hyperbolic speed–duration relationship observed is associated with the rate and capacity of energy provision from anaerobic and aerobic energy sources, which differ according to the required power output or velocity of the exercise being performed (Figure 4.1).

The energy that must be expended in order to sustain the physiological functioning of the skeletal muscles during exercise is provided by the hydrolysis of **adenosine-5′-triphosphate (ATP)**:

$$\text{ATP} + \text{H}_2\text{O} \overset{\text{ATPase}}{\rightarrow} \text{ADP} + \text{P}_i + \text{H}^+ \qquad\qquad \textbf{Eq. (4.1)}$$

where H_2O is water, ATPase is the enzyme that catalyzes the reaction, ADP is adenosine diphosphate, P_i is inorganic phosphate, and H^+ is hydrogen. There are three major sources of energy consumption within a muscle fiber during exercise:

- Na^+-K^+ pump. A difference in electrical charge exists across the sarcolemma, mainly due to the difference in the concentration of Na^+ and K^+ ions. The resting membrane potential of a muscle fiber (-90 mV) is due to the greater concentration of Na^+ outside of the cell and greater concentrations of K^+ in the interior. Transient change in the membrane potential that characterizes a muscle fiber action potential is caused by the movement of Na^+ and K^+ across the membrane down their concentration gradients; this change is required to

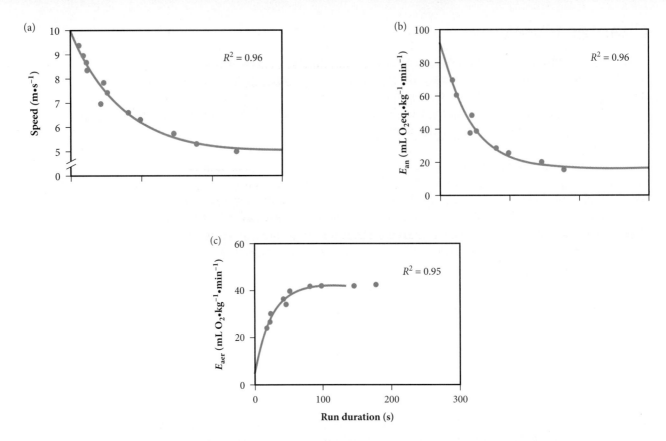

Figure 4.1 (a) The hyperbolic relationship between running speed and the duration that the speed is maintained. The estimated energy rates from anaerobic (b) and aerobic (c) sources required to sustain the running speeds.

Note: E_{an} is estimated rate of anaerobic energy release; E_{aer} is estimated rate of aerobic energy release.

Reproduced from Bundle, M. W., Hoyt, R. W., & Weyand, P. G. (2003). High-speed running performance: a new approach to assessment and prediction. *Journal of Applied Physiology, 95*, 1955–1962.

initiate the movement of Ca^{2+} into the cytosol. The hydrolysis of ATP via the Na^+-K^+ ATPase enzyme phosphorylates the pump and actively transports the Na^+ and K^+ ions against their concentration gradients to reestablish the resting membrane potential. It has been suggested that Na^+-K^+ ATPase consumes less than 5% of the total energy consumed during the activation of skeletal muscle (Spriet & Hargreaves, 2006).

Table 4.1
Times and Average Speeds for Record Holders in 100-m, 10,000-m, and Marathon Events

	100 m		10,000 m		Marathon (42,195 m)	
	Time (s)	Speed (m/s)	Time (s)	Speed (m/s)	Time (s)	Speed (m/s)
Men	9.58	10.44	1577.53	6.34	7418	5.69
Women	10.49	9.53	1771.78	5.64	8125	5.19

Note: Times accurate as of June 2013.

- Ca²⁺ pump. Recall that an action potential stimulates the release of Ca^{2+} from the terminal cisternae of the sarcoplasmic reticulum, resulting in the movement of Ca^{2+} down its concentration gradient and into the cytosol. The binding of Ca^{2+} to the regulatory protein troponin causes tropomyosin to undergo a structural change and expose the active binding sites on the actin molecule. The energized myosin crossbridge then binds to the actin molecule and undergoes a power stroke, generating the tension associated with muscle activation. The relaxation of the muscle fiber is caused by a reuptake of Ca^{2+} against its concentration gradient via the Ca^{2+} pump, returning the Ca^{2+} concentration in the cytosol to resting levels. It has been proposed that Ca^{2+}-ATPase, which harnesses the energy required by the Ca^{2+} pump, consumes 25–30% of the energy associated with muscle activation (Spriet & Hargreaves, 2006).

- Actomyosin crossbridge cycling. An ATP molecule that binds to the myosin crossbridge is hydrolyzed and provides energy for the myosin ATPase enzyme, thus "energizing" the crossbridge. However, actomyosin binding will not take place until Ca^{2+}-troponin binding exposes the active binding sites on the actin molecule via the structural change in tropomyosin. At this time, the energized crossbridge binds to actin and the initiation of the power stroke of the crossbridge and the dissociation of P_i occur. Following the power stroke, ADP dissociates from the crossbridge, but the actomyosin complex (the rigor complex) remains intact. The binding of an ATP molecule rapidly dissociates the actomyosin complex, and the myosin crossbridge is returned to its original, pre-power stroke position. It has been suggested that the enzyme myosin ATPase, which catalyzes the hydrolysis of ATP on the crossbridge, is responsible for approximately 70% of the energy consumed during muscle activation (Spriet & Hargreaves, 2006).

Maughan (2011) notes that approximately 31 kJ of energy is released as a result of the hydrolysis of 1 mole of ATP (**Worked Example 4.1**); the hydrolysis of 1.4 g of ATP is required per second for an individual who has an energy turnover at rest of 83 W (1.2 kcal/min). This high rate of hydrolysis just to meet the demands associated with the resting state should indicate that each ATP molecule provides a relatively small energy yield. As such, it would be inefficient for a cell to store ATP, yet the concentration of ATP within a muscle cell remains relatively constant even during exercise, when the energy demands of the cells can rise well above those associated with rest. Indeed, the total ATP content in the body at rest is typically 50 g (Maughan, 2011), so the required rate of ATP hydrolysis to sustain the resting state would last approximately 36 s before the ATP content of the body would be exhausted. However, even during exercise the concentrations of ATP within muscle fibers remain relatively constant, decreasing to only 20–40% below resting levels even following maximal sprint or repeated sprint bouts (Spriet, 2006). Therefore, the ATP that is hydrolyzed in the various ATPase-catalyzed reactions listed above must be resynthesized continually to match the energy demands of the muscle fiber. The energy demands of the muscle fiber will be largely determined by the intensity of the exercise undertaken by the athlete (e.g., power output, running speed) and will determine the duration that a given power output can be sustained (Figure 4.1). The type of muscle action will also influence the energy demands, with low-velocity, eccentric actions demanding a lower rate of energy provision than isometric actions, which in turn require a lower rate of energy provision than concentric actions (see Bioenergetics Concept 4.1).

Worked Example 4.1
Converting the units of energy

The metric unit of both work and energy is the joule, while power, the rate of performing work, has the unit of watts (joules per second). In discussions of energy provision from different substrates during exercise (e.g., carbohydrate, fats, proteins), the values are often expressed in calorie units, commonly referred to as the kilocalorie (kcal). For the purposes of converting between the units of energy, 1 kcal is equal to 4186 J.

The hydrolysis of 1 mole of ATP provides 31 kJ of energy. Convert this value to kilocalories.

i. Express kJ as J	31 kJ is 31,000 J
ii. Use the conversion factor	1 kcal is equal to 4186 J
iii. Answer	7.41 kcal

The hydrolysis of 1 mole of ATP provides 7.41 kcal of energy and represents the work that can be done as a result of the hydrolysis of ATP within the muscle fiber. Notice that not all of this energy is harnessed in the development of tension by the crossbridges, as the energy is also utilized to maintain ion concentrations within the cytosol (e.g., Ca^{2+}, Na^+, K^+). Furthermore, there will be a proportion of energy lost (usually to heat) in the conversion of chemical energy to mechanical energy during exercise, as dictated by the second law of thermodynamics. This is reflected in measures of **efficiency** associated with specific movements. Bangsbo (1996) reported the efficiency of high-intensity isolated muscle actions as between 22% and 26%, with the remaining energy (~75%) lost as heat. There is some evidence to suggest that heat loss is greater for aerobic ATP resynthesis compared to anaerobic resynthesis during exercise, implying a difference in efficiency (Krustrup, Ferguson, Kjær, & Bangsbo, 2003).

Resynthesizing ATP

There are three main metabolic pathways that are available for the resynthesis of hydrolyzed ATP:

- **Phosphagen system**
- **Glycolysis**
- **Oxidative phosphorylation**

The first two pathways are anaerobic and take place in the cytosol. They are collectively referred to as **substrate-level phosphorylation** and are able to resynthesize ATP at high rates, resulting in high power outputs during exercise, although their capacities for ATP resynthesis are limited and therefore the total amount of work performed is low. For example, the maximal power output for the phosphagen system has been estimated as 800 W/kg active skeletal muscle, that of glycolysis as 325 W/kg active skeletal muscle, and that of oxidative phosphorylation as 200 W/kg active skeletal muscle (Maughan, 2011). The high rates of ATP resynthesis associated with substrate-level phosphorylation render them ideal for energy provision at times when the ATP demand is high, such as during the transition from rest to exercise or during high-intensity work bouts. The third pathway, oxidative phosphorylation, takes place exclusively in the mitochondria within the muscle fibers and requires oxygen. Although this pathway has the lowest rate of ATP resynthesis, its capacity is much greater than that associated with substrate-level phosphorylation. For example, the phosphagen system

Bioenergetics Concept 4.1

ATP hydrolysis and Gibbs free energy

The energy released in a chemical reaction that can be used is known as the **Gibbs free energy** (ΔG) and is a measure of how far a given reaction is from equilibrium. The energy liberated from the hydrolysis of ATP comes from the high-energy phosphate bonds of the molecule. The ΔG for ATP hydrolysis is 31 kJ/mol under standard conditions ($\Delta G°$). However, such standard conditions are unlikely to be met within the muscle fiber. As such, the energy release from ATP hydrolysis can be more accurately written as follows (Hancock, Brault, & Terjung, 2006):

$$\Delta G = \Delta G° + R \times T \times \ln\left(\frac{[ADP] \times [P_i]}{[ATP]}\right) \qquad \text{Eq. (4.2)}$$

where ΔG is the Gibbs free energy released from the hydrolysis of ATP, $\Delta G°$ is the Gibbs free energy of ATP hydrolysis under standard conditions (31 kJ/mol), R is the ideal gas constant (~8.31 J/Kelvin), T is the temperature in Kelvin, [ADP] is the cytosolic concentration of adenosine diphosphate, $[P_i]$ is the cytosolic concentration of inorganic phosphate, and [ATP] is the cytosolic concentration of adenosine triphosphate.

Equation (4.2) is important because it informs us that the energy liberated by the hydrolysis of ATP will be dependent upon the phosphorylation potential of the cell (cytosolic [ATP]/[ADP] $[P_i]$). As a result of intense exercise, there is likely to be an increase in [ADP] and $[P_i]$ and a decrease in [ATP], reducing the Gibbs free energy associated with ATP hydrolysis. The ATPase reaction associated with the Ca^{2+} pump is particularly sensitive to a fall in the Gibbs free energy (Hancock et al., 2006), and a reduction in muscle relaxation due to a slowing in the reuptake of Ca^{2+} into the sarcoplasmic reticulum is likely to result.

has been estimated to have a resynthesis capacity of 400 J/kg active skeletal muscle, glycolysis has one of 1,000 J/kg active skeletal muscle, and oxidative phosphorylation has one of almost unlimited capacity (Maughan, 2011; see **Worked Example 4.2**). Furthermore, oxidative phosphorylation is able to metabolize carbohydrates, fats, and even proteins to provide the energy to resynthesize ATP. While it may be considered that the maximal power outputs during exercise are determined by the combined maximal rates of ATP resynthesis from the phosphagen system, glycolysis, and oxidative phosphorylation, the energy pathways do not achieve their maximal rates simultaneously.

Although many exercise intensities can be sustained with ATP provision via oxidative phosphorylation, there are many instances in sport where the required intensities cannot be achieved. Furthermore, it takes a finite time for the oxidative pathway to establish ATP resynthesis at the required rate due to the activation of associated enzymes and the mobilization of the substrates required or a limitation in O_2 supply to the mitochondria (Spriet, 2006). Exercise intensities in excess of the ATP provision via oxidative phosphorylation and the apparent lag in energy provision by this

Worked Example 4.2
Deriving mechanical power output from metabolic output

The energy derived from oxidative phosphorylation should provide a maximal power output of 200 W/ kg of active skeletal muscle (Maughan, 2011). Sloniger, Cureton, Prior, and Evans (1997) noted that an average lower-body muscle mass of 5.6 kg was activated in females with a body mass of approximately 60 kg during horizontal running. Farris and Sawicki (2012) used the ratio of mechanical power to metabolic power to determine that the efficiency of running at 3.25 m/s (~7.3 mph) was 41%. Use these values to determine the power output during running at a velocity of 3.25 m/s, which can be sustained by energy derived from oxidative phosphorylation.

i. Determine the power output associated with the active muscle mass	200×5.6
ii. Multiply the power output by the efficiency of running	1120×0.41
iii. Answer	459 W

The value of 459 W is above the average mechanical power output of 340 W reported by Farris and Sawicki (2012) recorded from subjects running at 3.25 m/s. Remember that the calculations above refer to the *maximal* power output that can be sustained via oxidative phosphorylation; clearly, higher velocities can be sustained when relying on energy provision from the oxidative system, although the efficiency of the movement will impact the mechanical power output observed. However, the values of 3,000 W that have been reported during sprint running (Lakomy, 2000) could not be achieved by energy provision from the oxidative phosphorylation system, requiring substrate-level phosphorylation to provide the necessary energy instead.

energy pathway would result in a mismatch between the demand and provision of ATP within the exercising muscle fiber, limiting the observed power output. However, the high rates of ATP resynthesis provided by the phosphagen and glycolytic pathways circumvent these issues. As such, substrate-level phosphorylation defends the ATP concentration of the muscle cell during high-intensity exercise and during the transition from rest to exercise (Spriet, 2006).

It should be noted that all pathways can contribute to ATP provision concurrently, but the intensity of the exercise will largely determine the relative contribution of each pathway to the overall provision of ATP (see **Bioenergetics Concept 4.2**). Referring to Figure 4.1, it can be seen that the contribution of the anaerobic energy pathways (substrate-level phosphorylation) is largest when the intensity of the sprints, determined by the running speed, is high, while the contribution of the aerobic pathway (oxidative phosphorylation) increases as the intensity of the sprint decreases. Notice also that there is an inverse relationship between the intensity and duration of the sprints; this inverse relationship is reflected in the rate and capacity of the energy pathways as mentioned above. Therefore, the maximal rate of ATP resynthesis sets an upper limit on exercise intensity, while the capacity of ATP resynthesis determines exercise duration at a given intensity (Sahlin, Tonkonogi, & Söderlund, 1998).

The specific profile of maximal power and exercise capacity at a given exercise intensity are determined by skeletal muscle mass, fiber-type composition, training, and nutritional status (Sahlin, 2006). For example, the substrates (e.g., phosphocreatine, glycogen) and enzymes controlling the rate of substrate flux (e.g., ATPase, creatine kinase, phosphofructokinase) will increase in proportion to the active muscle mass. In this respect, muscle hypertrophy and increased motor-unit recruitment will

Bioenergetics Concept 4.2

Is exercise intensity determined solely by ATP resynthesis rates?

The maximal rate of energy expenditure during exercise cannot exceed the maximal rate of ATPase activity (Sahlin, 2006); therefore, the provision of ATP via the metabolic pathways can be viewed as setting an upper limit on the intensity of exercise observed at any given time. However, power output is likely to fluctuate, even during exercise bouts performed under controlled laboratory conditions (Tucker et al., 2006), and these fluctuations are not necessarily caused by changing rates of energy provision associated with the different energy pathways. When interpreting the changes in power output observed during a given exercise bout, consideration should be given to the pace adopted by the athlete, particularly during "closed-loop" events where the athlete is required to complete a known distance in the shortest time possible (Abbiss & Laursen, 2008). Specifically, in a **teleoanticipatory model** of exercise regulation, it is proposed that the intensity of the exercise is regulated throughout a given bout, and a specific pace (e.g., power output, running speed) is adopted at any given time in anticipation of the end-point of the exercise to ensure that changes in physiological systems that could interfere with performance are limited (Tucker & Noakes, 2009). In this way, the athlete regulates the pace in advance of the attainment of catastrophic disturbances in the muscles and other organs, while a certain level of physiological disturbance is tolerated (e.g., decline in energy substrates, increase in metabolic byproducts, increased heat storage). For example, when exercising in conditions of increased ambient heat, a pacing strategy is selected whereby power output or running velocity is reduced soon after the initiation of the exercise as a means of preventing excessive heat storage and rise in body temperature (Tucker & Noakes, 2009). Therefore, the intensity observed in a given exercise bout is determined by a complex interaction of feedback and feed-forward mechanisms associated with the central nervous system, the duration of the event, as well as the ability of the energy pathways to resynthesize ATP.

be advantageous in increasing the rate of energy provision, likely improving performance in high-intensity activities. However, the increase in mass associated with muscle hypertrophy would not be beneficial for activities where energy expenditure is a limiting factor (e.g., endurance events). Furthermore, activities relying predominantly upon energy provision via oxidative phosphorylation are largely limited by O_2 delivery as opposed to intrinsic muscle characteristics (Bassett & Howley, 2000). The maximal ATP expenditure of type I, IIA, and IIX fibers is 6.5, 17.6, and 26.6 mM ATP/kg/s, respectively, and therefore the maximal power outputs achieved in a given exercise are strongly correlated with the proportion of fast fibers (Sahlin et al., 1998). The fiber-specific differences in the rates of energy expenditure arise from the differences in substrate and enzyme concentrations (Table 4.2). Training causes specific adaptations in muscle fiber types and will therefore dictate the specific profile of maximal power and exercise capacity at a given intensity (Wilson et al., 2012),

Table 4.2

Differences in Substrate and Enzyme Concentrations Between Type I and Type II Muscle Fibers

Substrate	Difference
Phosphocreatine	Type I < type II
Glycogen	Type I < type II
Triglycerides	Type I > type II
Enzyme	**Difference**
Creatine kinase	Type I < type II
Phosphorylase	Type I < type II
Phosphofructokinase	Type I < type II
Succinate dehydrogenase	Type I > type II
Citrate synthase	Type I > type II
Hormone sensitive lipase	Type I > type II

Reproduced from Jeukendrup, A. E., Saris, W. H. M., & Wagenmakers, A. J. M. (1998). Fat metabolism during exercise: a review. Part I: fatty acid mobilization and muscle metabolism. *International Journal of Sports Medicine, 19*, 231–244; Langfort, J., Ploug, T., Ihlemann, J., Saldo, M., Holm, C., & Galbo, H. (1999). Expression of hormone-sensitive lipase and its regulation by adrenaline in skeletal muscle. *Biochemistry Journal, 340*, 459–465; Schiaffino, S., & Reggiani, C. (2011). Fiber types in mammalian skeletal muscles. *Physiology Reviews, 91*, 1447–1531.

while supplementation of substrates (e.g., creatine, carbohydrate) has been shown to increase exercise intensity and ameliorate the reduction in exercise intensity associated with fatigue (Bemben & Lamont, 2005; Burke, Hawley, Wong, & Jeukendrup, 2011).

Phosphagen system

There are three reactions encompassed within the phosphagen system, the first of which is the **creatine kinase reaction** (Baker, McCormick, & Robergs, 2010):

$$PCr + ADP + H^+ \overset{\text{creatine kinase}}{\longleftrightarrow} ATP + Cr \qquad\qquad \textbf{Eq. (4.3)}$$

where PCr is phosphocreatine, ADP is adenosine diphosphate, H^+ is hydrogen, creatine kinase is the enzyme that catalyzes the reaction, ATP is adenosine triphosphate, and Cr is creatine. The creatine kinase (CK) reaction is very responsive to the energy requirements of the cell, as ADP is a substrate for CK; the reaction reaches a maximal rate 1.3 s after the initiation of maximal-intensity exercise (Sahlin, 2006). The capacity of the CK reaction is determined by the store of PCr within the muscle fiber, which typically amounts to 120–140 g in a 70-kg individual (Bemben & Lamont, 2005). Cr is derived from the diet by the ingestion of foods such as meats and fish or through supplementation (see Bioenergetics Concept 4.3), while training does little to the magnitude of PCr stores (Spriet, 2006). At rest, the total Cr pool is composed of approximately two-thirds PCr and one-third Cr (Walliman et al., 2011), but the PCr:Cr ratio decreases during exercise, with the decrease being greatest during high-intensity exercise. This is important, as Cr stimulates oxidative phosphorylation (Walsh et al., 2001). Moreover, the CK reaction

Bioenergetics Concept 4.3

Creatine monohydrate supplementation

Creatine can be synthesized endogenously, being obtained through the ingestion of foods such as meats and fish. However, supplemental creatine ingestion via creatine monohydrate can elevate total Cr and PCr pools within skeletal muscle by 5–20% (Wallimann, Tokarska-Schlattner, & Schlattner, 2011). A typical dosing regimen begins with 20 g Cr/day (4 doses of 5 g separated by 4 to 5 hours) for 4 to 6 days, followed by 3–5 g Cr/day for 1 to 6 months (Bemben & Lamont, 2005; Spriet, 2006).

Most of the ergogenic effects of creatine supplementation are related to energy provision, and it has been shown to be effective at improving performance in repeated, short bouts of high-intensity activity, where power output has been shown to be increased and there is a greater PCr resynthesis during the recovery periods (Bemben & Lamont, 2005). Therefore, creatine supplementation may be effective for athletes involved in repeated-sprint sports such as soccer, football, and basketball. Creatine supplementation has also been shown to promote glycogen loading, particularly in slow fibers (Hespel, Op't Eijnde, Derave, & Richter, 2001). However, it should be noted that improved performance following creatine supplementation is not a universal finding in the literature (Bemben & Lamont, 2005; Hespel et al., 2001). Furthermore, there is an increase in body mass associated with creatine supplementation, probably due to intracellular water retention (Bemben & Lamont, 2005), which may hinder performance in certain events.

It has been proposed that creatine supplementation may lower the production of reactive oxygen species in the intramitochondrial matrix (and thereby limit fatigue), activate signaling pathways involved in muscle cell differentiation, and reduce the appearance of inflammation markers and muscle damage during endurance exercises (Walliman et al., 2011), although further research is required to substantiate these claims. Aside from the proposed athletic performance benefits, creatine supplementation has been proposed to confer many health benefits, including improved glucose tolerance when combined with an exercise program, neuroprotective effects, and improved cognitive functioning (Wallimann et al., 2011). As with the purported performance benefits, however, further research is required to substantiate these claims.

---

also consumes H^+, which is likely to maintain the alkalinity of the cellular environment (Robergs, Ghiasvand, & Parker, 2004).

PCr is a high-energy molecule (with a higher free energy than even ATP) that serves a number of functions within the muscle fiber beyond providing immediate energy to resynthesize ATP (Greenhaff, 2001; Wallimann et al., 2011):

- PCr is an intracellular energy transporter that is able to transport the energy associated with ATP from the sites of resynthesis (i.e., glycolysis, mitochondria) to the sites of consumption (i.e., Na^+-K^+, Ca^{2+}, and actomyosin ATPase) in the **CK–PCr shuttle**. Specifically, Cr moves from the sites of ATP consumption to the sites of ATP resynthesis, with PCr moving in the opposite direction. This is important because ATP is not readily able to diffuse across the cell, so PCr acts as a spatial energy buffer.

■ PCr is a metabolic regulator. Notice that in the CK reaction, both ADP and H^+ are consumed; therefore, combining Equations (4.1) and (4.3), the net products of the ATPase and CK reactions results in the liberation of Cr and P_i. This is important because P_i is a substrate for phosphorylase, and therefore PCr degradation can exert an influence in controlling the rate of glycolysis within the cell.

■ Finally, Cr stimulates oxidative phosphorylation by increasing the ADP concentration in the locale of the mitochondria via the CK–PCr shuttle, so VO_2 is closely associated with the energy demand within the active muscles.

Although ATP concentrations within an active muscle cell remain relatively stable, stores of PCr can be almost completely degraded, with approximately 75–85% of the decline in PCr stores occurring in the first 10 s of maximal-intensity exercise (Gastin, 2001). The complete resynthesis of PCr can take between 5 and 15 minutes, depending upon the extent of the degradation of the stores during the exercise bout (Baker et al., 2010), and requires both glycolytic and mitochondrial ATP (Chung et al., 1998; Forbes, Paganini, Slade, Towse, & Meyer, 2009; Haseler, Hogan, & Richardson, 1999; Quistorff, Johansen, & Sahlin, 1993). Specifically, isoforms of CK are coupled with both the glycolytic and oxidative energy pathways that resynthesize some of the Cr within the cytosol to PCr. It appears that the resynthesis of PCr via mitochondrial ATP is particularly important following an exercise bout (Chung et al., 1998; Quistorff et al., 1993). Indeed, PCr resynthesis is used as a measure of mitochondrial functioning (Tarnopolsky & Raha, 2005; Tonkonogi & Sahlin, 2002). The recovery of PCr stores following exercise tends to follow a biexponential pattern, particularly following low-intensity exercise, being almost entirely dependent upon mitochondrial ATP (Haseler et al., 1999). Following high-intensity exercise, the response is more complicated, with an initial fast phase of recovery (< 15 s) dependent upon glycolytic ATP, and with the remaining resynthesis dependent upon mitochondrial ATP (Forbes et al., 2009). Because PCr degradation is very responsive to the energy demands of the muscle cell, resynthesis of PCr takes place during recovery as opposed to during work periods, a very important fact during activities involving the repetition of high-intensity work bouts such as the repeated-sprint activities associated with sports such as rugby, soccer, and tennis. Furthermore, incomplete resynthesis of PCr stores during the short recoveries associated with these sports (≤ 30 s) will compromise power output during the subsequent work bouts. These issues will be discussed later in this chapter.

The second reaction in the phosphagen system is the **adenylate kinase reaction** (Baker et al., 2010):

$$2ADP \overset{\text{adenylate kinase}}{\longleftrightarrow} ATP + AMP \qquad \text{Eq. (4.4)}$$

where ADP is adenosine diphosphate, adenylate kinase is the enzyme that catalyzes the reaction, ATP is adenosine triphosphate, and AMP is adenosine monophosphate. The production of AMP associated with the adenylate kinase (AK) reaction is important not only for resynthesizing ATP but also because AMP activates the enzymes phosphorylase and phosphofructokinase, stimulating ATP resynthesis via glycolysis (Spriet, 2006).

The third reaction in the phosphagen system is the **AMP deaminase reaction** (Baker et al., 2010):

$$AMP + H^+ \xrightarrow{\text{AMP deaminase}} IMP + NH_4^+ \qquad \text{Eq. (4.5)}$$

where AMP is adenosine monophosphate, H^+ is hydrogen, AMP deaminase is the enzyme that catalyzes the reaction, IMP is inosine monophosphate, and NH_4^+ is ammonium. Although the AMP deaminase reaction does not resynthesize ATP, the reaction is important in maintaining the activity of the AK reaction in generating ATP by reducing the concentration of AMP within the cytosol, as per Equation (4.4) (Spriet, 2006). Increases of IMP and NH_4^+ in the muscle cell are indicative of energy deficiency, so high levels of both may be expected in the blood of sprinters following high-intensity activities (Hancock et al., 2006; Sahlin, 2006). Collectively, the AK and AMP deaminase reactions act to limit the increase in ADP in times of high ATP demand, preserving the free energy of ATP hydrolysis (Hancock et al., 2006).

Glycolysis

Glycolysis involves the degradation of glucose 6-phosphate (G_6P) to pyruvate through a series of reactions in the cytosol to provide the energy to resynthesize ATP (Robergs et al., 2004). The process can be divided into two phases based upon the consumption of ATP (phase 1, Preparatory Reactions) and the generation of ATP (phase 2, Energy Harvesting Reactions) (Figure 4.2).

G_6P can be derived from either blood glucose or muscle glycogen with differences in the ATP yield. For example, the degradation of glucose to pyruvate yields three ATP for each pyruvate produced (Robergs et al., 2004):

$$Glucose + 2ADP + 2P_i + 2NAD^+ \rightarrow 2ATP + 2Pyruvate + 2NADH + 2H_2O + 2H^+$$

$$\text{Eq. (4.6)}$$

where ADP is adenosine diphosphate, P_i is inorganic phosphate, NAD^+ is the oxidized form of nicotinamide adenine dinucleotide, ATP is adenosine triphosphate, NADH is the reduced form of nicotinamide adenine dinucleotide, H_2O is water, and H^+ is hydrogen. Alternatively, the degradation of glycogen yields three ATP for each pyruvate produced (Robergs et al., 2004):

$$Glycogen + 3ADP + 3P_i + 2NAD^+ \rightarrow 3ATP + 2Pyruvate + 2NADH + 2H_2O + 1H^+$$

$$\text{Eq. (4.7)}$$

The reduced ATP yield associated with the degradation of glucose compared to glycogen comes from the hydrolysis of ATP required to phosphorylate glucose to G_6P, a step that is absent when glycogen is the substrate (Baker et al., 2010). Furthermore, there is a net release of two H^+ when glucose is the substrate, as opposed to only one when glycogen is degraded (Robergs et al., 2004). The protons associated with H^+ will increase the acidity of the cellular environment (decreased pH); degrading glucose as opposed to glycogen is therefore likely to result in a greater decrease in the cellular pH. During times of high energy demand when high rates of glycolysis are required, glycogen is the major substrate, as the uptake of glucose from the blood is limited and also the phosphorylation of glucose to G_6P within the cytosol is inhibited (Sahlin, 2006).

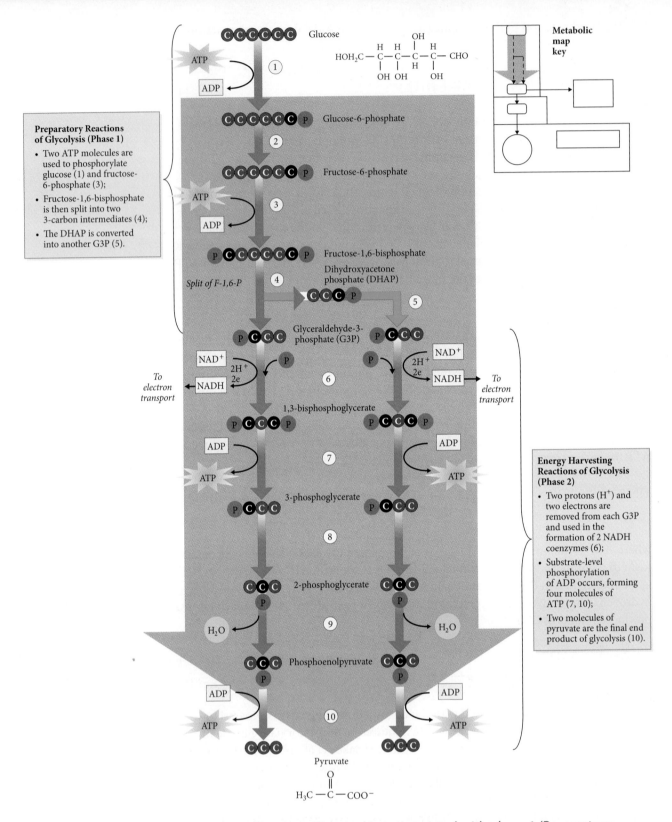

Figure 4.2 The reactions involved in glycolysis. The reactions associated with phase 1 (Preparatory Reactions) consume ATP whereas those in phase 2 (Energy Harvesting Reactions) resynthesize ATP such that there is a net gain in ATP as glucose 6-phosphate is degraded to pyruvate.

Muscle glycogen stores are greater in fast-muscle fiber types (De Bock, Derave, Ramaekers, Richter, & Hespel, 2007; Esbjörnsson-Liljedahl, Sundberg, Norman, & Jansson, 1999), and muscle glycogen stores can have a significant effect on exercise performance (see Bioenergetics Concept 4.4).

Bioenergetics Concept 4.4

Carbohydrate ingestion and exercise performance

Carbohydrate is a fuel source for both anaerobic (glycolysis) and aerobic (oxidative phosphorylation) energy pathways involved in the resynthesis of ATP. Carbohydrate stores are located in the muscle and liver as glycogen and in the blood as glucose, with the largest stores being those of muscle glycogen (see Table 4.3). Muscle glycogen is a very important source of fuel during exercise: Endurance performance is directly related to muscle glycogen stores at the initiation of the exercise bout, the perception of fatigue during prolonged exercise follows the decline in muscle glycogen stores, and high-intensity exercise is dependent upon muscle glycogen (Burke et al., 2011; Ivy, 2004). Therefore, recommendations have been made that ensure that the carbohydrate availability for both endurance and power athletes in relation to their workouts is appropriate (Burke et al., 2011; Stellingwerff, Maughan, & Burke, 2011). These recommendations vary between 3–5 g/kg body mass/day and 8–12 g/kg body mass/day, depending upon the intensity and duration of activities undertaken. Furthermore, carbohydrate loading prior to an activity and the ingestion of carbohydrate during an activity have been shown to improve performance in endurance events of both continuous and intermittent nature (Balsom, Wood, Olsson, & Ekblom, 1999; Hawley, Schabort, Noakes, & Dennis, 1997), while the ingestion of carbohydrate prior to and during a resistance training workout attenuates the reduction in muscle glycogen and results in a greater amount of work performed during a second resistance-training session later in the day (Haff et al., 1999; Haff et al., 2000).

Although both long-term endurance training and resistance training have been shown to increase muscle glycogen stores (Burgomaster, Hughes, Heigenhauser, Bradwell, & Gibala, 2005; Greiwe et al., 1999; MacDougall, Ward, Sale, & Sutton, 1977), the restoration following exercise is a relatively slow process. Therefore, supplementation with 1.2 g/kg body mass immediately post-exercise with the addition of a small amount of protein (~6–20 g) increases the rate of muscle glycogen repletion and also promotes protein synthesis while reducing protein degradation (Burke et al., 2011; Ivy, 2004). Somewhat paradoxically, there is recent evidence suggesting that the undertaking of some endurance workouts with low carbohydrate availability may promote greater adaptations (e.g., mitochondrial biogenesis) than when training with high carbohydrate availability (Hawley & Burke, 2010). However, further research is required to elucidate the specifics of the regimen (e.g., amount of carbohydrate depletion, number of sessions performed in the state of low carbohydrate availability), the cellular mechanisms behind this phenomenon, and indeed whether the increased adaptations translate into performance improvements.

The degradation of glycogen to G_6P requires that glycogen first be degraded to glucose 1-phosphate (glycogenolysis), the rate of which is controlled by the **phosphorylase** enzyme (see Figure 4.2). A rate-limiting step in glycolysis is the conversion of fructose 6-phosphate to fructose 1,6-bisphosphate (Figure 4.2), which is controlled by the enzyme **phosphofructokinase**. The activity of both of these enzymes is increased by ADP concentrations, while their activities are reduced by acidosis (Sahlin, 2006). Therefore, the high rates of ATP hydrolysis during times of high energy demands can stimulate glycolysis in a feed-forward manner through increased ADP concentrations; however, the H^+ produced by ATP hydrolysis and glycolysis inhibits glycolysis through feedback. Therefore, increases in intracellular H^+ buffering will augment the rate and capacity of the glycolytic energy pathway (Sahlin, 2006; see Bioenergetics Concept 4.5).

Pyruvate, which is the end product of glycolysis, can be converted to acetyl-CoA via **pyruvate dehydrogenase** (PDH) and oxidized in the mitochondria (Hargreaves, 2006). Alternatively, when the energy demand of the muscle cell is high, such as during high-intensity exercise, pyruvate and NADH accumulate, activating **lactate dehydrogenase** (LDH) via mass action to stimulate the conversion of pyruvate to lactate (van Hall, 2010):

$$\text{Pyruvate} + \text{NADH} \overset{\text{LDH}}{\longleftrightarrow} \text{Lactate} + \text{NAD}^+ \qquad \textbf{Eq. (4.8)}$$

where NADH is the reduced form of nicotinamide adenine dinucleotide, LDH is lactate dehydrogenase, the enzyme that catalyzes the reaction, and NAD^+ is the oxidized form of nicotinamide adenine dinucleotide. The LDH reaction is important as it oxidizes NADH, allowing NAD^+ to reenter glycolysis (see the glyceraldehyde-3-phosphate dehydrogenase reaction in phase 2, Figure 4.2). This allows glycolysis to continue to provide ATP at high rates. The fate of pyruvate gives rise to **alactic glycolysis** (pyruvate to acetyl-CoA conversion) or **lactic glycolysis** (pyruvate to lactate conversion). PDH that catalyzes the pyruvate to acetyl-CoA reaction has a limited capacity, and therefore the rapid formation of lactate is associated with a buildup of pyruvate and NADH. This occurs at times when the demand for ATP is high, such as during the transition from rest to exercise, with an associated oxygen deficit or when the exercise intensity is sufficiently high. When the demand for ATP is low, as during alactic glycolysis, the NADH produced by glycolysis is shuttled to the mitochondria via the malate–aspartate shuttle system for oxidative phosphorylation. NADH is the primary reducing equivalent in the electron transport chain where electrons are removed from H^+ before passing them to O_2 to provide energy to resynthesize ATP.

Lactate production has been shown to begin almost at the onset of muscle activation during maximal-intensity exercise efforts of ≤ 30 s, although there appears to be a lag of approximately 15 s before there is a rapid rise in lactate in the blood (Calbet, De Paz, Garatachea, Cabeza de Vaca, & Chavarren, 2003). Even during resting conditions, lactate is found in small quantities in the blood due to production by red blood cells (which lack mitochondria) and the activity of some glycolytic fast-muscle fibers. The quantity of lactate within the blood at any given time reflects the sum of the clearance from and the uptake by the muscles, although other tissues such as the heart, kidneys, and brain also take up lactate (van Hall, 2010). When blood lactate values increase, it can either reflect an increase in the production of lactate within the muscle fibers that effluxes to the blood or a decrease in the clearance of lactate from the blood via uptake by the muscle fibers. It should be noted that lactate is not the cause of fatigue; the high

Bioenergetics Concept 4.5

Buffering intracellular H⁺

H^+ ions are produced when ATP is hydrolyzed and as a result of the activation of the glycolytic energy pathway. At low exercise intensities, the H^+ would be transported to the mitochondria via the high-energy reducing equivalents NADH and $FADH_2$; however, during high-intensity exercise, H^+ ions accumulate in the cytosol. The accumulation of H^+ ions limits the rate of glycogenolysis/glycolysis via the inhibition of phosphorylase and phosphofructokinase. Furthermore, H^+ ions are associated with a reduction in crossbridge sensitivity as they compete with Ca^{2+} for the troponin C molecule (Fitts, 2008). Both of these situations would result in a reduced power output that is characteristic of fatigue.

Cellular buffering refers to processes that reduce the number of free H^+, thereby reducing fluctuations in cellular pH (Juel, 2008). At rest the pH within the muscle fibers is 7.0, while it can fall below 6.8 during exercise (McNaughton, Siegler, & Midgley, 2008). The mechanisms that act to maintain cellular pH include the following:

- Intracellular proteins and phosphates (e.g., carnosine, histidine, P_i)

- Metabolic buffering (e.g., CK, AMP deaminase, lactate dehydrogenase reactions)

- Extracellular fluid (plasma bicarbonate)

The movement of H^+ ions from the muscle fiber involves a series of transport proteins including the Na-H^+ and the monocarboxylic (MCT) transporters, both of which are increased following high-intensity training (Juel et al., 2004). Beyond training-induced increases in buffering, there have been a number of supplements that have been investigated in order to maintain muscle pH during exercise. The ingestion of **sodium bicarbonate** ($NaHCO_3$) is proposed to increase plasma bicarbonate concentrations, buffering H^+ through the formation of carbonic acid, eventually forming H_2O and CO_2, which are excreted via ventilation (nonmetabolic CO_2). The ingestion of 0.3 g/kg body mass of $NaHCO_3$ has been shown to maintain acid–base balance during exercise, resulting in an increased power output and time to exhaustion in events lasting between 1 and 5 minutes while also improving repeated sprint activities (Carr, Hopkins, & Gore, 2011; McNaughton et al., 2008; Stellingwerff et al., 2011). Gastrointestinal disturbances are often reported following $NaHCO_3$ supplementation, leading to the proposal that combining $NaHCO_3$ with **sodium citrate** or the ingestion of sodium citrate alone may be beneficial. However, sodium citrate has not been shown to be as effective as $NaHCO_3$ at improving performance (Carr et al., 2011). Supplementation with **β-alanine** in doses of 3–6 g/day has been shown to increase muscle carnosine content and increase buffering capacity, resulting in improvements in performance during events lasting 1 to 6 minutes (Stellingwerff et al., 2011).

blood lactate levels that are observed at exhaustion during exercise appear to be epi-phenomenal as opposed to causative, although lactate may result in slightly reduced Ca^{2+} release during muscle activation (Cairns, 2006). Furthermore, lactate can actually be considered to be ergogenic; given the reversible nature of the lactate dehydrogenase reaction, lactate can be transformed to pyruvate and used as a substrate for oxidative phosphorylation (van Hall, 2010), while lactate is also a gluconeogenic precursor via the Cori cycle in the liver (Cairns, 2006).

The movement of lactate across the sarcolemma requires facilitative transport via **monocarboxylate transporters** (MCTs), of which 14 variants have been identified (Bonen, 2006). MCT1 and MCT4 have been identified in skeletal muscle, and there is some evidence that the MCT1 variant, which is largely expressed in slow, oxidative muscle fibers, facilitates the uptake of lactate from the circulation and other fibers in close proximity. The MCTs also cotransport protons out from and in to the cytosol, and the activities of the MCT is dependent upon the pH and lactate gradients (Brooks, 2009; Thomas, Bishop, Lambert, Mercier, & Brooks, 2012). At times when both lactate and H^+ production increase in the cytosol (i.e., transitions from rest to exercise, high-intensity exercise), particularly in type II fibers, there may be an increased lactate and H^+ efflux from the muscle fibers via MCT1 and MCT4 and potentially an increased influx of lactate (and H^+) by MCT1 transporters of type I fibers (Thomas et al., 2012), although this has yet to be clearly established (Bonen, 2006). However, others have suggested a compartmentalization of lactate pools within muscle fibers—a myofibrillar pool of newly synthesized lactate derived from the conversion of pyruvate produced from glycolysis within the cytosol and an intermyofibrillar pool derived from extracel-lular lactate and pyruvate destined for the mitochondria (van Hall, 2010). Within the myofibrillar pool, lactate formation is catalyzed via the LDH reaction because of the high concentrations of both pyruvate and NADH associated with glycolysis, whereas pyruvate conversion from extracellular lactate is catalyzed in the intermyofibrillar pool given the low pyruvate and high NAD^+ associated with the close proximity to mitochondria. The existence of these distinct lactate pools within the muscle cell can explain the observation that skeletal muscle can simultaneously take up and release lactate (van Hall, 2010). To date, the specifics of lactate kinetics still remain an area of debate (Brooks, 2009; Cairns, 2006; Gladden, 2004; van Hall, 2010). However, the occurrence of lactate in the blood provides useful information to the strength and conditioning practitioner regarding the training status of athletes (see Bioenergetics Concept 4.6).

Bioenergetics Concept 4.6

What does blood lactate tell the practitioner?

Blood lactate concentrations are largely due to the interplay of production by the muscles that efflux to the blood and the clearance from the blood via skeletal muscle uptake. Lactate diffusion and carrier-mediated lactate exchange via monocarboxylic transporters (MCTs) occur down lactate gradients (Brooks, 2009). Mitochondrial respiration is important in maintaining glycolytic flux via the oxidation of NADH and pyruvate and therefore in determining the concen-tration of lactate; this will determine the lactate gradient across the sarcolemma and therefore the movement of lactate from or into the muscle fiber.

Type I muscle fibers, with their greater mitochondrial masses (Schiaffino & Reggiani, 2011) and greater concentration of MCT1 (Thomas et al., 2012), would tend to favor the influx of lactate from the blood into the cytosol. Endurance training has been shown to result in an increase in the oxidative capacity of muscle fibers and an increase in mitochondrial proteins (Yan, Okutsu, Akhtar, & Lira, 2011), as well as an up-regulation of MCT1 (Bonen, 2006), and an increase in capillarization (Juel et al., 2004). Furthermore, endurance training appears to increase lactate clearance from the blood as opposed to altering the production of lactate within the muscle fiber (Brooks, 2009). Type II muscle fibers, on the other hand, have a lower mitochondrial mass and greater glycogen stores (Schiaffino & Reggiani, 2011) and tend to produce greater amounts of lactate (Esbjörnsson-Liljedahl et al., 1999). Furthermore, these fibers have a lower concentration of MCT1 (Bonen, 2006). Therefore, type II fibers are likely to have lactate gradients and transport proteins that favor the efflux of lactate to the blood.

The recording of blood lactate values during exercise can provide an indication of the training status of the athlete. One would expect that power-trained and sprint-trained athletes, with their greater proportion of type II fibers, should produce high blood lactate values. This would be indicative of a high glycolytic rate and therefore a high rate of ATP resynthesis allowing the ATP-consuming reactions, and therefore exercise, to continue at a high rate. Conversely, endurance-trained athletes should produce low blood lactate concentrations, certainly at submaximal intensities, given their greater proportion of type I fibers. Indeed, this is the basis of establishing the **lactate threshold** of an endurance athlete. In this way, blood lactate informs the practitioner of the training status of an athlete.

Glycolysis is activated very rapidly but does not reach its maximal rate of ATP resynthesis until approximately 10 s after the initiation of exercise and sustains this rate for several seconds (Baker et al., 2010). Notice in Equations (4.6) and (4.7) that carbohydrate is the only substrate used in glycolysis. The typical energy yield is 3 mM ATP from carbohydrate during lactic glycolysis, in contrast to an energy yield of ~38 mM ATP from carbohydrate during oxidative phosphorylation (Spriet & Hargreaves, 2006). The higher rate of ATP provision when carbohydrate is metabolized anaerobically comes at a cost of a lower energy yield.

Oxidative phosphorylation

Oxidative phosphorylation is the final pathway that is able to provide the energy to regenerate ATP and takes place exclusively in the mitochondria. The energy is provided by the breakdown of mainly carbohydrates or lipid substrates, although protein catabolism can also provide energy but contributes less than 5% during exercise (Maughan, 2011). There are essentially two parts to oxidative phosphorylation, beginning with the degradation of acetyl coenzyme A (acetyl-CoA) to carbon dioxide and hydrogen ions in the **citric acid cycle** (CAC) (Maughan, 2011):

$$\text{Acetyl-CoA} + \text{ADP} + 3\text{NAD}^+ + \text{FAD} \rightarrow 2\text{CO}_2 + \text{ATP} + 3\text{NADH} + 3\text{H}^+ + \text{FADH}_2$$

Eq. (4.9)

where acetyl-CoA is acetyl coenzyme A, ADP is adenosine diphosphate, NAD^+ is the oxidized form of nicotinamide adenine dinucleotide, FAD is the oxidized form of flavin adenine dinucleotide, CO_2 is carbon dioxide, ATP is adenosine triphosphate, NADH is the reduced form of nicotinamide adenine dinucleotide, H^+ is hydrogen, and $FADH_2$ is the reduced form of flavin adenine dinucleotide. The various stages in the CAC are shown in **Figure 4.3**.

Acetyl-CoA can be derived from glucose or glycogen via the transformation of pyruvate, which is controlled by the enzyme pyruvate dehydrogenase (PDH) located in the mitochondria. PDH is important as it not only regulates glycolytic flux to the CAC, but it also determines the rate of glycolysis and lactate formation and is activated in response to high levels of pyruvate and cystolic Ca^{2+} as well as the phosphorylation and redox potentials of the cell (Brooks, Fahey, & Baldwin, 2005). Acetyl-CoA can also be derived from lipids via **beta-oxidation**, which takes place in the mitochondria (Jeukendrup, Saris, & Wagenmakers, 1998).

Notice in Equation (4.9) that O_2 does not participate in the degradation of acetyl-CoA in the CAC, and there is a low yield of ATP (strictly, it is guanosine triphosphate, which is energetically equivalent to ATP, that is generated). The importance of the CAC is the generation of high-energy reducing equivalents NADH and $FADH_2$, which transport H^+ to the **electron transport chain** (ETC). As shown in **Figure 4.4**, the ETC is a series of reactions that remove electrons from H^+, passing them to O_2 to ultimately form H_2O (Maughan, 2011).

The requirement of O_2 in the ETC renders oxidative phosphorylation an aerobic process, and the supply of O_2 to the working muscle via blood flow is likely to limit oxidative phosphorylation during exercise. The energy generated in the transfer of the electrons in the ETC is conserved as chemical potential energy in the form of ATP. The reactions of the ETC when starting with glucose can be summarized as follows (Maughan, 2011):

$$\text{Glucose} + 6O_2 + 38ADP + 38P_i \rightarrow 6CO_2 + 6H_2O + 38ATP \qquad \text{Eq. (4.10)}$$

where O_2 is oxygen, ADP is adenosine diphosphate, P_i is inorganic phosphate, CO_2 is carbon dioxide, and ATP is adenosine triphosphate. When a fatty acid such as palmitate (a saturated fatty acid) is oxidized, the reactions of the ETC can be summarized as follows (Maughan, 2011):

$$\text{Palmitate} + 23O_2 + 130ADP + 130P_i \rightarrow 16CO_2 + 146H_2O + 130ATP \quad \text{Eq. (4.11)}$$

where O_2 is oxygen, ADP is adenosine diphosphate, P_i is inorganic phosphate, CO_2 is carbon dioxide, H_2O is water, and ATP is adenosine triphosphate. When comparing Equations (4.10) and (4.11), it can be seen that the ATP yield from lipids greatly exceeds that from carbohydrate; fat contains 38 kJ/g (9 kcal/g) of energy compared to 18 kJ/g (4 kcal/g) of energy for carbohydrate (Jeukendrup et al., 1998; See **Worked Example 4.3**). Furthermore, the stores of fats in the body greatly exceed those of carbohydrates (**Table 4.3**) while carbohydrates must be stored in the presence of water, increasing the associated mass of the substrate when compared to fat (Jeukendrup et al., 1998).

The oxidation of fats provides the energy to resynthesize ATP at a rate less than twice of that associated with the oxidation of carbohydrate (Jeukendrup et al., 1998). This translates into a lower intensity of exercise being sustained by fat oxidation when compared to carbohydrate oxidation. For example, it has been estimated that

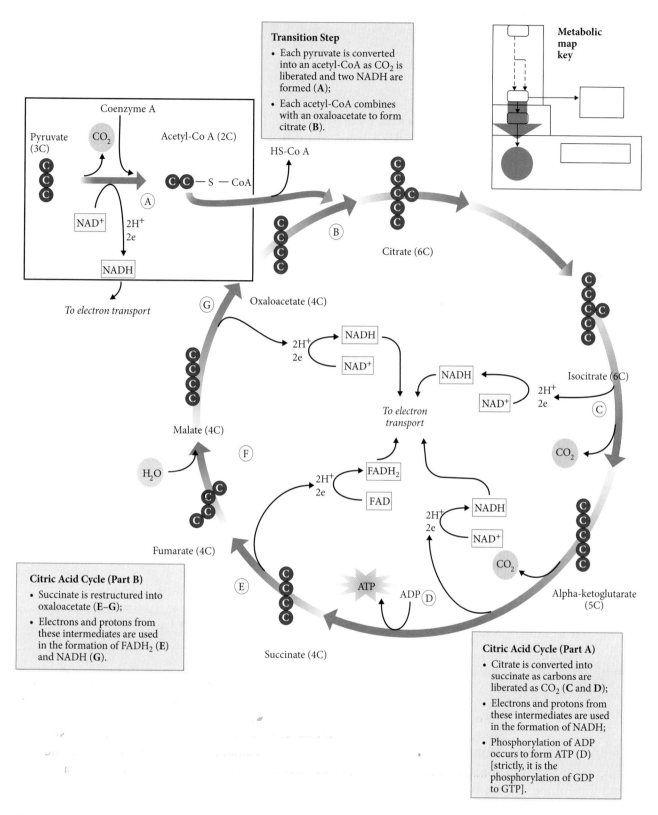

Transition Step
- Each pyruvate is converted into an acetyl-CoA as CO_2 is liberated and two NADH are formed (**A**);
- Each acetyl-CoA combines with an oxaloacetate to form citrate (**B**).

Metabolic map key

Coenzyme A

Pyruvate (3C)

CO_2

Acetyl-Co A (2C)

HS-Co A

NAD^+

$2H^+$
$2e$

NADH

To electron transport

Oxaloacetate (4C)

Citrate (6C)

$2H^+$
$2e$

NADH

NAD^+

NADH

NAD^+

Isocitrate (6C)

To electron transport

$2H^+$
$2e$

C

CO_2

Malate (4C)

H_2O

FADH₂ → FAD

$2H^+$
$2e$

NADH

NAD^+

$2H^+$
$2e$

CO_2

Fumarate (4C)

ATP

ADP D

Alpha-ketoglutarate (5C)

Citric Acid Cycle (Part B)
- Succinate is restructured into oxaloacetate (**E–G**);
- Electrons and protons from these intermediates are used in the formation of FADH₂ (**E**) and NADH (**G**).

Succinate (4C)

Citric Acid Cycle (Part A)
- Citrate is converted into succinate as carbons are liberated as CO_2 (**C** and **D**);
- Electrons and protons from these intermediates are used in the formation of NADH;
- Phosphorylation of ADP occurs to form ATP (D) [strictly, it is the phosphorylation of GDP to GTP].

Figure 4.3 The reactions in the citric acid cycle.

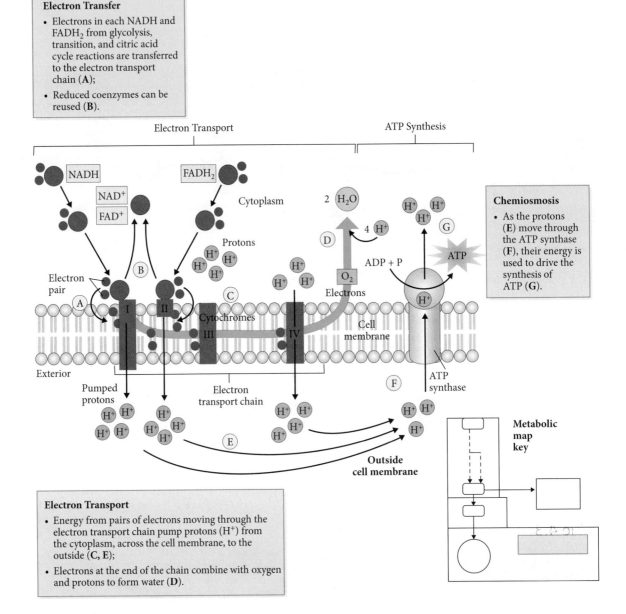

Electron Transfer
- Electrons in each NADH and FADH$_2$ from glycolysis, transition, and citric acid cycle reactions are transferred to the electron transport chain (**A**);
- Reduced coenzymes can be reused (**B**).

Chemiosmosis
- As the protons (**E**) move through the ATP synthase (**F**), their energy is used to drive the synthesis of ATP (**G**).

Electron Transport
- Energy from pairs of electrons moving through the electron transport chain pump protons (H$^+$) from the cytoplasm, across the cell membrane, to the outside (**C, E**);
- Electrons at the end of the chain combine with oxygen and protons to form water (**D**).

Figure 4.4 The reactions involved in the electron transport chain.

the oxidation of fats is only able to sustain exercise at intensities of approximately 55–75% VO$_{2max}$, while the oxidation of carbohydrates is able to sustain exercise at 100% VO$_{2max}$ (Spriet & Hargreaves, 2006). Carbohydrates are also able to be degraded anaerobically to provide energy for ATP resynthesis, whereas lipids (and proteins) are not. However, a common training adaptation is a shift to fats as a fuel source in the endurance-trained state, with the oxidation of intramuscular triglyceride stores as the main fat source via the activation of **muscle-specific hormone sensitive lipase** (Phillips, 2006). This shift to the oxidation of lipids in the endurance-trained state is largely caused by an increase in mitochondrial mass within the muscle fibers (see Bioenergetics Concept 4.7). Both muscle-specific hormone sensitive lipase and

Worked Example 4.3
Carbohydrate versus fat as a substrate for endurance activity

The energy cost associated with running has been shown to be 1 kcal/km/kg (Rapoport, 2010). Calculate the mass associated with the stores of carbohydrate and fat for a 60-kg athlete completing a marathon.

i. Calculate total energy requirement for athlete $1 \times 42.195 \times 60 = 2531.7$ kcal

ii. Convert kcal to kJ $2531.7 \times 4186 = 10,597.7$ kJ

iii. Calculate mass of carbohydrate to yield 10597.7 kJ $10,597.7/18 = 589$ g

iv. Calculate mass of fat to yield 10597.7 kJ $10,597.7/38 = 279$ g

Notice that the required carbohydrate mass actually exceeds that typically stored in the body (Table 4.3). Furthermore, every gram of carbohydrate retains 1–3 g of water (Maughan, 2011), meaning that the mass of the carbohydrate stores is actually increased. The greater energy yield associated with the oxidation of fats means that the mass of the fat stores required to complete a given endurance event is much lower than the mass of carbohydrate. However, the much lower rate of energy provision associated with fat oxidation would necessitate a lower running speed to complete the event.

stores of triglycerides are greater in type I muscle fibers than type II fibers (Jeukendrup et al., 1998; Langfort et al., 1999).

There is a difference in the energy yield between the oxidation of carbohydrates and fats when expressed relative to O_2 consumption, with carbohydrates yielding 21.1 kJ/L O_2 (5 kcal/L O_2) while the oxidation of fats yields 19.6 kJ/L O_2 (4.7 kcal/l O_2) (Maughan, 2011). This difference comes from the energy transfer associated with substrate-level phosphorylation in the complete oxidation of carbohydrate (glycolysis) compared to fat (Scott, 2005). There is also a difference in the stoichiometry of O_2 uptake to CO_2 production between the oxidation of the two substrates, as shown in

Table 4.3
Typical Carbohydrate and Lipid Stores of an 80-kg Man in a Fasted and Rested State

Substrate	Location of Store	Mass of Store (kg)	Energy of Store (kJ)
Carbohydrate	Plasma glucose	0.02	320
	Liver glycogen	0.10	1600
	Muscle glycogen	0.40	6400
	Total carbohydrate	**0.52**	**8000**
Fat	Plasma fatty acid	0.0004	16
	Plasma triglycerides	0.004	160
	Adipose tissue	12	404,000
	Intramuscular triglycerides	0.30	10,800
	Total fat	**12.3**	**440,000**

Note: Values are approximate and can vary among individuals and over time within individuals. The energy stored in protein is not mentioned but would equate to approximately 10 kg (160,000 kJ), mainly in skeletal muscle.

Reproduced from Jeukendrup, A. E., Saris, W. H. M., & Wagenmakers, A. J. M. (1998). Fat metabolism during exercise: a review. Part I: fatty acid mobilization and muscle metabolism. *International Journal of Sports Medicine, 19*, 231–244. © Georg Thieme Verlag KG.

Bioenergetics Concept 4.7

Changes in mitochondrial density affect substrate utilization

Endurance training has been shown to increase mitochondrial mass via **mitochondrial biogenesis** (Yan, Lira, & Greene, 2011), which is typically assessed by the increased activity of mitochondrial enzymes. Indeed, the increase in mitochondrial mass following endurance training is responsible for the enormous increases in oxidative enzymes, such as succinate dehydrogenase, citrate synthase, and cytochrome oxidase (Gollnick & Saltin, 1982). Recently, it has been proposed that endurance exercise may also promote the maintenance and clearance of dysfunctional and damaged mitochondria, thus not only increasing the quantity but also the quality of mitochondria in the muscle fibers (Yan et al., 2012).

The mitochondria within skeletal muscle appear to function as an interconnected network, as opposed to individual units. Two different populations of mitochondria have been identified within skeletal muscle, both with different metabolic properties (Elander, Sjöström, Lundgren, Scherstén, & Bylund-Fellenius, 1985). The subsarcolemmal (SS) mitochondria are located beneath the sarcolemma and comprise approximately 25% of total mitochondrial mass within a muscle fiber, while the intermyofibrillar (IM) mitochondria are located toward the muscle fiber center. The SS mitochondria tend to be characterized by a markedly lower maximal oxidative capacity than the IM mitochondria, although the SS mitochondria tend to respond with greater increases in oxidative capacity following endurance training (Chilibeck, Bell, Socha, & Martin 1998). Furthermore, it is proposed that SS mitochondria adapt together with capillarization following endurance training, suggesting an adaptive response to facilitate O_2 delivery (Inger, 1979).

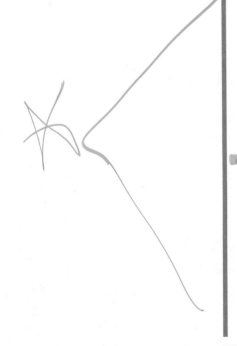

Mitochondrial activity is increased in response to increased cellular concentrations of ADP and Cr. Somewhat paradoxically, the sensitivity of an individual mitochondrion to changes in ADP is reduced, while there is a large increase in the sensitivity of a given mitochondrion to Cr. However, the increase in the mitochondrial mass of the endurance-trained muscle fibers means that there will be an increased mitochondrial ATP production for a given ADP concentration (Tonkonogi & Sahlin, 2002). This is referred to as **respiratory control** (Jones & DiMenna, 2011). Therefore, the capacity for the regulation of oxidative phosphorylation is greatly increased in an aerobically trained individual, and the phosphorylation potential (ATP:ADP concentrations) and redox potential (NAD^+:NADH concentrations) are defended during exercise. This is likely to have implications for the VO_2 kinetics, and therefore the O_2 deficit, during the transition from rest to exercise as well as work-to-work transitions associated with increasing intensity during continuous exercise bouts. The increased respiratory control exerted by the increased mitochondrial mass also reduces glycolytic flux, as the activation of phosphorylase and phosphofructokinase are sensitive to ADP concentrations, resulting in a reduced reliance on muscle glycogen in the endurance-trained muscle fiber (Phillips, 2006). This is also likely to reduce blood lactate in the endurance-trained athlete. Furthermore, the increase in oxidative enzymes that accompany the increase in mitochondrial mass following endurance training coupled with a constant supply of lipids as a substrate result in a greater reliance on fat oxidation following endurance training (Phillips, 2006).

Equations (4.10) and (4.11). The oxidation of carbohydrate produces 6 CO_2 for the consumption of 6 O_2, while that of palmitate produces 16 CO_2 for the consumption of 23 O_2. The ratio of CO_2 to O_2 is known as the **respiratory exchange ratio** (RER) and is lower for the oxidation of fats compared to carbohydrate due to the decarboxylation of pyruvate associated with carbohydrate oxidation (Scott, 2005). The RER therefore provides an indication of the substrate being oxidized during exercise.

Matching ATP Supply with Demand

The matching of ATP resynthesis to the ATP demand during exercise requires the activation of the specific energy pathways. The signals within the active cell that activate the energy pathways include the following (Spriet & Hargreaves, 2006):

- Ca^{2+} flux
- Phosphorylation potential of the cell expressed as the $[ATP]:[ADP][P_i]$ ratio
- Redox potential of the cell expressed as the $NAD^+:NADH$ ratio

These signals are important as they act as activators of, or substrates for, specific enzymes associated with the energy pathways. For example, Ca^{2+} activates phosphorylase, a rate-limiting enzyme involved in glycolysis, while ADP is a substrate for creatine kinase, the enzyme that catalyzes the breakdown of PCr to liberate energy. Both ADP and P_i activate phosphofructokinase, another rate-limiting enzyme of glycolysis. Increases in NADH activate lactate dehydrogenase to convert pyruvate, the end product of glycolysis, to lactate, while NADH is also a substrate for the electron transport chain associated with oxidative phosphorylation. Therefore, the signals listed above provide immediate feedback and feed-forward signals to the enzymes that ultimately control the energy pathways. Furthermore, the signals listed above also have consequences for long-term adaptations. For example, changes in Ca^{2+} flux during exercise such as would be experienced during low-intensity, long-duration exercise stimulate the activation of calcium-calmodulin kinase (CaMK), while alterations in the phosphorylation potential of the cell associated with higher intensity exercise stimulate the activation of AMP-activated protein kinase (AMPK). Both CaMK and AMPK signal the activation of PGC-1α, which is a key transcriptional cofactor in mitochondrial biogenesis (Adhihetty, Irrcher, Joseph, Ljubicic, & Hood, 2003). In this way, the alterations in the cellular milieu as a result of an exercise stimulus not only stimulate the energy pathways to ensure the matching of ATP supply with that of demand during the exercise bout, but they are also responsible for initiating the cellular adaptations observed following a training regimen.

Energy System Contributions During Exercise

An understanding of the contributions of the different energy pathways to the resynthesis of ATP during a given sporting performance is important for strength and conditioning practitioners as it allows the development of sport-specific tests and training programs. All pathways will contribute to the provision of ATP during most activities, but their relative contribution will largely depend upon the intensity and duration of the activity. Various methods have been used to establish the contribution of the energy pathways (see Bioenergetics Concept 4.8), each with their associated problems. The relative contributions to a given activity are further complicated by the mode of exercise and the training and nutritional status of the athlete under

Bioenergetics Concept 4.8

Assessing the contributions of energy systems during exercise

Indirect calorimetry techniques provide an estimate of energy expenditure via the quantities of respiratory gases O_2 and CO_2 in the inspired and expired air. The stoichiometry of the VO_2 to aerobic ATP production is known (see Equations 4.10 and 4.11), so the aerobic contribution to exercise can be easily determined. Furthermore, the respiratory exchange ratio can be used to determine the contribution of the oxidation of carbohydrates and fats in a given exercise bout. Some researchers have proposed that the anaerobic contribution to ATP resynthesis can also be expressed in units of O_2 consumption (Medbø et al., 1988). Indeed, it was proposed that the elevated VO_2 during the recovery following the completion of an exercise bout, the **oxygen debt** that is associated with the replenishment of myoglobin O_2 stores, PCr resynthesis, and the removal of metabolites (P_i, lactate) (Gaesser & Brooks, 1984), represented the anaerobic energy contribution using an application of energy conservation, although this was subsequently shown to be erroneous as it overestimates the anaerobic contribution to exercise (Scott, 2005). However, given the simple assumptions that (1) energy provision can be either anaerobic or aerobic, and (2) VO_2 represents the aerobic contribution to the exercise bout, the anaerobic contribution can be determined as the total energy release during the exercise less the aerobic contribution; that is, the total energy requirement expressed in units of O_2 minus the contribution of VO_2 during the bout (Medbø et al., 1988). Here, the contributions of anaerobic energy release are determined by the magnitude of the **oxygen deficit** and recorded in energy equivalents of O_2. Bundle, Hoyt, and Weyand, (2003) used this approach to determine the contribution of anaerobic and aerobic energy release to a series of maximal-effort runs of varying durations (see Figure 4.1). This method ignores O_2 bound to myoglobin and hemoglobin that can be consumed during the exercise bout, resulting in an overestimation of anaerobic contribution, although these O_2 stores are likely to be relatively small in comparison to the magnitude of the O_2 deficit during high-intensity exercise.

Although the oxygen deficit methods are noninvasive, they can be time consuming. Furthermore, they do not allow for the determination of the contributions of the different anaerobic pathways. **Muscle biopsies** can provide concentrations of both substrates and metabolites prior to and following exercise and therefore offer an indication of the contribution of each of the energy systems to the provision of energy during the exercise bout. However, the amount of muscle mass that is active during the exercise bout needs to be estimated to determine the overall anaerobic energy release. Furthermore, the timing at which the samples are taken relative to the exercise bout can have a significant impact on the observed concentrations, and of course, the collection of muscle biopsies is very invasive.

A noninvasive assessment of skeletal muscle metabolism *in vivo* can be obtained by **magnetic resonance spectroscopy** (MRS) techniques (Prompers et al., 2006). For example, ^{31}P MRS has been used to directly determine the concentrations of ATP, P_i, and PCr, as well as being used indirectly to establish intracellular pH values and ADP concentrations. From these data the glycogenolytic and oxidative flux and buffer capacity within the active muscles can be determined. ^1H MRS techniques are able to determine intramuscular lipid concentrations and lactate production, while ^{13}C MRS techniques can be used to quantify fluxes through specific energy pathways (e.g., ^{13}C-glucose) (Prompers et al., 2006). However, MRS techniques are currently limited to isolated muscle groups.

---

investigation. What follows is an overview of the contribution of the energy pathways to the provision of ATP during the transition from rest to exercise, during continuous exercise, and during repeated-sprint activities. This information can be used as a general guide to determine the metabolic requirements of different exercise activities.

Energy system contributions during the transition from rest to exercise

At the onset of exercise as the athlete transitions from rest to a given exercise intensity, the accumulation of metabolites associated with ATP hydrolysis (e.g., ADP, P_i) as well as increased Ca^{2+} flux stimulates the resynthesis of ATP via the CK reaction and glycolysis to meet the demands of the exercise. The activation of the phosphagen and glycolytic systems occurs during the transition from rest to exercise even when the intensity of the exercise can be met by the ATP resynthesis rate associated with oxidative phosphorylation. This is due to the finite time for the oxidative pathway to establish ATP resynthesis at the required rate or a limitation in O_2 supply (blood flow) to the mitochondria (Spriet, 2006). This gives rise to the oxygen deficit at the onset of an exercise bout (Figure 4.5).

Given the activation of substrate-level phosphorylation during the oxygen deficit, there will be an accumulation of metabolites associated with these systems (e.g., Cr, lactate, H^+) and a depletion of the substrates for these systems (e.g., PCr, muscle glycogen). This has important implications for subsequent exercise performance. The magnitude of the oxygen deficit will depend upon the required intensity of the exercise, with a greater intensity producing a greater deficit and therefore a greater contribution of the anaerobic energy systems, resulting in a greater accumulation of metabolites and a depletion of substrates. Moreover, the magnitude of the oxygen deficit is affected by the VO_2 kinetics, with a more rapid primary response of VO_2 (the initial rise in VO_2 at the onset of exercise; see Figure 4.5) reducing the oxygen deficit (Poole, Barstow, McDonough, & Jones, 2008). The primary response of VO_2 is largely dependent upon the respiratory control associated with the mitochondria, and it has been shown that endurance training results in a more rapid primary response of VO_2 (Poole et al., 2008). This would mean that an endurance-trained athlete is likely to incur a smaller oxygen deficit at the transition from rest to exercise and incur less metabolic disturbance from the reliance upon substrate-level phosphorylation during the transition.

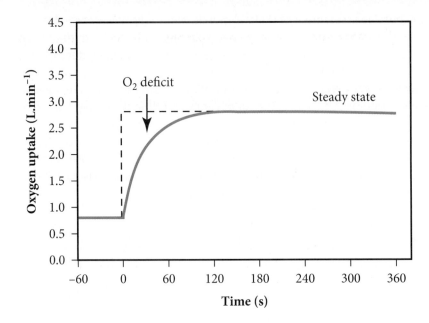

Figure 4.5 The oxygen deficit during the transition from rest to exercise. Note that VO$_2$, which reflects energy provision from oxidative phosphorylation, takes time to establish the required rate. The energy provision during this time is derived from substrate-level phosphorylation.

Reproduced from Burnley, M., & Jones, A. M. (2007). Oxygen uptake kinetics as a determinant of sports performance. *European Journal of Sport Science, 7*, 63–79.

Energy system contributions to continuous exercise

Continuous exercise refers to a single bout of exercise of a given intensity but finite duration, whether a maximal 5-s sprint or a submaximal 4-hour run. As one would expect, the contribution of the anaerobic energy systems (substrate-level phosphorylation) to an exhaustive bout of continuous exercise diminishes as the duration of the exercise increases (Table 4.4). Notice that in exhaustive exercise bouts lasting approximately 75 s there is an equal contribution from the anaerobic and aerobic energy systems, while even during exercise bouts as short as 10 s there is a contribution from the aerobic pathway, albeit a very small one.

The contributions from the reactions associated with the phosphagen system and glycolysis are not identified in Table 4.4. It was noted previously that the CK reaction reaches a maximal rate 1.3 s after the initiation of maximal-intensity exercise (Sahlin, 2006) and that a 75–85% decline in PCr stores occurs within the first 10 s of maximal-intensity exercise (Gastin, 2001). Gaitanos, Williams, Boobis, and Brooks, (1993) determined that 50% of the ATP provision during a single 6-s maximal sprint was derived from PCr degradation. It was also noted earlier that glycolysis is activated very rapidly but does not reach its maximal rate of ATP resynthesis until approximately 10 s after the initiation of maximal exercise, sustaining this rate for several seconds (Baker et al., 2010). Gaitanos et al. (1993) reported that glycolysis

Table 4.4

Estimated Contribution of the Anaerobic and Aerobic Energy Pathways to ATP Provision During Continuous Bouts of Exhaustive Exercise of Different Durations

Exercise Duration (s)	Anaerobic Contribution (%)	Aerobic Contribution (%)
0–10	94	6
0–5	88	12
0–20	82	18
0–30	73	27
0–45	63	37
0–60	55	45
0–75	49	51
0–90	44	56
0–120	37	63
0–180	27	73
0–240	21	79

Reproduced from Gastin, P. B. (2001). Energy system interaction and relative contribution during maximal exercise. *Sports Medicine, 31,* 725–741, with kind permission from Springer Science and Business Media.

contributed ~ 44% of the ATP provision during a single 6-s maximal sprint. Combining this information with the knowledge that there is a transition from predominantly anaerobic to predominantly aerobic energy provision after 75 s, we can determine the following:

- The PCr system contributes the largest energy provision during maximal bouts lasting ≤6 s.
- Glycolysis contributes the largest energy provision during maximal bouts lasting between 7 and 75 s.
- Oxidative phosphorylation contributes the largest energy provision during maximal bouts >75 s.

The relationship between the energy pathway contribution to total ATP provision and the duration of the exhaustive exercise bout is summarized in Figure 4.6.

The relative contribution of each energy system will vary with the training status of the individual athlete. Figure 4.7 shows the energy system contributions to ATP provision during maximal 90-s exercise bouts performed by sprint- and endurance-trained cyclists. Notice that the sprint-trained cyclists produced greater peak power outputs compared to the endurance-trained cyclists. However, the slope of the decline in power output is less in the endurance-trained cyclists, reflecting a lower fatigue in these athletes during the exercise bout. Furthermore, notice the greater PCr and glycolytic contributions early in the exercise bout for the sprint-trained cyclists compared to the endurance-trained cyclists, and contrast this with the greater aerobic contribution in the endurance-trained cyclists after approximately 20 s.

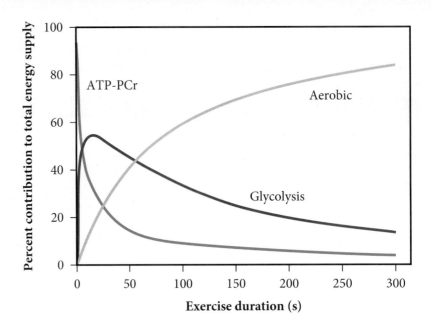

Figure 4.6 The relative energy pathway contribution to total ATP provision for a given duration of maximal-intensity exercise.

Reproduced from Gastin, P. B. (2001). Energy system interaction and relative contribution during maximal exercise. *Sports Medicine, 31*, 725–741, with kind permission from Springer Science and Business Media.

It has been shown that sprint-trained cyclists, who produce much greater maximal power outputs than endurance-trained cyclists during a maximal 30-s sprint effort, have a greater contribution to energy provision via the anaerobic pathways (Calbet et al., 2003). This greater anaerobic contribution is due to the greater percentage of fast-muscle fibers and the associated greater substrates (e.g., PCr, glycogen), enzymes (e.g., CK, PFK, LDH), and buffering capacity in the muscles of these athletes compared to their endurance-trained counterparts. The increased anaerobic contribution during short-duration maximal efforts by the sprint-trained athletes comes at a cost of greater fatigue during the effort.

The discussion of the energy pathway contributions during continuous exercise may imply a constant power output. Obviously, a constant power output is not achieved during maximal-intensity activity, as the mechanical power output will fluctuate; typically, maximal power output is achieved after approximately 5 s of maximal-intensity sprinting and then falls due to fatigue (Figure 4.7). However, there are likely to be fluctuations in power output during many longer-duration, submaximal activities, even when they are performed under controlled laboratory conditions. These fluctuations in power output are nonrandom (i.e., stochastic) and may reflect underlying control processes during the exercise activity (Tucker et al., 2006). It is probable that these fluctuations are even more likely during actual races where alterations in the terrain and the activity of opponents necessitate fluctuations in power output during the event. Such activity patterns can have significant implications for

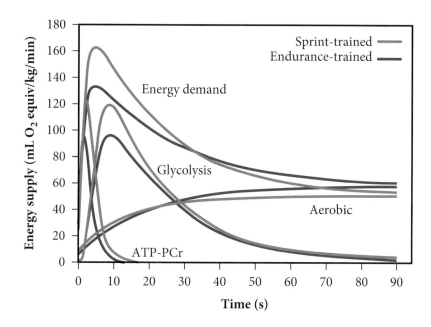

Figure 4.7 The energy system contribution to a maximal 90-s exercise bout in a group of sprint-trained and endurance-trained cyclists.

Reproduced from Gastin, P. B. (2001). Energy system interaction and relative contribution during maximal exercise. *Sports Medicine, 31,* 725–741, with kind permission from Springer Science and Business Media.

energy system utilization and therefore substrate utilization and metabolite accumulation within the muscle fibers that will ultimately influence the outcome in the event. Indeed, we can consider the stochastic fluctuations in power output during continuous activities as work-to-work transitions with the same metabolic consequences associated with the rest-to-exercise transition each time intensity is increased.

Energy system contributions to repeated-sprint activities

In many sports, athletes are required to perform short-duration, maximal sprints (≤ 10 s) and repeat them following a short recovery (≤ 60 s); these activity patterns characterize repeated sprints (Bishop & Girard, 2011) that are common in sports such as basketball, rugby, soccer, and tennis. Knowledge of the specific activity patterns in terms of the duration of the work and recovery periods is important because it can have a substantial effect on the contribution of the energy pathways to the activity. Specifically, as the number of short-duration, maximal sprints performed by the athlete increases, there is a decrease in the relative contribution of the anaerobic energy pathways, particularly glycolysis, and an increase in the aerobic energy pathway to ATP provision (Glaister, 2005). Power output during a 6-s maximal sprint relies predominantly on PCr degradation, which results in ~ 57% reduction in PCr stores (Gaitanos et al., 1993). Furthermore, the recovery of power output after maximal exercise follows the resynthesis of PCr stores (Glaister, 2005). However, during the short recovery periods associated with repeated-sprint activities, there will be incomplete PCr resynthesis, resulting in a reduced contribution from PCr degradation in successive sprints (Spencer, Bishop, Dawson, & Goodman, 2005). This will reduce the observed power output of the sprints. The decrease in power output across repeated sprints will depend upon the number of sprints undertaken as well as the duration of each sprint and the recovery period (**Figure 4.8**).

As the contribution of PCr degradation decreases with each successive sprint, so too does the contribution of glycolysis (Spencer et al., 2005), possibly due to a reduction in muscle glycogen and/or a decrease in intracellular pH (Glaister, 2005). Yet despite the reduced contribution of the anaerobic energy pathways to ATP provision during successive sprints, power output does not fall as precipitously as would be expected. This is due to the increased contribution from the aerobic pathway. Following a single sprint, there will be an elevation in VO_2 (oxygen debt) due to the requirement to replenish myoglobin O_2 stores, PCr resynthesis, and the removal of metabolites (e.g., P_i, lactate). A subsequent sprint will therefore be initiated from a higher O_2 level, providing a greater aerobic contribution to ATP provision during the sprint (Glaister, 2005).

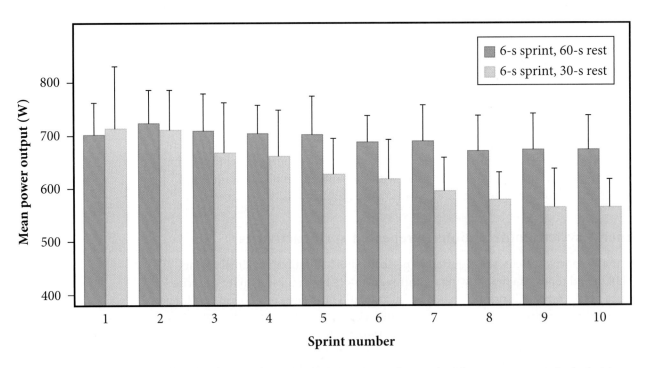

Figure 4.8 The power output during ten 6-s maximal sprints performed with a recovery period of either 60 s or 30 s. Notice the greater decline in power output when the recovery period is 30 s, most likely due to a reduced contribution of PCr degradation to each sprint as a result of incomplete resynthesis.

Bioenergetics and Fatigue

In the discussion of the energy pathways, it was noted that the maximal rate of ATP resynthesis sets an upper limit on exercise intensity, while the capacity of ATP resynthesis determines exercise duration at a given intensity (Sahlin et al., 1998). Therefore, the relationship between maximal running speed and the duration for which it can be sustained as depicted in Figure 4.1a is assumed to be largely due to the rate at which energy can be provided by the three energy pathways and their associated capacities. Figure 4.9 shows the power output achieved by individuals during a maximal 180-s exercise bout. What should be noted is that power output increases to a maximal value early in the bout (approximately 5 s) and then declines rapidly. Yet the rate at which power output declines as the exercise continues results in a hyperbolic relationship between power output and exercise time that qualitatively matches that in Figure 4.1a which was derived from separate exercise bouts performed at different intensities. The decline in power output in Figure 4.9 is fatigue, defined as a loss of muscle power output that is reversed with rest (Fitts, 2008).

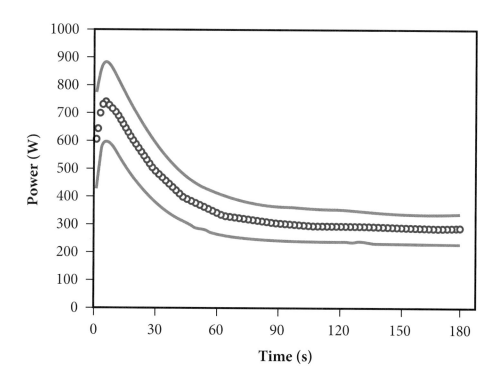

Figure 4.9 The mean (± standard deviation) power output from a group of participants performing a maximal 180-s exercise bout. Notice that peak power is achieved after approximately 5 s, then declines in a hyperbolic manner.

The cause of fatigue can be multifactorial, and the mechanisms responsible are largely dependent upon the intensity, duration, and mode of exercise as well as the training and nutritional status of the athlete and the environmental conditions associated with the exercise bout. However, the role of the energy pathways in fatigue is important. We have already shown here that performance is improved when the substrates for the resynthesis are increased as with creatine monohydrate and carbohydrate supplementation (Bemben & Lamont, 2005; Burke et al., 2011). Furthermore, increases in O_2 availability via hyperoxic breathing or increased blood volume can also improve performance (Sahlin, 2006). The converse is also true, and therefore we can assume that energy deficiency is a prime mechanism for fatigue. However, as Sahlin (2006) notes, total muscle ATP is well preserved during exercise, so it is not the lack of ATP that is responsible for fatigue but rather an increase in the products of ATP hydrolysis. For example, there is not a strong relationship between the decline in power output during maximal 30-s sprint and decline in ATP in either slow or fast fibers (Greenhaff et al., 1994). The energy pathways therefore contribute to fatigue by energy deficiency largely through product inhibition (increased ADP, P_i) rather than substrate limitation. Figure 4.10 summarizes the potential metabolic factors associated with fatigue.

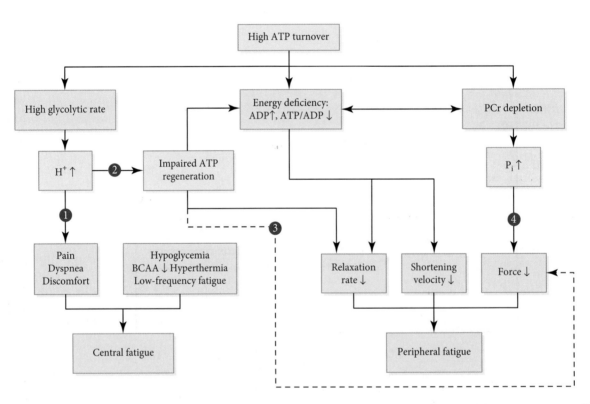

Figure 4.10 Metabolic factors associated with fatigue: (1) Reduced pH via H^+ accumulation causes central fatigue through sensation of pain and discomfort. (2) Reduced pH inhibits regulatory enzymes in glycolysis. (3) H^+ may reduce force via competition with Ca^{2+} for troponin. (4) P_i impairs crossbridge cycling and Ca^{2+} release.

Note: ATP is adenosine triphosphate; ADP is adenosine diphosphate; H^+ is hydrogen; PCr is phosphocreatine; P_i is inorganic phosphate.

Reproduced, with permission, from Sahlin, K. (2006). Metabolic factors in fatigue. In M. Hargreaves & L. L. Spriet (Eds.), *Exercise Metabolism* (pp. 163–186). Champaign, IL: Human Kinetics Publishers.

Chapter Summary

The energy required to sustain the physiological functioning of skeletal muscle during exercise is derived from the hydrolysis of ATP, with actomyosin, Ca^{2+}, and Na^+-K^+ ATPase being the major consumers of ATP. Each ATP molecule actually provides a relatively small energy yield, precluding the storage of the molecule within the muscle fibers. During exercise, the concentrations of ATP are defended by the resynthesis of the molecule via different metabolic pathways. The phosphagen system includes the reactions catalyzed by creatine kinase and adenylate kinase to resynthesize ATP. A further reaction catalyzed by AMP deaminase reduces the concentration of AMP within the cytosol, maintaining the activity of the adenylate kinase reaction. Glycolysis involves the degradation of G_6P to pyruvate in order to resynthesize ATP. The fate of pyruvate gives rise to alactic glycolysis, whereby pyruvate is converted to acetyl-CoA, and lactic glycolysis, whereby pyruvate is converted to lactate. Lactic glycolysis occurs at times when the demand for ATP is high, and the presence of lactate in the blood during exercise can provide the strength and conditioning practitioner with important information about the training status of the athlete. The reactions associated with the phosphagen system and glycolysis take place in the cytosol of the cell; they are referred to collectively as substrate-level phosphorylation and are anaerobic processes. In contrast, the reactions associated with oxidative phosphorylation to resynthesize ATP take place in the mitochondria and require O_2. Oxidative phosphorylation comprises the citric acid cycle and the electron transport chain. Acetyl-CoA is degraded to CO_2 and H^+ in the citric acid cycle, generating high-energy reducing equivalents NADH and $FADH_2$, which transport H^+ to the electron transport chain where the electrons are removed in a series of reactions to provide energy to resynthesize ATP. The phosphagen system has the highest rates of ATP resynthesis of the metabolic pathways, although its capacity is limited. Conversely, oxidative phosphorylation has the lowest rate of ATP resynthesis but the greatest capacity. Furthermore, oxidative phosphorylation can use carbohydrates, fats, or proteins as a fuel source, with the ATP yield from the oxidation of fats being much greater than that from carbohydrate, albeit at a lower rate. The requirement for ATP resynthesis is closely matched with the demand for ATP due to signals associated with the changes in the concentration of Ca^{2+} and the phosphorylation and redox potentials within the cytosol. All of the metabolic pathways will contribute to the resynthesis of ATP within a muscle fiber at any given time, although the relative contribution of each will largely be determined by the intensity if the exercise and the associated resynthesis rates of each pathway. The phosphagen system can be considered as contributing the largest energy provision during maximal exercise bouts lasting ≤ 6 s, with glycolysis contributing the largest energy provision during maximal bouts lasting 7–75 s, and oxidative phosphorylation contributing the largest energy provision during maximal-intensity bouts lasting > 75 s. During the transition from rest to exercise, there is a rapid increase in the demand for ATP. Even if the intensity of the exercise requires the supply of ATP be met by the activity of the oxidative pathway, the finite time for oxidative phosphorylation to establish ATP resynthesis gives rise to the oxygen deficit at the onset of exercise. The energy requirements during the oxygen deficit are met by substrate-level phosphorylation, resulting in an accumulation of metabolites (Cr, lactate, H^+) and a depletion in the substrates of PCr and muscle glycogen, potentially limiting subsequent exercise performance. Furthermore, increases in exercise intensity during continuous exercise bouts caused by tactical decisions or changes in the terrain will also invoke the oxygen deficit and the associated metabolic consequences. Each sprint performed during repeated-sprint activities relies predominantly on PCr degradation, and the recovery of sprint performance follows the resynthesis of PCr. The resynthesis of PCr relies largely upon mitochondrial ATP during the recovery periods, while the contribution of the oxidative system to each sprint increases with the number of sprints performed. The metabolic pathways contribute to the fatigue observed during many exercise bouts, and the energy deficiency within the muscle fibers can be related to the reduction in substrates within the fibers (e.g., PCr, glycogen) and also an increase in the products of ATP hydrolysis (ADP, P_i, H^+).

Review Questions and Projects

1. Describe the processes associated with the excitation–contraction coupling that consume ATP.

2. Place the processes identified in Question 1 in the order of their ATP consumption from the largest consumer to the smallest consumer.

3. What is the Gibbs free energy associated with the hydrolysis of ATP?

4. How do the metabolic byproducts of ATP hydrolysis affect the energy liberated from ATP hydrolysis?

5. Explain the difference between the phosphagen, glycolytic, and oxidative metabolic pathways that are used to resynthesize ATP in their rates of ATP provision.

6. Explain the differences between the phosphagen, glycolytic, and oxidative metabolic pathways that are used to resynthesize ATP in their capacity of ATP provision.

7. Which athletes may benefit from creatine monohydrate supplementation, and what are the mechanisms behind the proposed benefits?

8. What is the main contribution of the AMP deaminase reaction?

9. Discuss the cause of the increase in H^+ during exercise.

10. Explain the consequences of the increase in H^+ as well as the mechanisms to buffer the increase in H^+.

11. Explain some of the benefits associated with carbohydrate ingestion for different exercise bouts.

12. Explain the differences between the oxidation of glucose compared to the oxidation of glycogen in terms of the ATP yield and the metabolic byproducts.

13. What factors affect blood lactate values observed during exercise?

14. You test a group of sprint-trained athletes during a maximal sprint test. As well as recording their power output, you also record their blood lactate values and observe that they are very high following the completion of the sprint. What does this tell you about your athletes?

15. Explain why endurance-trained athletes are likely to have lower blood lactate values compared to their sprint-trained counterparts during a given exercise bout.

16. Why is the shift to the oxidation of fats rather than carbohydrates an important adaptation to endurance training?

17. Explain the signals that are activated within the muscle fiber that are responsible for matching the resynthesis of ATP with the demand.

18. Explain the bioenergetics associated with transitions from rest to exercise and also the work-to-work transitions when increasing exercise intensity during an exercise bout and the consequences for exercise performance.

19. Explain how the oxidative capacity of an athlete can influence his or her performance during a repeated-sprint test.

20. How might a reduction in substrates and an increase in metabolic byproducts induce fatigue during different exercise bouts?

References

Abbiss, C.R., & Laursen, P.B. (2008). Describing and understanding pacing strategies during athletic competition. *Sports Medicine, 38,* 239–252.

Adhihetty, P.J., Irrcher, I., Joseph, A.M., Ljubicic, V., & Hood, D.A. (2003). Plasticity of skeletal muscle mitochondria in response to contractile activity. *Experimental Physiology, 88,* 99–107.

Baker, J.S., McCormick, M.C., & Robergs, R.A. (2010). Interaction among skeletal muscle metabolic energy systems during intense exercise. *Journal of Nutrition and Metabolism, 2010,* 905612; doi: 10.1155/2010/905612.

Balsom, P.D., Wood, K., Olsson, P., & Ekblom, B. (1999). Carbohydrate intake and multiple sprint sports: with special reference to football (soccer). *International Journal of Sports Medicine, 20,* 48–52.

Bangsbo, J. (1996). Physiological factors associated with efficiency in high intensity exercise. *Sports Medicine, 22,* 299–305.

Bassett, D.R., & Howley, E.T. (2000). Limiting factors for maximum oxygen uptake and determinants of endurance performance. *Medicine and Science in Sports and Exercise, 32,* 70–84.

Bemben, M.G., & Lamont, H.S. (2005). Creatine supplementation and exercise performance. Recent findings. *Sports Medicine, 35,* 107–125.

Bishop, D., & Girard, O. (2011). Repeated-sprint ability (RSA). In M. Cardinale, R. Newton, & K. Nosaka (Eds.), *Strength and Conditioning. Biological Principles and Practical Applications* (pp. 223–241). West Sussex, UK: Wiley-Blackwell.

Bonen, A. (2006). Skeletal muscle lactate transport and transporters. In M. Hargreaves & L.L. Spriet (Eds.), *Exercise Metabolism* (pp. 71–87). Champaign, IL: Human Kinetics Publishers.

Brooks, G.A. (2009). Cell-cell and intracellular lactate shuttles. *Journal of Physiology, 587,* 5591–5600.

Brooks, G.A., Fahey, T.D., & Baldwin, K.M. (2005). *Exercise Physiology: Human Bioenergetics and its Application.* New York: McGraw-Hill.

Bundle, M.W., Hoyt, R.W., & Weyand, P.G. (2003). High speed running performance: a new approach to assessment and prediction. *Journal of Applied Physiology, 95,* 1955–1962.

Burgomaster, K.A., Hughes, S.C., Heigenhauser, G.J.F., Bradwell, S.N., & Gibala, M.J. (2005). Six sessions of sprint interval training increases muscle oxidative potential and cycle endurance capacity in humans. *Journal of Applied Physiology, 98,* 1985–1990.

Burke, L.M., Hawley, J.A., Wong, S.H.S., & Jeukendrup, A.E. (2011). Carbohydrates training and competition. *Journal of Sports Sciences, 29,* S17–S27.

Cairns, S.P. (2006). Lactic acid and exercise performance. Culprit or friend? *Sports Medicine, 36,* 279–291.

Calbet, J.A.L., De Paz, J.A., Garatachea, N., Cabeza de Vaca, S., & Chavarren, J. (2003). Anaerobic energy provision does not limit Wingate exercise performance in endurance-trained cyclists. *Journal of Applied Physiology, 94,* 668–676.

Carr, A.J., Hopkins, W.G., & Gore, C.J. (2011). Effects of acute alkalosis and acidosis on performance. A meta-analysis. *Sports Medicine, 41*, 801–814.

Chilibeck, P.D., Bell, G.J., Socha, T., & Martin, T. (1998). The effect of aerobic training on the distribution of succinate dehydrogenase activity throughout muscle fibers. *Canadian Journal of Applied Physiology, 23*, 74–86.

Chung, Y., Sharman, R., Carlsen, R., Unger, S.W., Larson, D., & Jue, T. (1998). Metabolic fluctuation during a muscle contraction cycle. *American Journal of Physiology, 274*, C846–C852.

De Bock, K., Derave, W., Ramaekers, M., Richter, E.A., & Hespel, P. (2007). Fiber type-specific muscle glycogen sparing due to carbohydrate intake before and during exercise. *Journal of Applied Physiology, 102*, 183–188.

Elander, A., Sjöström, M., Lundgren, F., Scherstén, T., & Bylund-Fellenius, A-C. (1985). Biochemical and morphometric properties of mitochondrial populations in human muscle fibers. *Clinical Sciences, 69*, 153–164.

Esbjörnsson-Liljedahl, M., Sundberg, C.J., Norman, B., & Jansson, E. (1999). Metabolic response in type I and type II fibers during a 30-s cycle sprint in men and women. *Journal of Applied Physiology, 87*, 1326–1332.

Farris, D.J., & Sawicki, G.S. (2012). The mechanics and energetics of human walking and running: a joint-level perspective. *Journal of the Royal Society Interface, 9*, 110–118.

Fitts, R.H. (2008). The cross-bridge cycle and skeletal muscle fatigue. *Journal Applied Physiology, 104*, 551–558.

Forbes, S.C., Paganini, A.T., Slade, J.M., Towse, T.F., & Meyer, R.A. (2009). Phosphocreatine recovery kinetics following low- and high-intensity exercise in human triceps surae and rat posterior hindlimb muscles. *American Journal of Physiology, 296*, R161–R170.

Gaesser, G.A., & Brooks, G.A. (1984). Metabolic bases of excess post-exercise oxygen consumption: a review. *Medicine and Science in Sports and Exercise, 16*, 29–43.

Gaitanos, G.C., Williams, C., Boobis, L.H., & Brooks, S. (1993). Human metabolism during intermittent maximal exercise. *Journal of Applied Physiology, 75*, 712–719.

Gastin, P.B. (2001). Energy system interaction and relative contribution during maximal exercise. *Sports Medicine, 31*, 725–741.

Gladden, L.B. (2004). Lactate metabolism: a new paradigm for the third millennium. *Journal of Physiology, 558*, 5–30.

Glaister, M. (2005). Multiple sprint work. Physiological responses, mechanisms of fatigue and the influence of aerobic fitness. *Sports Medicine, 35*, 757–777.

Gollnick, P.D., & Saltin, B. (1982). Significance of skeletal muscle oxidative enzyme enhancement with endurance training. *Clinical Physiology, 2*, 1–12.

Greenhaff, P.L. (2001). The creatine-phosphocreatine system: there's more than one song in its repertoire. *Journal of Physiology, 537*, 657.

Greenhaff, P.L., Nevill, M.E., Soderlund, K., Bodin, K., Boobis, L.H., Williams, C., & Hultman, E. (1994). The metabolic responses of human type I and II muscle fibres during maximal treadmill sprinting. *Journal of Physiology, 478*, 149–155.

Greiwe, J.S., Hickner, R.C., Hansen, P.A., Racette, S.B., Chen, M.M., & Holloszy, J.O. (1999). Effects of endurance exercise training on muscle glycogen accumulation in humans. *Journal of Applied Physiology, 87*, 222–226.

Haff, G.G., Stone, M.H., Warren, B.J., Keith, R., Johnson, R.L., Nieman, D.C., . . . Kirksey, K.B. (1999). The effects of carbohydrate supplementation on multiple sessions and bouts of resistance exercise. *Journal of Strength and Conditioning Research, 13*, 111–117.

Haff, G.G., Koch, A.J., Pottiger, J.A., Kuphal, K.E., Magee, L.M., Green, S.B., & Jakicic, J.J. (2000). Carbohydrate supplementation attenuates muscle glycogen loss during acute bouts of resistance training exercise. *International Journal of Sport Nutrition and Exercise Metabolism, 10*, 326–339.

Hancock, C.R., Brault, J.J., & Terjung, R.L. (2006). Protecting the cellular energy state during contractions: role of AMP deaminase. *Journal of Physiology and Pharmacology, 57*, S17–S29.

Hargreaves, M. (2006). Skeletal muscle carbohydrate metabolism during exercise. In M. Hargreaves & L.L. Spriet (Eds.), *Exercise Metabolism* (pp. 29–44). Champaign, IL: Human Kinetics Publishers.

Haseler, L.J., Hogan, M.C., & Richardson, R.S. (1999). Skeletal muscle phosphocreatine recovery in exercise-trained humans is dependent on O_2 availability. *Journal of Applied Physiology, 86*, 2013–2018.

Hawley, J.A., & Burke, L.M. (2010). Carbohydrate availability and training adaptation: effects on cell metabolism. *Exercise and Sport Science Reviews, 38*, 152–160.

Hawley, J.A., Schabort, E.J., Noakes, T.D., & Dennis, S.C. (1997). Carbohydrate-loading and exercise performance: an update. *Sports Medicine, 24,* 73–81.

Hespel, P., Op't Eijnde, B., Derave, W., & Richter, E.A. (2001). Creatine supplementation: exploring the role of the creatine kinase/phosphocreatine system in human muscle. *Canadian Journal of Applied Physiology, 26,* S79–S102.

Inger, F. (1979). Effects of endurance training on muscle fibre ATP-ase activity, capillary supply and mitochondrial content in man. *Journal of Physiology, 294,* 419–432.

Ivy, J.L. (2004). Regulation of muscle glycogen repletion, muscle protein synthesis and repair following exercise. *Journal of Sports Science and Medicine, 3,* 131–138.

Jeukendrup, A.E., Saris, W.H.M., & Wagenmakers, A.J.M. (1998). Fat metabolism during exercise: a review. Part I: fatty acid mobilization and muscle metabolism. *International Journal of Sports Medicine, 19,* 231–244.

Jones, A.M., & DiMenna, F.J. (2011). Cardiovascular adaptations to strength and conditioning. In M. Cardinale, R. Newton, & K. Nosaka (Eds.), *Strength and Conditioning. Biological Principles and Practical Applications* (pp. 165–177). West Sussex, UK: Wiley-Blackwell.

Juel, C. (2008). Regulation of pH in human skeletal muscle: adaptations to physical activity. *Acta Physiologica, 193,* 17–24.

Juel, C., Klarskov, C., Nielsen, J.J., Krustrup, P., Mohr, M., & Bangsbo, J. (2004). Effects of high-intensity intermittent training on lactate and H^+ release from human skeletal muscle. *American Journal of Physiology, 286,* E245–E251.

Krustrup, P., Ferguson, R.A., Kjær, M., & Bangsbo, J. (2003). ATP and heat production in human skeletal muscle during dynamic exercise: higher efficiency of anaerobic than aerobic ATP resynthesis. *Journal of Physiology, 549,* 255–269.

Lakomy, H.K.A. (2000). Physiology and biochemistry of sprinting. In J.A. Hawley (Ed.), *Running. Handbook of Sports Medicine* (pp. 1–13). Oxford, UK: Blackwell Science.

Langfort, J., Ploug, T., Ihlemann, J., Saldo, M., Holm, C., & Galbo, H. (1999). Expression of hormone-sensitive lipase and its regulation by adrenaline in skeletal muscle. *Biochemistry Journal, 340,* 459–465.

MacDougall, J.D., Ward, G.R., Sale, D.G., & Sutton, J.R. (1977). Biochemical adaptation of human skeletal muscle to heavy resistance training and immobilization. *Journal of Applied Physiology, 77,* 700–703.

Maughan, R.J. (2011). Bioenergetics of exercise. In M. Cardinale, R. Newton, & K. Nosaka (Eds.), *Strength and Conditioning. Biological Principles and Practical Applications* (pp. 53–61). West Sussex, UK: Wiley-Blackwell.

McNaughton, L.R., Siegler, J., & Midgley, A. (2008). Ergogenic effects of sodium bicarbonate. *Current Sports Medicine Reports, 7,* 230–236.

Medbø, J.I., Mohn, A., Tabata, I., Bahr, R., Vaage, O., & Sejersted, O. M. (1988). Anaerobic capacity determined by maximal accumulated O_2 deficit. *Journal of Applied Physiology, 64,* 50–60.

Phillips, S.M. (2006). Endurance training-induced adaptations in substrate turnover and oxidation. In M. Hargreaves & L.L. Spriet (Eds.), *Exercise Metabolism* (pp. 187–213). Champaign, IL: Human Kinetics Publishers.

Poole, D.C., Barstow, T.J., McDonough, P., & Jones, A.M. (2008). Control of oxygen uptake during exercise. *Medicine and Science in Sports and Exercise, 40,* 462–474.

Prompers, J.J., Jeneson, J.A.L., Drost, M.R., Oomens, C.C.W., Strijkers, G.J., & Nicolay, K. (2006). Dynamic MRS and MRI of skeletal muscle function and biomechanics. *NMR in Biomedicine, 19,* 927–953.

Quistorff, B., Johansen, L., & Sahlin, K. (1993). Absence of phosphocreatine resynthesis in human calf muscle during ischaemic recovery. *Biochemistry Journal, 291,* 681–686.

Rapoport, B.I. (2010). Metabolic factors limiting performance in marathon runners. *PLoS, 6,* e1000960.

Robergs, R.A., Ghiasvand, F., & Parker, D. (2004). Biochemistry of exercise-induced metabolic acidosis. *American Journal of Physiology, 287,* R502–R512.

Sahlin, K. (2006). Metabolic factors in fatigue. In M. Hargreaves & L.L. Spriet (Eds.), *Exercise Metabolism* (pp. 163–186). Champaign, IL: Human Kinetics Publishers.

Sahlin, K., Tonkonogi, M., & Söderlund, K. (1998). Energy supply and muscle fatigue in humans. *Acta Physiologica, 162,* 261–266.

Schiaffino, S., & Reggiani, C. (2011). Fiber types in mammalian skeletal muscles. *Physiology Reviews*, *91*, 1447–1531.

Scott, C.B. (2005). Contribution of anaerobic energy expenditure to whole body thermogenesis. *Nutrition and Metabolism*, *2*, 14.

Sloniger, M.A., Cureton, K.J., Prior, B.M., & Evans, E.M. (1997). Anaerobic capacity and muscle activation during horizontal and uphill running. *Journal of Applied Physiology*, *83*, 262–269.

Spencer, M., Bishop, D., Dawson, B., & Goodman, C. (2005). Physiological and metabolic responses of repeated-sprint activities. *Sports Medicine*, *35*, 1025–1044.

Spriet, L.L. (2006). Anaerobic metabolism during exercise. In M. Hargreaves & L.L. Spriet (Eds.), *Exercise Metabolism* (pp. 7–28). Champaign, IL: Human Kinetics Publishers.

Spriet, L.L., & Hargreaves, M. (2006). Overview of exercise metabolism. In M. Hargreaves & L.L. Spriet (Eds.), *Exercise Metabolism* (pp. 1–6). Champaign, IL: Human Kinetics Publishers.

Stellingwerff, T., Maughan, R.J., & Burke, L.M. (2011). Nutrition for power sports: middle-distance running, track cycling, rowing, canoeing/kayaking, and swimming. *Journal of Sports Sciences*, *29*, S79–S89.

Tarnopolsky, M.A., & Raha, S. (2005). Mitochondrial myopathies: diagnosis, exercise intolerance, and treatment options. *Medicine and Science in Sports and Exercise*, *37*, 2086–2093.

Thomas, C., Bishop, D.J., Lambert, K., Mercier, J., & Brooks, G.A. (2012). Effects of acute and chronic exercise on sarcolemmal MCT1 and MCT4 contents in human muscles: current status. *American Journal of Physiology*, *302*, R1–R14.

Tonkonogi, M., & Sahlin, K. (2002). Physical exercise and mitochondrial function in human skeletal muscle. *Exercise and Sport Science Reviews*, *30*, 129–137.

Tucker, R., Bester, A., Lambert, E.V., Noakes, T.D., Vaughan, C.L., & St Clair Gibson, A. (2006). Non-random fluctuations in power output during self-paced exercise. *British Journal of Sports Medicine*, *40*, 912–917.

Tucker, R., & Noakes, T.D. (2009). The physiological regulation of pacing strategies during exercise: a critical review. *British Journal of Sports Medicine*, *43*, e1–e9.

van Hall, G. (2010). Lactate kinetics in human tissue at rest and during exercise. *Acta Physiologica*, *199*, 499–508.

Wallimann, T., Tokarska-Schlattner, M., & Schlattner, U. (2011). The creatine kinase system and pleiotropic effects of creatine. *Amino Acids*, *40*, 1271–1296.

Walsh, B., Tonkonogi, M., Söderlund, K., Hultman, E., Saks, V., & Sahlin, K. (2001). The role of phosphorylcreatine and creatine in the regulation of mitochondrial respiration in human skeletal muscle. *Journal of Physiology*, *537*, 971–978.

Wilson, J.M., Loenneke, J.P., Jo, E., Wilson, G.J., Zourdos, M.C., & Kim, J.S. (2012). The effects of endurance, strength, and power training on fiber type shifting. *Journal of Strength and Conditioning Research*, *26*, 1724–1729.

Yan, Z., Lira, V.A., & Greene, N.P. (2012). Exercise training-induced regulation of mitochondrial quality. *Exercise and Sport Science Reviews*, *40*, 159–164.

Yan, Z., Okutsu, M., Akhtar, Y.N., & Lira, V.A. (2011). Regulation of exercise-induced fiber type transformation, mitochondrial biogenesis, and angiogenesis in skeletal muscle. *Journal of Applied Physiology*, *110*, 264–274.

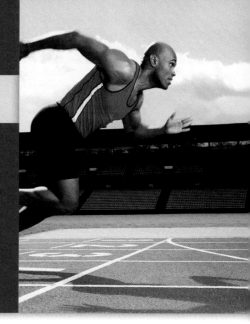

CHAPTER 5

Muscular Strength and Power

Chapter Objectives

At the end of this chapter, you will be able to:

- Define muscular strength
- Describe the different indices of muscular strength, including maximal muscular strength, speed-strength, explosive muscular strength, and reactive strength, and identify their importance in different sports
- Define muscular power and its importance in different sports
- Explain the determinants of muscular strength and power
- Explain the transformation of muscular forces to joint moments
- Explain the transformation of joint moments to external forces

Key Terms

Absolute maximum strength	High-load speed-strength	Ratio scaling	Stiffness
Allometric scaling	Low-load speed-strength	Reactive strength	Voluntary maximum strength
Bilateral deficit	Maximal dynamic strength	Reactive strength index	
Electromechanical delay	Maximal isometric strength	Repetition maximum testing	
Explosive muscular strength	Rate of force development	Sticking region	

Chapter Overview

Muscular strength is defined in terms of the magnitude of force developed during a specific movement task. The force generated by the activation of muscles is transformed into moments acting at the joints; these moments are then further transformed into an external force that changes the motion of the athlete's body or an object with which the athlete is in contact. As such, all sports rely on the application of force, and, therefore, muscular strength is important for all athletes. However, there are different indices of muscular strength (e.g., maximal strength, explosive strength), each of which has implications for different sporting activities. In this chapter, we describe these different indices of muscular strength and highlight their importance for specific sports. Furthermore, we describe the relationship between muscular strength and muscular power, and explore the important role of muscular power in sport. We begin the chapter by defining muscular strength.

Defining Muscular Strength

Muscular strength can be defined as the ability of a muscle or a group of muscles to produce a force against an external resistance (Moir, 2012). In most sporting situations, that external resistance is provided by the mass of a body—either the mass of the performer or the mass of an implement (e.g., soccer ball, baseball bat)—and success is often dependent upon the change in motion of the specific mass. A force is an agent that changes or tends to change the motion of a body. The relationship between the change in motion of a body of given mass and the applied force is provided by Newton's second law of motion, which can be written as follows:

$$a = \frac{F}{m}$$ **Eq. (5.1)**

where a is the linear acceleration of the body, F is the applied force, and m is the mass of the body.

Equation (5.1) informs us that the change in motion of a body is proportional to the applied force and acts in the same direction as the applied force, but is inversely proportional to the mass of the body. Therefore, a greater force must be applied to a 7.26-kg shot during the shot put event to achieve the same acceleration as that of an 800-g javelin. Furthermore, Equation (5.1) can be rearranged to allow us to determine the influence of the mass of the body on the magnitude of the applied force:

$$F = ma$$ **Eq. (5.2)**

where F is the applied force, m is the mass of the body, and a is the linear acceleration of the body. We can use Equation (5.2) to determine that the magnitude of the applied force, and therefore the expression of muscle strength, is largely dependent upon the magnitude of the mass being accelerated. For example, Figure 5.1 shows the peak vertical ground reaction force for two athletes during the performance of squat jumps performed with different external loads. Each athlete produces a greater peak force as the magnitude of the external load is increased; the greatest forces will be exerted against the greatest resistances.

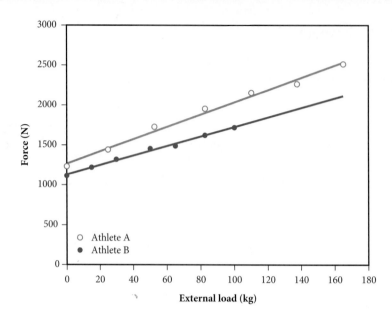

Figure 5.1 The peak vertical ground reaction force achieved by two athletes performing jump squats with different external loads on a force platform. The external loads were provided by a barbell and ranged from 0% to 85% of the load equivalent to each athlete's one-repetition maximum parallel back squat (1-RM). Athlete A has a body mass of 83.7 kg and a 1-RM of 195.0 kg; athlete B has a body mass of 83.2 kg and a 1-RM of 117.5 kg. For both athletes, the peak force achieved during the jump squats increases with the magnitude of the external load that provides resistance to the movement. Therefore, the maximal dynamic force generated by each athlete, and thus the maximal dynamic muscular strength, will be achieved under the heaviest external load that each could move in a single repetition. Athlete A is able to produce greater peak forces than athlete B under all loading conditions and, therefore, is the stronger athlete in this specific task.

The dependence of force upon the magnitude of the external mass being accelerated means that dynamic muscular strength can be determined from the load moved during a specific movement, forming the basis of **repetition maximum testing**. Specifically, the greatest load that can be lifted in a given movement for a single repetition is the one-repetition maximum (1-RM) for the athlete, which provides a measure of the **maximal dynamic strength** of the athlete. Such tests can involve concentric- or eccentric-only muscle actions, although typically they involve the stretch–shortening cycle. The greatest mass lifted during such tests is typically normalized to the mass of the athlete to account for the role of body size in confounding the measure (see Strength and Power Concept 5.1). Notice that the mass of the body to which the force is applied provides an inertial resistance to the movement. It is unlikely in any sporting situation that the resistance will be purely inertial, given that gravity (weight), friction, and drag forces may all contribute to the resistive force depending on the direction in which the mass is displaced, the surface across which the mass is displaced, and the fluid through which the mass is displaced, respectively.

Strength and Power Concept 5.1

Normalizing measures of muscular strength for body size

It is a common assumption that bigger athletes tend to be stronger than smaller athletes. This assertion leads us to consider what the physical criterion is for determining who is "bigger" and who is "smaller." Typically, the measure used is body mass. Body mass is a convenient measure that characterizes the size of the athlete, and evidence shows that more massive athletes tend to be stronger than their less massive counterparts (Crewther, Gill, Weatherby,& Lowe, 2009). To account for this body–size bias, the values representing a given measure of muscular strength are often normalized to the mass of the athlete:

$$\text{Normalized muscular strength} = \text{strength measure/body mass} \qquad \text{Eq. (5.3)}$$

This normalization method is known as **ratio scaling**. However, such normalization methods assume that muscular force is directly proportional to body mass and have actually been shown to bias the measure of muscular strength in the favor of the less massive athlete (Crewther et al., 2009).

Allometric scaling is predicated upon geometric similarity—namely, the notion that all human bodies have the same shape, differing only in size (Jaric, Mirkov, & Markovic, 2005). Consequently, all lengths are proportional to a characteristic length of the body, while all areas are proportional to the square of the characteristic length and all volumes are proportional to the cube of the characteristic length. If height is selected as the characteristic length measurement for a body, the area of the body is proportional to the square of the height (height^2), with the volume of the body being proportional to the cube of the height (height^3). Given that mass is related to the volume of a body, these simple relationships can be used to determine that any length characteristic of the body is proportional to $\text{mass}^{1/3}$ and any area characteristic of the body is proportional to $\text{mass}^{2/3}$. Given that muscle force is proportional to the cross-sectional area of the muscle, it should increase in proportion to $\text{mass}^{2/3}$. Therefore, the allometric scaling parameter of $\text{mass}^{2/3}$ should be used to normalize measures of muscular strength:

$$\text{Allometrically scaled muscular strength} = \text{strength measure/body mass}^{2/3}$$
$$\text{Eq. (5.4)}$$

This allometric scaling parameter has been recommended for tests of muscular force and power (Jaric et al., 2005). It has also been shown to effectively normalize muscular strength to body size (Crewther et al., 2009).

The magnitude of the muscular force generated voluntarily is limited by the level of muscular activation achieved by the athlete. Neural inhibitory mechanisms may limit the activation of muscles during voluntary contractions, such that the force generated voluntarily may not reflect the maximal capabilities of the individual. Protocols have been developed whereby an electrical stimulus (ES) is superimposed upon a maximal voluntary contraction to determine the maximal force of the stimulated muscles (Westing, Seger, & Thorstensson, 1990). Such protocols provide information about the intrinsic properties of the stimulated muscles; thus they have been termed measures of **absolute maximum strength** as opposed to **voluntary maximum strength** (Zatsiorsky, 1995). *In vivo* maximal force measurements using ES protocols have shown that absolute strength is greater than voluntary strength only during eccentric muscle actions (Westing et al., 1990). Electrically evoked measures of force are not always strongly associated with voluntary measures of muscle strength (Andersen & Aagaard, 2006), highlighting the importance of the activation dynamics on measures of muscular strength.

Returning to the data shown in Figure 5.1, notice that the regression line for athlete A is always above that for athlete B. From this fact, we can determine that athlete A is able to produce the greatest peak forces across a range of external loads; thus athlete A is the stronger of the two individuals in terms of this specific task. Indeed, even during the unloaded condition when the athlete's body weight provides the external resistance, athlete A is still able to generate the greater peak force. This demonstrates that stronger athletes are able to generate greater forces even against low external loads (Moss, Refsnes, Abildgaard, Nicolaysen, & Jensen, 1997).

Figure 5.2 shows the values of peak force generated during the jump squats when the external load is expressed as a percentage of the athlete's 1-RM. The vertical line at 30% 1-RM reflects the demarcation between measurements of **low-load speed-strength** and measurements of **high-load speed-strength** (Newton & Dugan, 2002). When the external load is relatively low (less than 30% 1-RM), the athlete is able to develop higher movement velocities than during conditions when the external load is higher (greater than 30% 1-RM) due to the lower mass involved, as per Equation (5.1). Notice in Figure 5.2 that athlete A has both greater low-load and high-load speed-strength than athlete B, although the differences are more pronounced as the external load increases. Identifying these different indices of speed-strength provides an insight into an athlete's ability to generate force under conditions characterized by different external loads. For example, in sports where athletes are required to exert forces against their own body weight, such as when sprinting and jumping, low-load speed-strength will be important. Conversely, during sports such as American football, rugby, and weight-lifting, where the external load against which athletes are required to exert a force is increased, high-load speed-strength becomes important. Furthermore, the different indices of speed-strength will respond to different specific training stimuli (Cormie, McCauley, & McBride, 2007).

The external force can also be measured as an athlete exerts a force against an immovable body. The measurement of the force exerted under such circumstances provides a measure of the athlete's muscular strength, with the peak force representing the **maximal isometric strength** of the athlete (Figure 5.3). In many sports, an athlete has limited time to develop force (Table 5.1). During tests of maximal isometric strength, the time taken to achieve peak force has been shown to be approximately 400 ms (Aagaard, Simonsen, Andersen, Magnusson, & Dyhre-Poulsen, 2002; Narici et al., 1996). Comparing this to the times shown in Table 5.1, we can see that in many sports an athlete is unable to generate maximal force; in such cases, measures of force generation during short time periods may be more revealing of the capability of an athlete.

The assessment of the magnitude of force generated during a given time period constitutes a measure of **explosive muscular strength** (Schmidtbleicher, 1992). The expression of explosive muscular strength is characterized by a high **rate of force**

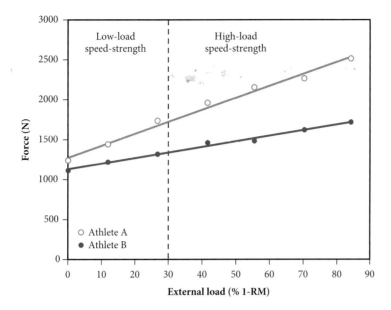

Figure 5.2 The peak vertical ground reaction force achieved by two athletes performing jump squats with different external loads on a force platform. Athlete A has a body mass of 83.7 kg and a 1-RM of 195.0 kg; athlete B has a body mass of 83.2 kg and a 1-RM of 117.5 kg. The external loads were provided by a barbell and ranged from 0% to 85% of the load equivalent to each athlete's one-repetition maximum parallel back squat (1-RM). The vertical line at the external load equivalent to 30% 1-RM represents the demarcation between low-load speed-strength (less than 30% 1-RM) and high-load speed-strength (more than 30% 1-RM). Athlete A is able to produce greater peak forces than athlete B under all loading conditions and so demonstrates greater low-load speed-strength and high-load speed-strength. The difference between the two athletes becomes more pronounced under high-load conditions; thus athlete A has much greater high-load speed-strength than athlete B.

development (RFD) and can be measured during both dynamic and isometric tasks (Haff et al., 2005; Haff et al., 1997; Moir, Garcia, & Dwyer, 2009). Various measures can be employed to quantify explosive muscular strength, all of which are derived from the force–time trace collected during specific tasks (Table 5.2). The time period over which the RFD is assessed has been divided into "early" (less than 50 ms) and "late" (150–250 ms) periods during tasks (Andersen & Aagaard, 2006). Such a demarcation is very informative (see Applied Research 5.1), as early RFD appears to reflect different neuromuscular qualities than late RFD, correlating more strongly with performance in different athletic tasks while also responding differently to different training regimens (Andersen, Andersen, Zebis, & Aagaard, 2010; Oliveira, Oliveira, Rizatto, & Denadai, 2013; Tillin, Pain, & Folland, 2013). The importance of explosive strength in sport is highlighted in **Worked Example 5.1**, while the calculations of the different force–time variables used to quantify explosive strength are shown in **Worked Example 5.2**.

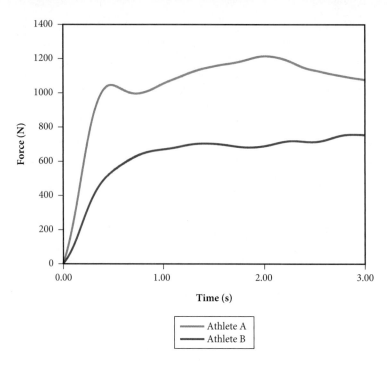

Figure 5.3 The net vertical ground reaction force for two athletes performing isometric back squats on a force plate. The squat was performed with an internal knee angle of 90° and each athlete was instructed to exert maximal force against an immovable resistance for a 3-s period. The body weight of each athlete has been removed from the respective force trace. Athlete A has a body mass of 84.3 kg and a 1-RM parallel back squat of 175.0 kg; athlete B has a body mass of 79.6 kg and a 1-RM parallel back squat of 110.0 kg. Athlete A is able to achieve a greater peak isometric force and, therefore, has greater maximal isometric strength than athlete B in this specific task.

The forces developed by an athlete in short time periods are below the peak force that an athlete is able to achieve during a given task. Thus maximal and explosive measures represent different indices of muscular strength, even though both are determined by the magnitude of the force generated. There is a relationship between measures of maximal and explosive strength, with maximal strength being strongly related to RFD (Andersen & Aagaard, 2006; Haff et al., 1997; Stone et al., 2003). (See Applied Research 5.1.) Researchers have proposed that maximal muscular strength forms the theoretical foundation upon which explosive strength is developed (Schmidtbleicher, 1992). Just as the magnitude of the force that an athlete is able to exert depends on the external mass being accelerated during dynamic tasks, so dynamic RFD depends on the magnitude of the external mass, with greater RFD values being achieved under conditions of low external loads (Haff et al., 1997; Stone et al., 2003).

Another expression of muscular strength is **reactive strength**, defined as the ability to tolerate high stretch-loads and rapidly transition from eccentric to concentric muscle actions in tasks involving the stretch–shortening cycle (Newton & Dugan, 2002).

Table 5.1
The Time Available for Force Development in Various Sporting Tasks

Sporting Task	Time for Force Development (s)
Countermovement jump takeoff	≤0.330
Long jump and high jump takeoff	≤0.220
Baseball delivery	≤0.170
Javelin delivery	≤0.140
Gymnastic tumbling takeoff	≤0.125
Stance phase of sprint running	≤0.120
Soccer kick (foot–ball contact)	≤0.010

Data from Dapena, J., & Chung, C. S. (1988). Vertical and radial motions of the body during the take-off phase of high jumping. *Medicine and Science in Sports and Exercise, 20,* 290–302; Escamilla, R. F., Fleisig, G. S., Barrentine, S. W., Zheng, N., & Andrews, J. R. (1998). Kinematic comparisons of throwing different types of baseball pitches. *Journal of Applied Biomechanics, 14,* 1–23; Feltner, M. E., Fraschetti, D. J., & Crisp, R. J. (1999). Upper extremity augmentation of lower extremity kinetics during countermovement vertical jumps. *Journal of Sports Sciences, 17,* 449–466; Kuitunen, S., Komi, P. V., & Kyröläinen, H. (2002). Knee and ankle joint stiffness in sprint running. *Medicine and Science in Sports and Exercise, 34,* 166–173; Liu, H., Leigh, S., & Yu, B. (2010). Sequence of upper and lower extremity motions in javelin throwing. *Journal of Sports Sciences, 13,* 1459–1467; Luhtanen, P., & Komi, P. V. (1979). Mechanical power and segmental contributions to force impulses in long jump take-off. *European Journal of Applied Physiology, 41,* 267–274; McNeal, J. R., Sands, W. A., & Shultz, B. B. (2007). Muscle activation characteristics of tumbling take-offs. *Sports Biomechanics, 6,* 375–390; Nunome, H., Lake, M., Georgakis, A., & Stergioulas, L. K. (2006). Impact phase of kinematics of instep kicking in soccer. *Journal of Sports Sciences, 24,* 11–22.

Table 5.2
Force–Time Variables That Can Be Used to Quantify Explosive Muscular Strength in a Given Task

Variable	Definition
Time of F_{peak}	The time associated with the occurrence of peak force during a specific task. Lower values reflect greater explosive muscular strength.
RFD	The slope of the force–time curve. Average RFD (RFD_{ave}) refers to the slope from the beginning of the force application to the occurrence of peak force. Peak RFD (RFD_{peak}) refers to the maximal slope of the force–time trace. Large values of both RFD_{ave} and RFD_{peak} reflect greater explosive muscular strength.
RFD across finite time periods	The slope of the force–time curve across finite time periods from the beginning of the force application. Typically, 50-ms time periods are used, with times less than 50 ms denoting "early" RFD and times greater than 150 ms denoting "late" RFD. Large RFD values within each time period reflect greater explosive muscular strength.

Note: RFD = rate of force development; F_{peak} = peak force; RFD_{ave} = average rate of force development; RFD_{peak} = peak rate of force development.

Applied Research 5.1
The relationship between measures of maximal and explosive muscular strength

The authors recorded the maximal voluntary and electrically evoked isometric RFD in a knee extension task during different time periods ranging from 0–10 ms to 0–250 ms. These time periods were used to define "early" (RFD < 50 ms) and "late" (RFD = 150–250 ms) phases of the muscle activity. Maximal strength was measured as the maximal force generated during an isometric knee extension task, and correlations were performed on the maximal strength and RFD data. Maximal voluntary RFD was moderately to strongly correlated with maximal isometric strength, and the magnitude of the relationship increased from early RFD ($r \approx$ 0.40) to late RFD ($r \approx$ 0.90). Furthermore, early voluntary RFD was more strongly related to electrically evoked characteristics of the active muscle ($r \approx$ 0.60) than was late voluntary RFD ($r \approx$ 0.30). The authors concluded that early voluntary RFD is more related to the intrinsic properties of skeletal muscle, while late voluntary RFD is more influenced by the maximal strength capabilities of the individual.

Andersen, L. L., & Aagaard, P. (2006). Influence of maximal muscle strength and intrinsic muscle contractile properties on contractile rate of force development. *European Journal of Applied Physiology, 96*, 46–52.

Worked Example 5.1
The importance of explosive strength in sprint running

Each stance phase of a 100-m sprint race represents the only time that the athlete is able to use the ground reaction force (GRF) to generate an impulse that increases the momentum of the center of mass (CM). When the athlete is sprinting at maximal velocity, the CM descends over the first half of the stance and ascends over the second half. At touchdown, the sprinter's CM possesses negative vertical momentum, which will be reduced to zero at mid-stance by the action of the vertical impulse associated with the GRF. Furthermore, the vertical component of the GRF must also exert an impulse equal to that associated with bodyweight during the stance phase because of gravity. The stance phases associated with maximal-velocity sprinting in well-trained sprinters are typically around 0.10 s (Bezodis, Kerwin, & Salo, 2008; Kuitunen, Komi, & Kyröläinen, 2002), so the vertical impulse must be generated in a very short period of time (half of the stance period), requiring a high rate of force development (RFD).

Calculate the RFD associated with the GRF required for a sprinter with a body mass of 75 kg to generate a vertical impulse to reduce the negative vertical momentum to 0 kg m/s over the first half of the stance. To do so, we will use a vertical velocity of the CM at touchdown of -0.50 m/s (Mero, Luhtanen, & Komi, 1986) and a total stance duration of 0.11 s. We will use the impulse–momentum relationship.

i. Calculate the vertical momentum of the CM at touchdown

$p = mv$

ii. Answer

$p = 75 \times -0.50 = -37.5$ kg m/s

iii. Calculate the GRF impulse required to reduce p to 0 kg m/s

$J_{\Delta p} = p_f - p_i$

iv. Answer

$J_{\Delta p} = 0 - -37.5 = 37.5$ Ns

v. Calculate the body weight impulse during half of stance

$J_{BW} = Ft$

vi. Answer

$J_{BW} = (75 \times -9.81) \times 0.055 = -40.5$ Ns

The value of -40.5 Ns represents the impulse acting downward due to body weight. This will be countered by the impulse associated with the GRF acting upward. Therefore, we will remove the negative sense from the value.

vii. Sum $J_{\Delta p}$ and J_{BW} to provide the total vertical GRF impulse $J_{GRF} = 78.0$ Ns

We now know that over the first half of the stance (0.055 s), the vertical impulse associated with the GRF needs to be 78.0 Ns to arrest the downward momentum of the CM and to support body weight. (Notice that the same magnitude of vertical GRF impulse is required over the second half of the stance to generate a vertical velocity of 0.50 m/s at takeoff to project the athlete into the flight phase.) We can use the trapezoid rule to determine the change in force that will provide an area under the force–time trace equal to 78.0 Ns. Assuming that the GRF begins at 0 N (F_i), this will then give the peak GRF (F_f) during the first half of stance.

viii. Use the trapezoid rule to determine the peak GRF (F_f) during the stance $J_{GRF} = [(F_i + F_f)/2] \times t$

ix. Rearrange the trapezoid rule $F_f = 2 \times (J_{GRF}/t)$

x. Answer $F_f = 2 \times (78.0/0.055) = 2836$ N

xi. Calculate the RFD required to develop 2836 N in 0.055 s $RFD = 2{,}836/0.055 = 51{,}564$ N/s

Therefore, to generate the required vertical impulse during the first half of the stance, the athlete must be able to produce a RFD of 51,564 N/s. Furthermore, notice that the magnitude of the peak vertical GRF required in this situation, which is approximately 4 times body weight, is being generated unilaterally.

This analysis is predicated on the vertical GRF rising at a constant rate over the first half of the stance (and then falling at the same rate over the second half of the stance), something that does not actually occur *in vivo*. Specifically, Figure 5.4 shows the vertical GRF generated when the RFD is a constant of 51,564 N/s and the rate of force relaxation is

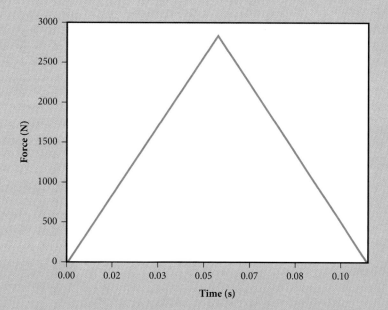

Figure 5.4 The vertical ground reaction force generated with a constant rate of force development of 51,564 N/s and a constant rate of force relaxation of −51,564 N/s.

(continues)

(continued)

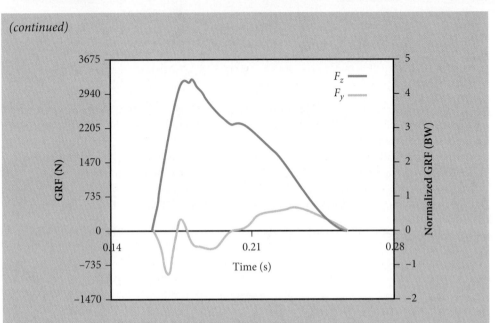

Figure 5.5 The vertical and horizontal components of the ground reaction force for an elite athlete sprinting at maximal velocity.

Reproduced from Bezodis, I. N., Kerwin, D. G., & Salo, A. I. T. (2008). Lower-limb mechanics during the support phase of maximum-velocity sprint running. *Medicine and Science in Sports and Exercise, 40,* 707–715.

a constant $-51,564$ N/s, as per our earlier example. Figure 5.5 shows the actual vertical GRF recorded from an elite sprinter running at maximal velocity.

Notice that while the magnitude of the peak GRF is similar between the two graphs, the overall shape differs greatly. The RFD recorded *in vivo* does not remain constant; indeed, it appears to be greater than that calculated in our example. However, despite the assumptions involved in the preceding analysis, we can determine that an elite sprinter is required to produce large peak vertical ground reaction forces during the stance phases associated with maximal-velocity sprinting and that the athlete must have high RFD to achieve these forces during the short durations of the stance phases. If the athlete is incapable of producing a high RFD, then he or she must remain in contact with the ground for a greater duration to reduce the negative vertical momentum of the CM to zero and to support body weight. This would result in a reduction in the athlete's running velocity. Therefore, explosive strength is very important for sprint athletes.

Worked Example 5.2
Quantifying explosive muscular strength during isometric back squats

Explosive muscular strength can be determined by calculating force–time variables collected from a force plate or a dynamometer during a given task. Here we calculate the rate of force development variables defined in Table 5.2 for two athletes performing isometric back squats on two force plates to provide the ground reaction force generated by each during a 3-s period. Athlete A has a body mass of 84.3 kg and a 1-RM parallel back squat of 175.0 kg; athlete B has a body mass of 79.6 kg and a 1-RM parallel back squat of 110.0 kg. The force–time traces for each athlete are shown in Figure 5.3. Table 5.3 shows

Table 5.3
Average Rate of Force Development, Peak Rate of Force Development, and Time of Peak Force Calculated for Two Athletes During an Isometric Back Squat

Athlete	F_{peak} (N)	Time F_{peak} (s)	RFD_{ave} (N/s)	RFD_{peak} (N/s)
A	1216	2.01	605	3482
B	759	2.89	263	1603

Note: F_{peak} = peak force; Time F_{peak} = time of peak force; RFD_{ave} = average rate of force development; RFD_{peak} = peak rate of force development.

the calculated values of peak force (F_{peak}), time of peak force (Time F_{peak}), average rate of force development (RFD_{ave}), and peak rate of force development (RFD_{peak}) derived from the force–time traces.

As per Table 5.2, RFD_{ave} is calculated as the ratio of F_{peak} and Time F_{peak}, while RFD_{peak} is calculated as the greatest value of the first derivative of force with respect to time. Notice that athlete A is able to produce a greater F_{peak} and achieves this force earlier in the task compared to athlete B; athlete A, therefore, has the greater RFD_{ave} of the two. Furthermore, the RFD_{peak} for athlete A is greater than that for athlete B. Table 5.4 shows the RFD values recorded during 50-ms time periods up to a time of 300 ms. These time periods include what some authors refer to as the early (<50 ms) and late (>150 ms) phases of RFD (Andersen & Aagaard, 2006). Notice that athlete A is able to achieve greater values of explosive muscular strength regardless of the measure used.

Table 5.4
Rate of Force Development Values Recorded During 50-ms Time Periods Calculated for Two Athletes During an Isometric Back Squat

Athlete	RFD_{50} (N/s)	RFD_{100} (N/s)	RFD_{150} (N/s)	RFD_{200} (N/s)	RFD_{250} (N/s)	RFD_{300} (N/s)
A	2032	2362	2640	2844	2929	2877
B	866	1011	1163	1271	1320	1317

Note: RFD_{50} = rate of force development in 50 ms; RFD_{100} = rate of force development in 100 ms; RFD_{150} = rate of force development in 150 ms; RFD_{200} = rate of force development in 200 ms; RFD_{250} = rate of force development in 250 ms; RFD_{300} = rate of force development in 300 ms.

Schmidtbleicher (1992) proposed that tasks involving the stretch–shortening cycle (SSC) can be divided into categories of fast and slow depending on the duration of the contraction times and the displacement of the joints during the task. Specifically, fast SSC tasks are characterized by short contraction times (<250 ms) and low joint displacements (e.g., drop jumps), whereas slow SSC tasks are characterized by longer contraction times and greater joint displacements (e.g., countermovement jumps). The fast SSC tasks produce high stretch-loads and constitute measures of reactive strength, an index of which can be quantified during a drop jump as follows (Flanagan & Comyns, 2008):

$$\text{Reactive strength index} = \frac{\left(\dfrac{v^2}{2g}\right)}{t} \qquad \text{Eq. (5.5)}$$

where v is takeoff velocity, g is the acceleration due to gravity, and t is the time of force application. Notice that the term $v^2/2g$ returns the jump height achieved during the drop jump, and that takeoff velocity is equal to the ratio of the net vertical impulse of the ground reaction force and body mass ($\int Fdt/m$). Thus, Equation (5.5) can be rewritten as follows:

$$\text{Reactive strength index} = \frac{\left(\int Fdt/m\right)^2/2g}{t} \qquad \text{Eq. (5.6)}$$

Inspection of Equation (5.6) informs us that the **reactive strength index** for an athlete will increase in proportion to the square of the net impulse that the individual is able to generate during the contact phase of the task and decrease in proportion to the square of body mass. Furthermore, the reactive strength index will decrease in proportion to the increase in contact time during the task. Therefore, a high reactive strength index is characterized by the application of a large relative impulse in a short period of time. Reactive strength would appear to be qualitatively similar to the measure of explosive strength discussed previously. However, the measurement of reactive strength is specific to tasks involving the stretch–shortening cycle, so it may have greater utility in sporting tasks such as sprint running, change of direction, and jumping activities.

The measure of reactive strength relates to the **stiffness** generated during a task involving the stretch–shortening cycle. Stiffness, which refers to the resistance of a body to a deformation (Brughelli & Cronin, 2008), can be calculated during a test of reactive strength such as a drop jump as follows:

$$k_{\text{vert}} = \frac{F}{\Delta s} \qquad \text{Eq. (5.7)}$$

where k_{VERT} is the vertical stiffness of the athlete, F is the peak vertical ground reaction force, and Δs is the change in displacement of the center of mass (CM) during the contact phase of the jump. During the performance of a drop jump, we could expect F and Δs to occur at the same time. We can compare Equation (5.7) with Equation (5.6) and identify the similarities. Specifically, Equation (5.6) informs us that an athlete who is able to generate a large relative vertical impulse during a short contact phase of a drop jump will demonstrate high reactive strength. It would also be expected that this athlete will achieve a large peak vertical ground reaction force while preventing the CM from descending over a large displacement due to the large force generation. This would result in a large k_{VERT} value for the athlete given the terms of Equation (5.7). The importance of vertical stiffness is highlighted in **Worked Example 5.3**.

Stiffness values can also be determined for the leg as follows:

$$k_{\text{leg}} = \frac{F}{\Delta l} \qquad \text{Eq. (5.8)}$$

Worked Example 5.3
The importance of vertical stiffness in sprint running

Vertical stiffness can be determined from the ratio of the ground reaction force acting on an athlete and the change in displacement of the individual's center of mass (CM) during the application of the ground reaction force. We will return to the data presented in Worked Example 5.1 for an athlete with a body mass of 75 kg sprinting at maximal velocity with a stance duration of 0.11 s. Figure 5.6 shows the hypothetical vertical ground reaction force data that we calculated for the athlete during the stance phase with a constant rate of force development of 51,564 N/s.

We can integrate the data shown in Figure 5.6 to provide the vertical velocity and the vertical displacement of the CM during the stance phase. These data are displayed in Figure 5.7.

We can determine that the CM falls 0.023 m during the stance phase and that this displacement coincides with the attainment of the maximal vertical ground reaction force of 2836 N (see Figures 5.6 and 5.7). Calculate the vertical stiffness for the athlete during the stance phase.

i. Calculate vertical stiffness using Equation (5.7)   Vertical stiffness = $F/\Delta s$

ii. Input the known variables   Vertical stiffness = $2836/0.023$

iii. Answer   Vertical stiffness = 123.3 kN/m

Notice how the vertical stiffness measure relates to the RFD of the athlete. Specifically, the RFD of 51,564 N/s allows the generation of 2836 N of force in 0.055 s. Given this RFD, the CM descends only 0.023 m during 0.055 s of the stance phase. If the athlete were unable to achieve this RFD, then the stance duration would have to be increased to accommodate the reduction in the vertical velocity of the CM. The high RFD required to achieve the acceleration of the CM may, in fact, be possible only because of the vertical stiffness of the athlete. If the athlete were unable to generate the required vertical stiffness of 123.3 kN/m, then his or her RFD would be reduced, requiring the athlete to increase the stance duration and, therefore, reduce the running velocity. The vertical stiffness of the athlete is largely determined by the interaction of the stiffness of the hip, knee, and ankle joints during the stance phase of sprinting.

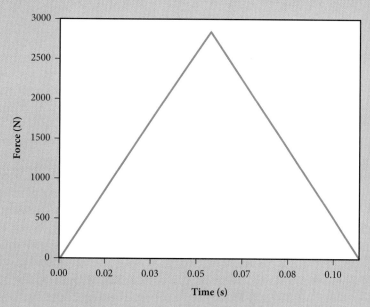

Figure 5.6 The vertical ground reaction force generated with a constant rate of force development of 51,564 N/s and a constant rate of force relaxation of −51,564 N/s.

(continues)

(continued)

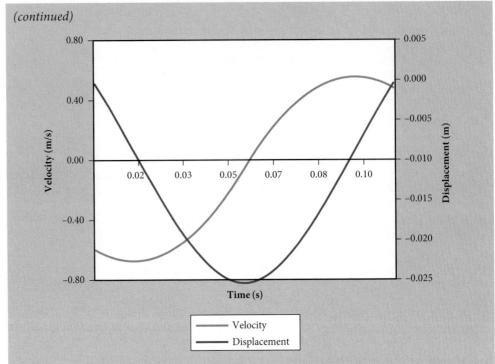

Figure 5.7 The vertical velocity and displacement of the center of mass during the stance phase of maximal-velocity sprint running.

where k_{leg} is the stiffness of the leg, F is the peak ground reaction force, and Δl is the change in the length of the leg during the force application. Leg stiffness will be determined from the interaction of the stiffness of the hip, knee, and ankle joints during the test of reactive strength:

$$k_{joint} = \frac{M}{\Delta\theta}$$

Eq. (5.9)

where k_{joint} is the joint stiffness, M is the peak joint moment, and $\Delta\theta$ is the change in joint angular displacement during force application. Stiffness has been identified as a modulator of RFD (Brughelli & Cronin, 2008).

The Importance of Muscular Strength in Sport

Measures of maximal muscular strength, both dynamic and isometric, have been shown to be important in a variety of sports, including baseball, basketball, American football, rugby, soccer, and sprint running; in all of these sports, the better athletes demonstrate the greater levels of maximal muscular strength (Baker & Newton, 2006; Bartlett, Storey, & Simons, 1989; Cometti, Maffiuletti, Pousson, Chatard, & Maffulli, 2001; Fry & Kraemer, 1991; Latin, Berg, & Baechle, 1994; Meckel, Atterbom, Grodjinovsky, Ben-Sira, & Rostein, 1995; Mero, Luhtanen, & Komi, 1983; Mero, Luhtanen, Viitasalo, & Komi, 1981; Wisløff, Castagna, Helgerud, Jones, & Hoff, 2004). RFD has been proposed as one of the most important variables to explain performance in activities where great acceleration is required (Aagaard et al., 2002; Cronin & Sleivert, 2005; González-Badillo & Marques, 2010), and high RFD has been associated with jumping performance (McLellan, Lovell, & Gass, 2011) and sprint running performance (Wilson, Lyttle, Ostrowski, & Murphy, 1995).

The time over which RFD is assessed affects the relationship with athletic tasks. Specifically, high values of RFD within 100 ms have been found to be strongly related to sprint performance, while high RFD values during times greater than 100 ms are more related to vertical jump performance (Tillin et al., 2013).

Low-load speed-strength, as measured by the force generated during an unloaded vertical jump, has been shown to be strongly correlated with sprinting performance (Mero, 1988; Mero et al., 1981; Young, McLean, & Ardagna, 1995), as has high-load speed-strength (Sleivert & Taingahue, 2004). Reactive strength, as measured by drop jump performance, has been shown to correlate strongly with sprinting performance (Cunningham et al., 2013; Mero, 1988; Mero et al., 1981; Smirniotou et al., 2008) and change of direction tasks (Young, James, & Montgomery, 2002). Finally, leg stiffness as measured in a hopping task has been shown to correlate strongly with maximal sprinting speed (Bret, Rahmani, Dufour, Messonnier, & Lacour, 2002; Chelly & Denis, 2001). Table 5.5 summarizes the different indices of muscular strength and their importance in sports performance.

Table 5.5
Indices of Muscular Strength

Strength Index	Description
Absolute maximal strength	The greatest force generated when an electrical stimulus is superimposed upon a maximal voluntary contraction during a given task.
	This index provides information about the intrinsic properties of the stimulated muscles.
Voluntary maximal dynamic strength	The greatest force generated voluntarily during a given dynamic task.
	Repetition maximum testing can be used to determine the maximal dynamic strength. The one-repetition maximum (1-RM) is the maximum load that can be lifted in a single repetition through an appropriate range of motion using the correct technique.
	The tasks can be concentric only or eccentric only, although they usually involve the stretch–shortening cycle.
	High maximal dynamic strength is strongly correlated with the level of sports performance.
Voluntary maximal isometric strength	The greatest external force exerted against an immovable body.
	High maximal isometric strength is strongly correlated with the level of sports performance.
Speed-strength	The force generated under conditions where the movement velocity is varied by altering the external load.
	An external load less than or equal to 30% 1-RM is used to determine low-load speed-strength; a load more than 30% 1-RM is used to determine high-load speed-strength.
	Both low-load and high-load speed-strength are strongly correlated with sprinting performance.
Explosive strength	The magnitude of force generated during a given time period characterized by high rates of force development (RFD).
	RFD is typically divided into "early" (less than 50 ms) and "late" (more than 150 ms) periods during dynamic and isometric tasks.
	RFD can be measured during both dynamic and isometric tasks.
	High RFD is strongly correlated with jumping and sprinting performance.
Reactive strength	The ability to tolerate high stretch-loads and rapidly transition from eccentric to concentric muscle actions in tasks involving the stretch–shortening cycle.
	This index is characterized by high vertical, leg, and joint stiffness.
	High reactive strength (stiffness) is strongly correlated with sprinting, change of direction, and jumping performance.

Defining Muscular Power

Power is defined as the rate at which work is done and can be determined from the product of the applied force and the velocity of the body. Alternatively, given that the work performed on a body changes the mechanical energy of the body (translational or rotational kinetic energy, gravitational potential energy, strain potential energy), net power can be determined from the rate of change of energy of the body to which the force is applied. Clearly, then, the variables of force and power are related. In turn, one should expect a relationship between muscular strength and power output. In the literature, numerous authors have shown that those athletes with greater levels of maximal dynamic muscular strength demonstrate greater muscular power output (Moss et al., 1997; Peterson, Alvar, & Rhea, 2006). However, while RFD and power are sometimes used interchangeably, it should be recognized that they are distinct mechanical variables (see Strength and Power Concept 5.2).

The relationship between power output and the force applied to a body can be expressed as follows:

$$\bar{P} = \frac{Fs}{t}$$

Eq. (5.10)

Strength and Power Concept 5.2

Rate of force development and mechanical power are distinct variables

Some practitioners use the terms "RFD" and "power" interchangeably. This tendency probably arises from the dependence of both variables on the application of a force onto a body as well as the use of a rate in the calculation of both variables; RFD is quantified as the rate at which a force is applied to a body, while mechanical power is the rate at which mechanical work is done by a force that is applied to a body. Given these definitions, mechanical power can be calculated only if the applied force actually performs mechanical work; that is, the point of application of the force must be displaced as the force is applied to the body. That the force does mechanical work is not a requirement when measuring RFD. Consider the situation during an isometric task where a force is applied to an immovable body. Under such mechanical constraints, the RFD can be determined but the force will not have performed any mechanical work, because the point of its application on the body is not displaced. (Metabolic work, however, is done during the isometric task to generate muscular force.)

Some authors have proposed RFD as one of a number of muscular qualities that contributes to mechanical power output developed during a given task (Newton & Dugan, 2002). From the mechanical expression of power given in Equation (5.10), it can be determined that the mechanical power output increases with the magnitude of the applied force, decreasing with an increase in the time over which the force acts. It follows that a large power output will be achieved if a large force is developed in a short period of time. In turn, a high RFD would allow the generation of a large mechanical power output. However, this relationship is valid only if the force developed does work on the body to which it is applied.

where P is the average mechanical power output, F is the average force applied, s is the displacement undergone by the body in the same direction as the force acts, and t is the time over which the force is applied to the body. Equation (5.10) informs us that power is the rate at which a force does mechanical work on a body and can be rewritten as follows:

$$P = Fv \hspace{4cm} \textbf{Eq. (5.11)}$$

where P is the mechanical power output, F is the magnitude of the applied force, and v is the linear velocity of the body. It follows that the mechanical power output during a given movement will depend on the mass of the body to which the athlete applies his or her force, given the effect this will have on the velocity of the body (see Equation 5.1). However, the magnitude of the external load that elicits maximal power output depends on the nature of the specific movements used, with a load equivalent to 0% squat 1-RM maximizing power output during the squat jump exercise, while a load of 50% 1-RM maximizes power output during the squat exercise (Cormie, McCauley, Triplett, & McBride, 2007). A load equivalent to 80% 1-RM has been shown to elicit maximal power output during the clean exercise (Cormie, McCauley, Triplett, & McBride, 2007). See Strength and Power Concept 5.3.

Strength and Power Concept 5.3

The external load that elicits maximal power output depends on the specific movement

Maximal power output for both isolated muscle fibers and single-joint movements is elicited when the external resistance is equivalent to 30% of the maximal isometric force (Cormie, McGuidan, & Newton, 2011). By comparison, for multiple-joint movements, the external load that maximizes power output varies between 0% and 80% of the maximal dynamic strength depending on the specific movement. For example, maximal power output occurs at 0% squat 1-RM during the squat jump, whereas a load of approximately 50% squat 1-RM maximizes power output during a squat (Cormie, McCauley, Triplett, & McBride, 2007). The differences in the load that elicits maximal power output between these two exercises likely reflects the ballistic nature of the squat jump: In this task, the load must possess positive vertical velocity at takeoff. In contrast, the squat has a non-ballistic nature, such that the velocity of the load is constrained to equal 0 m/s at the end of its ascent. The ballistic nature of the squat jump allows the generation of high forces under relatively low-load conditions because the duration of the acceleration of the load is greater.

Notice that body mass as well as the mass of the external load is being accelerated in the squat jump. This requirement is absent when performing the ballistic bench-throw exercise, which increases the relative load that elicits maximal power; loads equivalent to 30–45% bench press 1-RM have been identified in the research (Cormie et al., 2011). In weightlifting movements like the clean, the load that maximizes power output has been found to be 80% of 1-RM (Cormie, McCauley, Triplett, & McBride, 2007). Although this movement requires high

(continues)

(continued)

velocities of the load during the movement, the 1-RM for the clean is determined using the lift itself. It is likely that if the 1-RM load was determined from a non-ballistic exercise such as a deadlift, then the load that maximized power output in the clean would be a much lower percentage of the 1-RM (Cormie et al., 2011).

Equations (5.10) and (5.11) inform us that a given power output could be achieved by either the application of a large force or the achievement of a high movement velocity. For example, it is theoretically possible that the same power output might be produced in a specific movement either by the application of a large force with a relatively low movement velocity or by the application of a smaller force with a larger movement velocity. Furthermore, knowledge of the relative contributions of force and velocity to the power output generated by an athlete can guide the practitioner in determining the most appropriate training methods to develop power output (Samonzino, Rejc, Di Prampero, Belli, & Morin, 2012). A method to determine the contribution of force and movement velocity to power output is shown in Worked Example 5.4.

Worked Example 5.4
Quantifying the contributions of force and movement velocity to power output

Samonzino et al. (2012) propose that plotting the force against the velocity achieved during vertical jumps performed with different external loads can provide an indication of the relative contribution of force and velocity to each athlete's power output. Table 5.6 shows the values of the average normalized vertical ground reaction force (GRF), average vertical velocity, and the normalized average power output for two athletes recorded during squat jumps with external loads ranging from 0% to 85% of 1-RM back squat. The jumps were performed

Table 5.6
Average Normalized Vertical Force, Average Vertical Velocity, and Normalized Average Power Output for Two Athletes Recorded During Squat Jumps with External Loads Ranging from 0% to 85% of 1-RM Back Squat

Load	Force (N/kg)		Velocity (m/s)		Power Output (W/kg)	
	Athlete A	Athlete B	Athlete A	Athlete B	Athlete A	Athlete B
0% 1-RM	11.0	9.5	2.46	2.36	50.3	43.1
12% 1-RM	12.9	10.4	2.00	1.93	43.4	34.4
27% 1-RM	15.9	11.1	1.59	1.72	35.7	32.5
42% 1-RM	16.8	12.3	1.14	1.29	28.6	27.8
56% 1-RM	18.7	13.3	0.93	1.16	26.0	24.5
71% 1-RM	19.9	14.6	0.81	0.91	20.7	21.4
85% 1-RM	21.4	15.5	0.63	0.77	19.0	18.9

Note: 1-RM = one-repetition maximum.

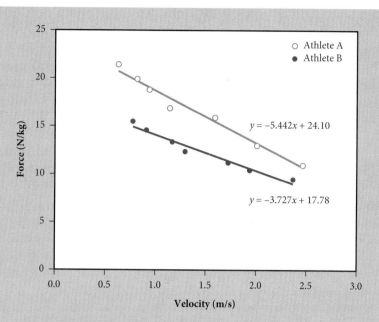

Figure 5.8 The force–velocity characteristics of two athletes calculated from the average vertical force and average vertical velocity values during jump squats performed under different load conditions from 0% to 85% of the load associated with their one-repetition maximum parallel back squat. The first term in each regression equation denotes the slope of the regression line, with a greater value reflecting a steeper slope and therefore a greater reliance on force. The second term in each regression equation denotes the maximal isometric force for each athlete.

on force plates to provide the GRF, while the velocity of the barbell was recorded from an opto-reflective motion analysis system. Athlete A has a body mass of 83.7 kg and a 1-RM back squat of 195.0 kg; athlete B has a body mass of 83.2 kg and a 1-RM back squat of 117.5 kg.

Both athletes achieve their maximal power output under the unloaded jumping condition. Athlete A tends to produce greater power outputs than athlete B under all of the loading conditions, although the difference becomes negligible at the higher percentages of 1-RM. Figure 5.8 shows the average vertical GRF plotted against the average vertical velocity for the two athletes. The regression equations for each athlete are displayed on the graph.

Notice that each graph in Figure 5.8 has a different slope, signifying a difference in the relative contributions of force and velocity to the production of power output for both athletes: Athlete A, who has the greatest dynamic strength, generates power through the application of large forces (as demonstrated by the larger slope of the regression), while athlete B, who is weaker, tends to rely on relatively greater velocity under the different load conditions (as demonstrated by the smaller slope of the regression line). Previous research has demonstrated that the slope of the force–velocity relationship assessed in such a manner can be altered through specific training (Cormie, McGuigan, & Newton, 2010); such an analysis, therefore, can be used to determine the training goals for the athlete. For example, improvements in power output for athlete A may be elicited by concentrating on training methods to increase velocity (e.g., low-load speed-strength training, overspeed training), while athlete B is likely to benefit from training methods that increase force production (e.g., high-load speed-strength training).

The Importance of Muscular Power in Sport

Given the relationship of mechanical power output to the change in mechanical energy of a body, it should be apparent that muscular power output can be used to distinguish between athletes with different performance levels. Indeed, researchers have demonstrated that elite rugby players have greater power output than lower-level players in both upper- and lower-body exercises (Baker, 2001; Hansen, Cronin, Pickering, & Douglas, 2011), while higher-level collegiate American football players demonstrate greater power outputs compared to their lower-level counterparts (Fry & Kraemer, 1991). Furthermore, starting football players are able to produce greater power outputs than nonstarters (Barker et al., 1993). Muscular power output has also been shown to be strongly correlated with sprint performance (Chelly & Denis, 2001; Sleivert & Taingahue, 2004). Vertical jump height is often used as a surrogate measure of muscular power output of the lower body; elite soccer players have been shown to jump higher than lower-level players (Cometti et al., 2001). Vertical jump height is also strongly correlated with sprint performance, with the fastest sprinters producing the greatest jump heights (Mero et al., 1983; Mero et al., 1981).

Determinants of Muscular Strength and Power

Usually what is measured during an assessment of muscular strength and/or muscular power output is a variable reflecting the mechanical output in a specific task (e.g., the mass lifted, the magnitude of the ground reaction force, the product of the force applied to the mass and the velocity of that mass), rather than a direct measurement of muscular forces being undertaken. Of course, any of these mechanical outputs will be largely determined by the forces generated by the active muscles during the specific task, but the practitioner requires an understanding of how muscle tension is transformed into the mechanical output measured to select an appropriate test of strength and power and to develop an appropriate training program to improve these variables. This requires an understanding of which factors determine muscle tension, how muscular tension is transformed into joint moments, and how joint moments are transformed into external forces.

Factors Determining Muscle Tension

The mechanical output developed by an active muscle depends on a number of factors. The influence of these factors on muscle tension, rate of force development, and power output is summarized in Table 5.7.

Although the various factors that affect the tension developed by a muscle are relatively well researched and understood, measuring individual muscle forces *in vivo* is a very difficult task. One approach is to take direct measurements of tendon forces (e.g., the Achilles tendon buckle; Finni, Komi, & Lukkariniemi, 1998), although such approaches are very invasive. Others have used imaging technologies (e.g., ultrasound, magnetic resonance imaging [MRI]; Maganaris, 2001) for this purpose (see Worked Example 5.5). While these techniques are certainly less invasive, the tasks that can be performed by the individual under investigation are necessarily single-joint movements. More recently, forward dynamic models of the human motor system have been used to allow the determination of individual muscle forces during more complex, multiple-joint movement tasks (Erdemir, McLean, Herzog, & van den Bogert, 2007).

Table 5.7
Factors Affecting the Tension Developed by a Muscle

Factor Affecting Muscle Tension	Explanation
Length of the muscle	Muscle tension is decreased when muscle fibers operate above or below the optimal length.
Velocity of dynamic muscle actions	Eccentric muscle tension > isometric tension > concentric muscle tension.
	Maximal power is achieved at 30% of maximal isometric tension.
	The force–velocity properties of skeletal muscle are largely determined by the predominant fiber type.
Fiber type	Tension per fiber cross-sectional area (specific tension) is greater in type II fibers.
	Maximal shortening velocities are greater in type II fibers.
	Rate of force development is greater in type II fibers.
	Power output per fiber cross-sectional area is greater in type II fibers.
Cross-sectional area	Muscle tension increases linearly with cross-sectional area (CSA).
	Increasing CSA is likely to increase power output.
Architecture	Greater pennation angles are associated with greater muscle tension.
	Greater pennation angles produce greater power output.
	Greater fiber length is associated with greater shortening velocities.
	Greater fiber lengths are associated with greater power output.
Activation dynamics	Greater motor unit recruitment produces greater muscle tension, rate of force development, and power output.
	Increased rate coding produces greater muscle tension, rate of force development, and power output.
	Timing and duration of activation of an individual muscle determine the tension, rate of force development, and power output during cyclical actions.
Spinal reflexes	Group Ia and II afferents make excitatory (agonist) and inhibitory (antagonist) connections with α-motoneurons.
	Group Ib afferents make inhibitory (agonist) and excitatory (antagonist) connections with α-motoneurons.
Contractile history	Greater muscle tension and power output occur when fibers are stretched before shortening (stretch–shortening cycle).
	Muscle fiber tension, rate of force development, and power output can be increased or decreased through previous activity via post-activation potentiation (PAP) and fatigue, respectively.
	Type II fibers demonstrate greater PAP and greater fatigue than type I fibers.

Reproduced from Cormie, P., McGuigan, M. R., & Newton, R. U. (2011). Developing maximal neuromuscular power. Part 1: Biological basis of maximal power production. *Sports Medicine, 41*, 17–38.

Worked Example 5.5
Calculating muscle forces using ultrasonography and magnetic resonance imaging

Maganaris (2001) had individuals perform electrically evoked contractions of the soleus muscle in a dynamometer at different joint angles to record the isometric moment at the ankle joint. Ultrasound-based measurements were also collected during the task to provide the pennation angle of the soleus, while MRI-based measurements were taken to provide the moment arm of the Achilles tendon. The data collected are shown in Table 5.8.

The author calculated the force at the Achilles tendon under each joint angle by dividing the moment by the moment arm. The soleus muscle force was then calculated by dividing the tendon force by the cosine of the pennation angle.

i. Calculate the tendon force (F_T) $\qquad$ $F_T = M/d$
ii. Calculate the muscle force (F_M) $\qquad$ $F_M = F_T/\cos\theta$

These calculations for the original data appear in Table 5.9. Note that the muscle force exceeds the tendon force due to the contribution of each fiber to the overall force being proportional to the cosine of the pennation angle. Moreover, both tendon and muscle force depend on the joint angle during the task.

Table 5.8
Isometric Moment, Achilles Tendon Moment Arm, and Pennation Angle During Electrically Evoked Contractions of the Soleus at Different Ankle Joint Angles

	Joint Angle (degrees)					
	−30	−15	0	15	30	45
Moment (Nm)	144	149	107	68	32	12
Tendon moment arm (m)	0.051	0.054	0.060	0.066	0.070	0.072
Pennation angle (degrees)	32	35	40	45	50	55

Note: Negative angles refer to dorsiflexion; 0° angle refers to the neutral (anatomic) position.

Table 5.9
Achilles Tendon and Soleus Muscle Forces During Electrically Evoked Contractions of the Soleus at Different Ankle Joint Angles

	Joint Angle (degrees)					
	−30	−15	0	15	30	45
Tendon force (N)	2824	2759	1783	1030	457	167
Muscle force (N)	3330	3368	2328	1457	711	291

Note: Negative angles refer to dorsiflexion; 0° angle refers to the neutral (anatomic) position.

Transforming Muscle Tension to Joint Moments

The force generated by a muscle is transmitted to the bones to which that muscle is attached to produce a moment about a joint. Recall that a moment of force is determined by the magnitude of the force and the moment arm of the force:

$$M = Fd$$ Eq. (5.12)

where M is the moment of force, F is the magnitude of the applied force, and d is the moment arm of the force (the perpendicular distance between the line of action of the force and the fulcrum). Equation (5.12) informs us that a given joint moment will be influenced not only by the magnitude of the muscular force developed, which is affected by numerous variables (Table 5.7), but also by the moment arm of the muscle. The muscle moment arm is greatly affected by the joint angle adopted during a given movement task (Dostal & Andrews, 1981; Tsaopoulos, Baltzopoulos, Richards, & Maganaris, 2009). One can therefore expect a given joint moment to be greatly affected by the posture adopted during the movement task. For example, performing a vertical jump with the trunk held in an upright position, thereby preventing rotation of the segment, results in reduction of the magnitude of the extensor moment at the hip joint, with a concomitant but smaller increase in the moment at the knee joint (Vanrenterghem, Lees, & De Clerque, 2008). Increasing the forward inclination of the trunk during a back squat reduces the moment at the knee joint, with a concomitant increase in the moment at the hip joint (Biscarini, Benventuti, Botti, Mastrandrea, & Zanuso, 2011). The joint angle assumed will also influence the length of the underlying muscles, and the magnitude of the joint moment will be further affected by the joint angle. In addition, the external load during a strength test produces a moment at a joint. Just as the moment arm associated with the muscular force changes with the joint angle, so, too, the moment arm associated with the external load used during a test of strength will differ as the joint is accelerated, thereby influencing the load that can be lifted and, in turn, the magnitude of muscular strength recorded (see Worked Example 5.6).

Worked Example 5.6
The moment arm of the external load affects the assessment of muscular strength

Consider the leg extension exercise performed in a weight machine to test the strength of an athlete. In this single-joint exercise, an external load is lifted by the athlete, exerting a knee extensor moment. Assume that the weight force associated with the mass added to the machine acts at a distance $l = 0.38$ m distal to the knee joint (Figure 5.9). Calculate the magnitude of the moment arm, d, associated with the weight force as the internal knee joint angle, θ, changes from 90° at the start of the movement to 180° at full extension.

  i. Calculate the moment arm associated with each knee angle $d = \cos(180 - \theta) \times l$
 ii. Answers are shown in Table 5.10

Notice that the magnitude of the moment arm associated with the weight force increases as the knee joint is accelerated into extension and reaches a maximum when the knee is fully extended. We can use the maximal moment arm to determine the maximal load that

(continues)

(continued)

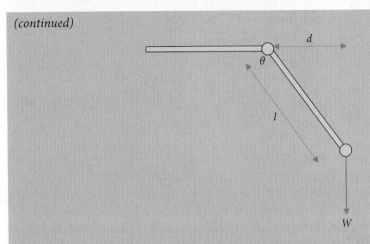

Figure 5.9 Free-body diagram of the knee extension task. *W* is the weight force associated with the load, *l* is the distance from the knee joint to the placement of the load, *d* is the moment arm associated with the load, and *θ* is the internal knee joint angle.

can be lifted assuming that the athlete is able to produce a maximal knee extensor moment of 250 Nm.

i. Calculate the maximal load that can be lifted at the point of maximal moment arm associated with the external load $M = Fd$

ii. Insert the known variables $250 = F \times 0.38$

iii. Rearrange for *F* $F = 250/0.38$

iv. Answer $F = 658\ \text{N}$

v. Remove gravitational acceleration to return the mass of the load $m = F/g$

vi. Answer $m = 67\ \text{kg}$

This value represents the maximal load that can be lifted by the athlete given a maximal knee extensor moment of 250 Nm. If the weight machine is changed such that the load is now placed 0.24 m distal to the knee joint, then the athlete will be able to lift a maximal load of 106 kg; the athlete's strength is substantially affected by the mechanics associated with the movement used during the assessment.

In this simple analysis, the mass of the body segments involved in the movement and the inertial forces have been ignored. Also, the magnitude of the knee extensor moment follows a curvilinear relationship *in vivo*, being greatest at a knee angle of approximately 100°, but decreasing by about 65% at 160° (Marginson & Eston, 2001). This means that the loads we have just calculated could only be lifted at certain knee joint angles.

Table 5.10
Magnitude of the Moment Arm Associated with the Weight Force Acting 0.38 m Distal to the Knee Joint at Selected Angles as the Internal Knee Joint Is Extended from 90° to 180° During the Movement

Internal Knee Joint Angle (degrees)	Load Moment Arm (m)
90	0.00
135	0.27
180	0.38

The effective mechanical advantage (EMA) of the active muscles can be determined from the ratio of the muscle moment arm to the moment arm of the external force. Alterations in the EMA during strength assessments have been proposed as the cause of the **sticking region**, defined as a period of decreasing vertical velocity during the ascent of the barbell that is evident when performing lifts with near maximal loads. Although the moment arm of the external load relative to the joints has not been shown to change during the sticking region of resistance exercise, the reduction in the moment arms associated with the active muscles crossing those joints appears to be a likely cause of the sticking region (Elliot, Wilson, & Kerr, 1989; Van den Tillaar, Sæterbakken, & Ettema, 2012). The sticking region, therefore, represents the weakest point during a given movement and provides a constraint on any measure of muscular strength.

The transformation of muscle tension to a joint moment is further complicated by the fact that there is unlikely to be a single muscle acting in isolation; rather, multiple muscles will be activated, some of which will act antagonistically. For example, we can update Equation (5.12) to determine the magnitude of the net flexor–extensor moment at the knee joint:

$$M_{NET} = F_{VI}d_{VI} + F_{VL}d_{VL} + F_{VM}d_{VM} + F_{RF}d_{RF} - F_{BF}d_{BF} - F_{ST}d_{ST} - F_{SM}d_{SM}$$

Eq. (5.13)

where M_{NET} is the magnitude of the net moment at the knee about the mediolateral axis, $F_{VI}d_{VI}$ is the moment produced by the vastus intermedius muscle, $F_{VL}d_{VL}$ is the moment produced by the vastus lateralis muscle, $F_{VM}d_{VM}$ is the moment produced by the vastus medialis muscle, $F_{RF}d_{RF}$ is the moment produced by the rectus femoris muscle at the knee joint, $F_{BF}d_{BF}$ is the moment produced by the biceps femoris muscle at the knee joint, $F_{ST}d_{ST}$ is the moment produced by the semitendinosus muscle at the knee joint, and $F_{SM}d_{SM}$ is the moment produced by the semimembranosus muscle at the knee joint. Notice in Equation (5.13) that the moments produced by the knee extensor muscle are positive while those produced by the knee flexors are negative. Consequently, the magnitude of the net moment about a given joint will be determined by the sum of the activity of the products of individual muscle forces and the moment arm associated with each muscle. It then becomes apparent that the net joint moment will be determined by the timing of activation of multiple muscles as well as their individual characteristics (e.g., muscle fiber length, muscle fiber type, physiological cross-sectional area, pennation angle, moment arm).

Notice that Equation (5.13) has an infinite number of solutions to return a given net joint moment due to unknown muscular forces and moment arms associated with each of the muscles. This situation arises when using inverse dynamics to calculate the net moment acting at a given joint; the contribution of individual muscles cannot be determined in such a case. Forward dynamic techniques overcome this problem and allow for the determination of the contribution of individual muscles to the joint moments during specific movements.

The expression of explosive strength will be affected by the mechanical characteristics of tendinous structures. A short delay (between 25 and 100 ms), known as an **electromechanical delay** (EMD), occurs following the activation of a muscle (measured via the electromyographic signal) until the force is detected; its source likely resides in an initial stretch of the connective tissue following crossbridge cycling (Zatsiorsky & Prilutsky, 2012). Indeed, the increased stiffness of tendinous structures increases the rate of torque development (Bojsen-Møller, Magnusson, Rasmussen, Kjær, & Aagaard, 2005). EMD is affected by the dynamic properties of the muscle (i.e., length–tension and force–velocity relationships). Specifically, the requirement to shorten rapidly during high-speed movements reduces the contractile elements' ability to generate force, so the mechanical response will further lag behind the activation dynamics (Caldwell & Li, 2000). The EMD is shorter for eccentric actions where the connective tissue is pre-stretched compared to concentric actions, and it decreases with an increase in lengthening velocity (Zatsiorsky & Prilutsky, 2012).

Transforming Joint Moments to an External Force

The net moments acting at the joints involved in a given task are transformed into external forces that are exerted on the environment. For example, the vertical ground reaction force during a vertical jump is largely determined by moments acting at the hip, knee, and ankle joints during the propulsive phase of the task (Figure 5.10).

The relationship between the joint moments and the external force produced in a given movement is further revealed in analyses showing the concomitant increase in the magnitude of the ground reaction force and the sum of the moments at the hip, knee, and ankle joints as the external load increases in both non-ballistic (back squat) and ballistic (squat jumps) movements (Flanagan & Salem, 2008; Moir, Gollie, Davis, Guers, & Witmer, 2012). However, despite the relationship that exists between the increase in the sum of the joint moments and the increase in the external force in response to increased external loads during the assessment of muscular strength, the contributions of the individual joint moments to the external force are more

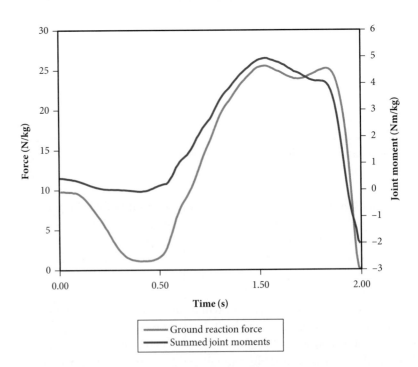

Figure 5.10 The vertical component of the ground reaction force and the sum of the hip, knee, and ankle joint moments during a vertical jump. Positive moments refer to extensor moments. Notice how the ground reaction force increases as the sum of the extensor moments at the joints increases.

complicated. For example, during the non-ballistic back squat, the largest moments are observed at the hip joint, and the lowest moments are found at the ankle joint, regardless of the external load (Flanagan & Salem, 2008). However, as the external load lifted increases, the hip and ankle joints increase their contributions to the external force while there is a concomitant decrease in knee joint moment (Flanagan & Salem, 2008). During a ballistic squat jump movement performed under different external loads, the power output at the knee and the ankle joints follows the power output of the external load, decreasing linearly as the mass of the external load increases (Moir et al., 2012). However, the power output at the hip joint actually increases with loads up to 42% of squat 1-RM, but then decreases thereafter (Figure 5.11). A similar response in joint power is observed during submaximal and maximal vertical jumps (Lees, Vanrenterghem, & De Clercq, 2004). Specifically, the ankle joint moment does not increase when jump height increases from 65% to 83% of maximal height, while the work at the knee and ankle joints remains unchanged during these efforts. The moment and work at the hip joint increase concomitantly with jump height. Therefore, submaximal jumping efforts may be sufficient to train the knee extensor and ankle plantarflexor muscle groups. However, maximal effort jumps are required to provide sufficient stimulus to train the hip extensor muscles.

What can be concluded from the preceding analysis is that the mechanical behavior of the joints contributing to a given multiple-joint movement can be summed to provide the mechanical output during the movement. At the same time, the contributions of the individual joints may not change in proportion to the mechanical output.

A number of constraints influence the transformation of joint moments into the generation of an external force—constraints that can be categorized as anatomic, geometric, and directional in nature (van Ingen Schenau, 1989). An *anatomic constraint*

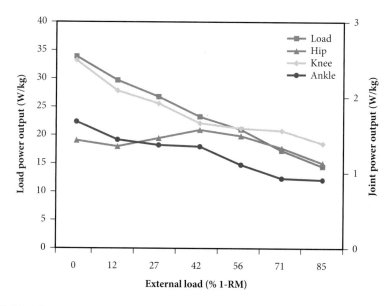

Figure 5.11 The power output of the external load and power outputs at the hip, knee, and ankle joints during vertical jumps performed with external loads from 0% to 85% squat 1-RM. Notice the decreases in the power output of the load and at the knee and ankle joints as the mass of the external load increases. The power output at the hip joint actually increases with the mass of the external load initially.

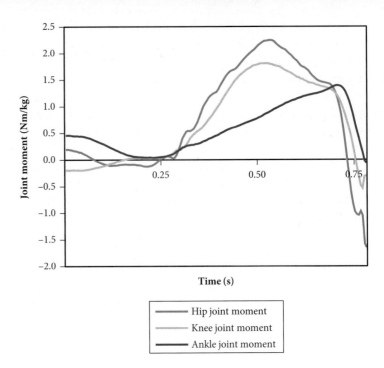

Figure 5.12 The flexor–extensor moments at the hip, knee, and ankle joints during the propulsive phase of a countermovement vertical jump. Positive values reflect extensor joint moments. As takeoff approaches, the magnitude of the extensor moment decreases at each of the joints and changes to a flexor moment to reduce the angular velocity of the joint to zero, thereby preventing damage to the joint structures.

is the requirement for zero angular velocity of a joint at the time of full extension. This constraint ensures that the joint structures are not damaged, but requires the reduction of the magnitude of a joint moment prior to full extension or the activation of antagonist muscles to decrease the angular velocity of the joint (**Figure 5.12**).

As a joint reaches the limits of its range of motion, the magnitude of the moment exerted in that direction decreases. For example, as the hip joint reaches full extension during the ascent of the load during a back squat, the magnitude of the extensor moment that can be generated is reduced; in turn, the contribution of the joint moment to the external force is reduced. This imposes a *geometric constraint* on the transformation of joint moments to an external force (see **Worked Example 5.7**).

The specific demands of the movement task that the athlete is performing will determine where the external force acts on the body and in which direction the external force acts, thereby imposing a *directional constraint* on the transformation of the joint moment to the external force. Many movements require that the athlete not only exert a large force against a body but also control the direction of the applied force throughout the movement (e.g., the direction of the ground reaction force during the stance phases of sprinting and during the contact phase of landing tasks). The location of the center of pressure associated with the external force and the direction in which the external force acts are affected by the relative magnitudes of the net joint moments associated with the joints of the limb in contact with the surface. For example, the

Worked Example 5.7
Geometric constraint imposed on the transformation of joint rotation to the translation of the center of mass

Consider a simple two-segment model of the lower body during a ballistic task that requires the center of mass (CM) to be accelerated vertically by the forceful extension of the joint (Figure 5.13).

The vertical velocity of the CM in this simple model depends on both the displacement and the velocity of the joint as expressed in the following equation (van Ingen Schenau, 1989):

$$v_{CM} = (l_1 \times l_2 \times \sin\theta / \sqrt{l_1^2 \times l_2^2 - 2l_1 \times l_2 \times \cos\theta}) \times d\theta/dt$$

where v_{CM} is the vertical velocity of the center of mass, l_1 is the length of segment 1, l_2 is the length of segment 2, θ is the angle between the segments, and $d\theta/dt$ is the derivative of the angle with respect to time (joint angular velocity). The term that appears in the parentheses in the equation reflects the transfer of the joint rotation to the translation of the CM; notice that this transfer will decrease to zero at the joint angle θ of 0°. This result can be demonstrated if we provide hypothetical values for the length of the segments in the model (0.45 m) and then determine the magnitude of the transfer function for joint angles between 90° and 180° (Table 5.11).

Notice from Table 5.11 that the magnitude of the transfer function decreases from its maximum when the joint angle is 90° to a value of 0 when the joint is in full extension. Therefore, the transformation of the rotation at the joint to the translation of the CM is reduced as the joint approaches full extension—a geometric constraint imposed upon joints *in vivo* that are required to generate a moment while they extend. This limits the transformation of the joint moment to the external force. Of course, in tasks where this situation might apply, such as during the vertical jump, multiple joints contribute to the vertical velocity of the CM. For example, as the knee joint approaches full extension and the transformation of its rotation to the translation of the CM is reduced, the ankle joint is

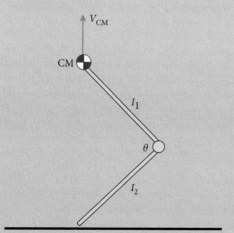

Figure 5.13 A simple two-segment model of the lower body during a vertical jump task. CM is the center of mass, v_{CM} is the vertical velocity of the CM, l_1 is the length of segment 1, l_2 is the length of segment 2, and θ is the joint angle.

(continues)

(continued)

Table 5.11
Magnitude of the Transfer Function for Joint Angles Between 90° and 180°

Joint Angle (degrees)	Transfer Function
90	1.00
120	0.36
150	0.16
180	0.00

able to rotate to continue the translation of the CM. However, all joints have this geometric constraint imposed upon them.

Notice in our example that the CM could still achieve high vertical velocity at the joint angles of 120° and 150° due to the transform function being multiplied by the angular velocity of the joint. However, the anatomic constraint imposed on the transformation of joint rotations to translations (as highlighted in the text) would limit these angular velocities as the full extension of the joint was approached.

application of a normal ground reaction force is achieved by the combination of net extensor moments acting at the hip, knee, and ankle joints. However, increasing the magnitude of the hip extensor moment while simultaneously changing the moment at the knee joint to a flexor moment induces a positive anterior–posterior component of the ground reaction force in addition to the normal component; producing a large knee extensor moment in combination with flexor moments at the hip and ankle joints changes the anterio-posterior component to a negative direction (Wells & Evans, 1987), as shown in **Table 5.12**.

Table 5.12
Effect of Net Joint Moments at the Hip, Knee, and Ankle Joints on the Direction of the Resultant Ground Reaction Force

Hip Moment (Nm)	Knee Moment (Nm)	Ankle Moment (Nm)	Direction of GRF (degrees)
41	−13	15	60
3	13	5	90
−31	33	−4	120

Notes: GRF = resultant ground reaction force. The direction of the ground reaction force is relative to the right horizontal. Positive moments refer to extensor moments; negative moments refer to flexor moments.

The task required individuals to lie on their side and apply an isometric force against a force platform with the hip, knee, and ankle joints in positions of slight flexion. Each individual was instructed to apply a constant force of equal magnitude (64 N) in the corresponding direction noted in the table.

Reproduced from Wells, R., & Evans, N. (1987). Functions and recruitment patterns of one- and two-joint muscles under isometric and walking conditions. *Human Movement Sciences, 6*, 349–372, with permission from Elsevier.

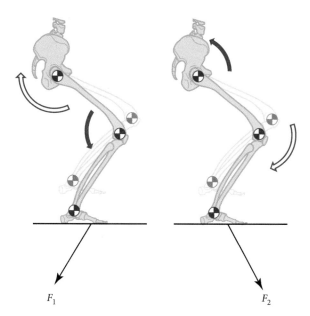

F_1 F_2

Figure 5.14 The changes in magnitude and direction of the joint moments at the hip and knee joints control the direction of the resultant force exerted by the foot onto the ground (F_1 and F_2). The open arrows refer to extensor moments. The curvilinear length of the arrow denotes the magnitude of the net moment. The generation of a large hip extensor moment combined with a smaller knee flexor moment directs the applied force down and back, while a hip flexor moment combined with a large knee extensor moment directs the applied force downward and forward. The resultant ground reaction force, which would produce an acceleration of the body, is simply a reaction to these applied forces.

During a ballistic movement such as the vertical jump, a similar alteration in the relative magnitude of the hip, knee, and ankle joint moments is observed as an attempt to control the direction of the resultant ground reaction force to satisfy the requirement of maximizing the vertical velocity of the CM (Jacobs & van Ingen Schenau, 1992a; van Ingen Schenau, 1989) (**Figure 5.14**). The relative magnitudes of the hip, knee, and ankle joint moments determine the location of the center of pressure associated with the external force as well as the direction in which the external force acts; these magnitudes are largely dependent upon the activation of the biarticular muscles crossing the joints (van Ingen Schenau, 1989). (See **Strength and Power Concept 5.4.**) Thus the patterning of muscle activation exerts a very great influence on the control of the direction of the external force generated in a given movement and, therefore, on the outcome of a specific task (Bobbert & van Soest, 1994; Nagano & Gerritsen, 2001). (See **Applied Research 5.2.**) As a consequence, the expression of muscular strength, defined by the mechanical output in a given task, is strongly influenced by the muscle activation pattern. Furthermore, the coactivation of monoarticular agonist and biarticular antagonists can serve a functional purpose in multijoint tasks, as it allows energy to be transported between joints while satisfying the anatomic and geometric constraints associated with transforming joint rotations into translations of the external load (van Ingen Schenau, 1989).

Strength and Power Concept 5.4

The muscle activation pattern determines the direction of the external force produced and, therefore, the outcome in ballistic tasks

During ballistic movements such as the vertical jump, the relative contributions of the hip, knee, and ankle joint moments are altered during the execution of the movement as the athlete attempts to control the location of the center of pressure associated with the ground reaction force and the direction that the ground reaction force acts, which will determine the acceleration of the center of mass (Bobbert & van Zandwijk, 1999). Specifically, early during propulsion, the magnitude of the hip joint moment is increased prior to and more rapidly than that of the knee and ankle joint moments, and the CM experiences an upward and forward acceleration. As the time of takeoff approaches, the magnitude of the knee and ankle joint moments increases, resulting in an almost purely vertical acceleration of the CM at takeoff.

A specific activation pattern of the monoarticular and biarticular muscles crossing the hip, knee, and ankle joints occurs to achieve the control of the ground reaction force. That is, the increase in the magnitude of the hip extensor moment is associated with the activation of the monoarticular hip extensor gluteus maximus, and the rise time in the activation of this muscle is strongly correlated with the rise in the vertical component of the ground reaction force (Bobbert & van Zandwijk, 1999). However, prior to this monoarticular muscle being activated, the biarticular hamstrings (biceps femoris, semitendinosus) are activated, increasing the magnitude of the hip extensor moment while concomitantly decreasing the extensor moment at the knee joint. Indeed, due to the early activation of the hamstrings, the horizontal component of the ground reaction force, which acts in the positive direction (forward), increases more rapidly than the vertical component.

The activation of the monoarticular gluteus maximus and the biarticular hamstrings reach maximal values relatively early in the propulsive phase, after which the hip extensor moment begins to decrease as the CM accelerates vertically. At the same time, the knee and ankle joint moments are increasing, so the direction of the ground reaction force vector changes from being upward and forward to being upward and backward such that the forward velocity of the CM is reduced as the point of takeoff approaches. During this latter part of the propulsive phase of the task, the ratio of the joint moments changes such that the combined knee and ankle joint moments exceed the hip joint moment. Furthermore, activation of the biarticular gastrocnemius couples knee extension with plantar flexion, allowing the ankle joint moment to contribute to the vertical acceleration of the CM late in the propulsive phase while also reducing the angular velocity of the knee joint. This combination compensates for the geometric and anatomic constraints associated with the transformation of joint rotations to translations (van Ingen Schenau, 1989).

If the jumping task were achieved only by the activation of the knee and/or ankle extensors, then there would be a tendency to rotate the body backward.

In that case, the joint rotations would not be effectively transferred into the vertical motion of the CM. Therefore, the increase in the knee and ankle joint moments must occur after the increase in the magnitude of the hip joint to ensure effective transfer from joint rotations to CM translation.

A proximal-to-distal sequencing of maximal activation of the monoarticular muscles is observed during the jumping task (Bobbert & van Zandwijk, 1999; Jacobs & van Ingen Schenau, 1992a). If the task were achieved simply by the simultaneous activation of monoarticular muscles crossing the lower-body joints, then the athlete would lose contact with the ground too early, limiting the energy of the CM at takeoff and, in turn, limiting performance in the task. The biarticular hamstrings and rectus femoris demonstrate reciprocal actions during propulsion, such that the hamstrings are activated early during the task, followed by the rectus femoris. Thus the monoarticular muscles increase their activation and increase the work performed while the biarticular muscles play a central role in controlling the distribution of joint moments, thereby controlling the location of the center of pressure and the direction of the external force (Bobbert & van Soest, 2000; Jacobs & van Ingen Schenau, 1992a; Mathiyakom, McNitt-Gray, & Wilcox, 2007; van Ingen Schenau, 1989). The reciprocal actions of the biarticular hamstrings and rectus femoris have also been observed during the acceleration phase of sprint running, where the requirement to control the direction of the resultant ground reaction force represents the key constraint on the task (Jacobs & van Ingen Schenau, 1992b). Successful execution in explosive tasks is not just determined by the generation of large forces, but also through the control of the direction in which the forces act.

Applied Research 5.2

Increased muscular strength requires concomitant changes in muscle activation patterns to realize improvements in performance

The authors developed a computer simulation using forward dynamic methods of the human motor system performing a vertical jump. The model comprised three joints representing the hip, knee, and ankle joints. They were served by actuators that reflected the force–velocity, length–tension, and activation dynamics of skeletal muscle *in vivo*. The kinematic and kinetic data generated from the model during simulated jumps were validated against the data collected from an elite athlete and were found to be representative. The authors used the simulation model to determine the effects of changing the mechanical parameters on the performance (jump height). It was found that increasing the strength of the lower-body muscles actually resulted in a reduced jump height. Furthermore, jump height increased with increased muscle strength only when the timing of the muscle activation was altered accordingly.

The findings of this simulation study can be interpreted as indicating that an increase in muscle strength will not necessarily be sufficient to increase performance in a task that relies on the generation of high muscular forces. Rather, an alteration in the activation pattern of the muscles is required to ensure that the muscular forces are combined appropriately to maximize the external force produced and, in turn, the performance in the specific task.

Bobbert, M. F., & van Soest, A. J. (1994). Effects of muscle strengthening on vertical jump height: A simulation study. *Medicine and Science in Sports and Exercise, 26,* 1012–1020.

The required direction of the external force has important implications for the mechanical factors that contribute to power output. For example, Samonzino et al. (2012) provide evidence that as the direction of the external force becomes more horizontal, the velocity capabilities of the athlete becomes more important than the force capabilities in developing large power outputs; the opposite is true when the external force is directed vertically. This relationship would have significant implications for athletes participating in tasks requiring large vertical power outputs (e.g., jumping, maximal-velocity sprinting) compared to those involved in tasks requiring large horizontal power outputs (e.g., accelerative sprinting, change of direction).

The mechanical output from both limbs acting concomitantly (bilateral tasks) is less than the sum of the output of the limbs acting separately (unilaterally), a phenomenon known as the **bilateral deficit** (Rejc, Lazzer, Antonutto, Isola, & di Prampero, 2010):

$$\text{Bilateral deficit} = \frac{\left(UL_{sum} - BL\right)}{UL_{sum}} \qquad \text{Eq. (5.14)}$$

where UL_{sum} is the sum of the mechanical output from each of the limbs assessed separately, and BL is the mechanical output from the limbs assessed concurrently. The bilateral deficit has been shown for both upper- and lower-body exercises and has been attributed to alterations of the force–velocity relationship of the active muscles (Bobbert, De Graaf, Jonk, & Casius, 2006) and neural inhibition during symmetrical bilateral muscle activation (Hay, de Souza, & Fukashiro, 2006; Howard & Enoka, 1991; Rejc et al., 2010). Recent experimental evidence has tended to support a change in the activation patterns of the muscles involved in the specific task as an explanation for the bilateral deficit (see Applied Research 5.3).

Applied Research 5.3
Unilateral tasks produce greater force and power at a given velocity than bilateral tasks

In this study, the authors had individuals perform an explosive pushing task for the lower body under both bilateral (BL) and unilateral (UL) conditions. Six resistances ranging from 50% to 200% of body weight were applied to each participant during the task to manipulate the force and velocity generated. The force applied by the participants and the resulting velocity of the movement were measured, allowing the calculation of power output under each of the loading conditions. The electromyographic activity of the vastus lateralis (VL), rectus femoris (RF), biceps femoris (BF), and the gastrocnemius medialis (GM) muscles were also measured.

The researchers found that the force and the power output developed by each leg under the six loading conditions were greater when the task was performed under the UL conditions compared to the BL conditions, precluding the alteration in the force–velocity relationship of the muscles as an explanation for the bilateral deficit. Greater EMG activity of VL and RF were recorded in the UL conditions compared to the BL conditions, with no differences observed in the activity of the BF and GM muscles. Furthermore, the coordination between these muscles was different in the BL and UL conditions. The authors concluded that the bilateral deficit resulted from changes in the activation pattern of the muscles during the task and not changes in the force–velocity relationships of the activated muscles.

Rejc, E., Lazzer, S., Antonutto, G., Isola, M., & di Prampero, P. E. (2010). Bilateral deficit and EMG activity during explosive lower limb contractions against different overloads. *European Journal of Applied Physiology, 108,* 157–165.

Specificity of Muscular Strength and Power

The preceding discussion should inform us that muscular strength and power are specific qualities, the magnitudes of which will depend on the mechanics of the task selected in the assessment. For example, maximal isometric force production and isometric RFD are influenced by the joint angle selected during the assessment task (Murphy, Wilson, Pryor, & Newton, 1995). The specificity of muscular strength and power has also been demonstrated in studies performed to investigate the effects of training modes in increasing measures of muscular strength and power. For example, gains in muscular strength and power have been shown to be greater in assessment tasks that were specific to the training exercises in terms of the type of muscle actions used (Abernethy & Jurimäe, 1996; Rutherford & Jones, 1986), bilateral compared to unilateral exercises Hakkinen et al., 1996; Häkkinen & Komi, 1983), and open-kinetic chain exercises compared to closed-kinetic chain exercises (Augustsson, Esko, Thomeé, & Svantesson, 1998; Carroll, Abernethy, Logan, Barber, & McEniery, 1998). Furthermore, the posture adopted during the movement task affects the ability of the athlete to generate force, which then influences the magnitude of strength recorded.

For example, when the assessment of maximal dynamic muscular strength is performed in a weight machine, the magnitude of the 1-RM load is different from that when the same exercise is performed with free weights, although there is a difference between upper- and lower-body exercises. Specifically, when the bench press exercise is performed using a Smith machine that constrains the movement of the barbell to purely vertical motion, the 1-RM load has been shown to be lower than that using free weights, while the reverse was found for 1-RM loads during the back squat exercise (Cotterman, Darby, & Skelly, 2005). Therefore, the strength and conditioning practitioner should consider the mechanical characteristics of any exercises selected to train or assess muscular strength and power.

Chapter Summary

Muscular strength is characterized by the ability of a muscle or a group of muscles to produce a force against an external resistance. Many indices of muscular strength exist. Maximal muscular strength is the ability to generate maximal force against a large external resistance and can be measured under dynamic (concentric, eccentric, stretch–shortening cycle) or isometric conditions. Speed-strength is measured as the peak force produced under dynamic conditions with varying external loads, providing low-load speed-strength (external load $\leq 30\%$ 1-RM) and high-load speed-strength (external load $> 30\%$ 1-RM). Explosive strength is characterized by high rates of force development and can be recorded under dynamic or isometric conditions. Reactive strength is the ability to tolerate high stretch-loads and rapidly transition from eccentric to concentric muscle actions. Muscular power output can be determined from the product of the force applied to a body and the movement velocity of the body, so the same power output can be produced by different combinations of force and velocity.

Measures of muscular strength and power output have been shown to be strongly correlated to successful performance in a number of sports and may be used to distinguish between athletes who compete at different levels. Muscular strength and power output are typically inferred from the mechanical output during a given movement task rather than assessing the force generated by the muscles directly. They are determined by a number of factors related to the intrinsic qualities of the musculotendinous units. However, the transformation of muscle tension to joint moments and the transformation of joint moments to external forces represent important determinants of muscular strength and power output. Given the transformations of muscle tension to joint moments and of joint moments to external forces, the assessment of muscular strength and power output are likely to be specific to the movements used.

Review Questions and Projects

1. Which information can be provided by measures of absolute dynamic muscular strength?

2. Explain the differences between ratio and allometric scaling methods for normalizing muscular strength to body mass.

3. Which tests could be performed to assess an athlete's ability in fast and slow stretch–shortening cycle tasks for the lower body?

4. Which muscular qualities influence early and late rates of force development?

5. Explain why a high rate of force development is important for a sprinter.

6. Explain the relationship between vertical stiffness and reactive strength.

7. Explain why there is likely to be a relationship between maximal dynamic muscular strength and power output.

8. Explain how the rate of force development can influence power output.

9. Why is the external load that maximizes power output different between the squat jump, the back squat, and the power clean exercises?

10. Describe a method to determine the contribution of force and movement velocity to power output during a multiple-joint movement.

11. Explain the implications of the bilateral deficit for the strength and conditioning practitioner.

12. Explain which factors influence the electromechanical delay and how they may affect the rate of force development.

13. Explain the difficulties that arise when one attempts to determine the force exerted by individual muscles during an assessment of muscular strength.

14. Explain the anatomic constraint associated with the transformation of a joint moment to an external force.

15. Explain the geometric constraint associated with the transformation of a joint moment to an external force.

16. Explain the directional constraint associated with the transformation of a joint moment to an external force.

17. Explain why the muscle activation pattern is important in influencing the outcome in an assessment of muscular strength or power.

18. How does the direction of the movement influence the contribution of force and velocity to power output?

19. How does the multijoint motor system accommodate the geometric constraint to the transformation of joint moments and turn it into an external force during ballistic movements?

20. Explain how the assessment of maximal dynamic muscular strength performed in a Smith machine may differ from that performed with free weights.

References

Aagaard, P., Simonsen, E. B., Andersen, J. L., Magnusson, P., & Dyhre-Poulsen, P. (2002). Increased rate of force development and neural drive of human skeletal muscle following resistance training. *Journal of Applied Physiology, 93,* 1318–1326.

Abernethy, P. J., & Jurimäe, J. (1996). Cross-sectional and longitudinal uses of isoinertial, isometric, and isokinetic dynamometry. *Medicine and Science in Sports and Exercise, 28,* 1180–1187.

Andersen, L. L., & Aagaard, P. (2006). Influence of maximal muscle strength and intrinsic muscle contractile properties on contractile rate of force development. *European Journal of Applied Physiology, 96,* 46–52.

Andersen, L. L., Andersen, J. L., Zebis, M. K., & Aagaard, P. (2010). Early and late rate of force development: Differential adaptive responses to resistance training. *Scandinavian Journal of Medicine and Science in Sports, 20,* 162–169.

Augustsson, J., Esko, A., Thomeé, R., & Svantesson, U. (1998). Weight training of the thigh muscles using closed vs. open kinetic chain exercises: A comparison of performance enhancement. *Journal of Sports Physical Therapy, 27,* 3–8.

Baker, D. (2001). Comparison of upper-body strength and power between professional and college-aged rugby league players. *Journal of Strength and Conditioning Research, 15,* 30–35.

Baker, D. G., & Newton, R. U. (2006). Discriminative analyses of various upper body tests in professional rugby-league players. *International Journal of Sports Physiology and Performance, 1,* 347–360.

Barker, M., Wyatt, T. J., Johnson, R. L., Stone, M. H., O'Bryant, H. S., Poe, C., & Kent, M. (1993). Performance factors, physiological assessment, physical characteristics, and football playing ability. *Journal of Strength and Conditioning Research, 7,* 224–233.

Bartlett, L. R., Storey, M. D., & Simons, B. D. (1989). Measurement of upper extremity torque production and its relationship to throwing speed in the competitive athlete. *American Journal of Sports Medicine, 17,* 89–91.

Bezodis, I. N., Kerwin, D. G., & Salo, A. I. T. (2008). Lower-limb mechanics during the support phase of maximum-velocity sprint running. *Medicine and Science in Sports and Exercise, 40,* 707–715.

Biscarini, A., Benventuti, P., Botti, F., Mastrandrea, F., & Zanuso, S. (2011). Modelling the joint torques and loadings during squatting at the Smith machine. *Journal of Sports Sciences, 29,* 457–469.

Bobbert, M. F., De Graaf, W. W., Jonk, J. N., & Casius, L. J. R. (2006). Explanation of the bilateral deficit in human vertical squat jumping. *Journal of Applied Physiology, 100,* 493–499.

Bobbert, M. F., & van Soest, A. J. (1994). Effects of muscle strengthening on vertical jump height: A simulation study. *Medicine and Science in Sports and Exercise, 26,* 1012–1020.

Bobbert, M. F., & van Soest, A. J. (2000). Two-joint muscle offer the solution, but what was the problem? *Motor Control, 4,* 48–52.

Bobbert, M. F., & van Zandwijk, J. P. (1999). Dynamics of force and muscle stimulation in human vertical jumping. *Medicine and Science and Sports and Exercise, 31,* 303–310.

Bojsen-Møller, J., Magnusson, S. P., Rasmussen, L. R., Kjær, M., & Aagaard, P. (2005). Muscle performance during maximal isometric and dynamic contractions is influenced by the stiffness of the tendinous structures. *Journal of Applied Physiology, 99,* 986–994.

Bret, C., Rahmani, A., Dufour, A. B., Messonnier, L., & Lacour, J. R. (2002). Leg strength and stiffness as ability factors in 100 m sprint running. *Journal of Sports Medicine and Physical Fitness, 42,* 274–281.

Brughelli, M., & Cronin, J. (2008). A review of research on the mechanical stiffness in running and jumping: Methodology and implications. *Scandinavian Journal of Medicine and Science in Sports, 18,* 417–426.

Caldwell, G. E., & Li, L. (2000). How strongly is muscle activity associated with joint moments? *Motor Control, 4,* 53–59.

Carroll, T. J., Abernethy, P. J., Logan, P. A., Barber, M., & McEniery, M. T. (1998). Resistance training frequency: Strength and myosin heavy chain responses to two and three bouts per week. *European Journal of Applied Physiology, 78,* 270–275.

Chelly, S. M., & Denis, C. (2001). Leg power and hopping stiffness: relationship with sprint running performance. *Medicine and Science in Sports and Exercise, 33,* 326–333.

Cometti, G., Maffiuletti, N. A., Pousson, M., Chatard, J.-C., & Maffulli, N. (2001). Isokinetic strength and anaerobic power of elite, subelite and amateur French soccer players. *International Journal of Sports Medicine, 22,* 45–51.

Cormie, P., McCauley, G. O., & McBride, J. M. (2007). Power versus strength-power jump squat training: Influence on the load–power relationship. *Medicine and Science in Sports and Exercise, 39,* 996–1003.

Cormie, P., McCauley, G. O., Triplett, T. N., & McBride, J. M. (2007). Optimal loading for maximal lower-body resistance exercises. *Medicine and Science in Sports and Exercise, 39,* 340–349.

Cormie, P., McGuigan, M. R., & Newton, R. U. (2010). Adaptations in athletic performance after ballistic power versus strength training. *Medicine and Science in Sports and Exercise, 42,* 1582–1598.

Cormie, P., McGuigan, M. R., & Newton, R. U. (2011). Developing maximal neuromuscular power. Part 1: Biological basis of maximal power production. *Sports Medicine, 41,* 17–38.

Cotterman, M. L., Darby, L. A., & Skelly, W. A. (2005). Comparison of muscle force production using the Smith machine and free weights for bench press and squat exercises. *Journal of Strength and Conditioning Research, 19,* 169–176.

Crewther, B. T., Gill, N., Weatherby, R. P., & Lowe, T. (2009). A comparison of ratio and allometric scaling methods for normalizing power and strength in elite rugby union players. *Journal of Sports Sciences, 27,* 1575–1580.

Cronin, J., & Sleivert, G. (2005). Challenges in understanding the influence of maximal power training on improving athletic performance. *Sports Medicine, 35,* 213–234.

Cunningham, D. J., West, D. J., Owen, N. J., Shearer, D. A., Finn, C. V., Bracken, R. M., . . . Kilduff, L. P. (2013). Strength and power predictors of sprinting performance in professional rugby players. *Journal of Sports Medicine and Physical Fitness, 53,* 105–111.

Dostal, W. F., & Andrews, J. G. (1981). A three-dimensional biomechanical model of the hip musculature. *Journal of Biomechanics, 14,* 803–812.

Elliott, B. C., Wilson, G. J., & Kerr, G. K. (1989). A biomechanical analysis of the sticking region in the bench press. *Medicine and Science in Sports and Exercise, 21,* 450–462.

Erdemir, A., McLean, S., Herzog, W., & van den Bogert, A. J. (2007). Model-based estimation of muscle forces exerted during movements. *Clinical Biomechanics, 22,* 131–154.

Finni, T., Komi, P. V., & Lukkariniemi, J. (1998). Achilles tendon loading during walking: Application of a novel optic fiber technique. *European Journal of Applied Physiology, 77,* 289–291.

Flanagan, E. P., & Comyns, T. M. (2008). The use of contact time and the reactive strength index to optimize fast stretch-shortening cycle training. *Strength and Conditioning Journal, 30,* 32–38.

Flanagan, S. P., & Salem, G. J. (2008). Lower extremity joint kinetic responses to external resistance variations. *Journal of Applied Biomechanics, 24,* 58–68.

Fry, A. C., & Kraemer, W. J. (1991). Physical performance characteristics of American collegiate football players. *Journal of Applied Sport Science Research, 5,* 126–138.

González-Badillo, J. J., & Marques, M. C. (2010). Relationship between kinematic factors and counter-movement jump height in trained track and field athletes. *Journal of Strength and Conditioning Research, 24,* 3443–3447.

Haff, G. G., Carlock, J. M., Hartman, M. J., Kilgore, J. L., Kawamori, N., Jackson, J. R., . . . Stone, M. H. (2005). Force–time curve characteristics of dynamic and isometric muscle actions of elite women Olympic weightlifters. *Journal of Strength and Conditioning Research, 19,* 741–748.

Haff, G. G., Stone, M. H., O'Bryant, H. S., Harman, E., Dinan, C., Johnson, R., & Han, K. H. (1997). Force–time dependent characteristics of dynamic and isometric muscle actions. *Journal of Strength and Conditioning Research, 11,* 269–272.

Häkkinen, K., Kallinen, M., Linnamo, V., Pastinen, U-M., Newton, R. U., & Kraemer, W. J. (1996). Neuromuscular adaptations during bilateral versus unilateral strength training in middle-aged and elderly men and women. *Acta Physiologica Scandinavica, 158,* 77–88.

Häkkinen, K., & Komi, P. V. (1983). Electromyographic changes during strength training and detraining. *Medicine and Science in Sports and Exercise, 15,* 455–460.

Hansen, K. T., Cronin, J. B., Pickering, S. L., & Douglas, L. (2011). Do force–time and power–time measures in a loaded jump squat differentiate between speed performance and playing level in elite and elite junior rugby union players? *Journal of Strength and Conditioning Research, 25,* 2382–2391.

Hay, D., de Souza, V. A., & Fukashiro, S. (2006). Human bilateral deficit during a dynamic multi-joint leg press movement. *Human Movement Science, 25,* 181–191.

Howard, J. D., & Enoka, R. M. (1991). Maximum bilateral contractions are modified by neutrally mediated interlimb effects. *Journal of Applied Physiology, 70,* 306–316.

Jacobs, R., & van Ingen Schenau, G. J. (1992a). Control of an external force in leg extensions in humans. *Journal of Physiology, 457,* 611–626.

Jacobs, R., & van Ingen Schenau, G. J. (1992b). Intermuscular coordination in a sprint push-off. *Journal of Biomechanics, 25,* 953–965.

Jaric, S., Mirkov, D., & Markovic, G. (2005). Normalizing physical performance tests for body size: A proposal for standardization. *Journal of Strength and Conditioning Research, 19,* 467–474.

Kuitunen, S., Komi, P. V., & Kyröläinen, H. (2002). Knee and ankle joint stiffness in sprint running. *Medicine and Science in Sports and Exercise, 34,* 166–173.

Latin, R. W., Berg, K., & Baechle, T. (1994). Physical and performance characteristics of NCAA Division I male basketball players. *Journal of Strength and Conditioning Research, 8,* 214–218.

Lees, A., Vanrenterghem, J., & De Clercq, D. (2004). The maximal and submaximal vertical jump: Implications for strength and conditioning. *Journal of Strength and Conditioning, 18,* 787–791.

Maganaris, C. N. (2001). Force-length characteristics of *in vivo* human skeletal muscle. *Acta Physiologica Scandinavica, 172,* 279–285.

Marginson, V., & Eston, R. (2001). The relationship between torque and joint angle during knee extension in boys and men. *Journal of Sports Sciences, 19,* 875–880.

Mathiyakom, W., McNitt-Gray, J. L., & Wilcox, R. R. (2007). Regulation of angular impulse during two forward translating tasks. *Journal of Applied Biomechanics, 23,* 149–161.

McLellan, C. P., Lovell, D. I., & Gass, G. C. (2011). The role of rate of force development on vertical jump performance. *Journal of Strength and Conditioning Research, 25,* 379–385.

Meckel, Y., Atterbom, H., Grodjinovsky, A., Ben-Sira, D., & Rostein, A. (1995). Physiological characteristics of female 100 metre sprinters of different performance levels. *Journal of Sports Medicine and Physical Fitness, 35,* 169–175.

Mero, A. (1988). Force–time characteristics and running velocity of male sprinters during the acceleration phase of sprinting. *Research Quarterly for Exercise and Sport, 59,* 94–98.

Mero, A., Luhtanen, P., & Komi, P. V. (1983). A biomechanical study of the sprint start. *Scandinavian Journal of Sports Science, 5,* 20–28.

Mero, A., Luhtanen, P., & Komi, P. V. (1986). Segmental contribution to velocity of center of gravity during contact at different speeds in male and female sprinters. *Journal of Human Movement Studies, 12,* 215–235.

Mero, A., Luhtanen, P., Viitasalo, J. T., & Komi, P. V. (1981). Relationships between the maximal running velocity, muscle fiber characteristics, force production and force relaxation of sprinters. *Scandinavian Journal of Sports Science, 3,* 16–22.

Moir, G. L. (2012). Muscular strength. In T. Miller (Ed.), *NCSA's guide to tests and assessments* (pp. 147–191). Champaign, IL: Human Kinetics.

Moir, G. L., Garcia, A., & Dwyer, G. B. (2009). Intersession reliability of kinematic and kinetic variables during vertical jumps in men and women. *International Journal of Sports Physiology and Performance, 4,* 317–330.

Moir, G. L., Gollie, J. M., Davis, S. E., Guers, J. J., & Witmer, C. A. (2012). The effects of load on system and lower-body joint kinetics during jump squats. *Sports Biomechanics, 11,* 492–506.

Moss, B. M., Refsnes, P. E., Abildgaard, A., Nicolaysen, K., & Jensen, J. (1997). Effects of maximal effort strength training with different loads on dynamic strength, cross-sectional area, load–power, and load–velocity relationships. *European Journal of Applied Physiology, 75,* 193–199.

Murphy, A. J., Wilson, G. J., Pryor, J. F., & Newton, R. U. (1995). Isometric assessment of muscular function: The effect of joint angle. *Journal of Applied Biomechanics, 11,* 205–215.

Nagano, A., & Gerritsen, K. G. M. (2001). Effects of neuromuscular strength training on vertical jumping performance: A computer simulation study. *Journal of Applied Biomechanics, 17,* 113–128.

Narici, M. V., Hoppeler, H., Kayser, B., Landoni, L., Claassen, H., Gavardi, C., . . . Cerretelli, P. (1996). Human quadriceps cross-sectional area, torque and neural activation during 6 months strength training. *Acta Physiologica Scandinavica, 157*, 175–186.

Newton, R. U., & Dugan, E. (2002). Application of strength diagnosis. *Strength and Conditioning Journal, 24*, 50–59.

Oliveira, F. B. D., Oliveira, A. S. C., Rizatto, G. F., & Denadai, B. S. (2013). Resistance training for explosive and maximal strength: Effects on early and late rate of force development. *Journal of Sports Science in Medicine, 12*, 402–408.

Peterson, M. D., Alvar, B. A., & Rhea, M. R. (2006). The contribution of maximal force production to explosive movement among young collegiate athletes. *Journal of Strength and Conditioning Research, 20*, 867–873.

Rejc, E., Lazzer, S., Antonutto, G., Isola, M., & di Prampero, P. E. (2010). Bilateral deficit and EMG activity during explosive lower limb contractions against different overloads. *European Journal of Applied Physiology, 108*, 157–165.

Rutherford, O. M., & Jones, D. A. (1986). The role of learning and coordination in strength training. *European Journal of Applied Physiology, 55*, 100–105.

Samonzino, P., Rejc, E., Di Prampero, P. E., Belli, A., & Morin, J.-B. (2012). Optimal force–velocity profile in ballistic movements: *Altius: citius* or *fortius*? *Medicine and Science in Sports and Exercise, 44*, 313–322.

Schmidtbleicher, D. (1992). Training for power events. In P. V. Komi (Ed.), *Strength and power in sport* (pp. 381–385). Oxford, UK: Blackwell.

Sleivert, G., & Taingahue, M. (2004). The relationship between maximal jump-squat power and sprint acceleration in athletes. *European Journal of Applied Physiology, 91*, 46–52.

Smirniotou, A., Katsikas, C., Paradisis, G., Argeitaki, P., Zacharogiannis, E., & Tziortzis, S. (2008). Strength–power parameters as predictors of sprinting performance. *Journal of Sports Medicine and Physical Fitness, 48*, 447–454.

Stone, M. H., Sanborn, K., O'Bryant, H. S., Hartman, M., Stone, M. E., Proulx, C., . . . Hruby, J. (2003). Maximum strength–power–performance relationships in collegiate throwers. *Journal of Strength and Conditioning Research, 17*, 739–745.

Tillin, N. A., Pain, M. T. G., & Folland, J. (2013). Explosive force production during isometric squats correlates with athletic performance in rugby union players. *Journal of Sports Sciences, 31*, 66–76.

Tsaopoulos, D. E., Baltzopoulos, V., Richards, P. J., & Maganaris, C. N. (2009). A comparison of different two-dimensional approaches for the determination of the patellar tendon moment arm length. *European Journal of Applied Physiology, 105*, 809–814.

Van den Tillaar, R., Sæterbakken, A. H., & Ettema, G. J. (2012). Is the occurrence of the sticking region the result of diminishing potentiation in bench press? *Journal of Sports Sciences, 30*, 591–599.

van Ingen Schenau, G. J. (1989). From rotation to translation: Constraints on multi-joint movements and the unique action of biarticular muscles. *Human Movement Sciences, 8*, 301–337.

Vanrenterghem, J., Lees, A., & De Clerque, D. (2008). Effect of forward trunk inclination on joint power output in vertical jumping. *Journal of Strength and Conditioning Research, 22*, 708–714.

Wells, R., & Evans, N. (1987). Functions and recruitment patterns of one- and two-joint muscles under isometric and walking conditions. *Human Movement Sciences, 6*, 349–372.

Westing, S. H., Seger, J. Y., & Thorstensson, A. (1990). Effects of electrical stimulation on eccentric and concentric torque–velocity relationships during knee extension in man. *Acta Physiologica, 140*, 17–22.

Wilson, G. J., Lyttle, A. D., Ostrowski, K. J., & Murphy, A. J. (1995). Assessing dynamic performance: A comparison of rate of force development tests. *Journal of Strength and Conditioning Research, 9*, 176–181.

Wisløff, U., Castagna, C., Helgerud, J., Jones, R., & Hoff, J. (2004). Strong correlation of maximal squat strength with sprint performance and vertical jump height in elite soccer players. *British Journal of Sports Medicine, 38*, 285–288.

Young, W. B., James, R., & Montgomery, I. (2002). Is muscle power related to running speed with changes of direction? *Journal of Sports Medicine and Physical Fitness, 42*, 282–288.

Young, W., McLean, B., & Ardagna, J. (1995). Relationship between strength qualities and sprinting performance. *Journal of Sports Medicine and Physical Fitness, 35*, 13–19.

Zatsiorsky, V. M. (1995). *Science and practice of strength training*. Champaign, IL: Human Kinetics.

Zatsiorsky, V. M., & Prilutsky, B. I. (2012). *Biomechanics of skeletal muscle*. Champaign, IL: Human Kinetics.

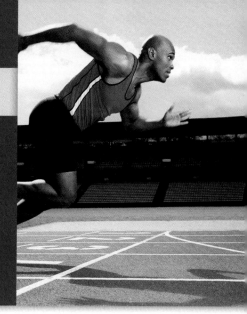

CHAPTER 6

Training Methods to Develop Muscular Strength and Power

Chapter Objectives

At the end of this chapter, you will be able to:

- Discuss the process of adaptation to an exercise stimulus
- Discuss the basic training principles that elicit adaptation
- Describe the neurogenic and phenotypic adaptations to resistance training
- Explain how the acute variables associated with a resistance training workout can be manipulated to elicit specific neuromuscular adaptations
- Explain how the acute variables associated with a plyometric workout can be manipulated to elicit specific neuromuscular adaptations
- Define the concept of periodization
- Develop a periodized resistance training program to elicit specific neuromuscular adaptations that enhance the indices of muscular strength

Key Terms

Agonist–antagonist pairs

Assistance exercises

Bilateral

Blocked periodization

Ca²⁺ calmodulin-dependent kinase/calcineurin

Cluster sets

Complex pairs

Core exercises

Double-split routines

Excitation–transcription coupling

Free weights

Functional overreaching

Insulin/insulin-like growth factor

Isoinertial

Isokinetic dynamometers

Machine weights

Nonfunctional overreaching

Overtraining syndrome

Post-activation potentiation

Pre-exhaustion

Primary messengers

Principle of overload

Principle of specificity

Principle of variation

Secondary messengers

Split routines

Supercompensation

Target repetition-maximum

Transfer of training effect

Undulating periodization

Unilateral

Chapter Overview

Given the importance of muscular strength in many sports, it is important that a strength and conditioning practitioner understand the methods used to develop the ability of muscles to generate force. The methods selected by the coach should elicit adaptations in the specific neuromuscular characteristics that underpin the different indices of muscular strength. This chapter introduces resistance training methods and the evidence relating to the adaptations in specific neuromuscular characteristics accrued from these methods. In so doing, it highlights the acute programming variables associated with a resistance training workout that can be manipulated to induce specific neuromuscular adaptations as well as modifications to traditional resistance training methods that can be implemented to elicit appropriate responses from the athletes. Plyometric exercises are also introduced and the associated acute programming variables discussed. Finally, we discuss the concept of periodization and the principles that the strength and conditioning coach can use to develop an effective training program to improve muscular strength and power. We begin, however, by describing the processes associated with adapting to an exercise stimulus.

[Handwritten margin note: → Methods used to develop the ability of muscles to generate force. % of that capacity]

The Adaptation Process

The demands associated with an exercise stimulus elicit transient neural, metabolic, hormonal, and mechanical alterations. The process of adaptation following an exercise stimulus relates to the cellular and molecular responses that lead to changes within the systems of the body (e.g., central nervous system, musculoskeletal system, cardiovascular system, endocrine system), resulting in functional enhancements in specific movement tasks such as lifting greater loads during a test of maximal muscular strength or being able to sustain exercise for a longer duration during an endurance test. In terms of neuromuscular adaptations to an exercise stimulus, the neural activation of skeletal muscles to generate tension during a given movement task (excitation–contraction coupling) disrupts cellular homeostasis. The resulting mechanical, metabolic, and hormonal responses initiate signaling pathways that ultimately create new cellular proteins (Coffey & Hawley, 2007). These signaling pathways appear to be specific to the mode of exercise undertaken, leading to the creation of specific proteins.

The relationship between the excitation of a muscle and the resulting transcription of specific cellular proteins in response to different modes of exercise has been termed the **excitation–transcription coupling** (Egan & Zierath, 2013); it is illustrated in Figure 6.1. For example, the adaptations following endurance training include mitochondrial biogenesis and substrate metabolism, whereas a regimen of heavy resistance training is likely to induce fiber hypertrophy (Coffey & Hawley, 2007). These disparate adaptations have very different functional consequences (increased endurance versus increased force production) and arise due to the different characteristics of the training exercises used (e.g., intensity, volume, frequency). Furthermore, long-term exposure to the specific exercise stimulus is required to allow the transient increases in proteins following each workout to settle into a new steady state through the cumulative effects of cellular processes, resulting in a new functional level of performance (Coffey & Hawley, 2007). For this reason, individual workouts need to be repeated to induce the positive adaptations that will result in an improved functional level.

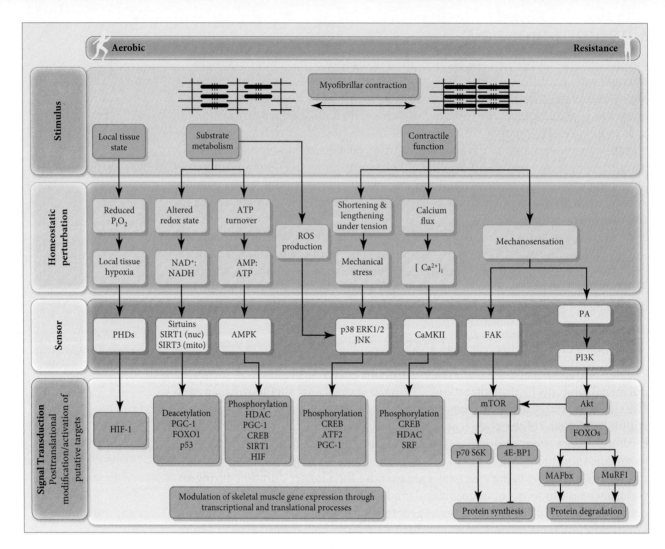

Figure 6.1 The schematic representation of the excitation–transcription coupling highlighting the different molecular pathways that are activated in response to different exercise stimuli (aerobic versus resistance training), and that lead to the transcription of specific proteins within a muscle cell. 4E-BP1 = eukaryotic translational initiation factor 4E binding protein; Akt = protein kinase B; AMP = adenosine diphosphate; AMPK = AMP kinase; ATF2 = activator of iron transcription protein 2; ATP = adenosine triphosphate; Ca^{2+} = calcium; CaMKII = calmodulin-dependent protein kinase; CREB = cyclic AMP response element binding protein; FAK = focal adhesion kinase; FOXO1 = forkhead transcription factor, O box subfamily 1; HDAC = histone deacetylase; HIF-1α = hypoxia-inducible factor 1α; MAFbx = muscle atrophy F box; mTOR = mammalian target of rapamycin; MuRF1 = muscle RING finger 1; NAD = nicotinamide adenine dinucleotide; p57 = cyclin-dependent kinase inhibitor; p70 S6K = ribosomal protein S6K; PA = phosphatidic acid; PGC-1α = peroxisome proliferator-activated receptor gamma coactivator 1α; PHD = prolyl hydroxylase enzyme; PI3K = phosphatidylinositol 3-kinase; P$_i$O$_2$ = partial pressure of oxygen; ROS = reactive oxygen species; SIRT = sirtuin; SIRT1 = sirtuin 1.

Reproduced from Egan, B., & Zierath, J. R. (2013). Exercise metabolism and the molecular regulation of skeletal muscle adaptation. *Cell Metabolism, 17,* 162–184, with permission from Elsevier.

Collectively, then, the functional responses following the adaptation to a given exercise regimen depend on the mode, intensity, volume, and frequency of exercises used and the duration of the training program. In addition, some other variables, including gender, age (chronological and training age), and nutritional status, act to modulate the adaptations to exercise (Coffey & Hawley, 2007; Hawley & Burke, 2010; Toigo & Boutellier, 2006). The general process of adaptation informs us that positive cellular responses are elicited when the stimulus applied exceeds the stimulus that the cell typically experiences, so long as an adequate period of recovery separates the applications of repeated stimuli. This forms the basis of the **principle of overload** associated with a training program, whereby the application of an exercise stimulus exceeding the level typically experienced by an athlete initiates the adaptive response (Stone, Plisk, & Collins, 2002). All exercise stimuli are associated with a particular intensity (rate of performing work/expending energy), duration (length of work periods), and frequency (number of repetitions, sets, training sessions, and so on). Collectively, the duration and frequency of the exercises provide the volume of the exercise stimulus. The variables of intensity and volume can be manipulated to allow the overload associated with an exercise stimulus to be altered accordingly, leading to specific adaptations.

Increases in muscular strength will require neuromuscular adaptations that allow greater force to be generated. Recall that the physiological and morphological adaptations required to enhance force generation include alterations in activation dynamics (e.g., motor unit recruitment, rate coding), timing and coordination of activation (e.g., coactivation of antagonistic muscles), changes in spinal reflexes (e.g., H-reflex), muscle fiber hypertrophy, and architectural changes (e.g., pennation angle, muscle fiber length). When the individual performs exercises that require the muscles to generate forces in excess of those typically experienced, these adaptations will accrue and result in a new functional level of performance. Large forces generated by the activation of skeletal muscle result in an upregulation of the **primary messengers** of the muscle cell that includes the mechanical stretch of the sarcolemma and calcium flux (Coffey & Hawley, 2007). These primary messengers activate numerous intracellular signaling cascades that mediate the response to the overload, known as **secondary messengers** (Coffey & Hawley, 2007). Important secondary messengers that have been implicated in adaptations increasing muscular strength include the **Ca^{2+} calmodulin-dependent kinase/calcineurin** and **insulin/insulin-like growth factor** signaling pathways (Coffey & Hawley, 2007). (See Strength and Power Training Concept 6.1.) Such pathways explain the transformation of a mechanical signal (muscular force) into a specific molecular response (synthesis of new proteins) during the adaptive process.

The exercises used in a training program will be effective only if they present sufficient overload to elicit an adaptation in the neuromuscular system. If the overload associated with a given exercise presents an insufficient stimulus, there is likely to be a reduction in the functional capacity of the neuromuscular system (e.g., detraining, involution, or reversibility). Such a response still constitutes an adaptation—but it is an adaptation that will not improve the functional capacity of the neuromuscular system. In contrast, if the overload associated with the specific exercises is too great and applied over prolonged periods such that the stimulus cannot be tolerated by the athlete, maladaptation is likely. This can result in a decrement in performance and possibly injury and overtraining. If the exercise stimulus remains unchanged, any further adaptations beyond those occurring in response to the initial stimulus will be minimal and the athlete will experience stagnation. The **principle of variation** proposes that appropriate manipulations in intensity and volume of the exercises within the training program are

Strength and Power Training Concept 6.1

The signaling pathways involved in the molecular adaptations of skeletal muscle to increased force

A training program comprising exercises involving the generation of high muscular forces would be characterized by high intensities and, therefore, low volumes. In response to high forces being generated, considerable stretch of the sarcolemma in each active muscle fiber will occur. Furthermore, short-duration cycles of high concentrations of Ca^{2+} within the cytosol will arise as a result of the excitation–contraction coupling. The mechanical stretch of the sarcolemma and the calcium flux associated with the generation of high forces represent primary messengers; they initiate a cascade of intracellular signaling pathways that can mediate the response to the exercise stimulus. The cascade of intracellular signaling pathways includes the Ca^{2+} calmodulin-dependent kinase/calcineurin and insulin/insulin-like growth factor pathways. Calcineurin is a coregulator of hypertrophy with insulin-like growth factor (IGF) and is also involved in the activation of satellite cells (Coffey & Hawley, 2007). IGF-I is involved in protein synthesis through its activation of the Akt-mTOR pathway, which concomitantly suppress the inhibitors of protein synthesis (TSC2, GSK3β) (Coffey & Hawley, 2007). The generation of high muscular force appears to be a potent mechanical variable that increases the activation of the Akt-mTOR pathway (Russ, 2008). In summary, the adaptive response that leads to an enhancement of the neuromuscular characteristics that increase the expression of muscular strength and power will be realized through exercises that require the generation of high muscular forces such as resistance training and plyometric exercises.

required for the prolongation of adaptations accrued from long-term training (Stone et al., 2002). Long-term adaptations, however, arise from the cumulative effects of each exercise stimulus leading to altered steady-state levels of specific proteins (Coffey & Hawley, 2007). Therefore, too much variation will not elicit appropriate adaptations.

When the neuromuscular system is overloaded through the application of exercises that require the generation of large forces, the subsequent cellular responses will confer functional enhancements—namely, an increase in the expression of muscular strength. The increases in muscular strength will be greater in those assessments of muscular strength that are most closely related to the exercises used in training. This response illustrates the **principle of specificity**, defined as the correspondence between the exercise stimulus and the movements being trained for in terms of the mechanical and bioenergetics characteristics (Stone et al., 2002). A high degree of specificity will increase the **transfer of training effect**, enhancing the functional consequences of the adaptation process.

Understanding the process of adaptation allows us to identify exercises and training methods that will produce enhancements in the different indices of muscular strength. The requirement for overload to be provided in the form of increased muscular force generation in the training exercises means that resistance and plyometric training methods are typically used to develop muscular strength and power. The basic training principles of overload, variation, and specificity can then be applied to develop an effective training program.

Resistance Training Methods

Resistance training methods include any exercises that use movements performed against resistance to elicit gains in muscular strength. This broad definition includes the use of any device that resists the movement of the athlete, including weight machines, free weights, elastic bands, chains, and even body mass. The resistance against which the athlete applies force provides a stimulus to which the neuromuscular system adapts as it is overloaded. This resistance is typically provided by a mass that is accelerated during the execution of the exercises (e.g., machine-weight and free-weight resistance exercises). Such exercises are termed **isoinertial** due to the constant external masses involved. However, resistance training exercises can also be performed using **isokinetic dynamometers**, whereby the resistance, which is provided by an electronic servo motor or a hydraulic valve (Baltzopoulos & Brodie, 1989), is manipulated such that the velocity remains constant over a specific range of the movement produced by the athlete. The resistance to movement can further be provided by the deformation of elastic structures (e.g., elastic bands) or the motion of fluids (e.g., pneumatic machines). It can also be provided by an immovable object that restricts any movement of the athlete (e.g., isometric resistance training exercises). The specific source of the resistance has a substantial effect on the biomechanics of the resistance training exercise, so the adaptations observed are likely to be largely influenced by the choice of resistance during the exercises used.

Resistance training programs have been shown to result in increases in measures of muscular strength including maximal dynamic and isometric strength, speed-strength, explosive strength, reactive strength, and muscular strength endurance (Abernethy, Jurimäe, Logan, Taylor, & Thayer, 1994; Stone et al., 2007). This increase in the expression of strength can be realized within weeks of beginning a resistance training program. Many neurogenic and phenotypic adaptations have been proposed to support the improvements in muscular strength following a period of resistance training (Abernethy et al., 1994; Baldwin & Haddad, 2001; Duchateau, Semmler, & Enoka, 2006; Folland & Williams, 2007; Kraemer, Fleck, & Evans, 1996); these adaptations are summarized in Table 6.1. In general, the increased muscular capabilities that are elicited within weeks of beginning a resistance training program appear to be due to neurogenic adaptations, with phenotypic adaptations such as fiber hypertrophy occurring later (Ratamess et al., 2009).

Activation Dynamics   _Neurogenic

The activation dynamics of skeletal muscle refers to motor unit recruitment and rate coding, both of which increase following a period of resistance training (Duchateau et al., 2006; Gardiner, Dai, & Heckman, 2006). These neurogenic adaptations increase the force-generating capabilities of the trained muscles, allowing for a greater expression of muscular strength in the absence of any phenotypic adaptations (e.g., fiber hypertrophy).

Timing and Coordination of Activation   — Neurogenic

Increased activation of the agonist muscle following a period of resistance training is accompanied by a decrease in the concomitant activation in the antagonist muscle group (Carolan & Cafarelli, 1992). This reduced coactivation can increase measures of muscular strength by increasing the net moment at a given joint.

Table 6.1

Neurogenic and Phenotypic Adaptations to Resistance Training That Support the Increases in Muscular Strength

Adaptation		Explanation
Neurogenic	Activation dynamics	Increased motor unit recruitment and rate coding
	Timing and coordination of activation	Reduced antagonist coactivation
	Spinal reflexes	Increased H-reflex
Phenotypic	Hypertrophy	Increased hypertrophy of all fiber types
		Greater hypertrophy in type II fibers
	Fiber type transformation	Shift from type IIx to IIa MHC isoforms
	Architectural adaptations	Increased pennation angle after heavy resistance training
		Increased fiber length after explosive resistance training

Note: MHC = myosin heavy-chain isoform.

[handwritten: Two major areas of adaptation to RT]

[handwritten: Neurogenic]

[handwritten: Phenotypic]

[handwritten: Phenotypic]

Spinal Reflexes

There is an increase in the H-reflex following a period of resistance training (Aagaard, Simonsen, Andersen, Magnusson, & Dyhre-Poulsen, 2002). The H-reflex is increased in response to an increase in the descending motor drive, an increase in the excitability of the α-motoneurons, or a reduction in the inhibition of Ia afferents (Aagaard, 2003). These factors would result in an increase in force developed by the trained muscles.

Fiber Hypertrophy

One of the most important adaptations to a period of resistance training is fiber hypertrophy, with the greatest increases being reported in type II fibers, although all fiber types are affected (Folland & Williams, 2007). The greater hypertrophy of the fast fibers is important because it results in a greater relative contribution to the cross-sectional area of the trained muscle by the fast fibers, substantially increasing the force-generating capacity of the muscle (Andersen & Aagaard, 2010). Increases in the cross-sectional area of the muscle fibers are measurable only after 4 to 6 weeks of resistance training when an individual begins a resistance training regimen from an untrained state (Seynnes, de Boer, & Narici, 2007). However, the processes that are responsible for hypertrophy (e.g., increased muscle protein synthesis, proliferation of satellite cells) are activated following the first exercise session (Atherton et al., 2005).

Fiber Type Transformation

Resistance training has generally been shown to induce type IIX to type IIA fiber transformations (Folland & Williams, 2007). This result would appear counterintuitive given the lower isometric tension that is associated with the IIA fibers compared to the IIX fibers (Linari et al., 2003). However, concomitant increases in muscular strength accompany these fiber transformations. In turn, other adaptations within a muscle fiber that accompany a period of resistance training (e.g., fiber hypertrophy, architectural changes) would likely be more important in affecting muscular strength than fiber type transformations. Indeed, some researchers have reported no change in the proportion of muscle fiber types despite substantial increases in muscular strength following a period of resistance training (Aagaard et al., 2001). In such studies, the increases in muscular strength were accompanied by increased fiber hypertrophy and pennation angle in the trained muscles.

Architectural Adaptations — *Phenotypic*

Heavy resistance training produces an increase in the pennation angle of skeletal muscle (Aagaard et al., 2001). This increased pennation angle allows for a greater increase in the physiological cross-sectional area of the trained muscle and, therefore, an increase in maximal muscular strength. When comparing the architectural adaptations following different resistance training regimens, Blazevich, Gill, Bronks, and Newton (2003) reported increased pennation angles in the vastus lateralis muscle of those athletes who completed heavy resistance exercises, while pennation angles decreased in the group undertaking jump training. However, jump training resulted in an increase in fascicle length in the vastus lateralis muscle. These disparate adaptations in architecture will lead to increased force-generating capacity (increased pennation angle) and increased velocity characteristics (increased fascicle length) in the trained muscles.

In addition to the neuromuscular adaptations that follow a period of resistance training, adaptations in the tendinous tissue occur. For example, increased tendon stiffness has been reported in a number of resistance training studies, with this effect arising from a combination of structural changes within the tissue as well as possible tendon hypertrophy (Folland & Williams, 2007). An increase in tendon stiffness following resistance training is likely to increase the rate of force development and decrease the electromechanical delay during voluntary muscle actions.

Resistance Training Program Design

The adaptive response associated with a resistance training workout depends on a number of acute training variables, including exercise selection, intensity and volume of the exercises, rest intervals between sets of exercises, the order in which the exercises are performed, and the frequency with which each workout is performed during each training week (Ratamess et al., 2009). The manipulation of these acute training variables is suspected to induce specific neuromuscular adaptations leading to the increased expression of muscular strength (Bird, Tarpenning, & Marino, 2005; Spiering et al., 2008). Unfortunately, the majority of research from which the recommended manipulations of the acute program variables are drawn has focused on only the response following the administration of single sets of a small number of resistance training exercises in untrained individuals; this focus makes the development of broader recommendations somewhat problematic (Crewther, Cronin, & Keogh, 2005). What follows is an overview of the general recommendations.

Exercise Selection

The resistance exercises that can be selected by a coach can differ in terms of muscle action, number of joints involved, bilateral or unilateral force production, and the method by which the resistance is provided. The exercise selection, therefore, determines the mechanical characteristics of the resistance training exercise. By matching the mechanical aspects of the resistance training exercises with those of the sporting movements, the coach can maximize the transfer of training effect, thereby enhancing

[handwritten margin notes: Further Research Needed on special populations i.e. Athletes Master's athletes Apparently Normal Healthy older people; carryover effect]

the athlete's ability to utilize muscular strength gained through training in his or her sporting performance. The increases in muscular strength following a period of resistance training are specific to the resistance training exercises used (see Strength and Power Training Concept 6.2), so the coach should consider the following factors to maximize mechanical specificity (Stone, Stone, & Sands, 2007):

- Accentuated region of force production
- Amplitude and direction of motion
- Dynamics of effort (e.g., static versus dynamic exercises)
- Rate and time of maximum force production
- Regimen of muscular work (e.g., eccentric, concentric, stretch–shortening cycle muscle actions)

Strength and Power Training Concept 6.2

Transfer of training effect depends the specificity of the resistance training exercises used

The principle of specificity proposes that the transfer of training effect is determined by the mechanical and bioenergetic correspondence between the resistance training exercises and the movements used by the athlete in his or her sport. The adaptations to resistance training have been shown to be specific to the muscle actions used. For example, Abernethy and Jürimäe (1996) reported that the gains observed in maximal muscular strength following a period of resistance training using isoinertial exercises were greater and occurred more rapidly when the assessment exercise was also isoinertial, compared to isometric and isokinetic assessments of maximal strength. Increases in muscular strength were greater following resistance training using bilateral exercises when the assessment of strength was also bilateral than when the assessment was unilateral, with the reverse also being true (Häkkinen & Komi, 1983). Carroll, Abernethy, Logan, Barber, and McEniery (1998) reported that increases in muscular strength following a period of training using a closed-kinetic chain movement (back squats) were greater when measured in a closed-kinetic chain movement than in an open-kinetic chain movement (leg extension). Moreover, the closed-kinetic chain resistance training exercises actually resulted in a decrease in the open-kinetic measure of muscular strength when the weekly frequency of training was increased, demonstrating a negative transfer effect of resistance training. Finally, a period of resistance training using heavy loads resulted in a greater increase in muscular strength assessed under high-load conditions compared to low-load conditions, while training with low-load exercises tended to induce the reverse effects (McBride, Triplett-McBride, Davie, & Newton, 2002).

These findings also have implications for evaluating the effectiveness of a given resistance training program. If the test of muscular strength is not specific to the resistance training exercises used in the training program, then improvements may not be realized and the coach may erroneously assume that the training program was ineffective. These findings also highlight the importance of understanding the mechanical requirements of the sport to allow the selection of appropriate exercises to use in a resistance training program.

Resistance training exercises can involve isolated eccentric, concentric, and isometric muscle actions, or a combination of these actions. Recall that the greatest muscle tensions are developed eccentrically, then isometrically, with the lowest forces generally being produced during concentric actions. As such, eccentric muscle actions have been proposed to provide a more potent stimulus for both hypertrophy and strength gains following a period of resistance training (Roig et al., 2009; Schoenfeld, 2010). Most sporting movements involve a combination of eccentric and concentric actions characterized by the stretch–shortening cycle (e.g., running, jumping, change of direction). Thus the principle of specificity would suggest that resistance training exercises utilizing the stretch–shortening cycle should increase the transfer of training effect to these activities. Ratamess et al. (2009) recommend that all types of muscle actions be used in the exercises selected in the design of an effective resistance training program.

Resistance training exercises can be categorized as single joint (e.g., biceps curls, leg extensions) or multijoint (e.g., bench press, back squat), depending on the number of joints involved in the movement. Some researchers use the terms **assistance exercises** to refer to single-joint resistance training exercises and **core exercises** to denote multijoint exercises (Baechle, Earle, & Wathen, 2008). Most sports involve multijoint movements, and Ratamess et al. (2009) recommend the use of both core and assistance exercises in an effective resistance training program.

Most resistance training exercises are **bilateral**, although many sporting tasks require **unilateral** force production (e.g., running, change of direction). The bilateral deficit is a phenomenon whereby the mechanical output from both limbs acting concomitantly (bilateral tasks) is less than the sum of the output of the limbs acting separately (unilateral task). There is evidence that the bilateral deficit is reduced following a period of resistance training comprising bilateral exercises (Kuruganti, Parker, Rickards, Tingley, & Sexsmith, 2005). Ratamess et al. (2009) recommend that bilateral and unilateral resistance exercises be included in an effective training program to develop muscular strength in an effective resistance training program.

Resistance training methods can include **machine weights** or **free weights**. Machine weights refer to plate-loaded and selectorizer devices, electronically braked devices, hydraulic devices, and rubber-band devices that offer resistance in a guided or restricted manner (Stone et al., 2002). Free weights refer to the use of freely movable masses to provide resistance, including barbells, dumbbells, associated benches and racks, medicine balls, throwing implements, body mass, and augmented body mass (e.g., weighted vests, limb weights) (Stone et al., 2002). A cursory examination of free-weight resistance exercises would suggest that they are more specific to most sporting movements than machine-weight exercises; for example, free-weight exercises are typically multijoint, have unrestricted range of motion, and can be performed explosively. Table 6.2 identifies a number of advantages and disadvantages associated with machine- and free-weight resistance exercises.

The use of machine- or free-weight resistance exercises is determined by the training status of the athlete, the location of the workouts in the training program, and the access to facilities. Ratamess et al. (2009) recommend both machine- and free-weight exercise be included in the training program of novice athletes (untrained individuals or those who have not engaged in resistance training for several years) and intermediate athletes (individuals with approximately 6 months of consistent resistance training experience), while advanced athletes (individuals with years of resistance training experience) are encouraged to focus on free-weight exercise with machine exercises being added to complement the needs of their program.

Table 6.2
Advantages and Disadvantages Associated with Machine- and Free-Weight Resistance Exercises

Advantages		Disadvantages	
Machine Weight	Free Weight	Machine Weight	Free Weight
Does not require spotters	Greater mechanical specificity with most sporting movements	Less mechanical specificity with most sporting movements	May require the use of spotters
Potentially less time consuming to change the resistance	Unlimited variations possible	Limited variations possible	May be more time consuming to change the resistance
Less time and effort required to learn the movements	Unrestricted range of motion and acceleration	Restricted range of motion and acceleration	Greater time and effort required to learn the movements
Less space taken up by equipment	Allows for motion in all three planes	Usually restricted to motion in a single plane	Potentially more space taken up by equipment
	Typically multijoint exercises that involve large muscle mass	Usually single-joint exercises that involve small muscle mass	
	Can target concentric, isometric, or eccentric muscle actions	Typically expensive and require more maintenance	
	Typically less expensive and require less maintenance		

Data from Ratamess, N. (2012). *ACSM's foundation of strength training and conditioning.* Philadelphia, PA: Lippincott Williams & Wilkins; Stone, M., Plisk, S., & Collins, D. (2002). Training principles: Evaluation of modes and methods of resistance training: A coaching perspective. *Sports Biomechanics, 1,* 79–103.

Exercise Intensity

The intensity of resistance training exercises is provided by the load used and is typically expressed relative to the maximal strength of the athlete (e.g., the percentage of the load equivalent to one-repetition maximum [1-RM] for the specific exercise). (See **Worked Example 6.1.**) This provides a measure of the relative exercise intensity. The intensity of resistance training exercises is generally considered as the most important acute programming variable to elicit gains in muscular strength (Kraemer, Fleck, & Deschenes, 1988). Heavier external loads are associated with greater forces, greater time under tension, and greater mechanical work performed during each repetition

Worked Example 6.1
One-repetition maximum test as an assessment of maximal dynamic muscular strength

The one-repetition maximum (1-RM) test can be used to establish the maximal dynamic muscular strength of an athlete. During the 1-RM protocol, the load that the athlete must lift is progressively increased until the greatest load that the individual can lift only once with the correct form is established. Although 1-RM tests are sometimes criticized for being unsafe, the use of these protocols with a variety of participants ranging from children to the elderly without any reported injuries testifies to their safety if the appropriate guidelines are followed (Moir, 2012). The protocols presented here use the free-weight bilateral back squat and free-weight bench press exercises (Baechle et al., 2008; Ratamess, 2012).

1-RM Free-Weight Bilateral Back Squat Protocol

Standard squat rack
Olympic barbell
Olympic plates

Barbell grasped with a closed, pronated grip slightly wider than shoulder width

Barbell is placed above the posterior deltoids

Feet slightly wider than shoulder width, toes pointing slightly out

Athlete descends until the thighs are parallel to the ground

Athlete rises from this position with a continuous motion without assistance

1. Athlete warms up by completing the exercise with a load that allows 5–10 repetitions
2. 1-min rest
3. Increase the load by 10–20% such that the athlete can complete only 3–5 repetitions
4. 2-min rest
5. Increase the load by 10–20% such that the athlete can complete only 2–3 repetitions
6. 2- to 4-min rest
7. Increase the load by 10–20% such that the athlete can complete only 1 repetition without assistance and using the appropriate technique
8. 2- to 4-min rest
9. Increase the load by 10–20% such that the athlete can complete only 1 repetition without assistance and using the appropriate technique
10. If the athlete is unable to lift the load, decrease it by 5–10% and perform again
11. 2- to 4-min rest
12. Continue to increase and decrease the load until the athlete can complete only 1 repetition without assistance and using the appropriate technique
13. The athlete's 1-RM should be achieved within five lifts from step 7

At least two spotters stand on either side of the barbell, following it during the descent and ascent without touching it

1-RM Free-Weight Bench Press Protocol

Equipment

Standard flat bench
Olympic barbell
Olympic plates

Technique

Athlete lies supine on the flat bench with the head, shoulders, and buttocks in contact with the bench, both feet on the floor

Barbell is grasped with a closed, pronated grip slightly wider than shoulder width

Spotters assist the athlete removing the barbell to the starting position

The athlete holds the barbell with the elbows extended

The barbell is lowered to the chest, where it touches at the level of the nipple

The athlete raises the barbell from this position with a continuous motion without assistance

Procedure

1. Athlete warms up by completing the exercise with a load that allows 5–10 repetitions
2. 1-min rest
3. Increase the load by 5–10% such that the athlete can complete only 3–5 repetitions
4. 2-min rest
5. Increase the load by 5–10% such that the athlete can complete only 2–3 repetitions
6. 2- to 4-min rest
7. Increase the load by 5–10% such that the athlete can complete only 1 repetition without assistance and using the appropriate technique
8. 2- to 4-min rest
9. Increase the load by 5–10% such that the athlete can complete only 1 repetition without assistance and using the appropriate technique
10. If the athlete is unable to lift the load, decrease it by 2.5–5% and perform again
11. 2- to 4-min rest
12. Continue to increase and decrease the load until the athlete can complete only 1 repetition without assistance and using the appropriate technique
13. The athlete's 1-RM should be achieved within five lifts from step 7

Spotters

A single spotter can be used, standing close to the athlete's head and holding the barbell with a closed, alternated grip

The spotter follows the barbell throughout the descent and ascent without touching it

(Crewther et al., 2005). High muscular forces are associated with greater motor unit recruitment as per the size principle (Henneman, Somjen, & Carpenter, 1965), the activation of specific intracellular signaling pathways (Russ, 2008), and muscle damage especially during eccentric actions (Proske & Morgan, 2001), all of which are proposed to be important in inducing fiber hypertrophy. A mean relative intensity of 85% 1-RM is required to elicit substantial gains in maximal muscular strength (Peterson, Rhea, & Alvar, 2004), and the greater the relative intensity of the resistance exercise, the greater the gains in maximal muscular strength (Fry, 2004).

There appears to be a greater fiber hypertrophy with greater relative intensities, with maximal muscle fiber growth being predicted from relative intensities between 80% and 95% 1-RM (Fry, 2004). However, relative intensity accounts for only a small proportion of the hypertrophic response. Thus other acute program variables (e.g., volume, frequency, rest periods) as well as other factors (e.g., nutritional status, genetics) may become more important. Researchers have demonstrated that performing resistance training with low-to-moderate intensities combined with vascular occlusion results in hypertrophy and gains in muscular strength comparable to those observed after conventional high-intensity workouts (Takarada, Sato, & Ishii, 2002; Wernbom, Augustsson, & Raastad, 2008). (See Applied Research 6.1.) It is believed that the ischemia associated with the vascular occlusion decreases the recruitment thresholds for the motor units (thereby increasing the recruitment of type II fibers), increases the response of hormones (e.g., growth hormone, IGF-I, noradrenaline), increases nitric oxide, and decreases reactive oxygen species. These

Applied Research 6.1
Low-intensity resistance training combined with vascular occlusion increases muscle hypertrophy and muscular strength

The authors divided male rugby players into one of three groups: (1) low-intensity resistance training with vascular occlusion (LIO); (2) low-intensity resistance training with no vascular occlusion (LI); and (3) a control group who maintained their normal activity. The two experimental groups followed an 8-week resistance training regimen comprising bilateral knee extension exercise with a load equivalent to 50% 1-RM, with two workouts per week. During each workout, the participants completed four sets of knee extensions separated by 30 s. The LIO group performed the exercises until volitional failure occurring during each set; the LI group was required to match their number of repetitions. The LIO group completed the resistance exercises with cuffs placed around both thighs that exerted a pressure of 196 mm Hg.

The authors reported that the LIO group demonstrated increases in maximal isometric knee extension torque and maximal isokinetic torque recorded at different velocities following the training period, whereas neither the LI nor the control group showed any changes in muscular strength. A 15% increase in muscle cross-sectional area of the midportion of the thighs, as determined by magnetic resonance imaging, was also observed in the LIO group. The increased thigh cross-sectional area was due to hypertrophy of the knee extensor muscles. As no changes in specific tension (isometric force/cross-sectional area) were observed, the authors concluded that the combination of low-intensity resistance training and vascular occlusion produced increased muscular strength through muscle hypertrophy.

Takarada, Y., Sato, Y., & Ishii, N. (2002). Effects of resistance exercise combined with vascular occlusion on muscle function in athletes. *European Journal of Applied Physiology, 86*, 308–314.

effects highlight the interplay between mechanical, metabolic, and hormonal factors in supporting the adaptive response to resistance training.

To elicit improvements in muscular power, researchers have proposed that resistance training should be performed with the load that maximizes power output (Kawamori & Haff, 2004). The load that maximizes power output varies depending on the exercise, with such loads varying from the equivalent of 56% 1-RM maximizing power output in the back squat, to 80% 1-RM in the power clean, to 0% 1-RM in the jump squat (Cormie, McCauley, Triplett, & McBride, 2007). However, the power output required in the respective sport should probably be considered when determining the load used to develop muscular power (Crewther et al., 2005), while the force–velocity characteristics of the athlete should guide the selection of the resistance training loads (Samonzino, Rejc, Di Prampero, Belli, & Morin, 2012). Furthermore, the expression of muscular power has been suggested to depend on a number of indices of muscular strength, including maximal strength, high-load speed-strength, low-load speed-strength, explosive strength, and reactive strength (Newton & Dugan, 2002). As such, the greatest training efficiency for power development will occur when the athlete's least developed qualities are targeted for training (Newton & Kraemer, 1994). Typically, loads ranging from 0% to 60% of 1-RM have been recommended to improve power output (Crewther et al., 2005; Ratamess et al., 2009). As the magnitude of the external load used during resistance exercises decreases, there is a greater reliance on rate of force development as opposed to maximal muscular strength.

A potential problem with using the relative intensity to establish training loads is the requirement to complete a 1-RM test for each exercise. This can be time consuming, and tests of maximal muscular strength are not recommended for single-joint resistance exercises. One way to circumvent this problem is to use the **target repetition-maximum** (RM) load, defined as the maximum number of repetitions that the athlete can perform with a given submaximal load. The establishment of target RM is achieved through trial and error. Figure 6.2 provides the general relationship between the number of repetitions completed before failure and the relative intensity used. The RM achieved for a

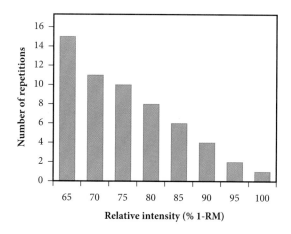

Figure 6.2 The general relationship between the intensity of the exercise and the number of repetitions completed before failure.

Data from Ratamess, N. (2012). *ACSM's foundation of strength training and conditioning.* Philadelphia, PA: Lippincott Williams & Wilkins.

given load can also be used in conjunction with prediction equations to determine the 1-RM values for the exercise (see **Worked Example 6.2**).

The values shown in Figure 6.2 are influenced by the type of exercise used (multijoint versus single-joint) as well as the training status of the athlete (Ratamess, 2012). Although the scheme presented in Figure 6.2 is linear, some evidence indicates that repetition-load schemes for the bench press performed utilizing the stretch–shortening cycle may actually be curvilinear (LeSuer, McCormick, Mayhew, Wasserstein, & Arnold, 1997). Moreover, repetitions performed to failure with lower relative intensities have been shown to induce greater fatigue than when repetitions are performed to failure with greater relative intensities (Behm, Reardon, Fitzgerald, & Drinkwater, 2002). Therefore, the practitioner should consider a set of 15 repetitions performed with a relative intensity of 65% 1-RM to be more demanding than a set comprising a single repetition performed with a relative intensity of 100%.

Worked Example 6.2
Using prediction equations to determine 1-RM from repetitions to failure with submaximal loads

Prediction equations can be used to establish the 1-RM for an athlete from the number of repetitions completed with a submaximal load. LeSuer et al. (1997) proposed the following regression equation to establish the 1-RM of college-aged men and women performing fewer than 10 repetitions to failure with a submaximal load in the back squat and bench press exercises:

$$1\text{-RM} = 100 \times l/[48.8 + 53.8 \times e(-0.075 \times r)]$$

where l is the load used, e is the base of the natural logarithm (approximately 2.71828), and r is the number of repetitions completed with appropriate form and without assistance. This regression equation tended to overestimate the true 1-RM value by less than 1% in the bench press (LeSuer et al., 1997).

Table 6.3 shows the number of repetitions in the free weight bench press until volitional fatigue in an athlete using loads of 108.0 kg and 121.5 kg. The 1-RM load predicted using LeSuer et al.'s equation is also shown. The athlete had a 1-RM of 135.0 kg established following the protocol outlined in Worked Example 6.1.

The data in Table 6.3 demonstrate that the accuracy of the prediction equation diminishes slightly as the load used decreases and, therefore, the number of repetitions completed increases. Furthermore, the strength and conditioning practitioner should recognize that each equation should be considered to be specific to the cohort and the exercise used in its development (Moir, 2012).

Table 6.3
Number of Repetitions Completed to Volitional Fatigue in the Free-Weight Bench Press with Submaximal Loads

Submaximal Load (kg)	Number of Repetitions	Predicted 1-RM (kg)	Actual 1-RM (kg)	Difference (%)
108.0	8	137.9	135.0	2
121.5	4	137.0	135.0	1

This distinction is important when using the target RM scheme to establish training loads. Furthermore, performing repetitions to volitional failure does not necessarily enhance the gains in muscular strength and may even be counterproductive (see **Strength and Power Training Concept 6.3**). Although the use of different target RMs has been shown to elicit specific neuromuscular adaptations (Campos et al., 2002), other researchers have reported no difference in the adaptations to disparate target RMs (Chestnut & Docherty, 1999).

Even when the resistance training exercises are performed against constant external loads with a maximal voluntary effort by an athlete, the velocity with which the external load is moved is likely to decrease with the number of repetitions completed. As a consequence, the intensity of each repetition is altered and, therefore, the external load may not provide an accurate measure of the intensities of the exercises. Recently researchers have suggested that the velocity at which the repetitions are performed can be used to determine the intensity of the resistance training exercises (González-Badillo & Sánchez-Medina, 2010). See **Worked Example 6.3**.

Strength and Power Training Concept 6.3

Is muscular fatigue necessary for muscular strength adaptations?

Fatigue can be defined as a reversible decline in the mechanical output associated with contractile activity that is marked by a progressive reduction in the contractile response of the active muscle (Allen, Lamb, & Westerblad, 2008). It has been proposed that the accumulation of metabolic by-products (H^+, lactate, P_i, Cr) may be a primary stimulus for the enhancements in muscle hypertrophy and strength following a period of resistance training (Crewther, Cronin, & Keogh, 2006). This posited relationship has led to the suggestions that (1) resistance training exercises should be performed to the point of volitional failure to maximize the adaptations or (2) forced repetitions should be performed, whereby further repetitions are completed with the assistance of a spotter once repetition failure has occurred. However, performing repetitions to the point of failure has not been shown to elicit gains in muscular strength beyond those demonstrated following nonfailure training (Folland, Irish, Roberts, Tarr, & Jones, 2002; Izquierdo et al., 2006). Meanwhile, the completion of forced repetitions has been shown to result in the same gains in strength as when repetitions beyond failure are not forced upon the athlete (Drinkwater, Pritchett, & Behm, 2007).

Fatigue has been proposed to be counterproductive to the development of certain indices of muscular strength. For example, the use of pre-exhaustion routines has been shown to reduce muscle activation (Augustsson et al., 2003). Moreover, it has been proposed that fatigue may promote a fast-to-slow fiber transition (Fry, 2004). Furthermore, incurring fatigue during resistance training workouts has been proposed to interfere with the development of muscular power output (Tidow, 1990). Fatigue, however, is a requirement of resistance training workouts designed to promote gains in muscular strength endurance.

Worked Example 6.3
Using repetition velocity to establish resistance training intensity

González-Badillo and Sánchez-Medina (2010) had a large number of participants complete an isoinertial bench press performed in a Smith machine with loads ranging from 30% to 100% 1-RM. The mean vertical velocity of the barbell was recorded during the ascent using a linear position transducer. The authors were able to establish a regression equation to predict the percentage of the 1-RM load that a given submaximal load represented from the mean vertical velocity:

$$\text{Percent of 1-RM represented by the load} = 7.5786 \times v^2 - 75.865 \times v + 113.02$$

where v is the mean vertical velocity (in m/s) of the barbell during the ascent. The standard error of the estimate using this equation was 3.77% of 1-RM. Furthermore, the values for mean vertical velocity during the bench press performed with a range of loads remained constant following a period of resistance training despite an average increase in 1-RM of 9.3%.

Table 6.4 shows the mean vertical velocity of the barbell for an athlete performing the bench press with loads of 67.5, 101.0, and 135.0 kg. The maximal dynamic muscular strength for this athlete, established using a 1-RM bench press test, was 135.0 kg. Mean vertical velocity was recorded during each lift using a linear position transducer attached to the barbell. Using González-Badillo and Sánchez-Medina's equation, the predicted percentage of 1-RM for the 67.5-, 101.0-, and 135.0-kg loads was calculated from the mean vertical velocity. As Table 6.4 shows, the equation is more accurate with heavier loads performed for fewer repetitions.

The use of the regression equation negates the requirement to perform a test of maximal muscular strength to determine the loads to be used during training and to monitor the intensity of the resistance training exercises (González-Badillo & Sánchez-Medina, 2010). However, the prediction equation may be specific to the bench press exercise and not appropriate for other resistance training exercises.

Table 6.4
Mean Vertical Velocity of the Barbell, Predicted 1-Repetition Maximum Value, Actual 1-Repetition, and Difference Between Predicted and Actual 1-Repetition Maximum Values for an Athlete Performing the Bench Press with Three Submaximal Loads

Test Load (kg)	Mean Velocity (m/s)	Predicted Percentage of 1-RM	Actual Percentage of 1-RM	Difference (%)
67.5	0.72	62	50	12
101.0	0.47	79	75	4
135.0	0.18	100	100	0

Note: 1-RM = one-repetition maximum.

Exercise Volume

The volume of resistance training exercises is expressed in terms of the number of repetitions and sets completed. There is an inverse relationship between the intensity and volume of resistance training exercises, with greater relative intensities necessitating lower volumes (Figure 6.2). However, stronger athletes are able to complete a greater number of repetitions at the same relative intensity compared to weaker athletes (Brown et al., 1990).

High exercise intensities are associated with the generation of greater forces. However, by reducing the intensity of the exercise such that the volume is increased during the workout, greater overall force is generated with the lower exercise intensity (Crewther et al., 2005). That is, the sum of the forces generated during a resistance training workout is greater when the intensity is lower due to the greater volume that can be achieved, and multiple sets are more effective at increasing muscular strength than single sets (Ratamess, 2012). The greater volumes associated with lower exercise intensities also result in a greater amount of work being performed during the workouts, which appears to be important for hypertrophy (Crewther et al., 2005).

Rest Intervals

The time for rest provided between the sets of resistance exercises can be manipulated to elicit alterations in the mechanics of the subsequent exercises, as the rest periods will determine the degree of fatigue or post-activity potentiation that exists at the beginning of subsequent sets. In general, the greater the relative exercise intensities used, the greater the rest periods between consecutive sets. Furthermore, greater gains in muscular strength have been reported with longer rest periods (2–3 min versus 30–40 s) (Ratamess, 2012).

The repetitions of the exercises within each set of a resistance training workout are typically completed in a continuous manner. This will result in fatigue during each set (Haff et al., 2003; Lawton, Cronin, & Lindsell, 2006; Rooney, Herbert, & Balnave, 1994). While the evidence for the beneficial influence of accumulated fatigue during resistance training contributing to the gains in muscular strength is conflicting (Folland, Irish, Roberts, Tarr, & Jones, 2002; Rooney et al., 1994; see also Strength and Power Training Concept 6.3), fatigue during resistance training exercises has been suggested to interfere with the development of muscular power output (Tidow, 1990). This has led to the development of **cluster sets**, in which short rest intervals (20–130 s) are inserted between consecutive repetitions to ameliorate the decreases in movement velocity and power output caused by fatigue (Haff, Hobbs, et al., 2008; Lawton et al., 2006; see also Applied Research 6.2). The use of cluster sets also provides an opportunity to undulate the load used during repetition to induce the post-activation potentiation effect through ascending clusters (Haff, Hobbs, et al., 2008). An example workout using cluster sets is shown in Table 6.5. Some evidence indicates that the effectiveness of cluster sets is likely to be influenced by the mechanics of the exercise, with the insertion of short inter-repetition rest intervals reducing power output in certain resistance training exercises by interfering with the stretch–shortening cycle (Moir, Graham, Davis, Guers, & Witmer, 2013). The strength and conditioning practitioner should therefore consider the mechanics of the exercise before implementing cluster sets.

Repetition Velocity

The speed with which each repetition of a resistance training exercise is performed will influence the neural, metabolic, and mechanical characteristics of the exercise (Ratamess et al., 2009). It is therefore likely that the repetition velocity will influence the adaptations to a resistance training stimulus. The external load used during a given resistance training exercise (exercise intensity) will affect the repetition velocity,

Applied Research 6.2
Cluster set configurations result in greater inter-repetition power outputs compared to repetitions performed continuously

Elite junior male basketball players performed the bench press with a load equivalent to 6-RM under one of three different conditions: (1) 6×1 repetition with an inter-repetition rest interval of 20 s (singles); (2) 3×2 repetitions with an inter-repetition rest interval of 50 s (doubles); or (3) 2×3 repetitions with an inter-repetition rest interval of 100 s (triples). These cluster set configurations were chosen such that the cumulative time for each set was equivalent (118 s). The power output during each cluster set configuration was compared to the traditional set configuration in which the repetitions were completed continuously. The authors reported that power output was significantly reduced during each repetition in the traditional configuration. However, significantly greater power outputs were reported during the later repetitions (4–6) of all cluster set configurations compared to the traditional configuration.

Lawton, T. W., Cronin, J. B., & Lindsell, R. P. (2006). Effects of interrepetition rest intervals on weight training repetition power output. *Journal of Strength and Conditioning Research, 20*, 172–176.

with greater external loads resulting in lower velocities for the same resistance training exercises (Cormie, McCauley, Triplett, et al., 2007). However, the athlete can intentionally move the load slowly or quickly. Generally, the performance of intentionally slow repetitions (e.g., 5-s or 10-s eccentric and concentric muscle actions) has been shown to result in lower muscle activation, lower energy expenditure, and lower force during each repetition despite a greater time under tension for the active muscles (Ratamess et al., 2009).

When the external load is large, the athlete can still intend to move it quickly, even if the actual movement velocity may be rather low. Behm and Sale (1993) reported similar neuromuscular adaptations to resistance training exercises where the motion of the limb was constrained but the participants intended to move the limb rapidly (explosive isometric task) compared to exercises where the participants were actually able to move their limbs rapidly (explosive concentric task). However,

Table 6.5
Example of a Strength/Power Workout Using Cluster Sets

Exercise	Sets × Repetitions	Set Type	Intensity (kg)	Inter-repetition Rest Interval (s)
Speed squat	3×3	Traditional	90	0
Power clean	$1 \times 3/1$	Ascending cluster	110, 115, 120	30
	$1 \times 3/1$	Ascending cluster	115, 120, 125	30
	$1 \times 3/1$	Ascending cluster	120, 125, 130	30
Push jerk	3×3	Traditional	120	0

Note: Based on 1-RM back squat of 180 kg, 1-RM power clean of 140 kg, and 1-RM push jerk of 135 kg.

Reproduced from Haff, G. G., Hobbs, R. T., Haff, E. E., Sands, W. A., Pierce, K. C., & Stone, M. H. (2008). Cluster training: A novel method for introducing training program variation. *Strength and Cond Journal, 30*, 67–76.

other researchers have reported that the actual movement velocity achieved during resistance training exercises is more important than the intention to move quickly. Specifically, the use of resistance training using heavy loads that result in low movement velocities does not result in improvements in high-velocity movement tasks, whereas the use of lower loads during the resistance training exercises, allowing the achievement of higher movement velocities, had a greater transfer to the high velocity movements tasks (McBride et al., 2002). It is important to note that the participants in this study were encouraged to move the external load as rapidly as possible regardless of the magnitude of the external load.

The repetition velocity achieved during a resistance training exercise is also influenced by the type of resistance training exercise performed. For example, greater velocities are achieved during a jump squat compared to a back squat with the same external load (Cormie, McCauley, McBride, 2007). This difference arises due to the ballistic nature of the jump squat, where the external load has positive velocity that allows the athlete to take off into the flight phase of the movement; in contrast, there is a requirement for zero velocity at the end of the movement in the back squat exercise. Low to moderate repetition velocities have been recommended for novice and intermediate athletes to develop hypertrophy and muscular strength, with high repetition velocities (intentional high velocities if using heavy external loads) recommended to develop muscular power output (Ratamess et al., 2009). A range of low, moderate, and high repetition velocities are recommended to develop hypertrophy and muscular strength, with high repetition velocities (intentional high velocities if using heavy external loads) recommended to develop muscular power in advanced athletes (Ratamess et al., 2009).

Exercise Order and Workout Structure

Each resistance training workout will comprise a number of different exercises to be completed by the athlete. The order in which high- and low-intensity exercises or single-joint and multijoint exercises are performed can be manipulated by the practitioner. Generally, the high-intensity resistance exercises are performed first during a workout so that they are performed in a nonfatigued state (Ratamess, 2012). This consideration is especially important when developing muscular power output. Tidow (1990) has proposed that a 10% reduction in power output caused by fatigue will negate any adaptations in power output. It is also recommended that multijoint resistance exercises be performed before single-joint exercises (Ratamess, 2012). Reversing this order and performing multijoint exercises at the end of the workout reduces the number of repetitions that are performed (Simão, Fleck, Polito, Monteiro, & Farinatti, 2005). In **pre-exhaustion** routines, single-joint exercises are performed to exhaustion before multijoint exercises involving similar muscles. Such routines have been shown to actually reduce the muscle activation during the multijoint exercise, however, so they are unlikely to be effective at improving muscular strength (Augustsson et al., 2003).

Other manipulations in the order of exercises include alternating **agonist–antagonist pairs** to provide a time-efficient method of developing muscular strength and power output (Robbins, Young, Behm, & Payne, 2010). Performing a high-intensity resistance exercise before performing a mechanically similar, but lower-intensity exercise following minutes of recovery has been shown to increase the power output during the lower-intensity exercise (Docherty, Robbins, & Hodgson, 2004). Such couplings between the mechanically similar high- and low-intensity

Table 6.6

Example of a Strength/Power Resistance Training Workout Using Agonist–Antagonist and Complex Pairs

Exercise	Sets and Repetitions	Intensity	Rest (min)
Bench pull	4 × 6	6-RM	4
Bench press	3 × 6	6-RM	4
Bench press throw	1 × 6	40% 1-RM	4

Note: RM = repetition maximum.

Modified from Robins, D. W., Young, W. B., Behm, D. G., & Payne, W. R. (2009). Effects of agonist–antagonist complex resistance training on upper body strength and power development. *Journal of Sports Sciences, 27,* 1617–1625.

resistance exercises are known as **complex pairs**. Their effectiveness is proposed to be due to the **post-activation potentiation** (Hodgson, Docherty, & Robbins, 2005). Table 6.6 shows an example of a resistance training workout using agonist–antagonist and complex pairs.

Frequency of Workouts

The frequency of resistance training workouts refers to the number of sessions completed within each training week. More importantly, the strength and conditioning practitioner should consider the number of times a given exercise is performed or a specific muscle group is trained each week. The frequency of the workouts will be determined by the intensity, volume, exercise selection, and training status of the athlete. The frequency will determine the fatigue experienced by the athlete. Generally, two or three workouts each week are recommended for novice athletes, with three workouts per week producing the greatest improvements in muscular strength (Ratamess, 2012). In more advanced athletes, four or five workouts per week are recommended (Ratamess, 2012). These recommendations relate to total-body workouts (i.e., workouts incorporating upper- and lower-body exercises). **Split routines**, where consecutive training days are undertaken with the focus of each day differing (i.e., day 1 involves lower-body exercises, day 2 involves upper-body exercises), would allow for increased training frequency. Likewise, **double-split routines**, involving two workouts per training day, each emphasizing different muscle groups, could increase the training frequency.

The recommendations for the acute program variables that can be manipulated by the coach to elicit specific adaptations are shown in Table 6.7.

The first task of developing an effective resistance training program aimed at improving strength and power is to complete analyses of the physiological and mechanical aspects of the specific sport as well as the current status of the athlete. Despite the recommendations for the manipulation of acute programming variables shown in Table 6.7, a coach can expect interindividual variation in the responses to the same resistance training workout, because the ability to exercise is distinct from the ability to adapt to an exercise stimulus (Toigo & Boutellier, 2006). For example, well-trained athletes demonstrate very different responses in testosterone to the

Table 6.7

Summary of the Acute Program Variables That Are Recommended to Elicit Increased Hypertrophy, Muscular Strength, Muscular Power Output, and Muscular Strength Endurance

	Hypertrophy	Muscular Strength	Muscular Power	Muscular Strength Endurance
Muscle action	Perform concentric, eccentric, and isometric muscle actions.	Perform concentric, eccentric, and isometric muscle actions.	Specific to the sporting movements.	
Intensity and volume	70–85% 1-RM for 8–12 repetitions/set for 1–3 sets/exercise for novice and intermediate athletes. 70–100% 1-RM for 1–12 repetitions/set for 3–6 sets/exercise for advanced athletes.	60–70% 1-RM for 8–12 repetitions/set for 1–3 sets/exercise for novice and intermediate athletes. 80–100% 1-RM for advanced athletes with variations in intensity and volume. Intensity should be progressed 2–10% (lower percentage for small muscle-mass exercises, higher percentage for larger muscle-mass exercises) for all athletes.	Various loads ranging from 85–100% 1-RM (to develop force capabilities) to 30–60% 1-RM (upper-body exercises) or 0–60% 1-RM (lower-body exercises) to develop velocity and RFD. 1–6 repetitions for 3–6 sets.	Relatively light loads (10–15 repetitions) with moderate to high volume for novice and intermediate athletes. Various loading strategies (10–25 repetitions) in a periodized manner for advanced athletes.
Exercise selection	Both single- and multijoint exercises for novice, intermediate, and advanced athletes.	Both single- and multijoint exercises for novice, intermediate, and advanced athletes.	Multijoint exercises (e.g., weightlifting exercises). Specific to the movements used in sporting activities.	Both single- and multijoint exercises for novice, intermediate, and advanced athletes.
Exercise order	Large muscle group exercises before small muscle group exercises, multijoint exercises before single-joint exercises, and higher-intensity exercises before lower-intensity exercises for novice, intermediate, and advanced athletes.	Large muscle group exercises before small muscle group exercises before single-joint exercises, and higher-intensity exercises before lower-intensity exercises for novice, intermediate, and advanced athletes.	Large muscle group exercises before small muscle group exercises, multijoint exercises before single-joint exercises, and higher-intensity exercises before lower-intensity exercises for novice, intermediate, and advanced athletes.	
Rest intervals	1- to 2-min rest between sets for novice and intermediate athletes. Between 1- to 2-min and 2- to 3-min rest between sets for advanced athletes depending on the intensity of the exercises.	2–3 min between sets of multijoint exercises for novice, intermediate, and advanced athletes. 1–2 min between sets of single-joint exercises for novice, intermediate, and advanced athletes.	2–3 min between sets.	1–2 min for high-repetition sets (15–20 repetitions). <1 min for moderate-repetition sets (10–15 repetitions).

(continues)

Table 6.7 (Continued)
Summary of the Acute Program Variables That Are Recommended to Elicit Increased Hypertrophy, Muscular Strength, Muscular Power Output, and Muscular Strength Endurance

	Hypertrophy	Muscular Strength	Muscular Power	Muscular Strength Endurance
Repetition velocity	Low to moderate velocities for novice and intermediate athletes. Low, moderate, and high velocities for advanced athletes depending on the intensity, repetition number, and goals of the program.	Low to moderate velocities for novice and intermediate athletes. Moderate velocities for intermediate athletes. A range from low to high velocities for advanced athletes with the intent to maximize the velocity during the concentric phase of the exercise.	High repetition velocities. Intend to perform the exercise with high velocities when load is high.	Intentionally slow velocity with moderate repetition sets (10–15 repetitions). Moderate to fast velocity with high repetition sets (15–25 repetitions).
Frequency	2–3 days/week for novice and intermediate athletes when each workout involves total body exercises. 4 days/week for intermediate athletes when using a split routine. 4–6 days/week for advanced athletes.	2–3 days/week for novice athletes when each workout involves total body exercises. 3–4 days/week for intermediate athletes using total body workouts or a split routine. 4–6 days/week for advanced athletes. Advanced athletes may train twice daily for 4–5 days/week.	2–3 days/week for novice athletes when each workout involves total body exercises. 3–4 days/week for intermediate athletes using total body workouts or a split routine. 4–5 days/week for advanced athletes using total body workouts or a split routine.	2–3 days/week for novice athletes using total body workouts. 3 days/week for intermediate athletes using total body workouts. 4 days/week for intermediate athletes using split routines. Higher frequency (4–6 days/week) for advanced athletes using split routines.
Modifications	Vascular occlusion (196 mm Hg pressure) may reduce the required load.	Vascular occlusion (196 mm Hg pressure) may reduce the required load.	Cluster sets (singles, doubles, triples) with inter-repetition rest intervals may allow greater power outputs to be achieved.	

Note: Novices are defined as untrained individuals or those who have not engaged in resistance training for several years; intermediate athletes are defined as individuals with approximately 6 months of consistent resistance training experience; and advanced athletes are defined as individuals with years of resistance training experience; 1-RM = 1-repetition maximum; RFD = rate of force development.

Data from Haff, G. G., Hobbs, R. T., Haff, E. E., Sands, W. A., Pierce, K. C., & Stone, M. H. (2008). Cluster training: A novel method for introducing training program variation. Strength and Conditioning Journal, 30, 67–76; Lawton, T. W., Cronin, J. B., & Lindsell, R. P. (2006). Effects of interrepetition rest intervals on weight training repetition power output. Journal of Strength and Conditioning Research, 20, 172–176; Ratamess, N. A., Alvar, B. A., Evetoch, T. K., Housh, T. J., Kibler, W. B., Kraemer, W. J., & Triplett, N. T. (2009). Progression models in resistance training for healthy adults. Medicine and Science in Sports and Exercise, 41, 687–708; Takarada, Y., Sato, Y., & Ishii, N. (2002). Effects of resistance exercise combined with vascular occlusion on muscle function in athletes. European Journal of Applied Physiology, 86, 308–314; Wernbom, M., Augustsson, J., & Raastad, T. (2008). Ischemic strength training: A low-load alternative to heavy resistance exercise? Scandinavian Journal of Medicine and Science in Sports, 18, 401–416.

Applied Research 6.3
Well-trained athletes demonstrated markedly different hormonal responses to the same resistance training workouts

Beaven, Gill, and Cook (2008) assessed the acute response in testosterone and cortisol following resistance training workouts comprising different intensity, volume, and rest periods in a group of elite rugby players. The athletes completed four different resistance training workouts: (1) 4 sets × 10 repetitions with a load equivalent to 70% 1-RM, 2-min rest between sets; (2) 3 sets × 5 repetitions with a load equivalent to 85% 1-RM, 3-min rest; (3) 5 sets × 15 repetitions with a load equivalent to 55% 1-RM, 1-min rest; and (4) 3 sets × 5 repetitions with a load equivalent to 40% 1-RM, 3-min rest. Each workout was separated by 2 days, and the order in which the workouts were completed was randomized.

The authors reported that the grouped data revealed a decrease in testosterone concentrations following the 3 sets × 5 repetitions workout, with no change in testosterone concentrations being observed following the other workouts. All four workouts resulted in a decrease in cortisol concentrations when the athletes' data were grouped. However, considerable individual variations were noted in testosterone responses. Specifically, different athletes responded with increased testosterone concentrations to different workouts. The authors suggested that these individual hormonal responses could modulate the adaptations to resistance training, such that athletes are likely to adapt differently to the same resistance training workout.

Beaven, C. M., Gill, N. D., & Cook, C. J. (2008). Salivary testosterone and cortisol responses in professional rugby players after four resistance exercise protocols. *Journal of Strength and Conditioning Research, 22,* 426–432.

same resistance training workouts (Beaven, Gill, & Cook, 2008; see also Applied Research 6.3). Furthermore, greater increases in muscular strength are achieved when following a resistance training program whose workouts elicit the greatest response in testosterone (Beaven, Cook, & Gill, 2008). This factor can complicate the development of a resistance training program, so the strength and conditioning practitioner should use the data presented in Table 6.7 as broad guidelines. Once the strength and power training program has been developed, it is then the responsibility of the strength and conditioning coach to continually monitor the athlete to assess his or her physiological and behavioral responses to the program. Through the monitoring process, appropriate changes in the program can be implemented when needed to ensure that the athlete continues to demonstrate positive adaptations.

Modifications to Traditional Resistance Training Methods

Resistance training exercises are those in which the movement of the athlete is resisted. Traditional resistance training exercises require the athlete to exert a force against an external resistance provided by an external mass. In such exercises, momentum is imparted to the mass (so long as the mass can be moved). This limits the length of the acceleration path when the exercise demands that the mass have no momentum at the end of the movement, such as during the traditional resistance training exercises including the squat and the bench press (see Worked Example 6.4). These types of resistance training exercises are known as non-ballistic. The reduction in the acceleration path limits the average force generated during the movement, potentially limiting the adaptations to the exercise. Although the use of heavier loads would increase the

Worked Example 6.4
The acceleration path during non-ballistic isoinertial bench press with different loads

During the non-ballistic bench press exercise, in which a constant mass is lifted, a constraint is imposed on the movement in that the barbell must not have any vertical momentum at the end of the ascent phase. Momentum is imparted to the barbell early during the ascent due to the impulse applied by the athlete; in turn, the barbell rises. However, due to the constraint of zero momentum at the end of the ascent, the force applied by the athlete to accelerate the barbell is applied over a short duration. This also means that the average force applied by the athlete to the barbell will be equal to the weight of the load lifted.

Frost, Cronin, and Newton (2008) recorded the kinematic variables associated with the non-ballistic isoinertial bench press performed with loads ranging from 15% to 90% 1-RM. Here, we use the data collected with loads equivalent to 15% and 75% 1-RM to highlight the potential shortcomings of non-ballistic resistance training exercises. Table 6.8 shows the kinematic data collected for the bench press performed with a load equivalent to 15% 1-RM.

The attainment of v_{peak} during the ascent denotes the end of the acceleration phase of the barbell; notice that the barbell is therefore decelerating for 44% of the ascent phase. We can use these data to calculate the vertical displacement of the barbell from the value of v_{peak}:

  i. Rearrange $v_f^2 = v_i^2 + 2as$ to solve for s $\qquad\qquad s = v_f^2 - v_i^2/2a$

 ii. Insert the known variables $\qquad\qquad\qquad\qquad s = 0^2 - 2.91^2/2 \times -9.81$

iii. Answer $\qquad\qquad\qquad\qquad\qquad\qquad\qquad\qquad s = 0.43$ m

The vertical displacement of 0.43 m is the displacement undergone by the barbell from the time of v_{peak} to the point where the vertical velocity has been reduced to 0 m/s due to gravitational acceleration. Notice from Table 6.8 that the barbell has already been displaced 0.33 m at the point of v_{peak}. By summing the values of 0.33 m and 0.43 m, we calculate the total vertical displacement of the barbell as 0.76 m. However, notice from Table 6.8 that the actual total vertical displacement of the barbell during the exercise was recorded as 0.58 m. This means that the athlete actually has to exert a downward force on the barbell after the attainment of v_{peak} to arrest its vertical motion, as the acceleration due to gravity is insufficient to reduce the momentum of the barbell to 0 kg m/s at the end of the ascent phase.

When the exercise is performed against a load equivalent to 75% 1-RM, the kinematic variables are very different (Table 6.9).

Table 6.8
Kinematic Data for the Non-ballistic Isoinertial Bench Press Performed with a Load Equivalent to 15% 1-RM

Ascent Time (s)	Ascent Displacement (m)	v_{peak} (m/s)	Time v_{peak} (s)	Displacement v_{peak} (m)
0.34	0.58	2.91	0.19	0.33

Note: v_{peak} = peak vertical velocity of the barbell during ascent; Time v_{peak} = time of peak vertical velocity; Displacement v_{peak} = vertical displacement of the barbell at time of v_{peak}.

Table 6.9
Kinematic Data for the Non-ballistic Isoinertial Bench Press Performed with a Load Equivalent to 75% 1-RM

Ascent Time (s)	Ascent Displacement (m)	v_{peak} (m/s)	Time v_{peak} (s)	Displacement v_{peak} (m)
0.95	0.47	0.77	0.74	0.36

Note: v_{peak} = peak vertical velocity of the barbell during ascent; Time v_{peak} = time of peak vertical velocity; Displacement v_{peak} = vertical displacement of the barbell at time of v_{peak}.

Notice that now the barbell is decelerating for only 22% of the ascent phase. Let us calculate the vertical displacement of the barbell from the value of v_{peak}:

i. Rearrange $v_f^2 = v_i^2 + 2as$ to solve for s $s = v_f^2 - v_i^2 / 2a$

ii. Insert the known variables $s = 0^2 - 0.77^2 / 2 \times -9.81$

iii. Answer $s = 0.03$ m

The sum of the displacement of the barbell at the point of v_{peak} (0.36 m) and the displacement that would be undergone by the barbell from v_{peak} to the point where gravity would reduce the velocity to 0 m/s returns a value of 0.39 m, some 0.08 m below the actual total vertical displacement of the barbell during the exercise. This means that the athlete is required to continue exerting a vertical force on the barbell to continue the vertical displacement, albeit a vertical force that is below the weight of the barbell. Therefore, both the magnitude of the force and the duration of force application are enhanced when heavier masses are lifted in non-ballistic exercises. However, it can be seen when comparing the v_{peak} values shown in Tables 6.8 and 6.9 that the increased external mass considerably reduces the velocity of the movement. These issues arise due to the momentum imparted to the external mass and the constraint of having to end the ascent phase with the mass possessing no vertical momentum. These issues can be mitigated by using variable resistance training methods, ballistic resistance exercises, or a pneumatic resistance during the exercise rather than a mass.

average force and the length of the acceleration path, the peak velocity of the movement is reduced, rendering these non-ballistic movements inappropriate for developing power (Frost, Cronin, & Newton, 2008).

To mitigate the kinematic and kinetic alterations that are associated with accelerating a constant mass while ending the movement with zero momentum, various modifications have been suggested to the typical isoinertial exercises. These changes include providing variable resistance during the acceleration of the mass through the addition of elastic bands or chains, performing the exercise ballistically, or replacing the mass with a pneumatic resistance.

Variable Resistance Training Methods

Variable resistance training exercises provide increased resistance to the athlete's motion during the exercise through either the addition of elastic bands to the load that resist the motion or the addition of chains to the load whereby the mass is increased as the load is lifted due to a greater proportion of chain links being supported by the athlete. The methods of achieving the variable resistance will likely influence the mechanics of the exercise and, therefore, the athlete's adaptive response (see Strength and Power Training Concept 6.4).

Strength and Power Training Concept 6.4

Mechanical differences in the resistance offered by elastic bands compared to chains

Although both elastic band and chain methods provide increased resistance to motion as the athlete raises the mass, in contrast to traditional isoinertial methods, some differences exist in the linearity of the increase in resistance offered by elastic bands versus chains. Specifically, the resistance offered by the chain method increases linearly with the increased displacement of the load as the number of chain links that is supported by the athlete increases proportionally (McMaster, Cronin, & McGuigan, 2009). In contrast, the resistance offered by elastic bands increases nonlinearly with the displacement of the load as a result of the viscous nature of the bands, such that there is a slight reduction in the resistance toward the end of the movement (McMaster et al., 2009). Furthermore, a mechanical analysis of these variable resistance methods highlights some important differences. When elastic bands are attached to the barbell, Equation (6.1) can be used to provide the magnitude of the resistive force:

$$F = mg + kx \qquad \text{Eq. (6.1)}$$

where F is the magnitude of the resistive force, m is the mass of the barbell, g is the acceleration due to gravity, k is the stiffness of the elastic band, and x is the displacement of the barbell ($x = 0$ m when the barbell is at the lowest point of the movement). When chains are attached to the barbell rather than elastic bands, the resistive force becomes

$$F = mg + wgx \qquad \text{Eq. (6.2)}$$

where F is the magnitude of the resistive force, m is the mass of the barbell, g is the acceleration due to gravity, w is the mass of each chain link, and x is the displacement of the barbell ($x = 0$ m when the barbell is at the lowest point of the movement). The term wgx, therefore, represents the mass per unit length of the chains. Equations (6.1) and (6.2) denote situations where the barbell is not moving—that is, static situations. In such static situations, if the stiffness of the elastic band, k, is chosen such that it is equal to the mass of the chain, wg, then the two types of loading become indistinguishable for the athlete (Arandjelović, 2010).

Under dynamic conditions, when the barbell is lifted by the athlete, these equations require modification. For the situation where elastic bands are attached to the barbell, the net force acting on the barbell becomes (Arandjelović, 2010)

$$F_{net} = F_{applied} - mg - kx \qquad \text{Eq. (6.3)}$$

where F_{net} is the magnitude of the net force acting on the barbell, $F_{applied}$ is the magnitude of the force applied by the athlete, m is the mass of the barbell, g is the acceleration due to gravity, k is the stiffness of the elastic band, and x is the displacement of the barbell. Thus, the net acceleration of the combined barbell and elastic bands becomes

$$a = \left(\frac{F_{applied} - kx}{m} \right) - g$$

Eq. (6.4)

where a is the net acceleration of the barbell, $F_{applied}$ is the magnitude of the force applied by the athlete, k is the stiffness of the elastic band, x is the displacement of the barbell, m is the mass of the barbell, and g is the acceleration due to gravity.

The situation is different when chains are attached to the barbell, because not only is the mass of the barbell accelerated, but links of the chain that were previously static are also accelerated to the velocity of the barbell (Arandjelović, 2010). Considering the change in both the gravitational potential and translational kinetic energy of the barbell as well as the gravitational potential and translational kinetic energy of each chain link during the movement, the net acceleration of the combined barbell and chains becomes (Arandjelović, 2010)

$$a = \left(\frac{F_{applied} - E_{TK}}{m + wx} \right) - g$$

Eq. (6.5)

where a is the net acceleration of the barbell, $F_{applied}$ is the magnitude of the force applied by the athlete, E_{TK} is the kinetic energy of the chain, m is the mass of the barbell, w is the mass of each chain link, x is the displacement of the barbell, and g is the acceleration due to gravity.

Comparing Equations (6.4) and (6.5), it can be determined that the variable resistance offered by the attachment of elastic bands to the barbell will result in a stimulus that is mechanically distinct from that offered by the attachment of chains to the barbell (Arandjelović, 2010); the athlete would have to exert a different force against the barbell to achieve the same net acceleration even if the stiffness of the elastic band were equal to the mass of the chains at each displacement. The practitioner may, therefore, expect different adaptations from these methods of variable resistance training given the potential roles played by these mechanical variables (Crewther et al., 2005), although there is a paucity of research to substantiate potential differences between the methods.

Elastic Bands

In one study, the use of elastic bands, which increased the resistance at the end of the ascent during a back squat exercise by 10% and reduced the resistance at the start of the ascent by 10%, allowed athletes to produce a greater peak force and power during the exercise compared to when the exercise was performed with an equivalent isoinertial load (85% 1-RM) (Wallace, Winchester, & McGuigan, 2006).

Furthermore, greater improvements in 1-RM loads in the bench press and back squat have been reported when resistance training exercises are combined with resistance offered by elastic bands compared to traditional resistance training (Anderson, Sforzo, & Sigg, 2008). In addition, greater improvements in maximal strength and power in both upper- and lower-body exercises have been reported when using elastic bands to provide additional resistance compared with traditional resistance training exercises (Bellar et al., 2010; Ghigiarelli et al., 2009; Joy, Lowery, Oliveira de Souza, & Wilson, 2013; Rhea, Kenn, & Dermody, 2009).

Chains

There have been fewer investigations to assess the effectiveness of chains on the kinematics and kinetics of resistance training exercises compared to elastic bands. Greater average barbell velocity is achieved during the bench press exercise when chains are added to the load, such that the resistance at the end of the ascent was equal to 75% 1-RM (with 15% of the load coming from chains), compared to the movement performed with an equivalent isoinertial load (Baker & Newton, 2009). This was possibly due to unloading during the end of the descent of the barbell, which is likely to facilitate a more rapid stretch–shortening cycle transition and greater velocities during the subsequent ascent phase. Greater improvements in maximal strength and power in upper-body exercises have been demonstrated when performing exercises where approximately 20% of the load came from chains compared with traditional resistance training exercises (Ghigiarelli et al., 2009).

The limited amount of research, particularly with chain-loaded exercises, makes it difficult to make recommendations for variable resistance training exercises. However, approximately 15–30% of the weight of the load should be provided by the tension of the elastic bands (Bellar et al., 2010; Joy et al., 2013), and approximately 15–20% of the load should come from chains (Baker & Newton, 2009; Ghigiarelli et al., 2009) to provide an effective stimulus.

Ballistic Resistance Training Methods

Ballistic resistance training exercises are those that require the external load to be projected or released at the end of the concentric phase. Such exercises remove the constraint of ensuring that the momentum of the load is zero at the end of the movement. As a result, greater force and power are generated during ballistic resistance training exercises compared to non-ballistic exercises (Crewther et al., 2005). The greater force produced during ballistic resistance training movements may reduce the intensity of the load required to elicit adaptations in muscular strength, with loads as low as 45% 1-RM or less being proposed in the literature (Crewther et al., 2005). Furthermore, ballistic resistance training methods are likely to be more specific to many sports than traditional, non-ballistic resistance training methods. However, ballistic resistance training exercises pose a potential risk for musculoskeletal injury given the requirement to catch the load after it has been projected. Examples of ballistic resistance training exercises include bench press throws and jump squats. Semi-ballistic resistance training exercises encompass the weightlifting exercises of the clean and snatch and their variations.

Pneumatic/Hydraulic Resistance Training Methods

With traditional resistance training exercises, the resistance is offered by an external mass that is accelerated. A limitation to these types of resistance training exercises is that momentum is imparted to the mass such that the external load will continue to move in the absence of a force being exerted by the athlete. This limitation is eliminated when the resistance is offered by a pneumatic/hydraulic element, such as the fluid contained within the cylinder found in resistance training machines (e.g., Keiser machines). When these machines are used, the force applied by the athlete is resisted by the motion of the fluid through an aperture, with the amount of resistance offered being determined by the size of the aperture. The resistance force can be expressed as follows:

$$F = dv^2$$

Eq. (6.6)

where F is the magnitude of the resistance force, d is the coefficient of fluid dynamics, and v is the velocity of the fluid. Notice in Equation (6.6) that no mass is being accelerated during these resistance training exercises.

Frost et al. (2008) reported that greater mean power outputs were recorded during the bench press performed against a pneumatic resistance than during either the traditional free-weight or ballistic free-weight exercises with the same relative intensities (60–90% 1-RM). The magnitude of the force, power output, and muscle activation were also greater during the last 10–20% of the ascent during the pneumatic exercise, probably due to the removal of the constraint associated with zero final momentum of the barbell (traditional bench press) and the momentum given to the barbell continuing its motion (ballistic bench press).

Eccentric Resistance Training Methods

It has been shown that 20–60% more force is produced eccentrically compared to that produced during concentric muscle actions (Cowell, Cronin, & Brughelli, 2012). However, the loads selected for resistance training exercises are typically based on those that can be raised; thus they are largely determined by the concentric force capabilities of the athlete. This factor is likely to minimize the eccentric adaptations to the exercises. When concentric-only and eccentric-only contractions are compared with the same external load, there is lower motor unit recruitment and hormonal response to the eccentric contractions (Crewther et al., 2005). Eccentric-only actions produce greater gains in eccentric strength but are more effective at inducing muscle fiber hypertrophy than concentric-only actions (Roig et al., 2009; Schoenfeld, 2010), which suggests the importance of eccentric resistance training methods. Two types of eccentric resistance training are used: supra-maximal eccentric training and augmented eccentric training.

Supra-maximal Eccentric Methods

Supra-maximal eccentric resistance training exercises involve movements performed against maximal or close-to-maximal eccentric loads. Such loads are greater than those associated with the concentric capabilities of the athlete—hence the term *supra-maximal*. Greater gains in strength have been reported following a resistance training program incorporating supra-maximal eccentric exercises, although the training program studied included overspeed exercises (Cook, Beaven, & Kilduff, 2013). It has been proposed that supra-maximal eccentric exercises increase motor unit recruitment and hypertrophy of fast muscle fibers (Bette et al., 2010). A limitation to this method of training may be the specificity of eccentric-only contractions given that many sports require the coupling of eccentric and concentric actions in the stretch–shortening cycle, while the potential for muscle damage is increased.

Augmented Eccentric Methods

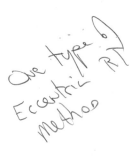

One type of Eccentric RT Method

Augmented eccentric resistance training exercises involve the completion of both eccentric and concentric muscle actions during the exercise, but the eccentric load is greater than the subsequent concentric load owing to the removal of some of the load at the end of the descent phase by releasing some of the weight. Peak power output has been shown to increase during jumps where eccentric overload was achieved by the use of dumbbells that were released by the athlete at the bottom of the countermovement (Sheppard et al., 2008). Others have used specialized weight releasers during the exercises and reported increased concentric force and power via augmented eccentric loading in bench presses and bench throws (Doan et al., 2002). The enhanced concentric capabilities resulting from augmented eccentric loading methods are proposed to include storage and return of strain potential energy from the musculotendinous unit, activation of stretch reflex, increased active state of the muscles, and an elongation of the tendon allowing the muscles to operate close to their optimal lengths (Moore & Schilling, 2005). However, there is a paucity of research into the effects of augmented eccentric training.

An issue with supra-maximal and augmented eccentric resistance training is the associated muscle damage that is sustained by the athlete (Proske & Morgan, 2001). While this damage will stimulate morphological adaptations, it will also limit the number of workouts that the athlete can complete. Thus the practitioner should insert these types of exercises into the training program carefully to avoid excessive damage and soreness that would compromise the ability of the athlete to complete the required training sessions. It is currently difficult to recommend specific load, repetition, and set schemes for eccentric-only resistance training exercises due to a lack of research in this area (see **Worked Example 6.5**).

Assisted Resistance Training Methods

An inverse relationship between force and velocity exists, such that as the magnitude of the external load increases, the velocity of the movement will decrease. This may compromise the transfer of training effect from the resistance training exercises to unloaded sporting movements, including jumping, sprint running, and change of direction. Assisted resistance training exercises allow the athlete to achieve supra-maximal movement velocities through the use of elastic bands attached to the athlete. In contrast to the use of elastic bands in variable resistance training methods, the bands in assisted resistance training are placed in such a way that they aid the movement of the barbell as opposed to resisting the movement.

Greater takeoff velocities are achieved when athletes jump with elastic bands assisting the movement compared to jumps performed with the elastic bands

Worked Example 6.5
Investigating the appropriate intensity and volume for eccentric-only bench press

Moir, Erny, et al. (2013) investigated athletes' kinematic and kinetic responses during a series of eccentric-only repetitions to failure during the bench press exercise performed with different supra-maximal loads (110%, 120%, and 130% traditional bench press 1-RM). Each lift consisted of a 2-s eccentric phase. The authors recorded the number of repetitions completed prior to volitional failure under each loading condition. Using these data, they were able to develop a regression equation to predict the number of repetitions to failure during the eccentric-only bench press under different supra-maximal loading conditions (Table 6.10). The regression equation predicted that the eccentric-only 1-RM would be 164.8% of the traditional bench press 1-RM.

The repetition-load scheme shown in Table 6.10 can be used to develop specific workouts using the eccentric-only bench press. Ratamess et al. (2009) recommend a program of 60–70% 1-RM performed for 8–12 repetitions progressing to loads equivalent to 80–100% 1-RM for 1–6 repetitions to develop muscular strength for an intermediate athlete. Using the eccentric-only repetition-load scheme, loads equivalent to 100–116% 1-RM for 8–12 repetitions would be performed initially, progressing to loads equivalent to 132–165% 1-RM for 1–6 repetitions. For muscular hypertrophy, Ratamess et al. (2009) recommend loads of 70–85% 1-RM performed for 8–12 repetitions. The corresponding loads for the eccentric-only bench would be 116–140% 1-RM, with equivalent repetitions expected to be completed. However, what remains to be determined is whether the rest periods, sets, and frequency of workouts recommended by Ratamess et al. (2009) are appropriate for the modified repetition-load schemes applied to the eccentric-only bench press.

Table 6.10
Actual Repetitions Completed Under Supra-maximal Load Conditions, Predicted Number of Repetitions Completed, and Supra-maximal Loading Conditions Expressed Relative to Predicted Eccentric-Only One-Repetition Maximum

Load Condition	100% 1-RM	110% 1-RM	120% 1-RM	130% 1-RM	140% 1-RM	150% 1-RM	160% 1-RM
Actual repetitions	—	14.2	11.4	9.4	—	—	—
Predicted repetitions	16.5	14.1	11.7	9.3	6.9	4.5	2.1
Loading (%1-RM$_{ECC}$)	60.7	66.7	72.8	78.9	85.0	91.0	97.1

Note: 1-RM is traditional bench press one-repetition maximum.

resisting the movement or jumps performed without elastic bands (Argus, Gill, Keogh, Blazevich, & Hopkins, 2011). The use of elastic bands during the assisted jumps was shown to reduce the bodyweight of the athlete by 10% (assessed with the athlete standing on a force plate). Furthermore, 4 weeks of assisted jump training resulted in greater improvements in countermovement vertical jump (CMJ) height in professional rugby players compared to resisted jumps or jumps performed without elastic bands (Argus et al., 2011). Cronin, McNair, and Marshall (2003) reported an 8.4% increase in peak velocity and a 14.3% increase in peak power during single-leg jumps following 10 weeks of assisted jump training, while other authors have reported an 11% increase in jump height following 5 weeks of assisted jump training in elite volleyball players (Sheppard et al., 2011). Elastic bands that reduce bodyweight by between 10% and 30% appear to be effective in increasing jumping performance. The proposed mechanisms underpinning the adaptations to assisted resistance exercises include reduced coactivation of antagonists during the movement and the increased recruitment of fast fibers during the exercises.

Unstable Surface and Unstable Load Resistance Training Methods

Recently there has been an interest in the utility of resistance training performed on unstable surfaces (e.g., physioballs, Bosu balls, wobble boards) for athletes. Exercises performed on unstable surfaces have been proposed to elicit greater neural adaptations as compared to resistance training performed on a stable surface, yielding improved balance, force production, and power (Behm, 1995; Behm & Anderson, 2006; Kibele & Behm, 2009). However, investigations of resistance training exercises performed on unstable surfaces have revealed a reduction in force and neural activity of the involved musculature when compared to the same exercises performed on a stable surface (Drinkwater et al., 2007; McBride, Cormie, & Deane, 2006; McBride, Larkin, Dayne, Haines, & Kirby, 2010). These effects occur independently of the loads used during the exercise. Specifically, McBride et al. (2010) reported a reduction in muscle activation during back squats performed on an unstable surface as compared to back squats performed on the ground despite using the same loads relative to the 1-RM achieved on each surface.

Unstable surfaces also preclude the generation of large forces and their rapid application (rate of force development) compared to stable surfaces (McBride et al., 2006). It has been reported that resistance training exercises performed on an unstable surface actually reduce the gains in jumping and sprinting performance compared to the response to the same exercises performed on a stable surface (Cressey, West, Tiberio, Kraemer, & Maresh, 2007; Oberacker, Davis, Haff, Witmer, & Moir, 2012).

It would appear that the reductions in force and muscle activation levels observed during resistance training exercises performed on unstable surfaces limit the adaptations to the training. However, this does not mean that resistance training exercises performed on an unstable surface should never be included in the training program of athletes. Rather, these exercises should be included during training periods where gains in muscular strength and power are not emphasized (see Strength and Power Training Concept 6.5).

An interesting alternative to performing resistance exercises on an unstable surface is to perform them on a stable surface with an unstable load (e.g., water-filled resistances). Such an approach may mitigate the decrements in mechanical variables such as rate of force development observed when exercises are performed on an unstable surface, although currently data to substantiate this claim are lacking (Langford, McCurdy, Ernest, Doscher, & Walter, 2007).

Strength and Power Training Concept 6.5

Should athletes perform resistance training on an unstable surface?

Because of the reduced force production and rate of force development that occur when resistance training exercises are performed on unstable surfaces, such exercises have not been recommended to improve athletic performance (Behm, Drinkwater, Willardson, & Cowley, 2010). The results of training studies would tend to confirm the lack of improvement in athletic performance following a period of resistance training performed on unstable surfaces (Cressey et al., 2007; Oberacker et al., 2012). Nevertheless, resistance training on an unstable surface has been proposed to serve both rehabilitative and even prehabilitative functions (Behm & Sanchez, 2012). For example, training performed on an unstable surface has been shown to improve measures of balance (Yaggie & Campbell, 2006), and poor balance has been associated with an increased risk of injury in a number of sports (Hrysomallis, 2007). Similarly, less injurious knee kinetics during cutting movements have been reported following a training intervention that involved resistance training exercises performed on unstable surfaces (Cochrane et al., 2010).

Given these findings, it seems likely that injury prevention can be enhanced through the use of resistance training exercises performed on unstable surfaces. In a periodized training program where training phases with specific emphasis are appropriately sequenced (Bompa & Haff, 2009), resistance training performed on unstable surfaces may be appropriate during off-season phases. However, such exercises should be used infrequently during phases where the development of muscular strength and power are emphasized.

Plyometric Training Methods

Plyometric exercises are those that involve the stretch–shortening cycle (SSC) during their execution (Markovic, 2007). The SSC is a special case of muscular actions whereby an eccentric action precedes a concentric action. This eccentric–concentric coupling allows the musculotendinous units to develop greater force and perform more mechanical work during the concentric action than if an initial eccentric action had not been performed.

Plyometric exercises have been shown to result in a number of neuromuscular adaptations, including muscle fiber hypertrophy, increased fiber shortening velocity, increased muscle fiber power output, increased fascicle length, and increased voluntary activation of muscles (Markovic & Mikulic, 2010). Furthermore, such exercises increase the ability of the tendinous structures to store strain potential energy (Markovic & Mikulic, 2010). These adaptations underpin the improvements in measures of muscular strength and power observed following a period of plyometric training and the associated improvements in measures of athletic ability including vertical jump, sprint

Applied Research 6.4
Effects of lower-body plyometric training on muscle fiber function and athletic performance

In a study conducted by Malisoux et al. (2006), eight recreationally active men followed an eight-week training program comprising the following jumps: static jumps (SJs), countermovement jumps (CMJs), drop jumps (0.40-m drop), double-leg triple jump, single-leg triple jump, double-leg hurdle jump, and single-leg hurdle jump. Each participant trained three times per week, completing 5,228 jumps across 24 workouts during the training period. The authors reported single-fiber hypertrophy of 23%, 22%, and 30% in fibers expressing type I, IIa, and IIa/x myosin heavy chain (MHC) isoforms, respectively, following training, and increases in maximal force in these fibers of 19%, 15%, and 16%, respectively. The unloaded shortening velocity of the fibers expressing type I, IIa, and IIa/x MHC increased by 18%, 29%, and 22%, respectively. The combined increases in force generation and shortening velocity resulted in substantial increases in single-fiber power output. The plyometric exercises led to an increase in maximal dynamic muscular strength and vertical jump performance, although the increase in CMJ performance following the training period (approximately 15%) was greater than that reported for SJ performance (7.5%), reflecting the specificity of adaptations to plyometric exercises. The authors concluded that plyometric training was able to induce favorable adaptations in all fiber types to enhance performance in measures of athletic performance.

Malisoux, L., Francaux, M., Nielens, H., & Theisen, D. (2006). Stretch-shortening cycle exercise: An effective training paradigm to enhance power output of single human muscle fibers. *Journal of Applied Physiology, 100*, 771–779.

running, and change of direction tasks (Markovic, 2007; Markovic & Mikulic, 2010). (See Applied Research 6.4.) The placement of plyometric exercises within an athlete's training program is important because these exercises are considered to expedite the transfer of muscular strength gained from traditional resistance training exercises to sporting movements (Young, 2006).

Plyometric Training Program Design

The strength and conditioning coach can manipulate the variables of exercise selection, exercise intensity, exercise volume, rest intervals, exercise order, and frequency of workouts associated with plyometric exercises to induce specific adaptations in their athletes. These variables are highlighted here; note that the recommendations provided in relation to them are for lower-body plyometric exercises.

Exercise Selection

Coaches have many plyometric exercises available to use with their athletes. The selection of exercises should be based on the specific demands of the sport.

Exercise Intensity   *for Plyometrics*

A number of factors associated with the selection of specific plyometric exercises as well as the execution of the exercises determine the intensity:

- Height of jump/drop
- Number of contact points (bilateral, unilateral)
- Requirement for vertical and/or horizontal motion

- Duration of contact time between jumps
- Number of jumps completed

The order of intensity for lower-body plyometric exercises, going from low intensity to high intensity, is shown in **Table 6.11**.

Table 6.11
Lower-Body Plyometric Exercises Ranked from Low Intensity to High Intensity

Plyometric Exercise	Description
Jumps-in-place	These exercises require the athlete to perform repeated vertical jumps.
	The athlete should avoid horizontal motion.
	Because multiple jumps are performed, the height attained during each jump, and therefore the intensity, is low.
	Example: bilateral repeated vertical jumps.
	Manipulating intensity: include an arms swing to increase jump height, increasing the intensity of the exercise.
Standing jumps	These exercises require the athlete to complete a single jump for maximal height and take appropriate rest before completing another jump.
	The rest period between the jumps allows the height attained, and therefore the intensity, to be higher than that associated with jumps-in-place.
	Example: bilateral countermovement vertical jump.
	Manipulating intensity: include an overhead goal that the athlete aims for to increase the jump height, thereby increasing the intensity of the exercise.
Multiple hops/bounds	These exercises include a horizontal component in addition to the vertical component associated with the jumps-in-place and standing jumps.
	Example: bilateral horizontal jumps.
	Manipulating intensity: include barriers to clear.
Bounding	These exercises are exaggerated running movements where the athlete uses an excessively long stride.
	Example: alternative bounding.
Box drills	These exercises require an athlete to jump on to or to drop from a box and hold the landing.
	By jumping to a box, the height that the athlete falls from, and therefore the forces associated with the landing, are reduced, limiting the intensity of these exercises.
	By dropping from a box and holding the landing rather than jumping, the forces associated with the landing are reduced, limiting the intensity of these exercises.
	Manipulating intensity: increase the height of the box; include an overhead goal that the athlete aims for to increase the jump height; use a contact mat or linear position transducer to provide height attained during each jump.
Drop jumps	These exercises require the athlete to step from a box, land, and then perform an immediate jump.
	By having the athlete immediately jump following the landing, the intensity of these exercises is increased relative to box drills.
	Manipulating intensity: increase the height of the box; include a barrier to clear; include an overhead goal that the athlete aims for to increase the jump height; use a contact mat or linear position transducer to provide height attained during each jump.

Modified from Ratamess, N. (2012). *ACSM's foundation of strength training and conditioning.* Philadelphia, PA: Lippincott Williams & Wilkins.

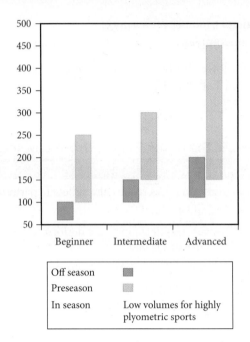

Figure 6.3 The recommended volumes (foot contacts) for lower-body plyometric exercises. Note: The exercises performed in the warm-up are not included in the volumes; the range in volumes reflects the variation in the intensities of the exercises, with lower volumes in the range corresponding to high-intensity exercises and the higher volumes corresponding to lower-intensity exercises.

Data from Chu, D. A. (1998). *Jumping into plyometrics.* Champaign, IL: Human Kinetics Publishers.

Exercise Volume

The volume of lower-body plyometric exercises is determined by the number of foot contacts per workout. On this basis, the volume of pylometric exercises is categorized according to the experience of the athlete and the placement of the workouts in the wider training program (Figure 6.3).

Rest Intervals

Increases in muscular power are expected after plyometric training, yet there have been suggestions that an athlete cannot increase power output when training in a fatigued state (Tidow, 1990). Furthermore, the coach needs to consider the effects of fatigue on the athlete's technique during the execution of plyometric exercises. For example, the largest forces are incurred during the most intense plyometric exercises, such as drop jumps. It would appear inappropriate to have an athlete perform these exercises at the end of a workout given the association between neuromuscular fatigue and injurious landing mechanics. Therefore, consideration needs to be given to the rest periods provided between exercises as well as between sets of plyometric exercises. The intensity of the plyometric exercise will determine both the inter-repetition and inter-set rest periods. For example, inter-repetition rest periods of 5–10 s have been recommended for submaximal-depth jumps, along with inter-set rest periods of

2–3 min (Ratamess, 2012). These durations are extended when maximal-drop jumps are performed, with inter-repetition rest periods of 2–4 min and inter-set periods of 5–10 min or more (Ratamess, 2012). A general guideline is to use a work-to-rest ratio of 1:5 for low- and moderate-intensity exercises, with a 1:10 ratio suggested for high-intensity exercises (Ratamess, 2012).

Exercise Order

The order in which the plyometric exercises are performed within a given workout will influence the accumulation of fatigue by the athlete. Fatigue can influence the adaptation to the exercises as well as increase the risk of the athlete incurring a musculoskeletal injury. This would preclude the performance of high-intensity plyometric exercises when the athlete is in a fatigued state, such as at the end of a workout. The phenomena of fatigue and potentiation, however, appear to operate at opposite ends of a continuum. Furthermore, the potential role of complex pairs in resistance training exercises must be considered, whereby a heavy resistance exercise is followed by the completion of a lower-intensity exercise to induce potentiation. Given all these factors, it may be appropriate to complete heavy resistance exercises prior to plyometric exercises.

The combination of heavy resistance training exercises with plyometric exercises has been shown to promote greater adaptation to a range of indices of muscular strength (e.g., maximal dynamic and isometric strength, low- and high-load speed-strength) than performing either type of exercise in isolation (Cormie, McCauley, & McBride, 2007; Harris, Stone, O'Bryant, Proulx, & Johnson, 2000). (See Applied Research 6.5.) An example of the sequencing of total-body resistance training and plyometric workouts during a training week is shown in Table 6.12.

Applied Research 6.5
Performing plyometric exercises and heavy resistance exercises in the same workout promotes strength gains across a greater range of strength indices

In their 2007 study, Cormie, McCauley, and McBride randomly assigned recreationally training men to one of three groups: (1) power training, (2) strength–power training, or (3) control group. The power training group completed 7 sets of 6 maximal-effort jump squats with no additional external load during each workout, with 3-min recovery periods between sets. The strength–power training group completed 5 sets of the same jump squats before completing 3 sets of 3 repetitions of back squats with a load equivalent to 90% 1-RM. The training program lasted 12 weeks and the amount of mechanical work completed by the experimental groups was not significantly different. The control group did not train.

The authors reported that the power training group increased low-load speed-strength, with no other changes in measures of muscular strength being reported. The strength–power training group, however, demonstrated increases in measures of maximal muscular strength (dynamic and isometric) as well as increases in measures of both low-load and high-load speed-strength. The authors concluded that the combination of heavy resistance exercises with plyometric exercises is likely to promote superior transfer to a wide variety of on-field demands associated with strength–power sports.

Cormie, P., McCauley, G. O., & McBride, J. M. (2007). Power versus strength–power jump squat training: Influence on the load–power relationship. *Medicine and Science in Sports and Exercise, 39*, 996–1003.

Table 6.12

Example of a Lower-Body Plyometric Workout for an Advanced Athlete During the Off-Season

Exercise	Intensity	Sets and Repetitions	Rest Intervals
Tuck jumps	Low	4×10	2–3 min (sets)
Split squat jumps (cycle)	Moderate	4×10	2–3 min (sets)
Drop jumps to box	High	3×8	2 min (jumps), 5 min (sets)
Multiple box jumps	Moderate	5×3	5–10 s (jumps), 2–3 min (sets)

Modifications to the session: The use of an overhead goal to increase jump height; the use of a contact mat or linear position transducer to provide a measure of the height attained during each jump to enhance jump height.

Note: Total foot contacts = 119.

Modified from Ratamess, N. (2012). *ACSM's foundation of strength training and conditioning.* Philadelphia, PA: Lippincott Williams & Wilkins.

Frequency of Workouts

The number of workouts completed each week determines the frequency. The number of workouts per week will be influenced by the intensity of the exercises selected, with higher-intensity exercises necessitating longer inter-workout recoveries and therefore lower weekly training frequency. Typically, a rest period of 48–72 hours between plyometric workouts is recommended (Ratamess, 2012). The location of the workouts within the wider training program will also influence the frequency, with fewer plyometric workouts being performed during the in-season period compared to preseason span. Workout frequencies between 1 and 4 per week have been recommended, with higher frequencies being used in the preseason and frequencies as low as 1–2 workouts per week during the in-season period (Ratamess, 2012). An example of a lower-body plyometric workout for an advanced athlete during the off-season following the guidelines discussed is presented in Table 6.12.

Periodization of Resistance Training

Periodization is defined as the planned variation in training methods and means on a cyclic or periodic basis (Plisk & Stone, 2003). A periodized training program is divided into the following hierarchical cycles:

- Macrocycle: the longest training cycle, typically lasting months
- Mesocycle: the intermediate training cycle, typically lasting weeks
- Microcycle: the shortest training cycle, typically lasting days

The variation in the resistance training methods used across these cycles comes from manipulations of the acute variables (e.g., exercise selection, intensity, volume, rest intervals, repetition velocity, exercise order and workout structure, frequency of workouts) throughout the training year, yet the variation is planned to elicit specific neuromuscular adaptations commensurate with the mechanical, metabolic demands of the sport. Variation in the training stimulus has been shown to be important in eliciting improvements in athletic performance (Haff, Jackson, et al., 2008; Smith, 2003; Suzuki, Sato, Maeda, & Takahashi, 2006; also see Applied Research 6.6), while also providing a means of managing the fatigue that accumulates throughout

Applied Research 6.6
Reductions in training volume are associated with favorable hormonal and mechanical responses in strength-trained athletes

Haff, Jackson, et al. (2008) recorded the training intensities and volumes of six elite female weightlifters during an 11-week period leading up to a major national competition. In addition to measuring the workouts completed by the athletes, the authors recorded isometric and dynamic force–time characteristics during mid-thigh pulls and testosterone:cortisol (T:C) ratio on a biweekly basis. During the 11-week period, the athletes completed a total of $3,593 \pm 606$ repetitions of varying resistance training exercises (clean, clean and jerk, snatch, clean pull, snatch pull, back squat, front squat) for a total volume load (repetitions × mass lifted) of $270,221 \pm 42,345$ kg. However, the weekly volume loads and intensities were varied throughout the 11-week period.

The authors reported very large negative correlations between the changes in volume load and the changes in force–time characteristics (peak force, peak rate of force development), with similarly large negative correlations observed between the changes in volume load and the changes in the T:C ratio. These changes in the T:C ratio were mainly caused by changes in cortisol. The authors concluded that reductions in the training volume load resulted in a more anabolic systemic environment, potentially promoting morphological adaptations and increased muscular performance in elite strength-trained athletes.

Haff, G. G., Jackson, J. R., Kawamori, N., Carlock, J. M., Hartman, M. J., Kilgore, J. L., . . . Stone, M. H. (2008). Force–time curve characteristics and hormonal alterations during an eleven-week training period in elite women weightlifters. *Journal of Strength and Conditioning Research, 22,* 433–446.

the training program and thereby potentially guarding against **overtraining syndrome** (Fry, Morton, & Keast, 1992; see also Strength and Power Concept 6.6).

In its original inception, a periodized approach to training subdivided the training cycle into smaller periods of preparation, competition, and transition, with the preparation phase then being further subdivided into general and specific subphases and the competition phase subdivided into the precompetition and main competition subphases (Bompa & Haff, 2009). There is a progression from general training exercises to sport-specific exercises and from high-volume, low-intensity workouts to low-volume, high-intensity workouts as the athlete moves from the preparation phase to the competition phase. Related specifically to resistance training, some researchers have proposed greater variation can be achieved in the training stimulus by manipulating the exercise intensity and repetitions during each workout performed within a microcycle, resulting in what is known as **undulating periodization** models (Kraemer & Fleck, 2007).

An example of a 10-week undulating periodization resistance training program for track and field athletes is shown in Table 6.13. Note that each workout has a different emphasis (strength/endurance, maximal strength, power) based on the exercise intensities selected, and that different exercises are used on each training day. Thus the undulating periodization model, as demonstrated in this example program, provides variation in the training stimulus within each microcycle (exercise selection, intensity, volume, rest intervals, repetition velocity). However, undulating periodization models typically rely on maximum repetitions for each exercise, requiring the athlete to exercise to failure in each set, which may result in a large accumulation of fatigue across the training program.

Other researchers have proposed an alternative approach to the periodization of training programs, whereby specialized mesocycles ("blocks"), each directed at a minimal number of physical capacities, are sequenced such that the adaptations

Strength and Power Concept 6.6

What is overtraining syndrome?

Overtraining syndrome (OTS) is characterized by chronic maladaptation to training that is manifested as performance decrements, disrupted physiological functions (increased resting heart rate and blood pressure, loss of body mass), and behavioral disturbances (decreased appetite, irritability, loss of sleep) (Meeusen et al., 2006). An athlete may take months and even years to recover once in the overtrained state. OTS is distinct from the **functional overreaching** that may accompany a short period of increased training volume, in which the athlete experiences performance decrements in the absence of severe psychological or other negative symptoms (Meeusen et al., 2006). When the training volume is reduced, the decrements in performance associated with functional overreaching dissipate, and the functional capacity of the athlete is enhanced through the adaptation response and the potential for **supercompensation**. However, if the stresses experienced by the athlete are not reduced (for the training stress, this would require a reduction in the training volume), then a state of **nonfunctional overreaching** (NFO) is attained—it is believed to be the precursor for overtraining syndrome.

The inclusion of the term "syndrome" in OTS acknowledges that the training stimulus may not represent the only stressor acting on the athlete. Rather, it is the accumulation of stress associated with training and/or nontraining sources that results in long-term maladaptation (Meeusen et al., 2006). The main treatment for OTS appears to be complete rest for the athlete.

There are currently no specific diagnostic criteria for OTS. The diagnosis is therefore one of exclusion—that is, excluding other illnesses (e.g., infectious mononucleosis, cancer, anemia, hypothyroidism) as an explanation for the symptoms demonstrated by the athlete in the overtrained state. However, Meeusen et al. (2010) recently developed a two-bout exercise protocol that could determine the presence of overtraining syndrome in a group of underperforming athletes from a variety of sports. Specifically, the hormonal response to two bouts of graded exercise performed to volitional failure that were separated by 4 hours differed between athletes diagnosed with NFO and OTS (the diagnoses were made in retrospect according to the severity and duration of the symptoms), with the athletes with OTS demonstrating a blunted response of adrenocorticotropic hormone and prolactin in the second exercise bout. Although such biochemical techniques are beyond the capabilities of most coaches, continual monitoring of the athlete (e.g., recording resting heart rate, body mass, and hours of sleep; psychological questionnaires; training logs) can provide information about the anthropometric, psychological, and behavioral disruptions associated with overtraining. Furthermore, the ability of the coach to change the training program in accordance with the results of such monitoring is very important. Finally, the most effective preventive strategy for OTS is to ensure that there is adequate provision of recovery/restitution periods in the athlete's training program when it is initially developed. Avoiding monotonous training has also been suggested as a preventive measure against OTS (Meeusen et al., 2006).

Table 6.13

Undulating Periodization Model Applied to a 10-Week Resistance Training Program Performed Three Times per Week

	Monday	Wednesday	Friday
Exercises	Back squat	Back squat	Quarter back squat
	Mid-thigh pull	Clean grip shrug	Mid-thigh pull
	Behind-neck press	Push press	Weighted jump (0–30% body mass)
	Bench press	Incline bench press	Push jerk
	Dumbbell row	Dumbbell row	Stiff-leg dead lift
Sets and repetitions	$3 \times 8–12$	$3 \times 5–7$	$3 \times 3–5$
Intensity	8–12 RM	5–7 RM	3–5 RM
Emphasis	Strength/endurance	Maximal strength	Power

Note: RM = repetition maximum.

Data from Painter, K. B., Haff, G. G., Ramsey, M. W., McBride, J., Triplett, T., Sands, W. A., . . . Stones, M. H. (2012). Strength gains: Block versus daily undulating periodization weight training among track and field athletes. *International Journal of Sports Physiology and Performance, 7*, 161–169.

in one mesocycle potentiate the adaptations in the following mesocycle (such as a maximal-strength mesocycle preceding a power mesocycle); such programs are said to follow **blocked periodization** models (Issurin, 2010). An example of a 10-week block periodization resistance training program for track and field athletes is shown in Table 6.14. This program includes three separate training blocks, each with a specific focus (strength/endurance, maximal strength, power) as determined by the intensity, repetitions, and sets used (as well as rest intervals and repetition velocity). The exercise intensities are increased within each of the training blocks to provide overload, but are reduced during the final microcycle in the maximal-strength block to promote recovery. Notice the inclusion of new exercises in the maximal-strength and power mesocycle (e.g., push press, push jerk, incline dumbbell press), which provides a new exercise stimulus for the athlete to adapt to. These manipulations provide variation in the training stimulus at the mesocycle level. Also notice that different exercises are performed on the second training day, while the intensity (and therefore the repetition velocity) differs between the three training days, providing variation in the exercise stimulus at the microcycle level. In a comparison between undulating and blocked periodization models of resistance training, Painter et al. (2012) reported that both resulted in improved measures of muscular strength, although the blocked periodized model was more efficient when the gains in muscular strength were normalized to the amount of work performed.

Many different periodization models are available to the strength and conditioning practitioner (Baker, 2007), although not all of them have experimental evidence to support their efficacy. Furthermore, adaptive responses to a given periodized model are likely to vary widely. Given this reality, Kiely (2012) notes that the strength and conditioning practitioner will be required to continuously monitor the response of the athlete to any specific program and make modifications as necessary to optimize the adaptive response. Examples of monitoring tools that are available to the strength and conditioner are shown in Table 6.15.

Table 6.14
Blocked Periodization Model Applied to a 10-Week Resistance Training Program Performed Three Times Per Week

	Monday	Wednesday	Friday
Exercises (block 1), 3 weeks	Back squat Behind-neck press Bench press	Power snatch Clean grip shrug Mid-thigh pull Stiff-leg dead lift Dumbbell row	Back squat Behind-neck press Bench press
Sets and repetitions	3×10	3×10	3×10
Intensity	Week 1: 75–80% 1-RM Week 2: 80–85% 1-RM Week 3: 85–90% 1-RM	Week 1: 70–75% 1-RM Week 2: 75–80% 1-RM Week 3: 75–80% 1-RM	Week 1: 65–70% 1-RM Week 2: 65–70% 1-RM Week 3: 70–75% 1-RM
Emphasis	Strength/endurance	Strength/endurance	Strength/endurance
Exercises (block 2), 5 weeks	Back squat Push press Incline press	Power snatch Clean grip shrug Mid-thigh pull Stiff-leg dead lift Dumbbell row	Back squat Push press Incline press
Sets and repetitions	Weeks 4, 5, and 8: 3×5 Week 6: 3×3 Week 7: 3×2	Weeks 4, 5, and 8: 3×5 Week 6: 3×3 Week 7: 3×2	Weeks 4, 5, and 8: 3×5 Week 6: 3×3 Week 7: 3×2
Intensity	Week 4: 75–80% 1-RM* Week 5: 80–85% 1-RM* Week 6: 85–90% 1-RM* Week 7: 90–95% 1-RM* Week 8: 75–80% 1-RM	Week 4: 75–80% 1-RM* Week 5: 80–85% 1-RM* Week 6: 85–90% 1-RM* Week 7: 85–90% 1-RM* Week 8: 85–90% 1-RM*	Week 4: 65–70% 1-RM* Week 5: 65–70% 1-RM* Week 6: 70–75% 1-RM* Week 7: 70–75% 1-RM* Week 8: 65–70% 1-RM*
Emphasis	Strength	Strength	Strength
Exercises (block 3), 2 weeks	Quarter back squat Weighted jumps (0–30% BM) Push jerk Incline dumbbell press	Power snatch Mid-thigh pull Stiff-leg dead lift	Quarter back squat Weighted jumps (0–30% BM) Push jerk Incline dumbbell press
Sets and repetitions	Week 9: 3×3 Week 10: 1×3	Week 9: 3×3 Week 10: 1×3	Week 9: 3×3 Week 10: 1×3
Intensity	Week 9: 85–90% 1-RM* Week 10: 90–95% 1-RM*	Week 9: 80–85% 1-RM* Week 10: 75–80% 1-RM*	Week 9: 70–75% 1-RM* Week 10: 70–75% 1-RM*
Emphasis	Power	Power	Power

*Workouts finished with a down set of 1×5 at approximately 60% of the load used during previous sets.

Note: 1-RM = 1-repetition maximum; BM = body mass.

Data from Painter, K. B., Haff, G. G., Ramsey, M. W., McBride, J., Triplett, T., Sands, W. A., . . . Stones, M. H. (2012). Strength gains: Block versus daily undulating periodization weight training among track and field athletes. *International Journal of Sports Physiology and Performance, 7*, 161–169.

Table 6.15
Tools Available to Strength and Conditioning Practitioners to Monitor Athletes' Responses to Periodized Resistance Training Programs

Monitoring Tool	Description
Physical tests	The scores attained on measures of muscular strength as well as measures of athletic performance.
Volume load	Product of the mass lifted and the number of repetitions and sets completed. Volume load provides information about the total work performed by the athlete.
Perceived training load	Modified rating of perceived exertion scale completed after the workout. Provides a measure of the subjective training load.
Monotony index	The weekly perceived training load divided by the standard deviation. Provides a measure of the variation in training, with a small monotony value indicating a large training variation.
Category ratio pain scale	Modified rating of perceived exertion scale completed after the workout. Provides a subjective measure of muscle soreness.
Total quality recovery	Modified rating of the perceived exertion completed each morning. Provides a subjective measure of recovery.
Heart rate variability	The autonomic nervous system (ANS) is involved in the functioning of many physiological systems within the body, including digestion, respiration, and heart rate. Given its importance in the control of numerous physiological systems, the responsiveness of the ANS has been suggested to provide information about the functional adaptations to stressors including exercise. The involvement of the ANS in the control of heart rate has led to the proposal that monitoring heart rate variability at rest and heart rate recovery following exercise can provide information about autonomic control and, therefore, the adaptation response to a training regimen.
Profile of mood states	Provides a measure of the mood states of the athlete. The fatigue–inertia scale is particularly informative.

Data from Bompa, T., & Haff, G. G. (2009). *Periodization: Theory and methodology of training.* Champaign, IL: Human Kinetics; Borresen, J., & Lambert, M. I. (2008). Quantifying training load: A comparison of subjective and objective methods. *International Journal of Sports Physiology and Performance, 3,* 16–30; Suzuki, S., Sato, T., Maeda, A., & Takahashi, Y. (2006). Program design based on a mathematical model using rating of perceived exertion for an elite Japanese sprinter: A case study. *Journal of Strength and Conditioning Research, 20,* 36–42.

Chapter Summary

The process of adaptation following an exercise stimulus relates to the cellular and molecular responses that lead to changes within the neuromuscular system, resulting in increases in indices of muscular strength. The general process of adaptation informs us that positive cellular responses are elicited when the stimulus applied exceeds the stimulus that the cell typically experiences, so long as an adequate recovery period is provided between the applications of repeated stimuli. Resistance training methods provide an appropriate stimulus to increase muscular strength and power. The improvements in strength and power following a resistance training program are the result of neurogenic and phenotypic adaptations, with early gains in strength primarily due to adaptations within the nervous system.

Resistance training programs should be based on the principles of overload, variation, and specificity. The adaptive response associated with a resistance training workout depends on a number of acute training variables, including exercise selection, intensity and volume of exercises, rest intervals between sets of exercises, the order in which exercises are performed, and the frequency with which each workout is performed during each training week. Manipulation of these acute training variables may induce specific neuromuscular adaptations leading to the increased expression of muscular strength.

Plyometric exercises incorporate the stretch–shortening cycle and have been shown to elicit a number of neurogenic and phenotypic adaptations that underpin improvements in measures of muscular strength and power. Plyometric exercises are considered to expedite the transfer of muscular strength gained from traditional resistance training exercises to sporting movements.

Periodization is the planned variation of training methods and means on a cyclic or periodic basis. Periodized resistance training programs are believed to be effective in enhancing performance at specific times and in reducing the potential for overtraining. Variation can be achieved across macrocycles, mesocycles, and microcycles within a training program by manipulating the acute training variables mentioned earlier. Many periodization models are available, and it is the responsibility of the strength and conditioning practitioner to continuously monitor the response of the athlete to a given program and to modify the program as necessary to optimize the adaptive response.

Review Questions and Projects

1. Describe the important characteristics of an exercise stimulus designed to elicit gains in muscular strength.

2. With reference to specific neuromuscular adaptations, explain the gains in muscular strength observed in a previously untrained individual two weeks after beginning a resistance training program.

3. List the acute programming variables associated with a resistance training workout that a strength and conditioning coach can manipulate to induce specific neuromuscular adaptations.

4. Why is the intensity of resistance training exercises proposed to be the most important variable for gains in muscular strength?

5. How might vascular occlusion during resistance training allow for strength gains from lower-intensity exercises?

6. Is exercising the muscle to the point of fatigue necessary to elicit gains in muscular strength?

7. Provide an explanation for the recommendations of acute programming variables to elicit gains in hypertrophy, muscular strength, muscular power output, and muscular strength endurance.

8. What are cluster sets, and why might the strength and conditioning practitioner want to use them?

9. Explain the limitations of traditional resistance training exercises in which a mass is accelerated by the athlete, and describe how these limitations may affect the neuromuscular adaptations.

10. Explain why the addition of elastic bands or chains to the barbell may influence the mechanics of a traditional back squat exercise.

11. Explain the mechanical alterations associated with pneumatic/hydraulic resistance training methods.

12. List the pros and cons associated with performing resistance training exercises on an unstable surface.

13. Explain the proposed benefits of plyometric exercises compared to traditional resistance training exercises.

14. Explain the benefits of combining heavy resistance training exercises with plyometric exercises within the same training week and also within the same workout.

15. What are some of the limitations of the guidelines presented for the development of resistance training and plyometric training workouts? Which steps can a strength and conditioning practitioner take to overcome these limitations?

16. You have been asked to develop a resistance training program for a soccer team. Outline the initial steps that you would follow in the development of the training program.

17. How might a strength and conditioning practitioner quantify the variation in a resistance training program?

18. What is overtraining syndrome, and how can it be measured?

19. Explain what block periodization is and where the variation in the training stimulus can be provided using this method.

20. Following a block of training characterized by high-volume load, an athlete is in a state of functional overreaching. Which manipulations should the coach implement in the subsequent training block and why?

References

Aagaard, P. (2003). Training-induced changes in neural function. *Exercise and Sport Sciences Reviews, 31*, 61–67.

Aagaard, P., Andersen, J. L., Dyhre-Poulsen, P., Leffers, A.-M., Wagner, A., Magnusson, S. P., . . . & Simonsen, E. B. (2001). A mechanism for increased contractile strength of human pennate muscle in response to strength training: Changes in muscle architecture. *Journal of Physiology, 534*, 613–623.

Aagaard, P., Simonsen, E. B., Andersen, J .L., Magnusson, P., & Dyhre-Poulsen, P. (2002). Neural adaptation to resistance training: Changes in evoked V-wave and H-reflex responses. *Journal of Applied Physiology, 92*, 2309–2318.

Abernethy, P. J., & J. Jürimäe, J. (1996). Cross-sectional and longitudinal uses of isoinertial, isometric, and isokinetic dynamometry. *Medicine and Science in Sports and Exercise, 28*, 1180–1187.

Abernethy, P. J., Jurimäe, J., Logan, P. A., Taylor, A. W., & Thayer, R. E. (1994). Acute and chronic response of skeletal muscle to resistance exercise. *Sports Medicine, 17*, 22–38.

Allen, D. G., Lamb, G. D., & Westerblad, H. (2008). Impaired calcium release during fatigue. *Journal of Applied Physiology, 104*, 296–305.

Andersen, J. L., & Aagaard, P. (2010). Effects of strength training on muscle fiber types and size; consequences for athletes training for high-intensity sport. *Scandinavian Journal of Medicine and Science in Sports, 20*, S32–S38.

Anderson, C. E., Sforzo, G. A., & Sigg, J. A. (2008). The effects of combining elastic and free weight resistance on strength and power in athletes. *Journal of Strength and Conditioning Research, 22*, 567–574.

Arandjelović, O. (2010). A mathematical model of neuromuscular adaptation to resistance training and its application in a computer simulation of accommodating loads. *European Journal of Applied Physiology, 110*, 523–538.

Argus, C. K., Gill, N. D., Keogh, J. W., Blazevich, A. J., & Hopkins, W. G. (2011). Kinetic and training comparisons between assisted, resisted and free countermovement jumps. *Journal of Strength and Conditioning Research, 25*, 2219–2227.

Atherton, P. J., Babraj, J. A., Smith, K., Singh, J., Rennie, M. J., & Wackerhage, H. (2005). Selective activation of AMPK-PGC-1α or PKB-TSC2-mTOR signaling can explain specific adaptive responses to endurance or resistance training-like electrical muscle stimulation. *FASEB Journal, 19,* 786–788.

Augustsson, J., Thomeé, R., Hörnstedt, P., Lindblom, J., Karlsson, J., & Grimby, G. (2003). Effect of pre-exhaustion exercise on lower-extremity muscle activation during a leg press exercise. *Journal of Strength and Conditioning Research, 17,* 411–416.

Baechle, T. R., Earle, R. W., & Wathen, D. (2008). Resistance training. In T. R. Baechle & R. W. Earle (Eds.), *Essentials of strength training and conditioning* (pp. 381–412). Champaign, IL: Human Kinetics.

Baker, D. (2007). Cycle-length variants in periodized strength/power training. *Strength and Conditioning Journal, 29,* 10–17.

Baker, D. G., & Newton, R. U. (2009). Effects of kinetically altering a repetition via the use of chain resistance on velocity during the bench press. *Journal of Strength and Conditioning Research, 23,* 1941–1946.

Baldwin, K. M., & Haddad, F. (2001). Effects of different activity and inactivity paradigms on myosin heavy chain gene expression in striated muscle. *Journal of Applied Physiology, 90,* 345–357.

Baltzopoulos, V., & Brodie, D. A. (1989). Isokinetic dynamometry: Applications and limitations. *Sports Medicine, 8,* 101–116.

Beaven, C. M., Cook, C. J., & Gill, N. D. (2008). Significant strength gains observed in rugby players after specific resistance exercise protocols based on individual salivary testosterone responses. *Journal of Strength and Conditioning Research, 22,* 419–425.

Beaven, C. M., Gill, N. D., & Cook, C. J. (2008). Salivary testosterone and cortisol responses in professional rugby players after four resistance exercise protocols. *Journal of Strength and Conditioning Research, 22,* 426–432.

Behm, D. G. (1995). Neuromuscular implications and applications of resistance training. *Journal of Strength and Conditioning Research, 9,* 264–274.

Behm, D. G., & Anderson, K. (2006). The role of instability with resistance training. *Journal of Strength and Conditioning Research, 20,* 716–722.

Behm, D. G., Drinkwater, E. J., Willardson, J. M., & Cowley, P. M. (2010). Canadian Society for Exercise Physiology position stand: The use of instability to train the core in athletic and non-athletic conditioning. *Applied Physiology, Nutrition and Metabolism, 35,* 11–14.

Behm, D. G., Reardon, G., Fitzgerald, J., & Drinkwater, E. (2002). The effects of 5, 10, and 20 repetitions maximums on the recovery of voluntary and evoked contractile properties. *Journal of Strength and Conditioning Research, 16,* 209–218.

Behm, D. G., & Sale, D. G. (1993). Intended rather than actual movement velocity determines velocity-specific training responses. *Journal of Applied Physiology, 74,* 359–368.

Behm, D., & Sanchez, J. C. C. (2012). The effectiveness of resistance training using unstable surfaces and devices for rehabilitation. *International Journal of Sports Physical Therapy, 7,* 226–241.

Bellar, D. M., Muller, M. D., Barkley, J. E., Kim, C-H., Ida, K., Ryan, E. J., . . . Glickman, E. L. (2010). The effects of combined elastic- and free-weight tension vs. free-weight tension on one-repetition maximum strength in the bench press. *Journal of Strength and Conditioning Research, 25,* 459–463.

Bette, F. B., Bauer, T., Kinscherf, R., Vorwald, S., Klute, K., Bischoff, D., . . . Billeter, R. (2010). Effects of strength training with eccentric overload on muscle adaptation in male athletes. *European Journal of Applied Physiology, 108,* 821–836.

Bird, S. P., Tarpenning, K. M., & Marino, F. E. (2005). Designing resistance training programmes to enhance muscular fitness: A review of the acute programme variables. *Sports Medicine, 35,* 841–851.

Blazevich, A. J., Gill, N. D., Bronks, R., & Newton, R. U. (2003). Training-specific muscle architecture adaptations after 5-wk training in athletes. *Medicine and Science in Sports and Exercise, 35,* 2013–2022.

Bompa, T., & Haff, G. G. (2009). *Periodization: Theory and methodology of training.* Champaign, IL: Human Kinetics.

Brown, S., Thompson, W., Bailey, J., Johnson, K., Wood, L., Bean, M., Thompson, D. (1990). Blood lactate response to weightlifting in endurance and weight trained men. *Journal of Applied Sport Science Research, 4,* 122–130.

Campos, G. E., Luecke, T. J., Wendeln, H. K., Toma, K., Hagerman, F. C., Murray, T. F., . . . Staron, R. S. (2002). Muscular adaptations in response to three different resistance-training regimens: Specificity of repetition maximum training zones. *European Journal of Applied Physiology, 88,* 50–60.

Carolan, B., & Cafarelli, E. (1992). Adaptations in coactivation after isometric resistance training. *Journal of Applied Physiology, 73*, 911–917.

Carroll, T. J., Abernethy, P. J., Logan, P. A., Barber, M., & McEniery, M. T. (1998). Resistance training frequency: Strength and myosin heavy chain responses to two and three bouts per week. *European Journal of Applied Physiology and Occupational Physiology, 78*, 270–275.

Chestnut, J. L., & Docherty, D. (1999). The effects of 4 and 10 repetition maximum weight-training protocols on neuromuscular adaptations in untrained men. *Journal of Strength and Conditioning Research, 13*, 353–359.

Cochrane, J. L., Lloyd, D. G., Bessier, T. F., Elliott, B. C., Doyle, T. L. A., & Ackland, T. R. (2010). Training affects knee kinematics and kinetics in cutting maneuvers in sport. *Medicine and Science in Sports and Exercise, 42*, 1535–1544.

Coffey, V. G., & Hawley, J. A. (2007). The molecular bases of training adaptations. *Sports Medicine, 37*, 737–763.

Cook, C. J., Beaven, M., & Kilduff, L. P. (2013). Three weeks of eccentric training combined with overspeed exercises enhances power and running speed performance gains in trained athletes. *Journal of Strength and Conditioning Research, 27*, 1280–1286.

Cormie, P., McCauley, G. O., & McBride, J. M. (2007). Power versus strength–power jump squat training: Influence on the load–power relationship. *Medicine and Science in Sports and Exercise, 39*, 996–1003.

Cormie, P., McCauley, G. O., Triplett, T. N., & McBride, J. M. (2007). Optimal loading for maximal lower-body resistance exercises. *Medicine and Science in Sports and Exercise, 39*, 340–349.

Cowell, J. F., Cronin, J., & Brughelli, M. (2012). Eccentric muscle actions and how the strength and conditioning specialist might use them for a variety of purposes. *Strength and Conditioning Journal, 34*, 33–48.

Cressey, E. M., West, C. A., Tiberio, D. P., Kraemer, W. J., & Maresh, C. M. (2007). The effects of ten weeks of lower-body unstable surface training on markers of athletic performance. *Journal of Strength and Conditioning Research, 21*, 561–567.

Crewther, B., Cronin, J., & Keogh, J. (2005). Possible stimuli for strength and power adaptation: Acute mechanical responses. *Sports Medicine, 35*, 967–989.

Crewther, B., Cronin, J., & Keogh, J. (2006). Possible stimuli for strength and power adaptation: Acute metabolic responses. *Sports Medicine, 36*, 65–78.

Cronin, J., McNair, P. J., & Marshall, R. N. (2003). The effects of bungy weight training on muscle function and functional performance. *Journal of Sports Sciences, 21*, 59–71.

Doan, B. K., Newton, R. U., Marsit, J. L., Triplett-McBride, T. N., Koziris, P. L., Fry, A. C., & Kraemer, W. J. (2002). Effects of increased eccentric loading on bench press 1RM. *Journal of Strength and Conditioning Research, 16*, 9–13.

Docherty, D., Robbins, D., & Hodgson, M. (2004). Complex training revisited: A review of its current status as a viable training approach. *Strength and Conditioning Journal, 26*, 52–57.

Drinkwater, E. J., Lawton, T. W., McKenna, M. J., Lindsell, R. P., Hunt, P. H., & Pyne, D. B. (2007). Increased number of forced repetitions does not enhance strength development with resistance training. *Journal of Strength and Conditioning Research, 21*, 841–847.

Drinkwater, E. J., Pritchett, E. J., & Behm, D. G. (2007). Effects of instability and resistance on unintentional squat-lifting kinetics. *International. Journal of Sports Physiology and Performance, 2*, 400–413.

Duchateau, J., Semmler, J. G., & Enoka, R. M. (2006). Training adaptations in the behavior of human motor units. *Journal of Applied Physiology, 101*, 1766–1775.

Egan, B., & Zierath, J. R. (2013). Exercise metabolism and the molecular regulation of skeletal muscle adaptation. *Cell Metabolism, 17*, 162–184.

Folland, J. P., Irish, C. S., Roberts, J. C., Tarr, J. E., & Jones, D. A. (2002). Fatigue is not a necessary stimulus for strength gains during resistance training. *British Journal of Sports Medicine, 36*, 370–374.

Folland, J. P., & Williams, A. G. (2007). The adaptations to strength training: Morphological and neurological contributions to increased strength. *Sports Medicine, 37*, 145–168.

Frost, D. M., Cronin, J. B., & Newton, R. U. (2008). A comparison of the kinematics, kinetics and muscle activity between pneumatic and free weight resistance. *European Journal of Applied Physiology, 104*, 937–956.

Fry, A. C. (2004). The role of resistance exercise intensity on muscle fibre adaptations. *Sports Medicine, 34*, 663–679.

Fry, R. W., Morton, A. R., & Keast, D. (1992). Periodisation and the prevention of overtraining. *Canadian Journal of Sport Science, 17*, 241–248.

Gardiner, P., Dai, Y., & Heckman, C. J. (2006). Effects of exercise training on α-motoneurons. *Journal of Applied Physiology, 101*, 1228–1236.

Ghigiarelli, J. J., Nagle, E. F., Gross, F. L., Robertson, R. J., Irrgang, J. J., & Myslinski, T. (2009). The effects of a 7-week heavy elastic band and weight chain program on upper-body strength and upper-body power in a sample of Division 1-AA football players. *Journal of Strength and Conditioning Research, 23*, 756–764.

González-Badillo, J. J., & Sánchez-Medina, L. (2010). Movement velocity as a measure of loading intensity in resistance training. *International Journal of Sports Medicine, 31*, 347–352.

Haff, G. G., Hobbs, R. T., Haff, E. E., Sands, W. A., Pierce, K. C., & Stone, M. H. (2008). Cluster training: A novel method for introducing training program variation. *Strength and Cond Journal, 30*, 67–76.

Haff, G. G., Jackson, J. R., Kawamori, N., Carlock, J. M., Hartman, M. J., Kilgore, J. L., . . . Stone, M. H. (2008). Force–time curve characteristics and hormonal alterations during an eleven-week training period in elite women weightlifters. *Journal of Strength and Conditioning Research, 22*, 433–446.

Haff, G. G., Whitley, A., McCoy, L. B., O'Bryant, H. S., Kilgore, J. L., Haff, E. E., . . . & Stone, M. H. (2003). Effects of different set configurations on barbell velocity and displacement during a clean pull. *Journal of Strength Conditioning Research, 17*, 95–103.

Häkkinen, K., & Komi, P. V. (1983). Alterations of mechanical characteristics of human skeletal muscle during strength training. *European Journal of Applied Physiology, 50*, 161–172.

Harris, G. R., Stone, M. H., O'Bryant, H. S., Proulx, C. M., & Johnson, R. L. (2000). Short-term performance effects on high power, high force, or combined weight-training methods. *Journal of Strength and Conditioning Research, 14*, 14–20.

Hawley, J. A., & Burke, L. M. (2010). Carbohydrate availability and training adaptation: Effects on cell metabolism. *Exercise and Sport Sciences Reviews, 38*, 152–160.

Henneman, E., Somjen, G., & Carpenter, D.O. (1965). Functional significance of cell size in spinal motoneurons. *Journal of Neurophysiology, 28*, 560-580.

Hodgson, M., Docherty, D., & Robbins, D. (2005). Post-activation potentiation. *Sports Medicine, 35*, 585–595.

Hrysomallis, C. (2007). Relationship between balance ability, training and sports injury risk. *Sports Medicine, 37*, 547–556.

Issurin, V. B. (2010). New horizons for the methodology and physiology of training periodization. *Sports Medicine, 40*, 189–206.

Izquierdo, M., Ibanez, J., González-Badillo, J. J., Häkkinen, K., Ratamess, N., Kraemer, W. J., . . . Gorostiaga, E.M. (2006). Differential effects of strength training leading to failure versus not to failure on hormonal responses, strength and muscle power gains. *Journal of Applied Physiology, 100*, 1647–1656.

Joy, J. M., Lowery, R. P., Oliveira de Souza, E., & Wilson, J. M. (2013). Elastic bands as a component of periodized resistance training. *Journal of Strength and Conditioning Research*. Epub ahead of print. doi: 10.1519/JSC.0b013e3182986ef

Kawamori, N., & Haff, G. G. (2004). The optimal training load for the development of muscular power. *Journal of Strength and Conditioning Research, 18*, 675–684.

Kibele, A., & Behm, D. G. (2009). Seven weeks of instability and traditional resistance training effects on strength, balance and functional performance. *Journal of Strength and Conditioning Research, 23*, 2443–2450.

Kiely, J. (2012). Periodization paradigms in the 21st century: Evidence-led or tradition driven? *International Journal of Sports Physiology and Performance, 7*, 242–250.

Kraemer, W. J., & Fleck, S. J. (2007). *Optimizing strength training: Designing non-linear periodization workouts*. Champaign, IL: Human Kinetics.

Kraemer, W. J., Fleck, S. J., & Deschenes, M. (1988). A review: Factors in exercise prescription of resistance training. *Strength and Conditioning Journal, 10*, 36–41.

Kraemer, W. J., Fleck, S. J., & Evans, W. J. (1996). Strength and power training: Physiological mechanisms of adaptation. *Exercise and Sport Sciences Reviews, 24*, 363–397.

Kuruganti, U., Parker, P., Rickards, J., Tingley, M., & Sexsmith, J. (2005). Bilateral isokinetic training reduces the bilateral leg strength deficit for both old and young adults. *European Journal of Applied Physiology, 94*, 175–179.

Langford, G. A., McCurdy, K. W., Ernest, J. M., Doscher, M. W., & Walter, S. D. (2007). Specificity of machine, barbell, and water-filled log bench press resistance training on measures of strength. *Journal Strength and Conditioning Research, 21*, 1061–1066.

Lawton, T. W., Cronin, J. B., & Lindsell, R. P. (2006). Effects of interrepetition rest intervals on weight training repetition power output. *Journal of Strength and Conditioning Research, 20*, 172–176.

LeSuer, D. A., McCormick, J. H., Mayhew, J. L., Wasserstein, R. L., & Arnold, M. D. (1997). The accuracy of predicting equations for estimating 1RM performance in the bench press, squat, and deadlift. *Journal of Strength and Conditioning Research, 11*, 211–213.

Linari, M., Bottinelli, R., Pellegrino, M. A., Reconditi, M., Reggiani, C., & Lombardi, V. (2003). The mechanism of the force response to stretch in human skinned muscle fibres with different myosin isoforms. *Journal of Physiology, 554*, 335–352.

Markovic, G. (2007). Does plyometric training improve vertical jump height? A meta-analytical review. *British Journal of Sports Medicine, 41*, 349–355.

Markovic, G., & Mikulic, P. (2010). Neuro-musculoskeletal and performance adaptations to lower-extremity plyometric training. *Sports Medicine, 40*, 859–895.

McBride, J. M., Cormie, P., & Deane, R. (2006). Isometric squat force output and muscle activity in stable and unstable conditions. *Journal of Strength and Conditioning Research, 20*, 915–918.

McBride, J. M., Larkin, T. R., Dayne, A. M., Haines, T. L., & Kirby, T. J. (2010). Effects of absolute and relative loading on muscle activity during stable and unstable squatting. *International Journal of Sports Physiology and Performance, 5*, 177–183.

McBride, J. M., Triplett-McBride, T., Davie, A., & Newton, R. U. (2002). The effect of heavy- vs. light-load jump squats on the development of strength, power, and speed. *Journal of Strength and Conditioning Research, 16*, 75–82.

McMaster, D. T., Cronin, J., & McGuigan, M. (2009). Forms of variable resistance training. *Strength and Conditioning Journal, 31*, 50–64.

Meeusen, R., Duclos, M., Gleeson, M., Rietjens, G., Steinacker, J., & Urhausen, A. (2006). Prevention, diagnosis and treatment of the overtraining syndrome. ECSS Position Statement "Task Force." *European Journal of Sports Science, 6*, 1–14.

Meeusen, R., Nderhof, E., Buyse, L., Roelands, B., de Schutter, G., & Piacentini, M. F. (2010). Diagnosing overtraining in athletes using the two-bout exercise protocol. *British Journal of Sports Medicine, 44*642–648.

Moir, G. L. (2012). Muscular strength. In T. Miller (Ed.), *NCSA's guide to tests and assessments* (pp. 147–191). Champaign, IL: Human Kinetics.

Moir, G. L., Erny, K. F., Davis, S. E., Guers, J. J., & Witmer, C. A. (2013). The development of a repetition-load scheme for the eccentric-only bench press exercise. *Journal of Human Kinetics, 38*, 23–31.

Moir, G. L., Graham, B. W., Davis, S. E., Guers, J. J., & Witmer, C. A. (2013). Effect of cluster set configurations on mechanical variables during the deadlift exercise. *Journal of Human Kinetics, 39*, 15–23.

Moore, C. A., & Schilling, B. K. (2005). Theory and application of augmented eccentric loading. *Strength and Conditioning Journal, 27*, 20–27.

Newton, R. U., & Dugan, E. (2002). Application of strength diagnosis. *Strength and Conditioning Journal, 24*, 50–59.

Newton, R. U., & Kraemer, W. J. (1994). Developing explosive muscular power: Implications for a mixed methods training strategy. *Strength and Conditioning, 16*, 20–31.

Oberacker, L. M., Davis, S. E., Haff, G. G., Witmer, C. A., & Moir, G. L. (2012). The Yo-Yo IR2 test: Physiological response, reliability, and application to elite soccer. *Journal of Strength and Conditioning Research, 26*, 2734–2740.

Painter, K. B., Haff, G. G., Ramsey, M. W., McBride, J., Triplett, T., Sands, W. A., . . . Stones, M. H. (2012). Strength gains: Block versus daily undulating periodization weight training among track and field athletes. *International Journal of Sports Physiology and Performance, 7*, 161–169.

Peterson, M. D., Rhea, M. R., & Alvar, B. A. (2004). Maximizing strength development in athletes: A meta-analysis to determine the dose-response relationship. *Journal of Strength and Conditioning Research, 18*, 377–382.

Plisk, S. S., & Stone, M. H. (2003). Periodization strategies. *Strength and Conditioning Journal, 25*, 19–37.

Proske, U., & Morgan, D. L. (2001). Muscle damage from eccentric exercise: Mechanism, mechanical signs, adaptation and clinical applications. *Journal of Physiology, 537*, 333–345.

Ratamess, N. (2012). *ACSM's foundation of strength training and conditioning.* Philadelphia, PA: Lippincott Williams & Wilkins.

Ratamess, N. A., Alvar, B. A., Evetoch, T. K., Housh, T. J., Kibler, W. B., Kraemer, W. J., & Triplett, N. T. (2009). Progression models in resistance training for healthy adults. *Medicine and Science in Sports and Exercise, 41*, 687–708.

Rhea, M. R., Kenn, J. G., & Dermody, B. M. (2009). Alterations in speed of squat movement and the use of accommodated resistance among college athletes training for power. *Journal of Strength and Conditioning Research, 23*, 2645–2650.

Robbins, D. W., Young, W. B., Behm, D. G., & Payne, W. R. (2010). Agonist–antagonist paired set resistance training: A brief review. *Journal of Strength and Conditioning Research, 24*, 2873–2882.

Roig, M., O'Brien, K., Kirk, G., Murray, R., McKinnon, P., Shadgan, B., & Reid, W. D. (2009). The effects of eccentric versus concentric resistance training on muscle strength and mass in healthy adults: A systematic review with meta-analysis. *British Journal of Sports Medicine, 43*, 556–568.

Rooney, K. J., Herbert, R. D., & Balnave, R. J. (1994). Fatigue contributes to the strength training stimulus. *Medicine and Science in Sports and Exercise, 26*, 1160–1164.

Russ, D. W. (2008). Active and passive tension interact to promote Akt signaling with muscle contraction. *Medicine and Science in Sports and Exercise, 40*, 88–95.

Samonzino, P., Rejc, E., Di Prampero, P. E., Belli, A., & Morin, J.-B. (2012). Optimal force–velocity profile in ballistic movements: *Altius: Citius* or *fortius? Medicine and Science in Sports and Exercise, 44*, 313–322.

Schoenfeld, B. J. (2010). The mechanisms of muscle hypertrophy and their application to resistance training. *Journal of Strength and Conditioning Research, 24*, 2857–2872.

Seynnes, O. R., de Boer, M., & Narici, M. V. (2007). Early skeletal muscle hypertrophy and architectural changes in response to high-intensity resistance training. *Journal of Applied Physiology, 102*, 368–373.

Sheppard, J. M., Dingley, A. A., Janssen, I., Spratford, W., Chapman, D. W., & Newton, R. U. (2011). The effect of assisted jumping on vertical jump height in high-performance volleyball players. *Journal of Science and Medicine in Sport, 14*, 85–89.

Sheppard, J. M., Hobson, S., Chapman, D., Taylor, K. L., McGuigan, M. R., & Newton, R. U. (2008). The effect of training with accentuated eccentric load counter-movement jumps on strength and power characteristics of high-performance volleyball players. *International Journal of Science and Coaching, 3*, 355–363.

Simão, R., Fleck, S. J., Polito, M., Monteiro, W., & Farinatti, P. (2005). Effects of resistance training intensity, volume, and session format on the postexercise hypotensive response. *Journal of Strength and Conditioning Research, 19*, 853–858.

Smith, D. J. (2003). A framework for understanding the training process leading to elite performance. *Sports Medicine, 33*, 1103–1126.

Spiering, B. A., Kraemer, W. J., Anderson, J. M., Armstrong, L. E., Nindl, B. C., Volek, J. S., & Maresh, C. M. (2008). Resistance exercise biology: Manipulation of resistance exercise programme variables determines the responses of cellular and molecular signaling pathways. *Sports Medicine, 38*, 527–540.

Stone, M., Plisk, S., & Collins, D. (2002). Training principles: Evaluation of modes and methods of resistance training: A coaching perspective. *Sports Biomechanics, 1*, 79–103.

Stone, M. H., Stone, M., & Sands, W. A. (2007). *Principles and practice of resistance training.* Champaign, IL: Human Kinetics.

Suzuki, S., Sato, T., Maeda, A., & Takahashi, Y. (2006). Program design based on a mathematical model using rating of perceived exertion for an elite Japanese sprinter: A case study. *Journal of Strength and Conditioning Research, 20*, 36–42.

Takarada, Y., Sato, Y., & Ishii, N. (2002). Effects of resistance exercise combined with vascular occlusion on muscle function in athletes. *European Journal of Applied Physiology, 86*, 308–314.

Tidow, G. (1990). Aspects of strength training in athletics. *New Studies in Athletics, 1*, 93–110.

Toigo, M., & Boutellier, U. (2006). New fundamental resistance exercise determinants of molecular and cellular muscle adaptations. *European Journal of Applied Physiology, 97*, 643–663.

Wallace, B. J., Winchester, J. B., & McGuigan, M. R. (2006). Effects of elastic bands on force and power characteristics during the back squat exercise. *Journal of Strength and Conditioning Research, 20*, 268–272.

Wernbom, M., Augustsson, J., & Raastad, T. (2008). Ischemic strength training: A low-load alternative to heavy resistance exercise? *Scandinavian Journal of Medicine and Science in Sports, 18*, 401–416.

Yaggie, J. A., & Campbell, B. M. (2006). Effects of balance training on selected skills. *Journal of Strength and Conditioning Research, 20*, 422–428.

Young, W. B. (2006). Transfer of strength and power training to sports performance. *International Journal of Sports Physiology and Performance, 1*, 74–83.

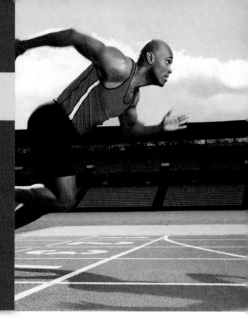

CHAPTER 7

Training Methods to Develop Flexibility

Chapter Objectives

At the end of this chapter, you will be able to:

- Define flexibility and discuss the different measures of flexibility
- Describe the factors that affect flexibility
- Discuss the importance of flexibility in athletic performance and injury prevention
- Discuss training methods to develop flexibility
- Develop protocols incorporating static stretching and proprioceptive neuromuscular facilitation techniques to increase flexibility

Key Terms

Agonist–contract technique

Autogenic inhibition

Computerized myotonometer

Contract–relax technique

Creep

Damped free oscillation

Dynamic flexibility

Hysteresis

Myofascial release techniques

Passive cooling

Passive heating

Real-time ultrasonography

Reciprocal inhibition

Static flexibility

Stiffness

Stress–relaxation

Torque–angle curve

Vibration

Chapter Overview

Flexibility is promoted as an important component of movements in everyday activities as well as sport (Protas, 2001), and many coaches instigate methods to assess and enhance the flexibility of their athletes (Ebben & Blackard, 2001; Ebben, Carroll, & Simenz, 2004; Ebben, Hintz, & Simenz, 2005). Methods that increase flexibility—particularly stretching techniques—are often promoted as enhancing athletic performance and preventing injuries (Fredette, 2001), yet the evidence supporting this position is often contradictory, and sometimes lacking altogether. The importance of flexibility to athletic performance and injury risk is complicated by the many factors that determine flexibility and our understanding of the mechanisms underpinning an increase in flexibility. In turn, the efficacy of specific methods promoted to enhance flexibility is largely limited by the measurements of flexibility employed by researchers. Furthermore, the requirements for flexibility are likely to be sport and injury specific, yet the optimal levels of flexibility for both remain unknown. In this chapter, we will identify the factors that affect flexibility and highlight the importance of flexibility in athletic performance and injury prevention. Different methods that can be used to develop flexibility will then be introduced. We will begin by defining flexibility and discussing the methods to measure flexibility.

Defining and Measuring Flexibility

Flexibility is typically defined as the range of motion available at a joint or group of joints without inducing an injury to the surrounding structures (Enoka, 2008; Siff, 2000). The concept highlighted in this definition is **static flexibility**, which is proposed to be an intrinsic property of the tissues and structures that surround a joint (Gleim & McHugh, 1997), although static flexibility is distinct from joint laxity (see Flexibility Concept 7.1). The range of motion available at a given joint is affected by the tissue and structures surrounding the joint and the joint movement attempted. Table 7.1 shows the typical ranges of motion available at specific joints.

Measurements of static flexibility are performed when the athlete is fully relaxed and the joint is moved to the limit of its range of motion. Examples of static flexibility tests include the toe-touch exercise, sit-and-reach, and the supine single-leg raise (Figure 7.1). The outcome measure in these tests is a kinematic description of the range of motion obtained using tape measures, goniometers, or inclinometers (see Flexibility Concept 7.2).

The end-point in measures of static flexibility is typically the sensation experienced by the athlete or the tester; thus static techniques provide a subjective measure of flexibility (Knudson, Magnusson, & McHugh, 2000). A variety of sensations are also cited in the literature as means to determine the end-point including the sensation of the "resistance" to the imposed stretch, or "discomfort," "tightness," "stiffness," or "pain" associated with the imposed stretch. The use of different subjective sensations can significantly affect the interpretation of the end-point associated with measures of static flexibility (Weppler & Magnusson, 2010). Furthermore, measures of static flexibility do not provide information about the properties of the MTU, as information regarding the force associated with the imposed stretch is not recorded (Magnusson, 1998; Weppler & Magnusson, 2010). This issue can be circumvented by applying stretch with a handheld dynamometer to record the passive resistance to the imposed stretch (see Applied Research 7.1).

Flexibility Concept 7.1

Difference between static flexibility and joint laxity

Static flexibility is related to extensibility of the musculotendinous unit (MTU) and the ability of the athlete to tolerate the stretch as the joint is moved toward its maximal range of motion (Gleim & McHugh, 1997). In contrast, joint laxity refers to a lack of stability of a joint and is more influenced by the ligaments and capsular structures that surround the joint (Nawata et al., 1999). Moreover, joint laxity is associated with a greater risk of injury—most notably, injuries to the anterior cruciate ligament (Myer, Ford, Paterno, Nick, & Hewett, 2008; Ramesh, VonArx, Azzopardi, & Schranz, 2005). Joint laxity certainly contributes to the outcome in typical measures of flexibility. Indeed, it is difficult to distinguish between a large range of motion at a joint resulting from an extensible MTU or heightened stretch tolerance and that from laxity in the ligamentous and capsular structures using simple measures of flexibility.

The Beighton criteria provide a measure of generalized joint laxity and require the completion of five maneuvers to determine the laxity of the joints, including the thumb, metacarpophalangeal joint, knee joint, elbow joint, and forward flexion of the trunk (palms-to-floor test). Four of the five maneuvers are performed on each side of the body, and a Beighton score greater than 4 is considered indicative of generalized joint laxity (Simpson, 2006).

Benign joint hypermobility syndrome (BJHS) is the occurrence of symmetric hypermobility of the joints of an individual in the absence of systemic rheumatologic disease; it is thought to be an inherited disorder of the connective tissue (Simpson, 2006). The hypermobility is accompanied by pain in the joints (arthralgia)—the major clinical criteria for BJHS—as a result of degradation of the joint surfaces (Remvig, Jensen, & Ward, 2007). Increased prevalence of hypermobility has been reported in ballet dancers compared to controls (McCormack, Briggs, Hakim, & Grahame, 2004). Other forms of heritable disorders of the connective tissue include Ehlers-Danlos syndrome (EDS), Marfan syndrome, and osteogenesis imperfecta; they are characterized by fragility of the connective tissues other than the joints, including the skin, bone, and eye (Malfait, Hakim, De Paepe, & Grahame, 2006). However, BJHS might be a mild form of EDS and may well be indistinguishable from the hypermobility type of EDS (Malfait et al., 2006; Ross & Grahame, 2011).

In contrast to the subjective nature of static flexibility, **dynamic flexibility** refers to the passive resistance to the range of motion available about a joint or group of joints (Gleim & McHugh, 1997). Measures of dynamic flexibility combine both kinematic and kinetic variables typically during the passive motion of a joint until a predetermined end-point (either a specified joint angle or the subjective sensation of pain) is reached. For example, through the measurement of torque–angle relationships attained from passive movements of isolated joints by means of a dynamometer,

Table 7.1
Movements at Specific Joints, Planes of Motion, and Typical Ranges of Motion

Joint	Joint Classification	Joint Movement	Plane of Motion	Range of Motion
Shoulder girdle (scapulothoracic)	Not a true joint	Elevation–depression	Frontal	55°
		Upward–downward rotation	Frontal	60°
		Protraction–retraction	Frontal	25°
Shoulder (glenohumeral)	Synovial (ball-and-socket)	Flexion–extension	Sagittal	170–180° flexion; 40–60° extension*
		Abduction–adduction	Frontal	170–180° abduction; 75° adduction*
		Horizontal abduction–adduction	Transverse	45° horizontal abduction; 140–150° horizontal adduction
		Internal–external rotation	Transverse	70–90°
Elbow (humeroulnar)	Synovial (hinge)	Flexion–extension	Sagittal	145–150° flexion; 5–10° hyperextension
Intervertebral	Cartilaginous	Flexion–extension	Sagittal	T1–T12: 12°; L vertebrae: ~13–15°
		Lateral flexion	Frontal	T1–T12: 8°; L vertebrae: ~3–6°
		Rotation	Transverse	T vertebrae: ~3–8°; L vertebrae: ~2–5°
Hip	Synovial (ball-and-socket)	Flexion–extension	Sagittal	0–130° flexion; 0–30° extension
		Abduction–adduction	Frontal	0–35° abduction; 0–30° adduction
		Medial–lateral rotation	Transverse	0–45° medial rotation; 0–50° lateral rotation
Knee	Synovial (modified hinge)	Flexion–extension	Sagittal	0–140° flexion; 10° extension
		Medial–lateral rotation	Transverse	0–15° medial rotation; 0–30° lateral rotation
Ankle (talocrural)	Synovial (hinge)	Flexion–extension†	Sagittal	15–20° flexion; 50° extension

*Includes shoulder girdle motion.

†These movements are typically referred to as dorsiflexion and plantarflexion, respectively.

Note: T = thoracic; L = lumbar.

Data from Floyd, R. T. (2009). *Manual of structural kinesiology.* New York, NY: McGraw-Hill; Mayer, J. M. (2007). Anatomy, kinesiology, and biomechanics. In W. R. Thompson, K. E. Baldwin, N. I. Pire, & M. Niederpruem (Eds.), *ACSM's resources for the personal trainer* (pp. 109–176). Baltimore, MD: Lippincott Williams & Wilkins; McGill, S. M. (2007). *Low back disorders.* Champaign, IL: Human Kinetics.

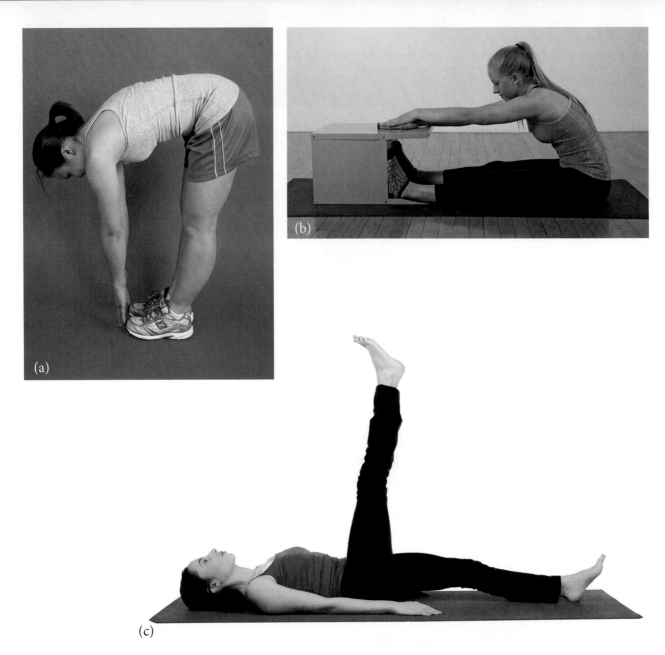

Figure 7.1 Tests of static flexibility. (a) Toe-touch exercise. (b) Sit-and-reach. (c) Supine single-leg raise.

Photo (c): © DenizA/iStockphoto.com

the viscoelastic properties of the MTU, including passive stiffness, stress–relaxation, and hysteresis, can be determined *in vivo* (Magnusson, 1998; Weppler & Magnusson, 2010). (See Flexibility Concept 7.3.) Measures of dynamic flexibility provide a more objective assessment of flexibility. Furthermore, the accuracy of measures of static and dynamic flexibility appears to be limited by different factors despite the inverse relationship that exists between the passive resistance during measures of dynamic flexibility and the maximal range of motion about a given joint (Gleim & McHugh, 1997).

Flexibility Concept 7.2

Measuring range of motion using a goniometer and an inclinometer

Goniometers provide an inexpensive method to measure the range of motion at a joint. A universal goniometer consists of two arms: One remains stationary against a body segment (stationary arm) while the other is moved through the arc of motion associated with the movement of the other body segment (mobile arm) (Figure 7.2). This method can produce reliable measurements with minimal user training (Konor, Morton, Eckerson, & Grindstaff, 2012). It requires that the anatomic reference points used to determine the center associated with the joint and those associated with the stationary and mobile arms of the goniometer remain consistent between testing occasions.

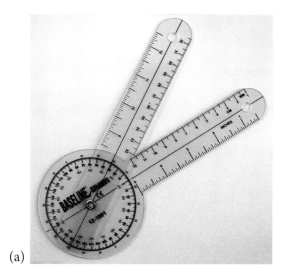

(a)

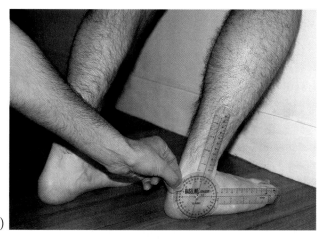

(b)

Figure 7.2 (a) A universal goniometer. (b) A goniometer being used to measure ankle dorsiflexion.

(continues)

(continued)

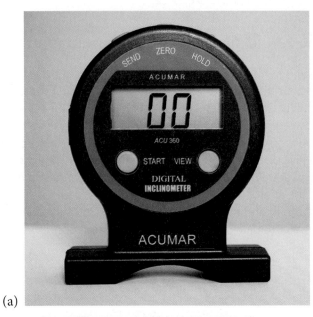

(a)

(b)

Figure 7.3 (a) An electronic inclinometer. (b) An electronic inclinometer being used to measure ankle dorsiflexion.

An inclinometer is an electronic device that is placed directly onto a body segment during a flexibility test (Figure 7.3). It compares the orientation of the body segment with the gravitational force to determine the segment angle, from which the joint angle can be determined. The use of an inclinometer has been shown to produce reliable joint angle measures when used by a novice practitioner, producing smaller errors than are associated with a goniometer (Konor et al., 2012). As with the use of a goniometer, the selection of the anatomic reference point for the placement of the inclinometer requires consistency between testing occasions.

Applied Research 7.1
Modifying measures of static flexibility to determine passive resistance to the imposed stretch

Bojsen-Møller et al. (2007) investigated the passive resistance of the knee extensors during an imposed stretch in two groups of women categorized as flexible and inflexible. A modified Ely's test was used, whereby the participant was placed in a prone position on a bench with the hip and knee joints of the right leg at full extension; the hip of the left leg was flexed at approximately 100°, with the foot placed on the floor. This posture produced posterior pelvic tilt. The knee of the right leg was passively flexed to the point that provoked a sensation of tightness in the anterior thigh. At this point, the knee angle was recorded from a goniometer and the force applied to the leg was determined by a handheld dynamometer. The force registered by the dynamometer was then corrected for the contribution of gravity on the leg segment and converted to a torque value.

The authors reported that the flexible participants were able to achieve a significantly greater knee flexion angle than the inflexible participants ($136 \pm 7°$ versus $76 \pm 16°$). Although the greater passive range of motion of the flexible participants was achieved with a greater torque applied to the leg compared to the inflexible participants (11.5 ± 5.5 Nm versus 8.4 ± 3.0 Nm), the difference was not statistically significant, likely due to the relatively large variations reported in the variables. This finding tends to lend support to the notion that the difference between flexible and inflexible participants is due to the ability to tolerate an imposed stretch as opposed to the extensibility of the MTU.

Bojsen-Møller, J., Brogaard, K., Have, M. J., Stryger, H. P., Kjær, M., Aagaard, P., & Magnusson, S. P. (2007). Passive knee joint range of motion is unrelated to the mechanical properties of the patellar tendon. *Scandinavian Journal of Medicine and Science in Sports, 17*, 415–421.

Flexibility Concept 7.3

Assessing the viscoelastic characteristics of muscle and connective tissue

The passive behavior of MTU during an imposed stretch is a combination of viscous and elastic properties. Viscosity represents a time- or rate-dependent property, whereas elasticity represents a force-dependent property. The viscous elements within the MTU will elongate in response to force that is applied slowly, while resisting a rapidly applied force. However, the force associated with the viscous elements that resist the elongation of the MTU will decrease over time if the length of the MTU is sustained, giving rise to a property known as **stress–relaxation**. If the force of elongation is held constant, then the length of the MTU gradually increases, giving rise to a property known as **creep**. The force required to elongate a passive MTU is mainly influenced by the elastic properties of the MTU. The elasticity of the MTU is determined from the slope of the force–elongation curve (analogous to a stress–strain curve): The greater the force required to elongate the MTU, the steeper the slope of the curve. The magnitude of the slope during the linear portion of the curve provides a measure of the **stiffness** of the MTU, known as the Young's modulus of the tissue. In this way, the elasticity of the MTU is defined by its stiffness. If the MTU is moved

(continues)

(continued)

passively through a given elongation and then returned to its original length, the difference between the force–elongation curve associated with lengthening and that associated with shortening provides a measure of another viscous property known as **hysteresis**. Hysteresis provides a measure of the strain potential energy that is dissipated (lost as heat) during elongation and shortening. These viscoelastic properties of the MTU underpin the measurement of dynamic flexibility.

The passive stiffness of the MTU can be measured using a number of techniques. The **damped free oscillation** technique uses the rate of decay in the oscillations of the perturbed MTU as a measure of the passive stiffness (McNair & Stanley, 1996; Wilson, Elliott, & Wood, 1992). Specifically, with the joint under investigation held in a relaxed position, a perturbing force is manually applied to the limb that results in an oscillation, observed as an acceleration of the limb or a force acting through the limb that decays over time. A stiffer MTU will produce a greater initial acceleration or force in response to the perturbing force and will oscillate at a higher frequency (Figure 7.4). The electromyographic (EMG) activity of the muscle is recorded throughout the protocol to ensure that the MTU remains passive.

By using a dynamometer that is able to record both the resistive torque acting at the joint and the angle of the joint, a **torque–angle curve** can be generated as the MTU is elongated passively (Magnusson, Simonsen, Aagaard, & Kjær, 1996; McHugh et al., 1999). The variable is a torque that arises as the

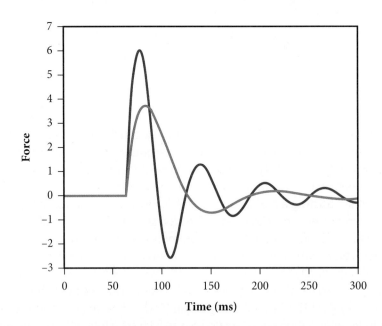

Figure 7.4 The response of two systems to an instantaneous force applied during the damped oscillation technique. The response of the stiffer system is given by the red line; the more compliant system is indicated by the blue line.

Reproduced from Gleim, G. W. & McHugh, M. P. (1997). Flexibility and its effects on sports injury and performance. *Sports Medicine, 24*, 289–299, with kind permission from Springer Science and Business Media.

force transducer of the dynamometer undergoes pure rotation during the movement. The EMG activity of the agonist muscle is recorded during the passive motion to reveal any involvement of the muscles (either voluntary or reflexive). The passive torque–angle curve allows the determination of the passive stiffness, stress–relaxation, creep, and hysteresis of the MTU (Figure 7.5). Although the elastic modulus (stiffness) of a material should be calculated based on the linear region of the stress–strain (torque–angle) curve, the torque–angle curves produced in typical measures of dynamic flexibility are nonlinear and are more similar to the "toe-region" of the relationship (Magnusson, Aagaard, Simonsen, & Bojsen-Møller, 2000). For this reason Magnusson et al. (2000) propose that the energy absorbed by the MTU during such *in vivo* measurements would actually be more appropriate.

The damped free oscillation and torque–angle curve methods do not allow the determination of which elements of the MTU contribute to the viscoelastic response observed. Through the use of **real-time ultrasonography**, the elongation of tendon, aponeurosis, and fascicles can be determined during isometric muscle actions (Kubo, Kanehisa, & Fukunaga, 2001), allowing the viscoelastic properties of the tendon–aponeurosis structures to be separated from those of the other elements of the MTU.

Muscle stiffness can be estimated by means of a **computerized myotonometer** (CMT). A CMT is placed above the tissue and exerts a small constant mechanical

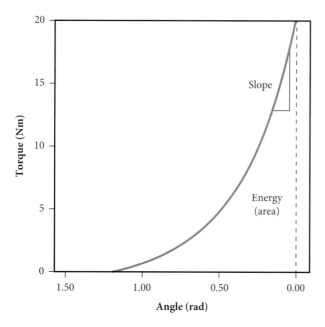

Figure 7.5 A schematic representation of the passive torque–angle curve during a measure of dynamic flexibility. The slope represents the stiffness of the MTU, while the area under the curve represents the energy absorbed by the tissue during elongation.

Reproduced from Magnusson, S. P. (1998). Passive properties of human skeletal muscle during stretch maneuvers. A review. *Scandinavian Journal of Medicine and Science in Sports, 8,* 65–77.

(continues)

(continued)

force via an indenter probe that moves at a constant speed until a predetermined force is achieved. From the force and tissue depth measurements recorded, the work done by the device on the tissue can be determined. The work done on the tissue correlates inversely with tissue stiffness (Ylinen et al., 2009).

It is only through the measurements discussed here that the factors affecting flexibility can be determined and the factors that contribute to the increases in flexibility observed following a specific intervention elucidated. Consequently, measures of static flexibility provide very limited information about the specific factors limiting flexibility.

Factors Affecting Flexibility

Many factors influence the range of motion available about a given joint and the resistance to an imposed stretch within the available range of motion. These factors, which are listed in Table 7.2, will affect measures of both static and dynamic flexibility. Researchers have typically focused their attention on the extensibility of the MTU, neuromuscular relaxation, and stretch tolerance as the major contributors to differences in flexibility between individuals (Enoka, 2008; Weppler & Magnusson, 2010). These factors are also proposed to be the sites of adaptation following training methods utilized to enhance flexibility (e.g., stretching techniques).

Table 7.2
Factors Affecting Measures of Static and Dynamic Flexibility

Factor	Description
Bony congruence of the articulating surfaces	Resistance provided by the contact between the bony surface areas.
	A close-packed position is defined by maximum surface area contact and provides a stable joint. This determines the degrees of freedom available at a joint.
Extensibility of the joint capsule and ligaments	Resistance of the joint capsule (synovial joint) and ligaments. Implicated in joint laxity.
Extensibility of the skin and neurovascular structures	Resistance of skin and blood vessels to length deformation associated with imposed stretch.
Extensibility of the musculotendinous units	Resistance of muscle and connective tissue to length deformation associated with imposed stretch.
Neuromuscular relaxation	Activation of group Ia and II afferents during an imposed stretch.
Stretch tolerance	Activation of group III and IV afferents during an imposed stretch.

Data from Enoka, R. M. (2008). *Neuromechanics of human movement*. Champaign, IL: Human Kinetic; Weppler, C. H., & Magnusson, S. P. (2010). Increasing muscle extensibility: A matter of increasing length or modifying sensation. *Physical Therapy, 90,* 438–449.

Extensibility of the MTU

The extensibility of the MTU refers to the ability of the tissue to be extended. When subjected to a tensile load, such as that associated with the length deformation of the tissue that accompanies a joint being moved through a range of motion, the MTU will increase the resistance (a tensile stress) that opposes the imposed stretch. The increase in this passive resistance is nonlinear, increasing markedly only after 30–50% of the maximal change in length, independent of whether the individual is flexible or inflexible (Magnusson et al., 2000). It is apparent that the MTUs of flexible individuals are exposed to greater change in length (strain) of the MTU at the maximal joint range of motion compared to inflexible individuals (Magnusson et al., 2000). In addition, inflexible individuals have greater passive stiffness of the MTU (Magnusson et al., 1997).

The passive resistance to an imposed stretch arises from a number of sources within the MTU. The MTU can be considered to comprise three components: a contractile component (actomyosin interaction), a series elastic component, and a parallel elastic component (Zatsiorsky & Prilutsky, 2012). During stretch of the MTU, the activity of the contractile components can be discounted if the individual is relaxed, although reflexive activation of these components may occur to oppose the stretch. The series and parallel elastic components have viscoelastic properties: Their resistance to lengthening depends on the magnitude and rate at which the deforming force is applied to the tissue and the time over which they are deformed. One of the outcomes is that the resistance offered by the MTU to passive stretch increases with the velocity of the imposed stretch—a property that has been confirmed by researchers (Nordez, Casari, & Cornu, 2008).

The tendon represents the major series elastic component in the MTU. Despite the similar contribution of muscle and tendon to the length change of the MTU during an imposed stretch (Morse, Degens, Seynnes, Maganaris, & Jones, 2008), the stiffness of the tendon does not make a major contribution to the overall passive stiffness of the MTU (Bojsen-Møller et al., 2007; Kubo, Kanehisa, & Fukunaga, 2001). Another series elastic component within the MTU is the titin molecule, which may be responsible for some of the passive tension that resists stretch of MTU (Horowits & Podolsky, 1987; Magid & Law, 1985). The parallel elastic component within the MTU comprises the endomysial, perimysial, and epimysial connective tissue; it has been determined that the perimysium makes a significant contribution to the passive stiffness of muscle (Purslow, 1989). The viscoelastic property (stress–relaxation) of the perimysium comes from the reorientation of the collagen fibers during length deformation as well as from relaxation processes in the matrix surrounding the fibers or within the fibers themselves (Purslow, Wess, & Hukins, 1998). The size of the muscle, determined by the cross-sectional area or volume, affects the extensibility of the MTU: A larger muscle would be expected to have greater amounts of contractile and connective tissue. Indeed, researchers have reported that the cross-sectional area of the hamstring muscles is inversely related to the resistance during passive stretching and to measures of static flexibility (Magnusson et al., 1997).

Neuromuscular Relaxation

During a stretch imposed on the MTU, there will be activation of the type Ia afferents associated with the muscle spindles that have excitatory connections with the α-motoneurons of the target muscle (Enoka, 2008). The result is an increase in the contractile activity of the stretched muscle via the stretch reflex, which would in turn increase the resistance of the MTU to the imposed stretch. This phenomenon explains why electromyographic activity of the stretched muscle is recorded during assessments of flexibility (Magnusson et al., 1997; Magnusson et al., 2000). However, the activation of the stretch reflex is likely to occur only if the rate of the imposed stretch is very high, the length change of the muscle is low, and the stretch is imposed with the muscle at the mid-range of its length (Chalmers, 2004). Such stretches are unlikely to be associated with measures of static or dynamic flexibility. Indeed, even during relatively high stretch rates, minimal EMG activity is reported (Gajdosik et al., 2005; Magnusson, Aagaard, Simonsen, & Bojsen-Møller, 1998; Nordez et al., 2008). During tests of flexibility, no differences in EMG activity of the stretched muscles were noted between flexible and inflexible individuals (Magnusson et al., 1997; Magnusson et al., 2000). It is therefore unlikely that the activation of the stretch reflex contributes substantially to measures of flexibility in healthy, uninjured individuals (Weppler & Magnusson, 2010).

Stretch Tolerance

As the MTU tissue is lengthened during an imposed stretch, the mechano-nociceptors (group III and IV afferents) within the MTU and joint are stimulated (Khals & Ge, 2004; Marchettini, 1993). This effect will result in the individual perceiving a sensation of pain and, therefore, will influence the maximal range of motion at a given joint. Evidence indicates that athletes have a greater threshold of the nociceptive reflexes than untrained individuals and that physical activity results in an increase in the threshold (Guieu, Blin, Pouget, & Serratrice, 1992). The perception of stretch can be modified by the posture adopted during the stretch (Laessøe & Voigt, 2004) and the completion of prior stretches of the MTU (Magnusson et al., 1998). Furthermore, evidence suggests that the difference between flexible and inflexible individuals resides in their ability to tolerate a greater stretch of the MTU (Bojsen-Møller et al., 2007; Magnusson et al., 1997; Magnusson et al., 2000; also see Applied Research 7.2).

Applied Research 7.2
The difference between flexible and inflexible athletes is due to stretch tolerance and the stiffness of the MTU

In this study, the authors investigated the difference between the mechanical characteristics of the hamstring muscles in endurance athletes categorized as either flexible or inflexible. Each athlete performed a test of static flexibility where the hamstring muscle was passively stretched until an end-point—defined as the initial onset of pain—was reached. At that point, the athletes were able to terminate the stretch. The test was performed in a dynamometer that extended the knee at a constant angular velocity (5°/s) and allowed the determination of the torque–angle curve during the stretching procedure.

The authors reported that the flexible athletes were able to achieve a greater maximal knee extension angle at the onset of pain compared to the inflexible athletes. However, the greater knee extension angle was achieved with a concomitantly greater passive torque at the knee joint and a greater stiffness of the MTU during the final 10° of the stretch. At the knee extension angles common to both groups during the passive stretch, the inflexible athletes produced greater stiffness values of the MTU. The authors concluded that the differences in flexibility were due to the greater ability of the flexible athletes to tolerate the passive stretch as well as a stiffer MTU in the inflexible athletes.

Magnusson, S. P., Simonsen, E. B., Aagaard, P., Boesen, J., Johannsen, F., & Kjær, M. (1997). Determinants of musculoskeletal flexibility: Viscoelastic properties, cross-sectional area, EMG and stretch tolerance. *Scandinavian Journal of Medicine and Science in Sports, 7,* 195–202.

Indeed, the outcome of measuring static flexibility when the joint is moved passively to an end-point determined by subjective sensations is likely to be largely influenced by the individual's ability to tolerate the stretch as opposed to the extensibility of the MTU. The importance of stretch tolerance as a limiting factor in flexibility is also highlighted by studies investigating the effects of increased range of motion observed following passive heating or cooling of the MTU, both of which induce analgesia (Shrier & Glossal, 2000).

It should be noted that the influence of the extensibility of the MTU, neuromuscular relaxation, and stretch tolerance on flexibility can be determined accurately only during measures of dynamic flexibility: With a simple measure of static flexibility, it is unclear which factors are specifically limiting the observed range of motion. However, given that the outcome in tests of static flexibility is determined by subjective sensations associated with the stretch, it is likely that stretch tolerance is the major limiting factor in inflexible individuals when these measures are used (Weppler & Magnusson, 2010).

Other factors that are often suggested to affect flexibility are age and sex. The evidence shows that these factors do influence measures of flexibility, albeit secondary to the extensibility of the MTU and stretch tolerance. For example, older soccer players are less flexible than their younger counterparts (McHugh, Magnusson, Gleim, Magnusson, & Nicholas, 1993), and younger individuals tend to have greater stretch tolerance and demonstrate lower resistance to passive stretch, which accounts for their greater flexibility (Magnusson, 1998). However, other researchers have reported that age is not correlated to passive stiffness of the elbow joint (Lin, Ju, & Huang, 2005); notably, older tennis players are not less flexible than their younger counterparts (Haywood & Williams, 1995). Furthermore, Roach and Miles (1991) noted that the difference in flexibility between young and older individuals was not clinically significant. Females have lower passive stiffness values compared to men during measures of dynamic flexibility (Blackburn, Riemann, Padua, & Guskiewicz, 2004; Morse, 2011), probably due to the smaller cross-sectional area of their MTU. Indeed, Lin et al. (2005) reported that men tended to demonstrate greater passive stiffness than women; however, these differences disappeared when the stiffness values were normalized to body weight. Note that neither age nor sex influences the response to methods employed to increase flexibility (Cipriani, Terry, Haiines, Tabibnia, & Lyssanova, 2012; Girouard & Hurley, 1995).

Flexibility and Athletic Performance

It is possible to develop theoretical arguments regarding the importance of flexibility in athletic performance. A large range of motion available at specific joints would appear to be advantageous for aesthetic sports such as gymnastics and dancing; consequently, these sports are characterized by extensive methods to develop flexibility (Guidetti et al., 2009; Reid, Burnham, Saboe, & Kushner, 1987). However, the role of large ranges of motion in other sports may be less clear, leading some authors to suggest that flexibility for a given athlete is a case of optimization rather than maximization (Sands, 2011). Unfortunately, the optimal levels of flexibility for specific sports are currently unknown despite established ranges for flexibility about specific joints promoted for health (Protas, 2001).

When attempting to establish the importance of flexibility in athletic performance, it is important to determine the measure of athletic performance that the researchers employed. Some studies have compared athletes of different performance levels or compared athletes with non-athletes. For example, flexibility is positively related to performance level in swimming (Sprague, 1976), tennis (Roetert, Brown, Piorkowski, & Woods, 1996), and wrestling (Yoon, 2002), while baseball pitchers have been shown to have greater flexibility than non-athletes (Magnusson, Gleim, & Nicholas, 1994). Conversely, flexibility does not differentiate between performance level in Australian Rules football players (Young & Pryor, 2007), track and field sprinters (Meckel, Atterbom, Grodjinovsky, Ben-Sira, & Rotstein, 1995), and professional soccer players (Arnason et al., 2004). Other researchers have employed surrogate measures of athletic performance that are common to many sports, such as speed, strength, and exercise economy. Flexibility has been shown to be positively related to swimming speed (Mookerjee, Bibi, Kenney, & Cohen, 1995) but is not strongly related to club-head speed in golfers (Gordon, Moir, Davis, Witmer, & Cummings, 2009). Somewhat surprisingly, inflexible runners have been shown to be more economical in their performance than the flexible runners (Craib, Mitchell, Fields, Hopewell, & Morgan, 1996; Gleim, Stachenfeld, & Nicholas, 1990; Hunter et al., 2011; Trehearn & Buresh, 2009). It is possible that the increased passive stiffness of the MTU requires less activation of the contractile element of the MTU or that a greater storage and return of strain potential energy by the MTU occurs during the running strides, resulting in a lower metabolic cost of locomotion.

Collectively, these findings imply that the importance of flexibility is sport specific. Indeed, tennis players have been shown to be more flexible than baseball players (Ellenbecker et al., 2007) and wrestlers less flexible than both weightlifters and gymnasts (Yoon, 2002). Furthermore, flexibility is likely to be position specific within a given sport, with linemen in football being shown to be less flexible than players filling other positions (Gleim, 1984) and soccer goalkeepers being more flexible than team members at other playing positions (Oberg, Ekstrand, Möller, & Gillquist, 1984). As mentioned earlier, these results imply that training flexibility may be more about optimization than maximization (Sands, 2011).

The studies highlighted here all employed a cross-sectional design and, therefore, do not allow the separation of genetic factors from those associated with adaptations to specific training regimens. Moreover, the previously mentioned studies used measures of static flexibility, which do not allow the determination of the MTU's properties. Previous authors have reported that a less stiff MTU is associated with greater performance on isometric and concentric strength tests that require rapid transmission of force (Wilson, Murphy, & Pryor, 1994). In one study, training that reduced the passive stiffness of the MTU resulted in improved performance during strength tests relying on the stretch–shortening cycle by means of increasing the contribution of strain potential energy to the movement (Wilson et al., 1992). Nevertheless, measures of flexibility provide little information about the ability of the athlete to actively accelerate a given joint through the available range of motion during sports performance—something that will be more influenced by muscular strength and skill (Sands, 2011). The value of flexibility assessment in predicting athletic performance is, therefore, likely to be limited.

Flexibility and Injury Risk

Sports injuries vary in their severity, and there is little reason to assume that flexibility will directly affect the risk of a traumatic injury (e.g., fracture, concussion). Although the causes of all sports injuries are likely to be multifactorial, certain injuries might be influenced by flexibility (e.g., strains, sprains). For example, the MTU might achieve a greater strain (change in length) before sustaining damage if a greater range of motion is available at a joint: A greater available range of motion at a joint may increase the "safety factor" about that joint for unaccustomed movements that may be experienced in a given sport. Furthermore, a greater available range of motion about a given joint may theoretically allow for lower forces acting across the tissue and structures associated with the joint for a given amount of energy absorbed (as per the work–energy theorem). However, increased laxity at the knee joint has been associated with greater knee energy absorption during landing tasks in female athletes but not males, a factor that may predispose the female athlete to injury during such movements (Shultz, Schmitz, Nguyen, & Levine, 2010). It has been suggested that deviations from optimal flexibility can contribute to muscle imbalances, unusual wear on capsular structures and articular surfaces, and dysfunctional movements (Weppler & Magnusson, 2010), though the optimal amounts of flexibility remain unknown. It is also likely that flexibility patterns that represent a risk factor in one sport do not apply to other sports (Gleim & McHugh, 1997).

Witvrouw, Mahieu, Daneels, and McNair (2004) propose a mechanism by which the compliance of the MTU may be implicated in athletic injuries during activities involving the stretch–shortening cycle. Specifically, when the contractile elements of a compliant MTU are active, more energy can be absorbed by the tendon structures, reducing the load experienced by the contractile elements. Conversely, in a MTU that has low compliance, greater energy will be transmitted to the contractile elements, increasing the likelihood of injury to the active muscle. While the proposed mechanism suggests a role for dynamic flexibility in mitigating the risk of incurring a muscle strain injury, it should be remembered that the compliance of the tendon does not make a major contribution to the overall passive stiffness of the MTU as measured during dynamic flexibility tests (Bojsen-Møller et al., 2007; Kubo, Kanehisa, & Fukunaga, 2001). Moreover, the mechanism proposed by Witvrouw et al. (2004) is an active mechanism that differs from any measures of dynamic flexibility that involve assessments of the passive MTU. However, it has been shown that those individuals who demonstrate less passive stiffness during dynamic flexibility incur less muscle damage following unaccustomed eccentric exercise (McHugh et al., 1999). To this end, training methods that increase flexibility (e.g., static stretching and proprioceptive neuromuscular facilitation techniques) have been shown to attenuate exercise-induced muscle damage (Chen et al., 2011).

To date, no prospective studies have been published demonstrating changes in flexibility concurrent with reductions in the occurrence of muscle strains. Abnormal repair to the MTU following nondisruptive strain injury (grade 1 and 2 strains) can adversely affect the viscoelastic properties of the MTU (Speer, Lohnes, & Garrett, 1993), and the restoration of both the strength and the flexibility of MTU are deemed important after injury of the MTU. However, rehabilitation programs that combine strengthening and stretching exercises have not always been shown to be effective at preventing reinjury. For example, a rehabilitation program that included strengthening and stretching activities was not as effective as a program combining agility and stabilization exercises for lowering the risk of reinjuring the hamstring muscles (de Visser, Reijman, Heijboer, & Bos, 2012). As a consequence, it is difficult to comment on the role of flexibility as a risk for injury as well as a mode of exercise to be included in a rehabilitation program.

Methods to Develop Flexibility

Stretching exercises are typically promoted to increase flexibility (Fredette, 2001), although all training methods should be aimed at taking the joints through the required range of motion (Siff, 2000). When interpreting the effects of different training methods on flexibility, the measure used to assess flexibility should be considered carefully, because the efficacy of the various methods largely depends on the test of flexibility used. For example, acute static stretching has been shown to significantly increase static flexibility with no change in dynamic flexibility, whereas 10 minutes of jogging resulted in an increase in dynamic flexibility with no change in static flexibility (McNair & Stanley, 1996). This again highlights the different qualities that underpin the different measures of flexibility.

Endurance Training

Endurance running (10-week program with a goal of running for 30 minutes continuously by the end) does not increase measures of static flexibility in beginning runners (Moore, Jones, & Dixon, 2012). Indeed, while the scores on the sit-and-reach test remained unchanged, measures of static flexibility of the ankle joint were actually decreased in such athletes, although the change was not statistically significant. Interestingly, the program resulted in an increase in running economy, again highlighting the inverse relationship between flexibility and running economy.

Resistance Training

A period of resistance training has been shown to increase measures of static flexibility (Junior, Leite, & Reis, 2011; Rodrigues Barbosa, Santarem, Filho, & Nunes Marucci, 2002). These improvements are likely due to an increased stretch tolerance, which is a major limitation to static flexibility. This supposition is further supported by measures of dynamic flexibility following resistance training, in which the passive resistance to the imposed stretch tends to increase (Klinge et al., 1997; Kubo, Kanehisa, & Fukunaga, 2002b), presumably due to the concomitant increase in the cross-sectional area of the trained muscles. Again, these findings highlight the fact that the effect of different training methods on flexibility is largely dependent upon the measure of flexibility used.

Stretching Techniques

Stretching exercises typically require the joint to be moved through a predetermined range of motion while the individual remains relaxed, rendering the MTU passive during the imposed stretch. The stress–relaxation response associated with the viscoelastic properties of the MTU produces a reduction in the passive resistance when the joint is held at a position that elongates the MTU (McHugh, Magnusson, Gleim, & Nicholas, 1992), with this reduction occurring within 20 s of the onset of the limit of the stretch (McNair, Dombroski, Hewson, & Stanley, 2000). The imposed elongation of the MTU also affects the mechanical response of the tendon, decreasing both the elasticity and viscosity (Kubo, Kanehisa, Kawakami, & Fukunaga, 2001). However, the altered passive mechanical properties of the MTU appear to be short lived, disappearing within minutes after the removal of the imposed stretch (Magnusson & Renström, 2006). Flexible and inflexible individuals do not appear to differ in this regard, with both groups demonstrating the same stress–relaxation response to a 90-s stretch, implying that both flexible and inflexible individuals are likely to respond similarly to stretching exercises (Magnusson et al., 1997).

The type of stretch imposed on the MTU will affect the mechanical changes in passive resistance of the tissue. For example, repetitive elongation and relaxation of the passive MTU for 60 s has been shown to produce greater reductions in passive stiffness compared to static stretches held for either 15 s (4 repetitions separated by 10 s) or 30 s (2 repetitions separated by 10 s) (McNair et al., 2000). The performance of an isometric muscle action of the target muscle prior to the stretch as part of a proprioceptive neuromuscular facilitation protocol does not induce any different changes in the passive mechanical properties of the MTU compared to those changes associated with static stretching techniques (Magnusson, Simonsen, Aagaard, Dyhre-Poulsen, et al., 1996), yet greater gains in static flexibility accompany these techniques compared to static stretching (Sharman, Cresswell, & Riek, 2006). However, we are interested in the response following the habitual performance of different stretching techniques.

Static Stretching Techniques

Static stretching techniques involve taking a joint to the maximal range of motion, usually determined by the onset of pain, and holding this position for a predetermined time before returning the joint to its resting position. The stretch is then repeated a number of times following a predetermined recovery period. In general, the habitual performance of static stretching techniques has been shown to increase measures of static flexibility (Gleim & McHugh, 1997). However, the effects of static stretching techniques on measures of dynamic flexibility are less clear. For example, there have been no changes in the passive resistance to an imposed stretch in many of the studies performed to date, despite increases in measures of static flexibility (Halbertsma & Goeken, 1994; Magnusson, Simonsen, Aagaard, Sorensen, & Kjær, 1996; Ylinen et al., 2009). These studies support the hypothesis that habitual static stretching increases stretch tolerance of the participants. An effective static stretching protocol to increase the range of motion during hip flexion is shown in Applied Flexibility Protocol 7.1.

That static stretching increases stretch tolerance appears indisputable. However, other researchers have reported measures of dynamic flexibility are enhanced following habitual performance of static stretches (Guissard & Duchateau, 2004; Kubo, Kanehisa, & Fukunaga, 2002a). The decrease in the passive resistance to the imposed stretch may result from an increase in the extensibility of the perimysial connective tissue (see Applied Research 7.3).

Proprioceptive Neuromuscular Facilitation Techniques

Proprioceptive neuromuscular facilitation (PNF) stretching techniques involve the performance of voluntary muscle actions immediately prior to or during an imposed stretch to increase the range of motion available at a given joint. The **contract-relax technique** requires that a joint be moved to a predetermined range of motion before the participant performs an isometric action of the target muscle (that being stretched), usually maximally, before the joint is slowly moved further. The **agonist-contract technique** requires that a joint be moved to a predetermined range of motion before the opposing muscle (the agonist of the joint motion) is activated by the participant while the joint is slowly moved further.

Applied Flexibility Protocol 7.1

Static stretching techniques to increase the range of motion during hip flexion

The following static stretching protocol—for a unilateral hamstring stretch—can be used to develop the flexibility of the hip joint (Figure 7.6).

1. The athlete sits on the floor with the right leg outstretched in front of the body and the sole of the left foot on the medial aspect of the right knee. The trunk remains upright.

2. The athlete reaches the right hand slowly down the right leg until the initial point where mild discomfort is experienced at the back of the leg.

3. This position is held for 45 s, after which the athlete returns slowly to the starting point.

4. Following a recovery of between 5 and 30 s, the stretch is repeated.

5. Between 3 and 6 repetitions of the stretch are performed.

6. Ensure that the posture of the athlete does not change substantially with each stretch, as this could impact the range of motion observed.

7. Consider methods to quantify the range of motion achieved during each stretch (e.g., tape measure, goniometer, inclinometer) so that progress can be determined.

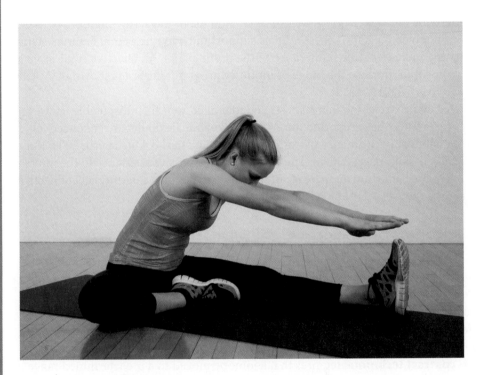

Figure 7.6 The unilateral hamstring stretch.

Applied Research 7.3
Effects of static stretching on measures of dynamic flexibility

In this study, the authors investigated the effects of habitual static stretching exercises on the dynamic flexibility of the ankle joint. Each participant completed five static stretches of the ankle plantarflexors on consecutive days over a 3-week period. Each stretch required the ankle to be dorsiflexed to 35° and held in that position for 45 s, with a 15-s inter-repetition recovery period. The stretches were performed twice daily: once in the morning and once in the afternoon. The measure of dynamic flexibility involved the application of a passive stretch of the ankle plantarflexors by a dynamometer at a constant velocity of 5°/s from the anatomic position through to 25° of dorsiflexion to provide a passive torque–angle curve. Real-time ultrasonography was used during a series of ramped isometric plantar flexion tasks up to the voluntary maximum to determine the viscoelastic properties of the tendon and aponeurosis of the medial gastrocnemius muscle.

The authors reported that the slope of the passive torque–angle curve decreased following the stretching intervention. Furthermore, the hysteresis of the tendon–aponeurosis structure was reduced, with no change in the elasticity of the tendon–aponeurosis being noted. The authors suggested that the reduced elasticity of the musculotendinous unit was as a result of the increased extensibility of the perimysial connective tissue rather than any changes associated with the tendon-aponeurosis structures.

Kubo, K., Kanehisa, H., & Fukunaga, T. (2002). Effects of stretching training on the viscoelastic properties of human tendon structures in vivo. *Journal of Applied Physiology, 92*, 595–601.

The habitual use of PNF stretching techniques has been shown to produce greater gains in the maximal range of motion available at a joint compared to static stretching techniques, with the improvements also occurring at a greater rate (Sharman et al., 2006). Furthermore, the agonist–contract technique appears to be more effective than the contract–relax technique (Sharman et al., 2006). The mechanisms proposed to underpin the responses to PNF techniques include an enhancement in neuromuscular relaxation via **autogenic inhibition** and **reciprocal inhibition** (see Flexibility Concept 7.4). Despite the promotion of these mechanisms in the strength and conditioning literature (e.g., Jefferys, 2008), there is no convincing evidence that neuromuscular relaxation contributes to the efficacy of PNF techniques (Sharman et al., 2006).

Other mechanisms to explain the greater increases in range of motion following PNF stretching techniques compared to static stretching include enhanced extensibility of the MTU, although this hypothesis again has received little experimental support (Sharman et al., 2006). Indeed, passive stiffness has been shown to increase following habitual PNF stretching techniques (Rees, Murphy, Watsford, McLachlan, & Coutts, 2007). This leaves an increase in stretch tolerance as the most likely explanation for the enhanced efficacy of PNF stretching techniques over static stretching methods (Chalmers, 2004; Sharman et al., 2006; also so Applied Research 7.4). An effective PNF stretching protocol to increase the range of motion during hip flexion is shown in Applied Flexibility Protocol 7.2.

Recommendations for Stretching Routines

This section highlights the duration of the stretches, the number of stretches performed in each session, the number of sessions per week, the progression of the stretches,

Flexibility Concept 7.4

Autogenic inhibition and reciprocal inhibition do not contribute to the effectiveness of PNF stretching techniques

Autogenic inhibition refers to the reduced excitability of an actively or passively stretched muscle as a result of the activation of Ib-inhibitory interneuron associated with Golgi tendon organs (GTOs). The activation of the GTO during the isometric action associated with the contract–relax PNF technique has been proposed to subsequently reduce the efferent drive to the target muscle and allow the MTU to undergo a greater elongation (Figure 7.7).

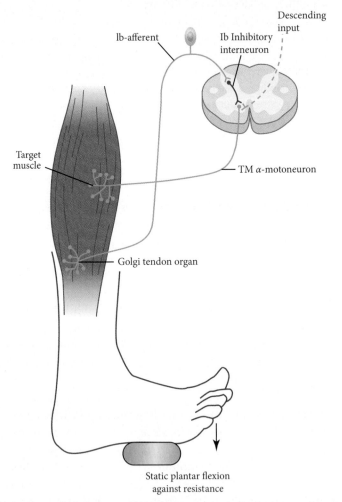

Figure 7.7 Autogenic inhibition is proposed to contribute to the neuromuscular relaxation of the target muscle during the contract–relax PNF stretching technique. A voluntary isometric action of the ankle plantarflexor is performed when the plantarflexors are at the limit of their range of motion. The isometric action activates the Golgi tendon organs (GTOs) within the target muscle (TM), which decreases the excitability of the TM via the Ib-inhibitory interneuron.

Reproduced from Sharman, M. J., Cresswell, A. G., & Riek, S. (2006). Proprioceptive neuromuscular facilitation stretching. Mechanisms and clinical implications. *Sports Medicine, 36*, 929–939, with kind permission from Springer Science and Business Media.

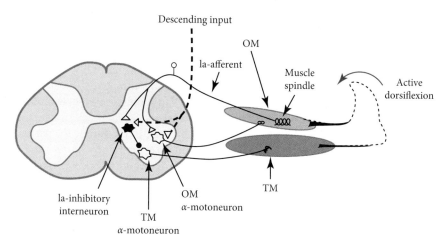

Figure 7.8 Reciprocal inhibition is proposed to contribute to the neuromuscular relaxation of the target muscle during the agonist–contract PNF stretching technique. A concentric action of the dorsiflexors (OM) during the stretch of the plantarflexors (TM) excites the Ia afferents and the associated Ia-inhibitory interneuron, which decreases the excitability of the TM.

Reproduced from Sharman, M. J., Cresswell, A. G., & Riek, S. (2006). Proprioceptive neuromuscular facilitation stretching. Mechanisms and clinical implications. *Sports Medicine, 36,* 929–939, with kind permission from Springer Science and Business Media.

The reduced excitability of the target muscle can also be achieved via reciprocal inhibition. Here activation of the opposing muscle (antagonist) during an imposed stretch of the target muscle as per the agonist–contract PNF technique excites the Ia-inhibitory interneurons; this effect inhibits the excitability of the target muscle, allowing it to be elongated further (Figure 7.8).

Evidence to support the contribution of these reflexes to an increased relaxation of the muscle during PNF techniques as identified via electromyographic recordings of the target muscle during the stretches is currently lacking (Chalmers, 2004; Sharman et al., 2006). Therefore, the efficacy of PNF techniques at increasing flexibility must be due to other mechanisms.

and the methods that can be used to enhance the response to the stretches used in stretching routines.

Duration of Stretches Within Each Session

Holding static stretches for 15 s appears to be less effective than holding them for 30 s (Bandy & Irion, 1994), probably due to the stress–relaxation response, which requires at least 20 s to stabilize (McNair et al., 2000). However, there appears to be no difference in the gains in flexibility when static stretches are held for 30 s compared to 1 min (Bandy, Irion, & Briggler, 1997). A duration of 45 s per static stretch is associated with alterations in the viscoelastic characteristics of the tendon structures (Kubo et al., 2002a). With PNF stretching techniques, it is the duration of the stretches and muscle activation that need to be considered. Typically, it is recommended that the stretches

Applied Research 7.4

Effects of PNF stretching on measures of static and dynamic flexibility

Rees et al. (2007) investigated the effects of the habitual performance of PNF stretches on measures of static and dynamic flexibility. The participants completed 4 weeks of training, in which a combination of the contract–relax and agonist–contract techniques were performed 3 times per week for the ankle plantarflexors. During each stretch, the ankle joint was moved to an end-point (prior to discomfort), at which time the participant performed a maximal isometric action for 6 s. The joint was then returned to neutral position for 2 s, after which it was returned to the end-point where a concentric action of agonist was performed for 6 s. The stretches were repeated 4 times with a 1-min recovery period. The force during the passive movement of the ankle joint to the end-point was assessed during each session to provide a measure of stretch tolerance. The stretching protocol was progressed by increasing the length of the isometric and concentric actions to 10 s and increasing the number of stretches to 6, with a concomitant increase in the recovery period to 2 min. Static flexibility was assessed using a goniometer, and dynamic flexibility was assessed using a damped free oscillation technique.

The authors reported that static flexibility was significantly increased, whereas the passive stiffness of the musculotendinous unit was also increased following the training period. Stretch tolerance was significantly increased as a result of the PNF stretches.

Rees, S. S., Murphy, A. J., Watsford, M. L., McLachlan, K. A., & Coutts, A. J. (2007). Effects of proprioceptive neuromuscular facilitation stretching on stiffness and force-producing characteristics of the ankle in active women. *Journal of Strength and Conditioning Research, 21*, 572–577.

Applied Flexibility Protocol 7.2

PNF stretching techniques to increase the range of motion during hip flexion

The contract–relax and agonist–contract PNF stretching techniques can be used to develop the flexibility of the hip joint.

Contract–Relax Technique (Figure 7.9)

1. The participant lies supine and raises the leg to be stretched.

2. The partner supports the leg at the knee and the ankle and moves the hip joint slowly into flexion.

3. At the point where the participant initially feels discomfort, the partner holds the leg stationary.

4. The participant then attempts to voluntarily extend the hip joint, and the partner resists the impending motion, producing an isometric action of the hip extensors. The level of activation by the participant during the isometric hip extension does not have to be at a maximal level, as values as low as 30% of the participant's maximum have been shown to be effective.

5. The isometric action is held for between 5 and 10 s, following which the participant relaxes.

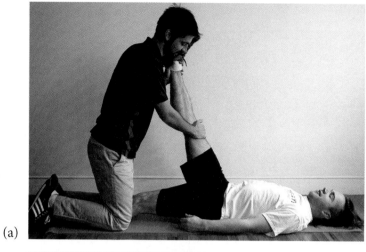

(a)

(b)

Figure 7.9 The contract–relax PNF stretching technique. (a) The partner moves the hip joint to the point where the participant initially feels discomfort. The participant then activates the hamstrings group to between 30% and 100% of maximal level, with the partner resisting this for 5–10 s. (b) Once the participant has relaxed, the partner moves the joint further until the point of discomfort and the position is held for 10–30 s.

6. The partner then slowly moves the joint further into flexion until the participant feels mild discomfort.

7. The new position is held for 10–30 s, following which the leg is lowered slowly to its starting position.

8. A recovery period of between 1 and 2 min is provided, and then another stretch is performed.

9. A total of 2–6 stretches are completed within each session.

10. Consider methods to quantify the range of motion achieved during each stretch (e.g., tape measure, goniometer, inclinometer) so that progress can be determined.

(continues)

(continued)

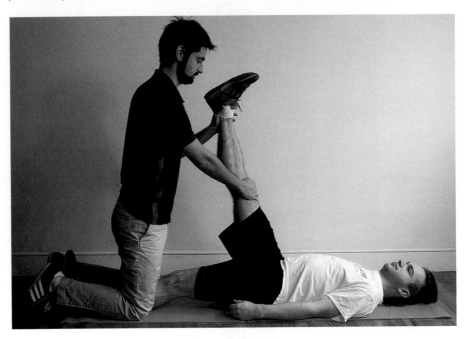

Figure 7.10 The agonist–contract PNF stretching technique. The partner moves the hip joint to the point where the participant initially feels discomfort. The participant then activates the agonist muscles (hip flexors) for 5 s, while the partner moves the joint further until the point of discomfort; this position is held for 10–30 s.

Agonist–Contract Technique (Figure 7.10)

1. The participant and partner assume the same starting positions as for the contract–relax technique.

2. The hip is moved slowly into flexion by the partner until the initial point of mild discomfort is experienced by the participant; the partner holds the leg stationary for 10 s.

3. The participant then activates the agonist (hip flexors) for 5 s as the partner slowly moves the hip joint into greater flexion until the point of mild discomfort is reached.

4. This position is held for 10–30 s, after which the leg is lowered slowly to its starting position.

5. A recovery period of between 1 and 2 min is provided, and then another stretch is performed.

6. A total of 2–6 stretches are completed within each session.

7. Consider methods to quantify the range of motion achieved during each stretch (e.g., tape measure, goniometer, inclinometer) so that progress can be determined.

with the joint held at the limit of the joint's range (determined by the sensation associated with the stretch) be held for between 10 and 30 s (Chen et al., 2011; Jefferys, 2008; Rowlands, Marginson, & Lee, 2003). The isometric action associated with the contract–relax technique and the activation of the agonist muscle during the agonist–contract technique are typically maintained between 5 and 10 s (Chen et al., 2011; Rees et al., 2007; Rowlands et al., 2003).

Number of Stretches Within Each Session

Static stretching techniques that involve 3–6 repetitions of the stretching exercise, with each repetition separated by a 5- to 30-s recovery period, have been shown to be effective in increasing flexibility (Bandy et al., 1997; Hunter & Marshall, 2002; Kubo et al., 2002b; Sands, McNeal, Stone, Russell, & Jemni, 2006; Ylinen et al. 2009). A single PNF stretch performed within each session has been shown to effectively increase flexibility (Sharman et al., 2006), although typically the stretches are repeated between 2 and 6 times, with a recovery period of between 1 and 2 min provided between stretches (Chen et al., 2011; Rees et al., 2007; Rowlands et al., 2003).

Number of Stretching Sessions per Week

Engaging in static stretching three times per week once daily has been shown to be effective at increasing flexibility, although the gains in flexibility were greater when the stretching sessions were performed more frequently (Cipriani et al., 2012). For PNF stretching techniques, two sessions per week appear to be effective at increasing flexibility (Sharman et al., 2006), although others have completed three sessions per week (Chen et al., 2011; Rees et al., 2007). The greatest gains for both static stretching and PNF techniques appear to occur within the first three weeks of the intervention, and it may be appropriate to reduce the frequency to once or twice per week to maintain these gains. However, the assessment of flexibility should occur relatively frequently to determine the effectiveness of the program.

Progression of Stretches

The stretching regimen can be progressed by increasing either the duration or the intensity of the stretches, or both. This obviously requires that the practitioner is able to determine the duration and intensity of each stretch. The duration of a stretch can be determined fairly easily, of course, and a 10-s increase in the duration of the static stretches every 2 weeks beginning from a 20-s stretch has been shown to be effective at increasing flexibility in a 10-week study (Hunter & Marshall, 2002).

Measuring the intensity of the stretch may be more problematic. The practitioner can record the joint angle attained through either linear or angular measurements, or he or she can assess the sensation associated with different magnitude of stretch to determine the associated intensity. Stretches should be performed at or below the pain threshold of the individual. However, the sensation used (e.g., "onset of mild discomfort," "onset of stiffness," "onset of stretch") should be consistent between stretching sessions, as the end-range joint angles differ depending on the specific sensation used (Weppler & Magnuson, 2010). Furthermore, the perception of stretch can be modified by the posture adopted during the stretch (Laessøe & Voigt, 2004); thus the posture should remain consistent between stretching sessions.

In a study using static stretches, the intensity of each stretch was increased every 2–3 days for 4 weeks by increasing the starting joint angle at the beginning of each movement (Ylinen et al., 2009). For PNF techniques, progressively increasing the intensity of the isometric action from 30% of the individual's maximal voluntary contraction (MVC) to 70% MVC over a 2-week period results in greater gains in range of motion than maintaining a constant intensity MVC (50%) (Schmitt, Pelham, & Holt, 1999). Note that the intensity of the muscle activation does not have to be maximal for PNF techniques to be effective.

Methods to Enhance the Response to Stretching

There is no difference in the change in static flexibility when stretching exercises are performed after an exercise session (Cornelius, Hagermann, & Jackson, 1988; de Weijer, Gorniak, & Shamus, 2002). Indeed, 10 minutes of jogging followed by 5×30-s static stretches has been found to be no more effective than the completion of a static-stretching-only protocol in increasing static flexibility; the combination of running and stretching was not as effective at increasing dynamic flexibility as a running-only protocol, but was more effective than the stretching-only protocol (McNair & Stanley, 1996). Nevertheless, it may be practical to perform stretching routines after a workout, although the practitioner should be aware that the visco-elastic properties of MTU can be altered by exercise-induced fatigue, with stiffness under relatively high passive loads increasing (Noda, Shibayama, Ishige, & Fukashiro, 2000). PNF stretches are sometimes performed after the completion of low-intensity dynamic activities (e.g., jogging) and following the completion of static stretches for the target muscles (Chen et al., 2011; Rowlands et al., 2003).

The use of **passive heating** or **passive cooling** methods applied during the imposed stretch has been shown to enhance the range of motion following static stretches but not PNF techniques (Shrier & Glossal, 2000). A **vibration** stimulus (30 Hz, 2-mm displacement) applied to target muscle during static stretches has been shown to enhance the gains in static flexibility beyond those associated with static stretches over a 4-week period (Sands et al., 2006). These increases are likely due to an increase in the MTU temperature associated with the vibration stimulus, which may increase the stretch tolerance and/or the extensibility of the tissue.

Myofascial release techniques, including foam rolling of the target tissue, are becoming common in both strength and conditioning and athletic training. These techniques are proposed to increase the extensibility of the MTU by relieving spasms, breaking adhesions, and increasing blood flow and lymphatic drainage (Paolini, 2009). However, evidence of changes in MTU extensibility as assessed through measures of dynamic flexibility is currently lacking. Furthermore, well-designed comparisons of the effectiveness of myofascial release techniques and the traditional methods of static stretching and PNF remain to be performed.

Individualization of the Stretching Routine of Athletes

The recommendations for a stretching routine will necessarily be generic as opposed to specific to any particular athlete. It is the responsibility of the strength and conditioning coach to determine which protocols work for each athlete and to individualize the routine accordingly. This requires practitioners to test their athletes regularly. Table 7.3 summarizes the recommendations for the use of static and PNF techniques within a stretching routine to enhance flexibility.

Table 7.3
Recommendations for Effective Stretching Routines Using Static and PNF Techniques

Variable	Static Stretching Routine	Proprioceptive Neuromuscular Facilitation
Duration of stretches	45 s	Contract–relax technique: hold stretch for 10 s; relax for 10 s; isometric action for 6–10 s; further stretch for 10 s Agonist–contract technique: 5-s activation of agonist; hold stretch for 10 s
Number of stretches per session	3–6 stretches with 5- to 30-s recovery	2–6 stretches with 1- to 2-min recovery
Number of sessions per week	3 × week	2–3 × week
Progression of stretches	Determine intensity from sensation (e.g., "point of mild discomfort") Increase duration by 10 s every 2 weeks	Determine intensity from sensation (e.g., "point of mild discomfort") Increase the number of stretches (1 per week) Increase the length of muscle activation (2 s per week) Increase the intensity of muscle activation (10–20% per week)
Methods to enhance stretches	Application of passive heating, cooling, or vibration stimulus	Low-intensity dynamic activities (e.g., jogging) and static stretches performed prior to PNF stretches
Individualize the routine	Test athletes to determine the most effective routine	Test athletes to determine the most effective routine

Combining Training Modes

It is unlikely that any athlete will engage in only one mode of training at any time during his or her training program. While stretching techniques are effective methods to increase flexibility and are widely promoted, the athlete will be engaging in other modes of training concurrently. It is pertinent, then, to consider the effects of combined training modes on measures of flexibility as well as measures of performance.

Klinge et al. (1997) reported that 13 weeks of isometric resistance training resulted in a 43% increase in isometric strength. However, passive stiffness and resistance during a test of dynamic flexibility also increased, presumably due to the increase in cross-sectional area of the trained muscles. The combination of the resistance training with flexibility training (static stretching) did not alter the adaptations.

Kubo et al. (2002b) found that 8 weeks of resistance training resulted in an increase in maximal isometric force and muscle volume. These responses were not attenuated when the resistance training was combined with a regimen of static stretching. However, the reduction in dynamic flexibility following the resistance training was abolished when it was combined with the stretching exercises. Furthermore, the combination of resistance training and static stretches was shown to reduce the hysteresis of the tendon while maintaining the increase in tendon stiffness. This may allow greater storage and return of strain potential energy.

Thus stretching exercises performed habitually may potentiate the performance adaptations gained from a period of resistance training (see Flexibility Concept 7.5).

Flexibility Concept 7.5

Does the addition of stretching exercises potentiate the response of other training modes?

In a systematic review of the literature, Shrier (2004) concluded that regular stretching exercises improved performance in activities requiring high force and power, and sprinting speed, although the research on running and walking economy was equivocal. Wilson et al. (1992) reported that the combination of resistance training and flexibility exercises (static stretching) reduced the passive stiffness of the MTU, resulting in improved performance during strength tests relying on the stretch–shortening cycle by means of increasing the contribution of strain potential energy to the movement. Hunter and Marshall (2002) reported that 10 weeks of plyometric training increased countermovement (CMJ) and drop jump performance between 2.3% and 3.7%; when this training was combined with a static stretching regimen, the improvements ranged from 3.4% to 4.9%. The stretching regimen by itself resulted in a slight improvement in CMJ performance only.

The mechanisms underlying this apparent potentiation of the response of resistance training as a result of the inclusion of regular stretching exercises are currently unknown. Perhaps the stretching regimen aids the repair and recovery of the MTU following the resistance training stimulus, although the research to support this contention is limited (Robson-Ansley, Gleeson, & Ansley, 2009; Torres, Ribeiro, Duarte, & Cabri, 2012). Or perhaps the stretching exercises attenuate the negative adaptations that accompany resistance training, such as the hysteresis of the tendinous structures (Kubo et al., 2002b), or perhaps they induce adaptations that are not associated with resistance training, such as increasing the extensibility of the perimysial connective tissue (Kubo et al., 2002a). Although the mechanism of action is currently unknown, it would appear that the inclusion of a stretching regimen is likely to potentiate the response of resistance and power training, particularly in activities that involve the stretch–shortening cycle.

For this reason, methods of enhancing flexibility need to be integrated with other training components to optimize performance in a given sporting task (Sands, 2011).

Chapter Summary

Flexibility is defined as the range of motion available at a joint or group of joints without inducing an injury to the surrounding structures. Flexibility is influenced by a number of factors, with the main differences in flexibility between individuals being noted in the extensibility of the MTU, neuromuscular relaxation, and stretch tolerance. Static flexibility is measured when an individual moves a joint to the limit of the range of motion, with the end-point of the assessment defined by a subjective sensation. Flexibility is then quantified by a kinematic descriptor. Measures of static flexibility do not provide information about the mechanical characteristics of the MTU that limit the range of motion about a joint. In contrast, dynamic flexibility tests allow the direct assessment of the viscoelastic properties of the MTU. Such assessments have shown that the difference between flexible and inflexible individuals is largely due to the greater pain tolerance in the flexible individuals.

Flexibility would appear to be important for aesthetic sports, but its importance in other sports is less clear. It is therefore likely that flexibility for a given athlete is a case of optimization rather than maximization. The importance of flexibility as a risk factor in sports injuries is difficult to ascertain, although flexibility training has been shown to attenuate exercise-induced muscle damage.

Stretching techniques are commonly employed to develop flexibility. Static stretching involves taking a joint to the limit of the available range of motion and holding the stretch for a predetermined time. PNF stretching techniques have been proposed to promote the relaxation of the target muscle via either autogenic inhibition (contract–relax technique) or reciprocal inhibition (agonist–contract technique). Habitual PNF techniques are more effective at increasing flexibility compared to static techniques, although there is currently no convincing evidence that this effect arises due to the neuromuscular relaxation that is proposed to accompany these techniques; rather, PNF techniques may simply promote a greater tolerance to the imposed stretch of the MTU during tests of flexibility. Evidence indicates that the inclusion of stretching exercises may potentiate the responses to a resistance training regimen by attenuating the reduction in tendon hysteresis or by increasing the extensibility of the perimysial connective tissue, thereby enhancing performance in activities incorporating the stretch–shortening cycle.

Review Questions and Projects

1. Provide a definition of static flexibility.

2. Provide a definition of dynamic flexibility.

3. Identify the factors that most likely differ between flexible and inflexible athletes.

4. Explain the difference between flexibility and joint laxity.

5. Explain the contributions of the contractile components to the extensibility of musculotendinous units.

6. Explain the contributions of the series and parallel elastic components to the extensibility of musculotendinous units.

7. Describe how the viscoelastic characteristics of stress–relaxation, creep, and stiffness affect the flexibility of musculotendinous units.

8. What is a torque–angle curve?

9. What information can a torque–angle curve provide about the flexibility of an athlete?

10. Explain why female athletes may be more flexible than their male counterparts.

11. Explain why older athletes may be less flexible than their younger counterparts.

12. Discuss the potential role of flexibility in athletic performance.

13. Identify the sports in which performance is most likely to be influenced by an increase in flexibility.

14. Identify the sports in which performance might be adversely affected by increased flexibility.

15. Discuss the potential role of flexibility in injury risk.

16. Do age and sex influence the response to the methods to increase flexibility?

17. Develop a stretching regimen for a tennis player that includes static stretches. Consider how the program would be progressed.

18. Which athletes are most likely to benefit from the inclusion of a regular regimen of stretching in their training program?

19. Develop a stretching regimen for a 100-m sprint athlete that includes PNF stretches. Consider how the program would be progressed.

20. Discuss the methods that could be employed to enhance the effects of stretching exercises.

References

Arnason, A., Sigurdsson, S. B., Gudmundsson, A., Holme, I., Engerbresten, L., & Bahr, R. (2004). Physical fitness, injuries, and team performance in soccer. *Medicine and Science in Sports and Exercise*, *36*, 278–285.

Bandy, W. D., & Irion, J. M. (1994). The effect of time of static stretch on the flexibility of the hamstring muscles. *Physical Therapy, 74*, 845–852.

Bandy, W. D., Irion, J. M., & Briggler, M. (1997). The effect of time and frequency of static stretching on flexibility of the hamstring muscles. *Physical Therapy, 77*, 1090–1096.

Blackburn, J. T., Riemann, B. L., Padua, D. A., & Guskiewicz, K. M. (2004). Sex comparison of extensibility, passive, and active stiffness of the knee flexors. *Clinical Biomechanics, 19*, 36–43.

Bojsen-Møller, J., Brogaard, K., Have, M. J., Stryger, H. P., Kjær, M., Aagaard, P., & Magnusson, S. P. (2007). Passive knee joint range of motion is unrelated to the mechanical properties of the patellar tendon. *Scandinavian Journal of Medicine and Science in Sports, 17*, 415–421.

Chalmers, G. (2004). Re-examination of the possible role of Golgi tendon organ and muscle spindle reflexes in proprioceptive neuromuscular facilitation muscle stretching. *Sports Biomechanics, 3*, 159–183.

Chen, C-H., Nosaka, K., Chen, H-L., Lin, M-J., Tseng, K-W., & Chen, T. C. (2011). Effects of flexibility training on eccentric exercise-induced muscle damage. *Medicine and Science in Sports and Exercise, 43*, 491–500.

Cipriani, D. J., Terry, M. E., Haiines, M. A., Tabibnia, A. P., & Lyssanova, O. (2012). Effect of stretch frequency and sex on the rate of gain and rate of loss in muscle flexibility during a hamstring-stretching program: A randomized single-blind longitudinal study. *Journal of Strength and Conditioning Research, 26*, 2119–2129.

Cornelius, W. L., Hagermann, R. W., & Jackson, A. W. (1988). A study on the placement of stretching within a workout. *Journal of Sports Medicine and Physical Fitness, 28*, 234–236.

Craib, M. W., Mitchell, V. A., Fields, K. B., Hopewell, R., & Morgan, D. W. (1996). The association between flexibility and running economy in sub-elite male distance runners. *Medicine and Science in Sports and Exercise, 28*, 737–743.

de Visser, H. M., Reijman, M., Heijboer, M. P., & Bos, P. K. (2012). Risk factors of recurrent hamstring injuries: A systematic review. *British Journal of Sports Medicine, 46*, 124–130.

de Weijer, V. C., Gorniak, G. C., & Shamus, E. (2002). The effects of static stretch and warm-up exercise on hamstring length over the course of 24 hours. *Journal of Orthopaedic and Sports Physical Therapy, 33*, 727–733.

Ebben, W. P., & Blackard, D. O. (2001). Strength and conditioning practices of National Football League strength and conditioning coaches. *Journal of Strength and Conditioning Research, 15*, 48–58.

Ebben, W. P., Carroll, R. M., & Simenz, C.J. (2004). Strength and conditioning practices of National Hockey League strength and conditioning coaches. *Journal of Strength and Conditioning Research, 18,* 889–897.

Ebben, W. P., Hintz, M. J., & Simenz, C. J. (2005). Strength and conditioning practices of Major League Baseball strength and conditioning coaches. *Journal of Strength and Conditioning Research, 19,* 538–546.

Ellenbecker, T. S., Ellenbecker, G. A., Roetert, E. P., Silva, R. T., Keuter, G., & Sperling, F. (2007). Descriptive profile of hip rotation range of motion in elite tennis players and professional baseball pitchers. *American Journal of Sports Medicine, 35,* 1371–1376.

Enoka, R. M. (2008). *Neuromechanics of human movement.* Champaign, IL: Human Kinetic.

Fredette, D. M. (2001). Exercise recommendations for flexibility and range of motion. In J. L. Roitman (Ed.), *ACSM's resource manual for guidelines for exercise testing and prescription* (pp. 468–477). Baltimore, MD: Lippincott Williams & Wilkins.

Gajdosik, R. L., Vander Linden, D. W., McNair, P. J., Riggin, T. J., Albertson, J. S., Mattick, D. J., & Wegley, J. C. (2005). Viscoelastic properties of short calf muscle–tendon units of older women: Effects of slow and fast passive dorsiflexion stretches in vivo. *European Journal of Applied Physiology, 95,* 131–139.

Girouard, C. K., & Hurley, B. F. (1995). Does strength training inhibit gains in range of motion from flexibility training in older adults? *Medicine and Science in Sports and Exercise, 27,* 1444–1449.

Gleim, G. W. (1984). The profiling of professional football players. *Clinical Sports Medicine, 3,* 185–197.

Gleim, G. W., & McHugh, M. P. (1997). Flexibility and its effects on sports injury and performance. *Sports Medicine, 24,* 289–299.

Gleim, G. W., Stachenfeld, N. S., & Nicholas, J. A. (1990). The influence of flexibility on the economy of walking and jogging. *Journal of Orthopedic Research, 8,* 814–823.

Gordon, B. S., Moir, G. L., Davis, S. E., Witmer, C. A., & Cummings, D. M. (2009). An investigation into the relationship of flexibility, power, and strength to club head speed in male golfers. *Journal of Strength and Conditioning Research, 23,* 1606–1610.

Guidetti, L., Di Cagno, A., Chiara Gallotta, M., Battaglia, C., Piazza, M., & Baldari, C. (2009). Precompetition warm-up in elite and subelite rhythmic gymnastics. *Journal of Strength and Conditioning Research, 23,* 1877–1882.

Guieu, R., Blin, O., Pouget, J., & Serratrice, G. (1992). Nociceptive threshold and physical activity. *Canadian Journal of Neurological Sciences, 19,* 69–71.

Guissard, N., & Duchateau, J. (2004). Effect of static stretch training on neural and mechanical properties of human plantar-flexor muscles. *Muscle and Nerve, 29,* 248–255.

Halbertsma, J. P. K., & Goeken, L. N. H. (1994). Stretching exercises: Effects of passive extensibility and stiffness in short hamstrings of healthy subjects. *Archives of Physical Medicine and Rehabilitation, 75,* 976–981.

Haywood, K. M., & Williams, K. (1995). Age–gender and flexibility differences in tennis serving among experienced older adults. *Journal of Aging and Physical Activity, 3,* 54–66.

Horowits, R., & Podolsky, R. J. (1987). The positional stability of thick filaments in activated skeletal muscle depends on sarcomere length: Evidence for the role of titin filaments. *Journal of Cell Biology, 105,* 2217–2223.

Hunter, G. R., Katsoulis, K., McCarthy, J. P., Ogard, W. K., Bamman, M. M., Wood, D. S., . . . Newcomer, B. R. (2011). Tendon length and joint flexibility are related to running economy. *Medicine and Science in Sports and Exercise, 43,* 1492–1499.

Hunter, J. P., & Marshall, R. N. (2002). Effects of power and flexibility training on vertical jump technique. *Medicine and Science in Sports and Exercise, 34,* 478–486.

Jefferys, I. (2008). Warm-up and stretching. In T. R. Baechle & R. W. Earle (Eds.), *Essentials of strength training and conditioning* (pp. 295–324). Champaign, IL: Human Kinetics.

Junior, R. S., Leite, T., & Reis, V. M. (2011). Influence of the number of sets at strength training in the flexibility gains. *Journal of Human Kinetics, supplement,* 47–52.

Khals, P. S., & Ge, W. (2004). Encoding of tensile stress and strain during stretch by muscle mechano-nociceptors. *Muscle and Nerve, 30,* 216–224.

Klinge, K., Magnusson, S. P., Simonsen, E. B., Aagaard, P., Klausen, K., & Kjær, M. (1997). The effect of strength and flexibility training on skeletal muscle EMG activity, stiffness and viscoelastic stress relaxation response. *American Journal of Sports Medicine, 25,* 710–716.

Knudson, D. V., Magnusson, P., & McHugh, M. (2000). Current issues in flexibility fitness. *President's Council on Physical Fitness and Sports Research Digest, 3,* 1–6.

Konor, M. M., Morton, S., Eckerson, J. M., & Grindstaff, T. L. (2012). Reliability of three measures of ankle dorsiflexion range of motion. *International Journal of Sports Physical Therapy, 7,* 279–287.

Kubo, K., Kanehisa, H., & Fukunaga, T. (2001). Is passive stiffness in human muscles related to the elasticity of tendon structures? *European Journal of Applied Physiology, 85,* 226–232.

Kubo, K., Kanehisa, H., & Fukunaga, T. (2002a). Effects of stretching training on the viscoelastic properties of human tendon structures in vivo. *Journal of Applied Physiology, 92,* 595–601.

Kubo, K., Kanehisa, H., & Fukunaga, T. (2002b). Effects of resistance and stretching training programmes on the viscoelastic properties of human tendon structures *in vivo. Journal of Physiology, 538,* 219–226.

Kubo, K., Kanehisa, H., Kawakami, Y., & Fukunaga, T. (2001). Influence of static stretching on viscoelastic properties of human tendon structures in vivo. *Journal of Applied Physiology, 90,* 520–527.

Laessøe, U., & Voigt, M. (2004). Modifications of stretch tolerance in a stooping position. *Scandinavian Journal of Medicine and Science in Sports, 14,* 239–244.

Lin, C.-C. K., Ju, M.-S., & Huang, H.-W. (2005). Gender and age effects on elbow joint stiffness in healthy subjects. *Archives of Physical Medicine and Rehabilitation, 86,* 82–85.

Magid, A., & Law, D. J. (1985). Myofibrils bear most of the resting tension in frog skeletal muscle. *Science, 230,* 1280–1282.

Magnusson, S. P. (1998). Passive properties of human skeletal muscle during stretch maneuvers: A review. *Scandinavian Journal of Medicine and Science in Sports, 8,* 65–77.

Magnusson, S. P., Aagaard, P., Simonsen, E. B., & Bojsen-Møller, F. (1998). A biomechanical evaluation of cyclic and static stretch in human skeletal muscle. *International Journal of Sports Medicine, 19,* 310–316.

Magnusson, S. P., Aagaard, P., Simonsen, E. B., & Bojsen-Møller, F. (2000). Passive tensile stress and energy of the human hamstring muscles *in vivo. Scandinavian Journal of Medicine and Science in Sports, 10,* 351–359.

Magnusson, S. P., Gleim, G. W., & Nicholas, J. A. (1994). Shoulder weakness in professional baseball pitchers. *Medicine and Science in Sports and Exercise, 26,* 5–9.

Magnusson, S. P., & Renström, P. (2006). The European College of Sports Sciences Position statement: The role of stretching exercises in sports. *European Journal of Sport Science, 6,* 87–91.

Magnusson, S. P., Simonsen, E. B., Aagaard, P., Boesen, J., Johannsen, F., & Kjær, M. (1997). Determinants of musculoskeletal flexibility: Viscoelastic properties, cross-sectional area, EMG and stretch tolerance. *Scandinavian Journal of Medicine and Science in Sports, 7,* 195–202.

Magnusson, S. P., Simonsen, E. B., Aagaard, P., Dyhre-Poulsen, P., McHugh, M. P., & Kjær, M. (1996). Mechanical and physiological responses to stretching with and without preisometric contraction in human skeletal muscle. *Archives of Physical Medicine and Rehabilitation, 77,* 373–378.

Magnusson, S. P., Simonsen, E. B., Aagaard, P., & Kjær, M. (1996). Biomechanical responses to repeated stretches in human skeletal muscle *in vivo. American Journal of Sports Medicine, 24,* 622–628.

Magnusson, S. P., Simonsen, E. B., Aagaard, P., Sorensen, H., & Kjær, M. (1996). A mechanism for altered flexibility in human skeletal muscle. *Journal of Physiology, 497,* 291–298.

Malfait, F., Hakim, A. J., De Paepe, A., & Grahame, R. (2006). The genetic basis of the joint hypermobility syndromes. *Rheumatology, 45,* 502–507.

Marchettini, P. (1993). Muscle pain: Animal and human experimental and clinical studies. *Muscle and Nerve, 16,* 1033–1039.

McCormack, M., Briggs, J., Hakim, A., & Grahame, R. (2004). Joint laxity and the benign joint hypermobility syndrome in student and professional ballet dancers. *Journal of Rheumatology, 31,* 173–178.

McHugh, M. P., Connolly, D. A. J., Eston, R. G., Kremenic, I. J., Nicolas, S. J., & Gleim, G. W. (1999). The role of passive muscle stiffness in symptoms of exercise-induced muscle damage. *American Journal of Sports Medicine, 27,* 594–599.

McHugh, M. P., Magnusson, S. P., Gleim, G. W., Magnusson, S. P., & Nicholas, J. A. (1993). A cross-sectional study of age-related musculoskeletal and physiological changes in soccer players. *Medicine Exercise Nutrition and Health, 2,* 261–268.

McHugh, M. P., Magnusson, S. P., Gleim, G. W., & Nicholas, J. A. (1992). Viscoelastic stress relaxation in human skeletal muscle. *Medicine and Science in Sports and Exercise, 24,* 1375–1382.

McNair, P. J., Dombroski, E. W., Hewson, D. J., & Stanley, S. N. (2000). Stretching at the ankle joint: Viscoelastic responses to holds and continuous passive motion. *Medicine and Science in Sports and Exercise, 33*, 354–358.

McNair, P. J., & Stanley, S. N. (1996). Effect of passive stretching and jogging on the series elastic muscle stiffness and range of motion of the ankle joint. *British Journal of Sports Medicine, 30*, 313–318.

Meckel, Y., Atterbom, H., Grodjinovsky, A., Ben-Sira, D., & Rotstein, A. (1995). Physiological characteristics of female 100 metre sprinters of different performance levels. *Journal of Sports Medicine and Physical Fitness, 35*, 169–175.

Mookerjee, S., Bibi, K. W., Kenney, G. A., & Cohen, L. (1995). Relationship between isokinetic strength, flexibility, and flutter kicking speed in female collegiate swimmers. *Journal of Strength and Conditioning Research, 9*, 71–74.

Moore, I. S., Jones, A. M., & Dixon, S. J. (2012). Mechanisms for improved running economy in beginner runners. *Medicine and Science in Sports and Exercise, 44*, 1756–1763.

Morse, C. I. (2011). Gender differences in the passive stiffness of the human gastrocnemius muscle during stretch. *European Journal of Applied Physiology, 111*, 2149–2154.

Morse, C. I., Degens, H., Seynnes, O. R., Maganaris, C. N., & Jones, D. A. (2008). The acute effects of stretching on the passive stiffness of the human gastrocnemius muscle tendon unit. *Journal of Physiology, 586*, 97–106.

Myer, G. D., Ford, K. R., Paterno, M. V., Nick, T. G., & Hewett, T. E. (2008). The effects of generalized joint laxity on risk of anterior cruciate ligament injury in young female athletes. *American Journal of Sports Medicine, 36*, 1073–1080.

Nawata, K., Teshima, R., Morio, Y., Hagino, H., Enokida, M., & Yamamoto, K. (1999). Anterior–posterior knee laxity increased by exercise: Quantitative evaluation of physiological changes. *Acta Orthopaedica Scandinavica, 70*, 261–264.

Noda, M., Shibayama, A., Ishige, Y., & Fukashiro, S. (2000). Change of viscoelastic properties in human triceps surae after isometric endurance exercise. *Japanese Journal of Biomechanics in Sports and Exercise, 4*, 232–242.

Nordez, A., Casari, P., & Cornu, C. (2008). Effects of stretching velocity on passive resistance developed by the knee musculo-articular complex: Contributions of frictional and viscoelastic behaviours. *European Journal of Applied Physiology, 103*, 243–250.

Oberg, B., Ekstrand, J., Möller, M., & Gillquist, J. (1984). Muscle strength and flexibility in different positions of soccer players. *International Journal of Sports Medicine, 5*, 213–216.

Paolini, J. (2009). Review of myofascial release as an effective massage therapy technique. *Athletic Therapy Today, 14*, 30–34.

Protas, E. J. (2001). Flexibility and range of motion. In J. L. Roitman (Ed.), *ACSM's resource manual for guidelines for exercise testing and prescription* (pp. 381–390). Baltimore, MD: Lippincott Williams & Wilkins.

Purslow, P. P. (1989). Strain-induced reorientation of an intramuscular connective tissue network: Implications for passive muscle elasticity. *Journal of Biomechanics, 22*, 21–31.

Purslow, P. P., Wess, T. J., & Hukins, D. W. L. (1998). Collagen orientation and molecular spacing during creep and stress-relaxation in soft connective tissues. *Journal of Experimental Biology, 201*, 135–142.

Ramesh, R., VonArx, O., Azzopardi, T., & Schranz, P. J. (2005). The risk of anterior cruciate ligament rupture with generalized joint laxity. *Journal of Bone and Joint Surgery, 87-B*, 800–803.

Rees, S. S., Murphy, A. J., Watsford, M. L., McLachlan, K. A., & Coutts, A. J. (2007). Effects of proprioceptive neuromuscular facilitation stretching on stiffness and force-producing characteristics of the ankle in active women. *Journal of Strength and Conditioning Research, 21*, 572–577.

Reid, D. C., Burnham, R. S., Saboe, L. A., & Kushner, S. F. (1987). Lower extremity flexibility patterns in classical ballet dancers and their correlation to lateral hip and knee injuries. *American Journal of Sports Medicine, 4*, 347–352.

Remvig, L., Jensen, D. V., & Ward, R. C. (2007). Epidemiology of general joint hypermobility and basis for the proposed criteria for benign joint hypermobility syndrome: Review of the literature. *Journal of Rheumatology, 34*, 804–809.

Roach, K. E., & Miles, T. P. (1991). Normal hip and knee active range of motion: The relationship to age. *Physical Therapy, 71*, 656–665.

Robson-Ansley, P. J., Gleeson, M., & Ansley, L. (2009). Fatigue management in the preparation of Olympic athletes. *Journal of Sports Sciences, 27*, 1409–1420.

Rodrigues Barbosa, A., Santarem, J. M., Filho, W. J., & Nunes Marucci, M. D. F. (2002). Effects of resistance training on the sit-and-reach test in elderly women. *Journal of Strength and Conditioning Research, 16*, 14–18.

Roetert, E. P., Brown, S. W., Piorkowski, P. A., & Woods, R. B. (1996). Fitness comparisons among three different levels of elite tennis players. *Journal of Strength and Conditioning Research, 3*, 139–143.

Ross, J., & Grahame, R. (2011). Joint hypermobility syndrome. *British Medical Journal, 342*, 275–277.

Rowlands, A. V., Marginson, V. F., & Lee, J. (2003). Chronic flexibility gains: Effect of isometric contraction duration during proprioceptive neuromuscular facilitation stretching techniques. *Research Quarterly for Exercise and Sport, 74*, 47–51.

Sands, W. A. (2011). Flexibility. In M. Cardinale, R. Newton, & K. Nosaka (Eds.), *Strength and conditioning: Biological principles and practical applications* (pp. 389–398). West Sussex, UK: Wiley-Blackwell.

Sands, W. A., McNeal, J. R., Stone, M. H., Russell, E. M., & Jemni, M. (2006). Flexibility enhancement with vibration: Acute and long-term. *Medicine and Science in Sports and Exercise, 38*, 720–725.

Schmitt, G. D., Pelham, T. W., & Holt, L. E. (1999). A comparison of selected protocols during proprioceptive neuromuscular facilitation stretching. *Clinical Kinesiology, 53*, 16–21.

Sharman, M. J., Cresswell, A. G., & Riek, S. (2006). Proprioceptive neuromuscular facilitation stretching: Mechanisms and clinical implications. *Sports Medicine, 36*, 929–939.

Shrier, I. (2004). Does stretching improve performance? A systematic and critical review of the literature. *Clinical Journal of Sport Medicine, 14*, 267–273.

Shrier, I., & Glossal, K. (2000). Myth and truths of stretching: Individualized recommendations for healthy muscles. *Physician and Sports Medicine, 28*, 57–63.

Shultz, S. J., Schmitz, R. J., Nguyen, A., & Levine, B. J. (2010). Joint laxity is related to lower extremity energetics during a drop jump landing. *Medicine and Science in Sports and Exercise, 42*, 771–780.

Siff, M. C. (2000). *Supertraining.* Denver, CO: Supertraining Institute.

Simpson, M. R. (2006). Benign joint hypermobility syndrome: Evaluation, diagnosis, and management. *Journal of the American Osteopathic Association, 106*, 531–536.

Speer, K. P., Lohnes, J., & Garrett, W. E. (1993). Radiographic imaging of muscle strain injury. *American Journal of Sports Medicine, 21*, 89–96.

Sprague, H. A. (1976). Relationship of certain physical measurements to swimming speed. *Research Quarterly, 47*, 810–814.

Torres, R., Ribeiro, F., Duarte, J. A., & Cabri, J. M. H. (2012). Evidence of the physiotherapeutic interventions used currently after exercise-induced muscle damage: Systematic review and meta-analysis. *Physical Therapy in Sport, 13*, 101–114.

Trehearn, T. L., & Buresh, R. (2009). Sit-and-reach flexibility and running economy of men and women collegiate distance runners. *Journal of Strength and Conditioning Research, 23*, 158–162.

Weppler, C. H., & Magnusson, S. P. (2010). Increasing muscle extensibility: A matter of increasing length or modifying sensation. *Physical Therapy, 90*, 438–449.

Wilson, G. J., Elliott, B. C., & Wood, G. A. (1992). Stretch-shortening cycle performance enhancement through flexibility training. *Medicine and Science in Sports and Exercise, 24*, 116–123.

Wilson, G. J., Murphy, A. J., & Pryor, J. F. (1994). Musculotendinous stiffness: Its relationship to eccentric, isometric and concentric performance. *Journal of Applied Physiology, 76*, 2714–2719.

Witvrouw, E., Mahieu, N., Daneels, L., & McNair, P. (2004). Stretching and injury prevention: An obscure relationship. *Sports Medicine, 34*, 443–449.

Ylinen, J., Kankainen, T., Kautiainen, H., Rezasoltani, A., Kuukkanen, T., & Häkkinen, A. (2009). Effect of stretching on hamstring muscle compliance. *Journal of Rehabilitative Medicine, 41*, 80–84.

Yoon, J. (2002). Physiological profiles of elite senior wrestlers. *Sports Medicine, 32*, 225–233.

Young, W., & Pryor, L. (2007). Relationship between pre-season anthropometric and fitness measures and indicators of playing performance in elite junior Australian Rules football. *Journal of Science and Medicine in Sport, 10*, 110–118.

Zatsiorsky, V. M., & Prilutsky, B. I. (2012). *Biomechanics of skeletal muscle.* Champaign, IL: Human Kinetics.

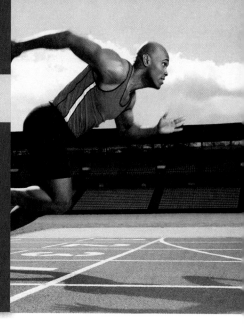

CHAPTER 8

Warm-up Methods

Chapter Objectives

At the end of this chapter, you will be able to:

- Explain the physiological and mechanical benefits of engaging in specific warm-up activities prior to exercise
- Assess the suitability of performing different warm-up activities for specific athletes
- Explain the structure of an effective warm-up routine
- Develop effective warm-up routines for specific sports

Key Terms

Active methods	Massage	Priming exercise	Stretching
Diathermy	Passive heating methods	Q_{10}	Thixotropy
Hot water immersion	Post-activation potentiation	Stress relaxation	Whole-body vibration

Chapter Overview

Prior to undertaking physical activity, whether during a training session or during a competition, athletes will perform a routine to prepare themselves both physically and mentally. This warm-up routine will typically include activities that are employed in the belief that the physical capacity of the motor system can be enhanced and the risk of injury reduced. The methods available to a strength and conditioning coach for preparing athletes for exercise are numerous, and many of the acute methods that have been suggested for use in preparing the athlete for physical activity are reviewed in this chapter. The physiological and mechanical mechanisms underpinning the efficacy of each method as revealed in the scientific literature are assessed, and suggestions are made regarding how these methods can be employed on a practical level with different athletes. We finish the chapter by highlighting the development of effective warm-up routines.

Warm-up Methods

An athlete can engage in a number of activities immediately prior to a training session or an athletic competition in an attempt to perform at an optimal level while also reducing the risk of subsequent injury. Although the influence of warm-up activities on athletic performance is relatively straightforward to determine, their role in preventing injuries is more difficult to ascertain (see Warm-up Concept 8.1). Typically, warm-up activities involve volitional movements performed by the athlete, where the methods are described as **active methods**. However, many disparate activities can be incorporated into the period of preparation immediately preceding

Warm-up Concept 8.1

The effects of warm-up routines on sports injuries: interpreting the evidence

Although the completion of many activities in a warm-up routine is proposed to elicit a prophylactic effect, establishing a causal link between warm-up activities and sports injuries is very difficult. This problem arises not only because of the diversity of the activities included in many warm-up routines but also because of methodological issues in the extant literature. Conceptually, an injury occurs when the stress applied to a biological tissue exceeds that tissue's ability to withstand the stress either acutely or chronically (McBain et al., 2012a). Providing an operational definition, however, is more difficult. An event is classified as an injury if it results in time missed from the sport or activity, it affects the level of play, or it is diagnosed by a medical professional (Woods, Bishop, & Jones, 2007). When reviewing the literature, it is very important to interpret the type of injury being assessed and the severity of the injury; while some evidence indicates that warm-up activities can reduce the incidence of musculotendinous unit (MTU) strains and ligamentous sprains (Woods et al., 2007), it would be inappropriate to expect such activities to provide protective effects against traumatic injuries such as fractures or concussions.

(continues)

(continued)

Some studies focus on interventions aimed at reducing the risk factors associated with specific injuries as opposed to actual injury rates themselves (McBain et al., 2012b). Furthermore, the design of the studies is important. In a review of the current literature, McBain et al. (2012b) reported that only 40% were randomized-controlled trials (RCTs), although the number of RCTs has increased in recent years. This trend suggests that researchers are more widely adopting an evidence-based approach to identify the prophylactic effects of specific interventions. However, RCTs are not always appropriate to study the effects of interventions on injuries. For example, cohort studies are recommended if an intervention is highly unlikely to increase the risk for injury; such study designs have been used to confirm the NFL's and NHL's bans on same-day return to play following a concussive event (McBain et al., 2012b).

Even when RCTs are performed, methodological limitations abound. Aaltonen, Karjalainen, Heinonen, Parkkari, and Kujala (2007) performed a systematic review of RCTs designed to investigate the effects of various interventions on sports injuries. Of the 32 studies (with a total of 24,931 participants) that were reviewed, only 5 provided convincing evidence that the allocation of the treatment was adequately concealed from the participants. Most studies also suffered from inadequate blinding of the care providers and assessors (i.e., researchers, trainers, physicians), which can potentially result in performance and detection bias. Furthermore, attrition bias was noted in 20 of the 32 studies because of failure to perform an intention-to-treat analysis. Aaltonen et al. (2007) noted that none of the three RCTs that were designed to examine the effects of stretching and other physical activities performed prior to exercise on the rate of lower-extremity injuries showed preventive effects; all of these studies also contained methodological issues.

Recently, researchers have begun to investigate the efficacy of specific exercises focusing on jumping and agility movements prior to soccer training sessions in reducing the incidence of anterior cruciate ligament (ACL) injuries in female adolescent soccer players (Kiani, Hellquist, Ahlqvist, Gedeborg, & Michaëlson, 2010; Mandelbaum et al., 2005; Soligard et al., 2010; Steffen, Myklebust, Olsen, Holme, & Bahr, 2008; Waldén, Atroshi, Magnusson, Wagner, & Hägglund, 2012). These studies were all performed on a large number of athletes over entire seasons. They typically required the athletes in the experimental groups to complete 15 min of exercises emphasizing stability, balance, and dynamic stabilization before training and/or competitive matches; the players in the control group completed traditional warm-up routines. Although not all of the interventions were successful in reducing the injury rate (Steffen et al., 2008), some were reported to reduce injury risk in those players who completed the specific exercises (Kiani et al., 2010; Mandelbaum et al., 2005), particularly when compliance with the program was high (Soligard et al., 2010). Waldén et al. (2012) completed a large-scale RCT and found that a modified warm-up routine consisting of dynamic exercises including single-leg squats, lunges, and jumping/landing techniques that progressed in level of difficulty throughout the soccer season was able to reduce the rate of ACL injuries incurred by participants compared to a typical warm-up routine. It appeared to be long-term adaptations to the warm-up activities that elicited the protective effect in these studies (e.g., altered knee joint and trunk mechanics during landing and cutting tasks) as opposed to any acute responses.

> In conclusion, evidence supporting a prophylactic effect from performing warm-up activities prior to exercise is limited. However, many methodological issues surround the extant literature, so further investigation is warranted. In future studies, the research questions should be more specific; that is, the type of injury and the activities used in the warm-up routine should be clearly defined. The strength and conditioning practitioner should establish which injuries are common in a specific sport and the risk factors associated with those injuries, and then determine which warm-up activities might exert a prophylactic effect.

exercise, some of which are **passive heating methods** (Table 8.1). Whether the warm-up activity is active or passive, the associated performance benefits are derived from either the induction of acute metabolic and cardiovascular changes or a change in the mechanical properties of the biologic tissue (e.g., skeletal muscle, tendon). The induction of such responses is often underpinned by an increase in the temperature of the body that accompanies the activity—hence the use of the term "warm-up" to describe these activities. However, some activities rely on an initial decrease in temperature to exert their influence on subsequent physical performance, with others inducing an acceleration of VO_2 kinetics, a change in the mechanical properties of the musculotendinous units (MTU), or an alteration in motoneuron excitability independent of substantial temperature changes.

Table 8.1
Warm-up Activities That Can Be Used to Enhance Physical Performance

Activity	Description	Proposed Mechanism of Performance Enhancement
Aerobic activities	Active method	Acute increase in temperature
		Acute metabolic and cardiovascular changes
Post-activity potentiation	Active method	Acute changes in mechanical properties of musculotendinous units
Vibration	Active method	Acute metabolic and cardiovascular changes
		Acute changes in mechanical properties of musculotendinous units
Stretching	Active or passive method	Acute changes in mechanical properties of musculotendinous units
Pre-cooling	Passive method	Acute decrease in body temperature
		Acute metabolic and cardiovascular changes
Massage	Passive method	Acute increase in temperature
		Acute changes in mechanical properties of musculotendinous units
Hot water immersion	Passive method	Acute increase in body temperature
Diathermy	Passive method	Acute increase in temperature

Thermal Effects of Warm-up Activities

While the body core temperature is maintained within a narrow homeostatic range during exercise, skin and skeletal muscle temperature can experience much greater variations (Drinkwater, 2008). Intramuscular temperatures at rest (approximately 35°C) tend to be lower than the body core temperature (approximately 37°C) (Kenny et al., 2003). Exercising muscle generates considerable heat; this heat occurs in proportion to the intensity of the exercise, rising rapidly with the onset of exercise before stabilizing after approximately 10–20 min (Bishop, 2003a). Rectal temperature—a measure of the temperature of the body core—is independent of the ambient temperature and rises during exercise only once the muscle temperature has exceeded the rectal temperature, whereas the skin temperature tends to drop during the first 10 min of exercise (Bishop, 2003a). Ten minutes of running at an intensity of 70% VO_{2max} has been shown to elevate intramuscular temperature from 35°C to 38°C (Magnusson, Aagaard, Larsson, & Kjær, 2000). By comparison, 15 min of isolated bilateral knee extension exercise at an intensity equivalent to 60% VO_{2max} produced an increase in intramuscular temperature of between 2°C and 3°C (with the greatest increase seen in the superficial muscles); these temperatures remained elevated above baseline values for up to 1 hour after the exercise bout (Kenny et al., 2003).

The intensity of the muscle actions influences the magnitude of the increase in muscle temperature, with greater increases occurring following isometric actions (8–20 s in duration) at intensities between 30% and 70% of the maximal force (Saugen & Vøllestad, 1995). Furthermore, the increase in intramuscular temperature observed following the completion of an exercise bout at a given intensity is affected by the ambient temperature. Specifically, greater increases in muscle temperature can be expected with a given exercise intensity (70% VO_{2peak}) in higher ambient temperatures (approximately 5°C change at an ambient temperature of 40°C) compared to normothermic (approximately 4°C change at an ambient temperature of 20°C) and even cold ambient temperatures (approximately 4°C change at an ambient temperature of 3°C), despite the muscle temperature being no different at the beginning of the exercise session (Parkin, Carey, Zhao, & Febbraio, 1999). The same trend is seen with rectal temperature, although the magnitude of the changes is lower (approximately 3°C at 40°C, and approximately 2°C at both 20°C and 3°C).

The influence of temperature on performance can be gleaned from the variations in rectal temperature and measures of muscle force and power throughout the day. Rectal temperature follows a circadian rhythm, reaching its highest point in the late afternoon compared to the morning hours; this diurnal variation in rectal temperature is similar to that followed by muscle force and power output, such that short-duration (less than 1 min) maximal efforts yield a better performance in the afternoon compared to the morning hours (Racinais, 2010). Interestingly, performance in longer-duration events is less affected by diurnal variations.

Temperature can affect almost every process in the excitation–contraction coupling associated with voluntary muscle actions. However, certain mechanical aspects of muscle performance appear to be more strongly influenced by temperature variations compared to others. For example, maximal force appears to be largely unaffected by temperature changes around physiological values, decreasing in response to more extreme reductions in temperature (de Ruiter, Jones, Sargeant, & de Haan, 1999; Dewhurst et al., 2010). (See Warm-up Concept 8.2.) By comparison, other mechanical characteristics of muscle, such as rate of force development and rate of relaxation, are much more sensitive to temperature variations and demonstrate progressive decreases and increases,

Warm-up Concept 8.2

Thermal dependence of the mechanical behavior of skeletal muscle

The thermal dependence of biological and chemical processes can be established by calculating the temperature coefficient known as Q_{10} (the rate of change in a given variable in response to a 10°C temperature change). A Q_{10} greater than 1.0 indicates a positive thermal dependence for the variable under investigation. Most skeletal muscle enzymes have a value of 2.0–3.0 (Bishop, 2003a), meaning that a 10°C increase in muscle temperature will double or triple enzyme activity. The rate-dependent mechanical variables associated with muscle actions (e.g., rate of force development and relaxation) have a Q_{10} of approximately 2, reflecting their dependence upon enzyme activities, while maximal force generation is characterized by low thermal dependence (Bennett, 1985).

Q_{10} values are not linear, because they depend on the initial temperature of the tissue. For example, Q_{10} for the maximal rate of force development and the rate of relaxation between 37°C and 25°C is approximately 2, while the corresponding value between 25°C and 22°C is approximately 4 (de Ruiter et al., 1999). The practical implication of this variability is that these mechanical properties are more sensitive to an increase in muscle temperature when the initial temperature is relatively low. The effects of warm-up activities are therefore likely to be greater in conditions characterized by low ambient temperatures.

respectively, when muscle temperature begins to fall from physiological values (de Ruiter et al., 1999). Muscle fiber conduction velocity has also been shown to have a positive linear relationship with muscle temperature (Gray, De Vito, Nimmo, Farina, & Ferguson, 2006). Thus, while measures of maximal strength may be influenced only by extreme muscle temperature changes, power output is much more readily affected by small alterations. Measures of strength endurance appear to be adversely affected by increased muscle temperatures (Hoffman, Williams, & Lind, 1985; Holewijn & Heus, 1992). Racinais and Oksa (2010) propose that a 1°C increase in muscle temperature can enhance performance in short-term, maximal-intensity activities; this magnitude of intramuscular temperature elevation persists for as long as an hour after completing a 15-min exercise session of moderate intensity (Kenny et al., 2003).

A number of passive methods have been shown to be effective at increasing intramuscular temperature (e.g., hot water immersion, massage, diathermy techniques). (See Warm-up Concept 8.3.) However, despite the increases in muscle temperatures achieved through these passive methods, they fail to produce the other physiological alterations that accompany active methods (e.g., post-activation potentiation, altered VO$_2$ kinetics). Consequently, active methods are recommended to increase muscle temperature prior to athletic performance (Bishop, 2003b).

The metabolic characteristics of skeletal muscle are also affected by temperature. While an increase in muscle temperature can cause a small increase in maximal force production, the increase in the consumption of adenosine-5′-triphosphate (ATP) is much greater in this scenario (Steinen, Kiers, Bottinelli, & Reggiani, 1996), resulting

Warm-up Concept 8.3

Passive methods to increase skeletal muscle temperature

Intramuscular temperature can be increased using passive methods including immersion in hot water, thermal clothing, massage, or diathermy.

Hot water immersion (e.g., a hot bath/shower) is probably the simplest form of passive heating that can be undertaken by an athlete prior to exercise. Cochrane, Stannard, Sargeant, and Rittweger (2008) reported that immersion in hot water (41°C) for approximately 17 min elevated intramuscular temperature by a value of approximately 1.5°C. This magnitude of increase was similar to that observed following cycling for 10 min. Furthermore, the increase in vertical jump height (approximately 4%) was similar following both conditions.

Massage involves a mechanical manipulation of body tissue that is applied in a rhythmical manner. Classic Western massage techniques that are often used by therapists include effleurage, petrissage, friction, and tapotement (Weerapong, Hume, & Kolt, 2005). The application of 5–15 min of effleurage has been shown to be effective at increasing intramuscular temperature, albeit only at superficial (less than 30 mm) depths (Drust, Atkinson, Gregson, French, & Binningsley, 2003). The use of massage techniques in a warm-up routine has not been shown to be effective in improving sprint running performance (Fletcher, 2010; Goodwin, Glaister, Howatson, Lockey, & McInnes, 2007).

Diathermy techniques use high-frequency electromagnetic waves to elicit a thermal response in biologic tissue. Short-wave diathermy techniques typically use a frequency of approximately 27 MHz with a wavelength of 11 m, whereas microwave diathermy employs shorter wavelengths applied at much higher frequencies. Ultrasound diathermy relies on acoustic vibrations that are transmitted through the tissue to induce a thermal effect. Nosaka, Sakamoto, Newton, and Sacco (2004) reported that microwave diathermy increased muscle temperature at a 20-mm depth by approximately 4°C. The muscle temperature remained elevated by approximately 3°C for 10 min after the application of the diathermy intervention. Ultrasound diathermy has been reported to increase muscle temperature at 10- and 30-mm depths by approximately 3.5°C (Draper et al., 1998). Despite increases in intramuscular temperature following diathermy techniques, no changes have been reported in measures of maximal strength following acute applications (Mitchell, Trowbridge, Fincher, & Cramer, 2008). Moreover, these techniques have no effect on O_2 kinetics during subsequent exercise bouts (Fukuba et al., 2012).

Although these passive methods may be effective at increasing the temperature of the muscle tissue beyond the 1°C that is required for an improved mechanical response (Racinais & Oksa, 2010), they will not induce the physiological alterations that are seen when active methods are used and that can enhance exercise performance (e.g., post-activation potentiation, accelerated O_2 kinetics). For this reason, active methods are recommended as more effective means of improving subsequent exercise performance (Bishop, 2003b). However, thermal clothing (e.g., heated trousers) appears to be effective at maintaining the elevated muscle temperatures achieved through execution of the active methods (Faulkner et al., 2013). This novel passive method of heating was shown to minimize the drop in muscle temperature over a 30-min recovery period between the completion of the active exercises and a maximal sprint effort, resulting in greater peak power outputs being produced.

in an increased metabolic cost of force generation at higher muscle temperatures. Furthermore, increased muscle temperature increases the degradation of phosphocreatine (PCr) during exercise (Febbraio et al., 1996). This increased degradation of high-energy phosphates (ATP, PCr) associated with increased temperature of the working muscle is greater in type IIA muscle fibers (Gray, Söderlund, & Ferguson, 2008); thus it would tend to favor improved performance in events characterized by maximal efforts of short duration.

Muscle glycogen use is also augmented following an increase in muscle temperature of approximately 7°C, independent of high-energy phosphate degradation (Starkie, Hargreaves, Lambert, Proietto, & Febbraio, 1999). Furthermore, submaximal exercise (70% VO_{2peak}) performed in lower ambient temperatures (3°C) results in a reduced glycogenolytic rate compared to similar exercise performed in normothermic (20°C) or high (40°C) ambient temperatures (Parkin et al., 1999). This lower glycogenolytic rate is associated with greater times to exhaustion during exercise.

An increase in temperature also results in an increased dissociation of O_2 from hemoglobin and, to a lesser extent, from myoglobin while simultaneously stimulating vasodilation (Bishop, 2003a). These changes increase the O_2 delivery to the working muscles and might potentially improve performance in activities where the athlete's achievement is otherwise limited by O_2 delivery, such as short-term, high-intensity activities. When exercise takes place in a hot environment, the thermal strain experienced by the athlete is increased such that fatigue is exacerbated in both continuous and repeated-sprint activities (Drust, Rasmussen, Mohr, Nielsen, & Nybo, 2005; Tucker, Marle, Lambert, & Noakes, 2006). Under such circumstances, an increase in temperature resulting from the athlete's warm-up activities may increase the thermal stress experienced during subsequent exercise. Therefore, in contrast to sprint and explosive activities, the athlete's performance in endurance events may be enhanced by a *reduction* in the temperature of the body core and the exercising muscle during the warm-up routine as a result of reducing the thermal load prior to exercise and the sparing of muscle glycogen during the exercise bout (see Warm-up Concept 8.4).

Some evidence indicates that an increase in temperature can alter the viscoelastic characteristics of the MTU (Bishop, 2003a). For example, the force required to damage muscle and the length at which the muscle failed were greater in isolated animal specimens that had their temperature increased by approximately 1°C as a result of a 15-s maximal isometric action performed immediately before the muscle was stretched to failure (Safran, Garrett, Seaber, Glisson, & Ribbeck, 1988). Such a finding may have significant implications for the thermally induced prophylactic effect associated with warm-up activities, although it is unclear whether the effects in the experiment were due to the increase in muscle temperature or to factors associated with the initial isometric action (e.g., stress relaxation, post-activation potentiation, thixotropic

Warm-up Concept 8.4

The use of pre-cooling methods

While intramuscular temperature may increase by approximately 3°C after 15 min of exercise at an intensity equivalent to 60% VO_{2max} performed in a normothermic environment, the temperature of the body core appears to be elevated by less than 1°C under the same circumstances (Kenny et al., 2003). By comparison, exercise in hot ambient conditions can result in greater increases in body core temperatures. El Helou et al. (2012) reported optimal ambient temperatures of between 6.2°C and 6.8°C for elite male and female marathon runners, respectively, with a 0.03% reduction in performance for every 1°C above the optimal temperatures. When the ambient temperature exceeds these optimal values by 20°C, the authors predicted a 12% to 17% reduction in performance. The increase in the body core temperature is proposed to be responsible for this drop in endurance exercise performance; an increase in the body core temperature to more than 39.7°C ± 0.15°C has been associated with exhaustion during exercise (Nielsen et al., 1993). This whole-body hyperthermia leads to impaired cardiovascular functioning that limits arterial O_2 delivery to the working muscles; this factor, in turn, impairs performance during short-duration, high-intensity exercise. By comparison, during prolonged exercise, elevated body core temperatures induce central fatigue that is manifested as a reduction in neural drive to the active musculature (Nybo, 2008). Given that one result of engaging in dynamic exercises as part of a warm-up routine is an increase in thermoregulatory strain of the athlete (Bishop, 2003a), investigators have sought to identify the effects of reducing the temperature of the body core or skin prior to exercise through various pre-cooling methods on subsequent endurance performance.

Methods of pre-cooling include lowering of the ambient temperature, cooling fans, evaporative cooling garments, ice vests, cold drink ingestion, or cold water immersion. The most practical of these methods is likely to be the use of cooling vests and cold drink ingestion (Wegmann et al., 2012), although cold water immersion might be the most effective method (Jones, Barton, Morrisey, Maffulli, & Hemmings, 2012). In general, pre-cooling methods yield their greatest improvements in endurance exercise performed in hot (greater than 26°C) environments (Wegmann et al., 2012). In addition, greater effects are observed in those individuals with the highest aerobic capacities. A reduction in body core temperature of 1.5°C prior to exercise appears to be effective at enhancing performance, whereas reducing the temperature by 1.9°C may diminish performance (Wegmann et al., 2012).

The mechanisms that underpin the effectiveness of pre-cooling methods have yet to be elucidated. Exercising in a hot environment is associated with an increased glycogenolytic rate and accumulation of blood lactate, while exercising in reduced ambient temperatures has been reported to reduce the glycogenolytic rate of the working muscle as a result of a blunted epinephrine response to the exercise stimulus (Parkin et al., 1999). Therefore, a reduction in temperature prior to exercise would seem to spare muscle glycogen stores and enhance performance in prolonged, submaximal exercise bouts. However, fatigue can occur during long-term exercise in hot environments in the presence of adequate muscle glycogen stores (Bishop, 2003a). The thermal stress experienced by the athlete is reduced following the application of pre-cooling methods due to the reduction in stored heat, allowing more heat to be absorbed during the exercise bout (Wegmann et al., 2012). This reduced thermal stress would be evident as a lower heart rate during exercise and a lower rate of sweating. Furthermore, an increase in central blood volume caused by the reduced skin temperature, resulting in peripheral vasoconstriction, has been reported following pre-cooling (Wegmann et al., 2012). This effect is predicted to increase the perfusion of the working muscles and enhance exercise performance.

Because of the heterogeneity of research designs employed in the extant literature, it is currently difficult to provide specific guidelines for the application of pre-cooling methods (Jones et al., 2012; Wegmann et al., 2012). For example, cooling duration and the time between the pre-cooling protocol and the initiation of the exercise bout require determination.

effect). Indeed, alterations in the viscoelastic properties of the MTU are not apparent when humans perform submaximal warm-up exercises (running at 70–75% VO_{2max} for 10–30 min) despite an approximate 3°C increase in intramuscular temperature (Magnusson et al., 2000).

Evidence also shows that increases in temperature increase the extensibility of tendons in animals (Lehmann, Masock, Warren, & Koblanski, 1970). These findings have potential implications for athletic performance and injury risk. However, the temperature changes induced by researchers are beyond the physiological temperatures that one would find in an exercising human. *In vivo* measurements taken during maximal isometric actions or passive movements indicate that there is little change in the mechanical behavior of tendons following temperature changes induced by hot and cold water immersion (Kubo, Kanehisa, & Fukunaga, 2005). In summary, the mechanical properties of tendons appear to have a much lower thermal dependency than skeletal muscle.

The thermal dependence reported in the mechanical properties of skeletal muscle tends to be much greater than the changes observed in measures of performance (e.g., vertical jump height, sprinting time). It seems that the increases in muscle temperature that arise from completing voluntary activities during a warm-up routine (active methods) largely contribute to increased performance in events requiring short-term (10 s or less) maximal efforts (Bishop, 2003b). The mechanisms underlying this thermal dependence include increased nerve conduction velocity, increased high-energy phosphate degradation (ATP, PCr), and increased glycogenolytic rate. However, the elevation of temperature is unlikely to contribute to improved performance in longer-duration events (5 min or more); indeed, it may actually impair performance in these events via an increased glycogenolytic rate, an increased thermal load at the onset of performance, and/or impaired thermoregulatory mechanisms (Bishop, 2003b). It is unclear how temperature changes within physiological ranges influence the viscoelastic properties of the MTU *in vivo*.

Nonthermal Effects of Warm-up Activities

Up to this point, we have discussed the thermally mediated effects associated with activities performed by an athlete during a warm-up routine and considered how these may influence subsequent exercise performance. However, a number of non-thermal effects resulting from activities performed during the warm-up routine may potentially influence performance. For example, muscle activity results in an acute reduction in motor unit recruitment thresholds (Adam & De Luca, 2003; Carpentier, Duchateau, & Hainaut, 2001), which could enhance subsequent force production. The completion of a prior exercise session also elevates the baseline VO_2, thereby promoting a greater aerobic contribution to subsequent work bouts (Bishop, 2003a). This effect would limit the involvement of the finite anaerobic energy systems (substrate-level phosphorylation) early in the exercise bout and potentially improve performance. Finally, stable bonds between actin and myosin molecules may develop when a muscle remains inactive, increasing the stiffness of the tissue (Enoka, 2008). This stiffness can be reduced by moving the muscle through a range of motion by either active or passive means—a mechanical property of skeletal muscle known as **thixotropy**. Specific activities and methods can also be executed as part of a warm-up routine that elicit acute alterations in spinal reflexes, accelerate VO_2 kinetics, and change the viscoelastic properties of the MTU so as to influence subsequent athletic performance independent of any thermal responses.

Post-activation Potentiation

Post-activation potentiation (PAP) is an acute increase in the mechanical output of a muscle induced by the completion of maximal or near-maximal voluntary muscle actions (Tillin & Bishop, 2009). In practical terms, the PAP response can be induced by having an athlete complete a set of back squats with a load equivalent to 90% of the one-repetition maximum (1-RM), after which the athlete performs a mechanically similar exercise without any additional external load, such as a vertical jump. In this example, the heavy back squats represent the conditioning exercise and the vertical jump is the performance exercise that is expected to be enhanced as a result of the PAP process.

The mechanical output of a muscle in response to prior activity depends on the interaction between the processes of fatigue (which acts to reduce the expected output) and PAP (which acts to increase the expected output). Whether the output is reduced, is increased, or remains unchanged will depend on the coexistence and decay of these two processes (Robbins, 2005), so the timing between the conditioning and performance exercises becomes a determining factor in the outcome. Evidence suggests that the PAP response may develop at a faster rate than fatigue after the conditioning exercise (Tillin & Bishop, 2009). Although PAP is proposed operate during long-duration activities, its influence is countered by fatigue processes (Sale, 2002). Therefore, the use of acute PAP methods to enhance performance is limited to short-duration, explosive-type activities (Hodgson, Docherty, & Robbins, 2005). The mechanisms by which the PAP process operates remain to be determined conclusively, with increased Ca^{2+} sensitivity and/or altered structure of the myosin crossbridge due to phosphorylation of the myosin light chains and an increase in motoneuron excitability being the most common mechanisms cited in the literature (Hodgson et al., 2005; Tillin & Bishop, 2009).

The practical application of PAP protocols as part of a warm-up routine remains a subject of debate. Practical issues to be considered include the mechanical specificity of the conditioning and performance exercises (e.g., muscle groups, muscle actions), the intensity and volume of the conditioning exercise (e.g., external load, repetitions and sets), and the timing of the conditioning and performance exercises (Robbins, 2005). There appears to be considerable variation in these parameters that would induce the PAP response in different athletes, rendering generalized PAP protocols impractical in the view of some (Robbins, 2005). Moreover, the PAP response dissipates rapidly (4–6 min) following the conditioning exercise (MacIntosh, Robillard, & Tomaras, 2012), further limiting the utility of the method. The relative increases in electrically evoked twitch force are greater following conditioning exercises performed in a PAP protocol than the increases in voluntary measures of muscle performance, which may also limit the effectiveness of PAP protocols for improving measures of athletic performance (Hodgson, Docherty, & Zeher, 2008). Indeed, PAP protocols have been shown to enhance electrically evoked muscle force and reflexes of the previously activated muscle without changing measures of voluntary muscle force (Folland, Wakamatsu, & Fimland, 2008).

Most of the extant research has investigated the PAP response in lower-body exercises. Because of the methodological heterogeneity in the extant studies (i.e., conditioning and performance exercises, timing of exercises, participants) it is difficult to establish an effective PAP protocol. However, the following recommendations can be used to guide the development of a lower-body PAP protocol:

- Conditioning exercises should be performed close to maximal intensity with loads of 90% 1-RM or greater for dynamic activities (Comyns, Harrison, Hennessey, & Jensen, 2007; McBride, Nimphius, & Erickson, 2005).
- A passive recovery period of 4 min between the conditioning and performance exercises appears to be effective (Comyns et al., 2007; McBride et al., 2005), although this period is likely to differ between individuals (Comyns, Harrison, Hennessey, & Jensen, 2006).
- Athletes should be able to back squat 2 (or more) times their body mass to benefit from the PAP protocol (Ruben et al., 2010).

An effective PAP protocol to be used in a warm-up routine is described in Applied Warm-up Protocol 8.1.

Stretching

Stretching activities have typically been included in the warm-up routine for many athletes. The primary goal of stretching is to increase the range of motion about a joint and the compliance of the MTU, which may in turn enhance performance or reduce the risk of injury (McHugh & Cosgrave, 2010). Three types of stretching can be used to this end:

- Static stretch. The target joint is slowly moved to the limit of its range of motion (identified by the mild discomfort experienced by the athlete). This position is held for a predetermined time (typically more than 10 s) before returning the joint to its original position.
- Dynamic stretch. The target muscle group is elongated in a controlled manner through the range of motion before returning to its original length. The elongated position is not held for any substantial time.

Applied Warm-up Protocol 8.1

Practical use of lower-body PAP in a warm-up routine

The following protocol is based on the one used by Comyns et al. (2007). The conditioning exercise is a free-weight back squat, and the performance exercise is a drop jump for maximal height.

1. Have the athlete engage in low-intensity dynamic activities for 5 min.

2. Perform five repetitions of the conditioning exercise with a load equivalent to 50% 1-RM.

3. Perform three repetitions with a load equivalent to 60% 1-RM.

4. Perform three repetitions with a load equivalent to 93% 1-RM.

5. Provide a passive recovery period of 4 min between the conditioning exercise and the performance exercise.

6. Modify the protocol for each athlete to determine the relationship to improvements in the performance exercise.

- Proprioceptive neuromuscular facilitation (PNF). PNF techniques require the movement of the target joint to the limit of the range of motion before the muscles involved are activated to inhibit the reflex activity of the target muscle, reducing the passive stiffness of the muscle and allowing a greater change in the length of the muscle.

In response to a stretch, a decrease in the excitability of spinal reflexes and the passive resistance of the MTU occurs (Guissard & Duchateau, 2006; McHugh & Cosgrave, 2010). Due to the slow lengthening motions applied during these stretches, the stretch reflex is unlikely to be initiated. The decrease in passive resistance induced by the completion of stretches, which can last up to 1 hour, is known as **stress relaxation**. Aerobic activities (e.g., 10 min of jogging) do not always induce the stress relaxation response in MTU, whereas passive resistance is reduced when stretches are performed following jogging exercises (McHugh & Cosgrave, 2010). The duration of the stress relaxation effect depends on the duration of the stretch. Specifically, short-duration static stretches (e.g., 4×30 s) with a total duration of 2 min reduce passive stiffness for less than 10 min after the completion of the stretches, whereas 6 min of total stretching (e.g., 4×90 s) on each target muscle reduces passive stiffness for up to 1 hour after the stretches (McHugh & Cosgrave, 2010). In practical terms, such a protocol would require more than 60 min of the warm-up routine to be dedicated to stretching. However, reductions in passive stiffness lasting up to 1 hour can occur after only 2 min total duration of PNF stretches (McHugh & Cosgrave, 2010). Stretching activities may be more important to complete prior to activities that require large ranges of motion, such as gymnastics. Indeed, coaches in these sports utilize static stretches as part of the warm-up routine of their athletes (Guidetti et al., 2009).

Evidence exists demonstrating a decrease in measures of muscle strength immediately following static stretches and PNF stretching techniques (Kay & Blazevich, 2012; McHugh & Cosgrave, 2010; Rubini, Costa, & Gomes, 2007). The underlying mechanism appears to be neural in nature (McHugh & Cosgrave, 2010). Decrements in measures of athletic performance (e.g., jump height, sprint time) have also been reported in the literature, although they tend to be smaller than the decrements in measures of muscular strength (McHugh & Cosgrave, 2010). Such interference effects have prompted a number of authors to recommend that static stretches not be included in a warm-up routine (Faigenbaum, 2011; Magnusson & Renström, 2006). (See Warm-up Concept 8.5.) However, there appears to be a dose-response effect in that stretch durations of less than 30 s have no detrimental effect on measures of strength and performance, whereas stretch durations of 60 s or greater are likely to induce significant reductions in these measures (Kay & Blazevich, 2012). This dose-response effect appears to be independent of the performance task or muscle group.

Long-duration stretches are rarely used in warm-up routines. For example, strength and conditioning coaches report using average stretch durations of between 12 s and 18 s (Ebben & Blackard, 2001; Ebben, Hintz, & Simenz, 2005). Furthermore, most evidence indicating impaired performance following static stretches has

Warm-up Concept 8.5

Should static stretching be included in a warm-up routine?

Reductions in measures of muscular strength and performance are only likely following the completion of long-duration static stretches (60 s or more), with short-duration stretches (less than 30 s) being unlikely to diminish these measures (Kay & Blazevich, 2012). Therefore, the inclusion of short-duration stretches in a warm-up routine performed prior to exercise should not interfere with subsequent performance. However, such short-duration stretches are unlikely to induce any substantial mechanical changes in the MTU: Stretch durations of 60 s are required to induce the stress relaxation response (decreased passive resistance of the MTU), with this response then lasting approximately 1 hour (McHugh & Cosgrave, 2010). The interference of these longer duration stretches with athletic performance can be removed by having the athlete engage in moderate-intensity aerobic exercises after the stretches (Kay & Blazevich, 2009; Murphy, Di Santo, Alkanani, & Behm, 2010). This may have implications for the use of long-duration stretches in protecting the athlete against muscle strain injuries, although the evidence of a prophylactic effect of stretching prior to exercise is currently limited (McHugh & Cosgrave, 2010).

At present, there is little evidence to support the use of stretching prior to exercise either from a performance enhancement standpoint or an injury risk prevention perspective. However, if the strength and conditioning coach decides that stretching exercises are to be removed from the warm-up routine of an athlete, the coach must consider the potential psychological effects on an athlete who has a history of using such exercises and believes in their efficacy (Young, 2007).

come from studies that have failed to include any other activities that would typically be included in a warm-up routine along with stretching exercises (Young, 2007). Indeed, the inclusion of moderate-intensity aerobic exercise performed after static stretches has been shown to eliminate the detrimental effects of the stretches (Kay & Blazevich, 2009; Murphy, Di Santo, Alkanani, & Behm, 2010); however, this effect is not apparent when the stretches are followed by sport-specific drills (Taylor, Weston, & Portas, 2013; Young & Behm, 2003). The performance of aerobic activity following short-duration static stretches (6×6 s) also produces a greater increase in the range of motion about the target joints than stretching alone, and the effects persist for 30 min (Murphy, Di Santo, Alkanani, & Behm, 2010). Dynamic stretches do not appear to interfere with subsequent exercise performance (Behm & Chaouachi, 2011). There is also evidence to suggest that passive cyclic stretches of MTU, where the elongated position is not held for prolonged periods, can reduce the passive stiffness of the MTU (McNair, Dombroski, Hewson, & Stanley, 2000).

Priming Exercise

Evidence suggests that performing an exercise session at an intensity above the lactate threshold (LT) can improve performance during subsequent exercise bouts. Specifically, the completion of 6 min of exercise at an intensity of 70%Δ (the power output equivalent to 70% of the difference between LT and VO_{2peak}) can substantially increase the time to failure in a subsequent exercise bout performed at 80%Δ when a 9- or 20-min recovery period is inserted between the two sessions (Bailey, Vanhatalo, Wilkerson, DiMenna, & Jones, 2009). The improvements derived from the initial **priming exercise** bout are due to an increased primary response of VO_2 kinetics and a reduced amplitude of the slow component. The accelerated VO_2 kinetics are proposed to result from an increase in muscle O_2 availability, increased muscle oxidative enzyme activation, and altered motor unit recruitment patterns during the exercise performed after the priming bout (Jones & Burnley, 2009).

The accelerated VO_2 response will reduce the contribution of substrate-level phosphorylation (e.g., PCr hydrolysis, muscle glycogen utilization) during the exercise bout, thereby limiting the accumulation of metabolites that would otherwise contribute to the fatigue process (e.g., H^+, ADP, P_i) (Jones & Burnley, 2009). The acceleration of VO_2 kinetics with priming exercise occurs independently of the thermal effect (Burnley, Doust, & Jones, 2002), but does reflect the intensity of the priming exercise as well as the duration of the recovery period. Low-intensity priming exercises (40%Δ) do not alter VO_2 kinetics during subsequent exercise bouts, whereas higher intensities (50%Δ, 70%Δ, 30-s all-out sprint) have been shown to be effective in this respect (Bailey et al., 2009; Burnley, Doust, Carter, & Jones, 2001). A recovery period of 9 min or longer between the priming session and the performance exercise bout has been shown to be effective at accelerating the VO_2 kinetics and improving exercise tolerance (Bailey et al., 2009). Taken together, the interaction between the intensity of the priming exercise and the duration of the intervening recovery period should allow the maintenance of accelerated VO_2 kinetics and the restoration of muscle homeostasis (e.g., PCr resynthesis; H^+, ADP, and P_i concentrations).

A useful marker is the blood lactate concentration prior to the performance exercise, with values of between 3 mM and 5 mM being associated with improved performance following priming (Bailey et al., 2009; Jones, Wilkerson, Burnley, & Koppo, 2003; Miura et al., 2009). Lower blood lactate values (2 mM or less) do not

Applied Warm-up Protocol 8.2

Practical use of priming exercises in a warm-up routine

The following protocol was developed by Ingham, Fudge, Pringle, and Jones (2013), who showed that the priming exercise would elicit an average blood lactate value of 3.6 mM prior to the performance of an 800-m running time-trial. Performance in the time-trial was improved and the total O_2 consumed during the time-trial was increased. The inclusion of 20 min of seated rest in the protocol simulated the athlete "call-up" procedures that are typically followed in major track and field competitions.

1. The athlete performs 10 min of self-paced jogging and dynamic exercises.

2. The athlete performs 2×50-m strides at the estimated 800-m race-pace with a walk-back recovery (45–60 s).

3. Following a 45- to 60-s recovery, the athlete performs a 200-m sprint at the estimated 800-m race-pace.

4. The athlete remains seated for 20 min.

5. The athlete performs 2×50-m strides at the estimated 800-m race-pace with a walk-back recovery (45–60 s).

6. The athlete completes the 800-m time-trial.

7. Modify protocol for each athlete to identify the protocol characteristics that optimize performance.

---

alter VO_2 kinetics (Burnley, Doust, & Jones, 2006), while higher values (7 mM or more) are associated with impaired exercise performance despite accelerated VO_2 kinetics (Bailey et al., 2009).

A priming protocol to be used in a warm-up routine is shown in Applied Warm-up Protocol 8.2.

Whole-Body Vibration

Vibration is a mechanical stimulus defined by the frequency and amplitude of a sinusoidal wave form imparted on a dynamic surface (Maffiuletti & Cardinale, 2011). Whole-body vibration (WBV), dependent upon the device, can produce vertical, frontal plane, and sagittal plane oscillations through a vibrating platform. The athlete can assume a variety of functional positions on top of the platform, while performing activities that are either dynamic or static in nature (Figure 8.1). The athlete experiences the vibration as an acceleration transmitted through the body that is proposed to elicit an improvement in subsequent motor performance.

WBV protocols have been shown to enhance performance in short-duration events requiring high power outputs (Maffiuletti & Cardinale, 2011), with the improvements being elicited within minutes of completing the protocol. The acute effects of WBV include a proposed reflex potentiation as a result of damping the rapid changes in muscle length that accompany the vibrations being transmitted to

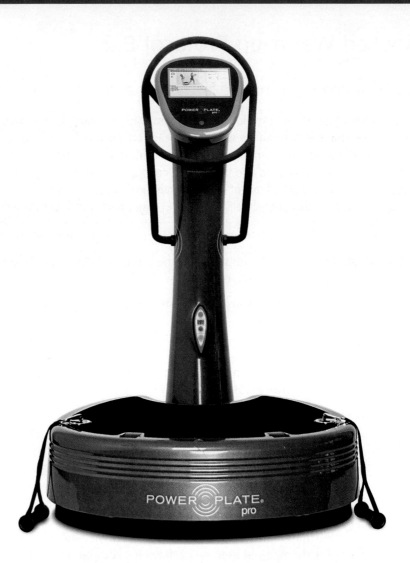

Figure 8.1   A commercially available vibrating platform used during whole-body vibration protocols.

Photo courtesy of Performance Health Systems, LLC.

the body (Maffiuletti & Cardinale, 2011). Specifically, the vibration stimulus activates the muscle spindles, causing inhibition of the antagonistic muscles (reciprocal inhibition). However, such reflex potentiation is unlikely to occur due to the long exposures to the low-frequency stimulus that are typically used in vibration protocols as well as the reduction in the frequency and amplitude of the oscillations as they are transmitted superiorly up the body (Norlund & Thorstensson, 2007). Another physiological response to a WBV protocol is an increase in muscle temperature resulting from increased blood flow and muscle perfusion (Fuller, Thompson, Howe, & Buckley, 2013). Indeed, WBV has been shown to increase muscle temperature more rapidly than both passive heating (hot-water immersion) and cycling exercise (Cochrane et al., 2008). WBV has also been shown to induce the PAP response (Cochrane, Stannard, Firth, & Rittweger, 2010).

The following practical recommendations have been suggested for a WBV protocol to elicit acute enhancements in performance (Maffiuletti & Cardinale, 2011):

- Vibration frequency of between 20 and 50 Hz
- Oscillations of 3 to 10 mm (peak-to-peak displacement)
- Duration of no more than 5 min per set to minimize the potential for fatigue
- Combination of WBV with loaded static and dynamic activities performed on the platform

An example of a WBV protocol to be used in a warm-up routine is shown in Applied Warm-up Protocol 8.3.

The proposed physiological and mechanical responses to active methods performed during a warm-up routine are shown in Table 8.2. These responses have been shown to improve performance in maximal-effort events of short duration (10 s or less), provided that the intensity of the exercises is sufficiently high without causing fatigue, and

Applied Warm-up Protocol 8.3

Practical use of whole-body vibration in a warm-up routine

The following protocol is based upon one developed by McBride et al. (2010) using a commercially available vibration plate (Power Plate International, Irvine, California) operating with a frequency of 30 Hz at the high-amplitude setting (approximately 3.5 mm). The individual is required to perform 6 sets of static, body-weight squats, both bilaterally and unilaterally, with each set lasting 30 s. Peak force has been shown to be significantly elevated above baseline immediately after the completion of the final set of the protocol and to remain elevated for 8 min.

1. The athlete removes his or her shoes and stands on the plate.
2. With the plate operating, the athlete assumes a bilateral static squatting position with an internal knee angle of 100°.
3. The position is held for 30 s.
4. A 60-s passive recovery period is provided (quiet sitting).
5. Repeat two more times.
6. With the plate operating, the athlete assumes a unilateral static squatting position on the right leg with an internal knee angle of 100°.
7. The position is held for 30 s.
8. A 60-s passive recovery period is provided (quiet sitting).
9. With the plate operating, the athlete assumes a unilateral static squatting position on the left leg with an internal knee angle of 100°.
10. The position is held for 30 s.
11. A 60-s passive recovery period is provided (quiet sitting).
12. Repeat two more times.
13. Modify the protocol for each athlete to identify a dose-response relationship.

Table 8.2
The Proposed Acute Alterations Resulting from the Execution of
Dynamic Exercises Prior to Performance

Thermal Responses
Greater release of O_2 from hemoglobin and myoglobin
Increased rates of high-energy phosphate degradation
Increased glycogenolytic rates
Increased nerve conduction velocity
Increased blood flow to working muscles
Reduced stiffness of musculotendinous structures

Nonthermal Responses
Increased blood flow to working muscles
Accelerated O_2 kinetics
Altered spinal reflexes
Increased Ca^{2+} sensitivity of actin–myosin interaction
Reduced stiffness of musculotendinous structures
Psychological effects

with sufficient recovery provided between the completion of the exercises and the subsequent athletic performance to avoid a reduction in high-energy phosphates and/or the buildup of metabolites (Bishop, 2003b). For maximal-effort events of intermediate duration (more than 10 s, but less than 5 min) and long-term fatiguing efforts (5 min or longer), the accelerated VO_2 kinetics resulting from the dynamic exercises have been shown to improve performance so long as the subsequent performance begins from a relatively nonfatigued state, muscle glycogen stores are not depleted, and the athlete does not experience increased thermoregulatory strain (Bishop, 2003b).

Designing a Warm-up Routine

The general structure for a warm-up routine executed prior to short-duration (10 s or less) maximal-intensity activities comprises three phases (Behm & Chaouachi, 2011; Bishop, 2003b; Jefferys, 2008):

- Phase I: An initial bout of 5–10 min of submaximal aerobic activity (40–60 VO_{2max}), as this will limit the depletion of high-energy phosphates while raising intramuscular temperatures.
- Phase II: The completion of large-amplitude dynamic stretches that are specific to the movements typical of those in the sport (e.g., lunge walk, high-knee walk, straight-leg kicks).
- Phase III: The completion of sport-specific dynamic activities of increasing intensity (e.g., sprint drills, jumping and bounding activities) and the rehearsal of sport-specific skills.

The combined duration of Phases II and III has been recommended as between 8 and 12 min (Jefferys, 2008), although the duration may be increased for warm-up routines executed prior to sports involving multiple activities performed at a variety of intensities such as soccer (see Applied Warm-up Protocol 8.4). A sufficient recovery period (5 min is recommended) should be provided between the completion of the warm-up routine and the initiation of the athletic performance, so as to allow the restoration of high-energy phosphates and the clearance of metabolites that may induce fatigue (Bishop, 2003b).

Prior to intermediate-intensity (maximal efforts for more than 10 s but less than 5 min) and long-term sports activities (fatiguing efforts for 5 min or longer), a warm-up routine comprising 5–10 min of exercise at an intensity of 60–70% VO_{2max} with a 5-min recovery before the performance has been recommended (Bishop, 2003b). This routine is proposed to increase baseline VO_2 while limiting muscle glycogen depletion and thermal stress experienced by the athlete prior to performance.

Applied Warm-up Protocol 8.4

A warm-up routine for soccer

The following protocol is based on the work of Devore and Hagerman (2006).

Phase I: 5 min of Submaximal Aerobic Activity
- Jogging around field

Phase II: 15 min of Large-Amplitude Dynamic Stretches

General mobility exercises for the upper extremities
- Neck clock
- Shoulder rolls
- Windmills

General mobility exercises for the midsection
- Trunk circles
- Trunk twists

General mobility exercises for the lower extremities
- Body-weight squats
- Lateral lunges

Transit mobility exercises
- Crossover toe touches
- Forward lunges with trunk rotations
- Trail leg walking
- Forward skipping
- Backward skipping
- Carioca

Phase III: 20 min of Sport-Specific Dynamic Activities of Increasing Intensity
- Ball juggling
- Cutting drills
- Dribbling drills
- Shots on goal
- 2-on-2 drills; 3-on-3 drills
- Full-speed sprints

The development of an effective warm-up routine requires the strength and conditioning coach to determine the typical movements that characterize the sport. Such information can be gleaned from a performance analysis of the sport. Furthermore, the strength and conditioning coach should consider individualizing the warm-up routines for athletes to optimize their performance. Another consideration when developing a warm-up routine is that many sports are separated into distinct playing periods, such as halves or quarters (e.g., soccer, rugby, football, basketball, lacrosse). In these sports, the break between playing periods can be long enough that a reduction in athletic performance may be expected (Mohr, Krustrup, & Bangsbo, 2003). Warm-up activities may, therefore, need to be performed during the interval between playing periods (see Warm-up Concept 8.6). However, the duration of the break constitutes a considerable constraint on the time available to the strength and conditioning coach to facilitate these activities (e.g., 15 min between halves in soccer, 10 min in rugby).

Warm-up Concept 8.6

Half-time warm-up routines in soccer

Researchers have demonstrated a reduction in high-intensity activities performed during the second half of soccer matches (Mohr, Krustrup, & Bangsbo, 2003). Although the reasons for this outcome are unclear, it may be due to the activities of the players during the 15-min half-time interval. As such, researchers have investigated the effects of different interventions performed during the half-time interval and their effect on subsequent soccer-specific performance.

Mohr, Krustrup, Nybo, Nielsen, and Bangsbo (2004) had soccer players perform 7 min of passive recovery at the beginning of the half-time interval, then do 7 min of moderate-intensity running and other dynamic activities (average heart rate approximately 135 bpm), ceasing 1 min before the beginning of the second half. This active half-time routine resulted in a 2.1°C increase in muscle temperature during the break compared to a passive half-time recovery condition and attenuated the reduction in 30-m sprint time.

Zois, Bishop, Fairweather, Ball, and Aughey (2013) reported that a half-time warm-up routine comprising a 5-RM leg-press exercise improved physical performance (e.g., repeated-sprint ability), while a 3-min small-sided game during the half-time interval enhanced skill execution (e.g., passing performance). Athletes who undertook WBV or intermittent agility drills were able to maintain performance measures during the second half of a simulated soccer match in comparison to a passive half-time interval (Lovell, Midgley, Barrett, Carter, & Small, 2013).

Price, Boyd, and Goosey-Tolfrey (2009) investigated the physiological response of soccer players during a simulated match-play test performed during elevated ambient temperatures. These researchers reported that cooling achieved by wearing an ice vest during the half-time period reduced the thermal stress experienced by the athletes during the second half. Although performance measures were not recorded, these findings have implications for the physical capacities of the players during the second half of a soccer game.

Chapter Summary

Warm-up routines involve activities executed prior to a workout or an athletic competition so as to help the athlete perform at an optimal level and reduce the risk of incurring an injury. Although improvements in measures of athletic performance are readily observed following a warm-up routine, determining the ability of a warm-up to reduce injury risk is more difficult.

The activities in a warm-up may be classified as active, whereby the individual engages in volitional movements, or passive, whereby an external agent is used to acutely improve performance/reduce injury risk. Many of the acute enhancements in performance accrued from the completion of a warm-up routine are derived from an increase in the temperature of the MTU. The rate of force development and force relaxation demonstrate high thermal dependence largely due to an associated increase in the degradation of high-energy phosphates and enzyme activity; performance in explosive athletic activities is likely to be enhanced following warm-up routines that increase muscular temperatures by 1°C. Not all of the physiological and mechanical responses associated with a warm-up routine are due to an increase in temperature, however. Increased Ca^{2+} sensitivity and/or altered structure of the myosin crossbridge, the stress relaxation response of the MTU, and accelerated VO_2 kinetics and reduced VO_2 slow components have been reported following post-activation potentiation (PAP), stretching, and priming exercise protocols, respectively, completed as part of a warm-up routine. Whole-body vibration administered during a warm-up routine has been shown to be effective at improving measures of athletic performance, although the mechanisms underlying these improvements are not clear. Performing exercise in hot environments can increase the thermal strain experienced by athletes, limiting their performance in endurance activities; to avoid this problem, pre-cooling methods have been proposed whereby the body core temperature or skin temperature is reduced prior to the exercise.

A warm-up routine completed prior to short-duration (10 s or less) maximal-intensity activities should include 5–10 min of low-intensity activities followed by 8–12 min of large-amplitude dynamic stretches and sport-specific activities of increasing intensity. Such routines should increase muscle temperature, although a sufficient recovery period between the completion of the warm-up routine and the initiation of the athletic performance should be provided to allow the restoration of high-energy phosphates and the clearance of metabolites that may cause fatigue. The warm-up routine prior to intermediate- and long-duration activities should comprise exercises performed at an intensity of 60–70% VO_{2max} for 5–10 min, finishing 5 min prior to the event. This will increase the baseline VO_2 while minimizing glycogen depletion and thermal stress. While many activities can be selected when developing a warm-up routine, the strength and conditioning practitioner should individualize these routines for athletes by determining which exercises and structures are most effective for each athlete.

Review Questions and Projects

1. Explain why it is difficult to establish a causal link between the completion of a warm-up routine and a reduction in injuries based upon the extant literature.

2. Which musculoskeletal injuries might an appropriate warm-up routine guard against and why?

3. Which mechanical characteristics of skeletal muscle are likely to be improved by the increases in muscle temperature that result from completion of the activities in a warm-up routine?

4. Describe the role of hot water immersion, massage, and diathermy in a warm-up routine.

5. Why might passive heating methods not be as effective in improving athletic performance as active methods?

6. Why would a traditional warm-up routine implemented to raise temperature be likely to improve performance during high-intensity, short-duration events?

7. Why do measures of maximal power output demonstrate diurnal variations?

8. Explain what is meant by the Q_{10} of a physiological process.

9. What are the implications of the nonlinearity of Q_{10} values associated with many physiological processes?

10. What are the consequences of a body core temperature of 39.7°C or greater on performance during prolonged-endurance exercise?

11. A distance runner is planning to participate in a marathon in a region where the ambient temperatures are typically greater than 20°C. Which pre-workout warm-up methods might you suggest that the athlete try in training to improve his or her performance during this event?

12. What are the arguments against the use of static stretches in a warm-up routine?

13. What are the arguments for the use of static stretches in a warm-up routine?

14. Describe the physiological mechanisms underpinning the efficacy of priming exercises.

15. Develop a warm-up routine for an 800-m athlete who is about to perform a training session that involves 3×400-m and 6×600-m repetitions with a 3-min recovery period.

16. How would you modify the warm-up routine of the 800-m sprint athlete in Question 15 so that it can be implemented prior to a major track and field competition where the athlete will be held for 20 min prior to the race as part of the "call-up" procedure?

17. Develop a warm-up routine for an Olympic weightlifter incorporating a whole-body vibration protocol.

18. Develop a warm-up routine for an Olympic weightlifter to use during competitions.

19. Develop a warm-up routine for a group of collegiate basketball players to implement prior to a competitive game.

20. Which activities would you implement for the basketball players in Question 19 during the breaks between the playing periods of the game?

References

Aaltonen, S., Karjalainen, H., Heinonen, A., Parkkari, J., & Kujala, U. M. (2007). Prevention of sports injuries: Systematic review of randomized controlled trials. *Archive of Internal Medicine, 167*, 1585–1592.

Adam, A., & De Luca, C. J. (2003). Recruitment order of motor units in human vastus lateralis muscle is maintained during fatiguing contractions. *Journal of Neurophysiology, 90*, 2919–2927.

Bailey, S. J., Vanhatalo, A., Wilkerson, D. P., DiMenna, F. J., & Jones, A. M. (2009). Optimizing the "priming" effect: Influence of prior exercise intensity and recovery duration on O_2 uptake kinetics and severe-intensity exercise tolerance. *Journal of Applied Physiology, 107*, 1743–1756.

Behm, D. G., & Chaouachi, A. (2011). A review of the acute effects of static and dynamic stretching on performance. *European Journal of Applied Physiology, 111*, 2633–2651.

Bennett, A. F. (1985). Temperature and muscle. *Journal of Experimental Biology, 115*, 333–344.

Bishop, D. (2003a). Warm up I: Potential mechanisms and the effects of passive warm up on exercise performance. *Sports Medicine, 33*, 439–454.

Bishop, D. (2003b). Warm up II: Performance changes following active warm up and how to structure the warm up. *Sports Medicine, 33*, 483–498.

Burnley, M., Doust, J. H., Carter, H., & Jones, A. M. (2001). Effects of prior exercise and recovery duration on oxygen uptake kinetics during heavy exercise in humans. *Experimental Physiology, 86*, 417–425.

Burnley, M., Doust, J. H., & Jones, A. M. (2002). Effects of heavy exercise, prior sprint exercise and passive warming on oxygen uptake kinetics during heavy exercise in humans. *European Journal of Applied Physiology, 87*, 424–432.

Burnley, M., Doust, J. H., & Jones, A. M. (2006). Time required for the restoration of normal heavy exercise VO_2 kinetics following prior heavy exercise. *European Journal of Applied Physiology, 101*, 1320–1327.

Carpentier, A., Duchateau, J., & Hainaut, K. (2001). Motor unit behavior and contractile changes during fatigue in the human first dorsal interosseus. *Journal of Physiology, 534*, 903–912.

Cochrane, D. J., Stannard, S. R., Firth, E. C., & Rittweger, J. (2010). Acute whole-body vibration elicits post-activation potentiation. *European Journal of Applied Physiology, 108*, 311–319.

Cochrane, D. J., Stannard, S. R., Sargeant, A. J., & Rittweger, J. (2008). The rate of muscle temperature increase during acute whole-body vibration exercise. *European Journal of Applied Physiology, 103*, 441–448.

Comyns, T. M., Harrison, A. J., Hennessey, L. K., & Jensen, R. L. (2006). The optimal complex training rest interval for athletes from anaerobic sports. *Journal of Strength and Conditioning Research, 20*, 471–476.

Comyns, T. M., Harrison, A. J., Hennessey, L. K., & Jensen, R. L. (2007). Identifying the optimal resistive load for complex training in male rugby players. *Sports Biomechanics, 6*, 59–70.

de Ruiter, C. J., Jones, D. A., Sargeant, A. J., & de Haan, A. (1999). Temperature effects on the rates of isometric force development and relaxation in the fresh and fatigued human adductor pollicis muscle. *Experimental Physiology, 84*, 1137–1150.

Devore, P., & Hagerman, P. (2006). A pregame soccer warm-up. *Strength and Conditioning Journal, 28*, 14–18.

Dewhurst, S., Macaluso, A., Gizzi, L., Felici, F., Farina, D., & De Vitto, G. (2010). Effects of altered muscle temperature on neuromuscular properties in young and older women. *European Journal of Applied Physiology, 108*, 451–458.

Draper, D. O., Harris, S. T., Schulthies, S., Durrant, E., Knight, K. L., & Ricard, M. (1998). Hot-pack and 1-MHz ultrasound treatments have an additive effect on muscle temperature increase. *Journal of Athletic Training, 33*, 21–24.

Drinkwater, E. J. (2008). Effects of peripheral cooling on characteristics of local muscle. In F. E. Marino (Ed.), *Thermoregulation and human performance: Physiological and biological aspects* (pp. 74–88). Basel, Switzerland: Karger.

Drust, B., Atkinson, G., Gregson, W., French, D., & Binningsley, D. (2003). The effects of massage on intra muscular temperature in the vastus lateralis in humans. *International Journal of Sports Medicine, 24*, 395–399.

Drust, B., Rasmussen, P., Mohr, M., Nielsen, B., & Nybo, L. (2005). Elevations in core and muscle temperature impairs repeated sprint performance. *Acta Physiologica Scandinavica, 183*, 181–190.

Ebben, W. P., & Blackard, D. O. (2001). Strength and conditioning practices of National Football League strength and conditioning coaches. *Journal of Strength and Conditioning Research, 15*, 48–58.

Ebben, W. P., Hintz, M. J., & Simenz, C. J. (2005). Strength and conditioning practices of Major League Baseball strength and conditioning coaches. *Journal of Strength and Conditioning Research, 19*, 538–546.

El Helou, N., Tafflet, M., Berthelot, G., Tolaini, J., Marc, A., Guillaume, M., Hausswirth, C., & Toussaint, J. F. (2012). Impact of environmental parameters on marathon running performance. *PLoS One, 7*, e37407.

Enoka, R. M. (2008). *Neuromechanics of human movement*. Champaign, IL: Human Kinetics.

Faigenbaum, A. D. (2011). Dynamic warm-up. In J. Hoffman (Ed.), *NSCA's guide to program design* (pp. 51–70). Champaign, IL: Human Kinetics.

Faulkner, S. H., Ferguson, R. A., Gerrett, N., Hupperets, M., Hodder, S. G., & Havenith, G. (2013). Reducing muscle temperature drop after warm-up improves sprint cycling performance. *Medicine and Science in Sport and Exercise, 45*, 359–365.

Febbraio, M. A., Murton, P., Selig, S. E., Clark, S. A., Lambert, D. L., Angus, D. J., & Carey, M. F. (1996). Effects of CHO ingestion on exercise metabolism and performance in different ambient temperatures. *Medicine and Science in Sports and Exercise, 28*, 1380–1387.

Fletcher, I. M. (2010). The effects of precompetition massage on the kinematic parameters of 20-m sprint performance. *Journal of Strength and Conditioning Research, 24*, 1179–1183.

Folland, J. P., Wakamatsu, T., & Fimland, M. S. (2008). The influence of maximal isometric activity on twitch and H-reflex potentiation, and quadriceps femoris performance. *European Journal of Applied Physiology, 104*, 739–748.

Fukuba, Y., Shinhara, Y., Houman, T., Endo, M. Y., Yamada, M., Miura, A., . . . Yoshida, T. (2012). VO_2 response at the onset of heavy exercise is accelerated not by diathermic warming of the thigh muscles but by prior heavy exercise. *Research in Sports Medicine, 20*, 13–24.

Fuller, J. T., Thompson, R. L., Howe, P. R. C., & Buckley, J. D. (2013). Effect of vibration on muscle perfusion: A systematic review. *Clinical Physiology and Functional Imaging, 33*, 1–9.

Goodwin, J. E., Glaister, M., Howatson, G., Lockey, R. A., & McInnes, G. (2007). Effect of performance lower-limb massage on thirty-meter sprint running. *Journal of Strength and Conditioning Research, 21*, 1028–1031.

Gray, S. R., De Vito, G., Nimmo, M. A., Farina, D., & Ferguson, R. A. (2006). Skeletal muscle ATP turnover and muscle fiber conduction velocity are elevated at higher muscle temperatures during maximal power output development in humans. *American Journal of Physiology, 290*, R376–R382.

Gray, S. R., Söderlund, K., & Ferguson, R. A. (2008). ATP and phosphocreatine utilization in single human muscle fibers during the development of maximal power output at elevated muscle temperatures. *Journal of Sports Sciences, 26*, 701–707.

Guidetti, L., Di Cagno, A., Chiara Gallotta, M., Battaglia, C., Piazza, M., & Baldari, C. (2009). Precompetition warm-up in elite and subelite rhythmic gymnastics. *Journal of Strength and Conditioning Research, 23*, 1877–1882.

Guissard, N., & Duchateau, J. (2006). Neural aspects of muscle stretching. *Exercise and Sport Sciences Reviews, 34*, 154–158.

Hodgson, M., Docherty, D., & Robbins, D. (2005). Post-activation potentiation: Underlying physiology and implications for motor performance. *Sports Medicine, 35*, 585–595.

Hodgson, M. J., Docherty, D., & Zeher, E. P. (2008). Postactivation potentiation of force is independent of H-reflex excitability. *International Journal of Sports Physiology and Performance, 3*, 219–231.

Hoffman, M. D., Williams, C. A., & Lind, A. R. (1985). Changes in isometric function following rhythmic exercise. *European Journal of Applied Physiology, 54*, 177–183.

Holewijn, M., & Heus, R. (1992). Effects of temperature on electromyogram and muscle function. *European Journal of Applied Physiology, 65*, 541–545.

Ingham, S. A., Fudge, B. W., Pringle, J. S., & Jones, A. M. (2013). Improvement of 800-m running performance with prior high-intensity exercise. *International Journal of Sports Physiology and Performance, 8*, 77–83.

Jefferys, I. (2008). Warm-up and stretching. In T. R. Baechle & R. W. Earle (Eds.), *Essentials of strength training and conditioning* (pp. 295–324). Champaign, IL: Human Kinetics.

Jones, A. M., & Burnley, M. (2009). Oxygen uptake kinetics: An underappreciated determinant of exercise performance. *International Journal of Sports Physiology and Performance, 4*, 524–532.

Jones, A. M., Wilkerson, D. P., Burnley, M., & Koppo, K. (2003). Prior heavy exercise enhances performance during subsequent perimaximal exercise. *Medicine and Science in Sports and Exercise, 35*, 2085–2092.

Jones, P. R., Barton, C., Morrisey, D., Maffulli, N., & Hemmings, S. (2012). Pre-cooling for endurance exercise performance in the heat: A systematic review. *BMC Medicine, 10*, 166.

Kay, A. D., & Blazevich, A. J. (2009). Isometric contractions reduce plantar flexor moment, Achilles tendon stiffness and neuromuscular activity but remove the subsequent effects of stretch. *Journal of Applied Physiology, 107*, 1181–1189.

Kay, A. D., & Blazevich, A. J. (2012). Effect of acute static stretch on maximal muscle performance: A systematic review. *Medicine and Science in Sports and Exercise, 44*, 154–164.

Kenny, G. P., Reardon, F. D., Zaleski, W., Reardon, M. L., Haman, F., & Ducharme, M. B. (2003). Muscle temperature transients before, during, and after exercise measured using an intramuscular multisensory probe. *Journal of Applied Physiology, 94*, 2350–2357.

Kiani, A., Hellquist, E., Ahlqvist, K., Gedeborg, R., & Michaëlson, K. (2010). Prevention of soccer-related knee injuries in teenaged girls. *Archives of Internal Medicine, 170*, 43–49.

Kubo, K., Kanehisa, H., & Fukunaga, T. (2005). Effects of cold and hot water immersion on the mechanical properties of human muscle and tendon in vivo. *Clinical Biomechanics, 20*, 291–300.

Lehmann, J. F., Masock, A. J., Warren, C. G., & Koblanski, J. N. (1970). Effect of therapeutic temperatures on tendon extensibility. *Archives of Physical Medicine and Rehabilitation, 51*, 481–487.

Lovell, R., Midgley, A., Barrett, S., Carter, D., & Small, K. (2013). Effects of different half-time strategies on second half soccer-specific speed, power and dynamic strength. *Scandinavian Journal of Medicine and Science in Sports, 23*, 105–113.

MacIntosh, B. R., Robillard, M-E., & Tomaras, E. K. (2012). Should postactivation potentiation be the goal of your warm-up? *Applied Physiology, Nutrition and Metabolism, 37*, 546–550.

Maffiuletti, N. A., & Cardinale, M. (2011). Alternative modalities of strength and conditioning: Electrical stimulation and vibration. In M. Cardinale, R. Newton, & K. Nosaka (Eds.), *Strength and conditioning: Biological principles and practical applications* (pp. 193–208). Chichester, UK: John Wiley & Sons.

Magnusson, S. P., Aagaard, P., Larsson, B., & Kjær, M. (2000). Passive energy absorption by human muscle-tendon unit is unaffected by increase in intramuscular temperature. *Journal of Applied Physiology, 88*, 1215–1220.

Magnusson, P., & Renström, P. (2006). The European College of Sports Sciences position statement: The role of stretching exercises in sports. *European Journal of Applied Sport Science, 6*, 87–91.

Mandelbaum, B. R., Silvers, H. J., Watanabe, D. S., Knarr, J. F., Thomas, S. D., Griffin, L. Y., Kirkendall, D. T., & Garrett, W. (2005). Effectiveness of a neuromuscular and proprioceptive training program in preventing anterior cruciate ligament injuries in females athletes. *American Journal of Sports Medicine, 33*, 1003–1010.

McBain, K., Shrier, I., Shultz, R., Meeuwisse, W. H., Klügl, M., Garza, D., & Matheson, G. O. (2012a). Prevention of sports injury I: A systematic review of applied biomechanics and physiology outcomes research. *British Journal of Sports Medicine, 46*, 169–173.

McBain, K., Shrier, I., Shultz, R., Meeuwisse, W. H., Klügl, M., Garza, D., & Matheson, G. O. (2012b). Prevention of sports injury II: A systematic review of clinical science research. *British Journal of Sports Medicine, 46*, 174–179.

McBride, J. M., Nimphius, S., & Erickson, T. M. (2005). The acute effects of heavy-load squats and loaded countermovement jumps on sprint performance. *Journal of Strength and Conditioning Research, 19*, 893–897.

McBride, J. M., Nuzzo, J. L., Dayne, A. M., Israetel, M. A., Nieman, D. C., & Triplett, N. T. (2010). Effect of an acute bout of whole body vibration exercise on muscle force output and motor neuron excitability. *Journal of Strength and Conditioning Research, 24*, 184–189.

McHugh, M. P., & Cosgrave, C. H. (2010). To stretch or not to stretch: The role of stretching in injury prevention and performance. *Scandinavian Journal of Medicine and Science in Sports, 20*, 169–181.

McNair, P. J., Dombroski, E. W., Hewson, D. J., & Stanley, S. N. (2000). Stretching at the ankle joint: Viscoelastic responses to holds and continuous passive motion. *Medicine and Science in Sports and Exercise, 33*, 354–358.

Mitchell, S. M., Trowbridge, C. A., Fincher, A. L., & Cramer, J. T. (2008). Effect of diathermy on muscle temperature, electromyography, and mechanomyography. *Muscle and Nerve, 38*, 992–1004.

Miura, A., Shiragiku, C., Hirotoshi, Y., Kitano, A., Endo, M. Y., Barstow, T. J., . . . Fukuba, Y. (2009). The effect of prior heavy exercise on the parameters of the power–duration curve for cycle ergometry. *Applied Physiology, Nutrition and Metabolism, 34*, 1001–1007.

Mohr, M., Krustrup, P., & Bangsbo, J. (2003). Match performance of high-standard soccer players with special reference to development of fatigue. *Journal of Sports Science, 21*, 439–449.

Mohr, M., Krustrup, P., Nybo, L., Nielsen, J. J., & Bangsbo, J. (2004). Muscle temperature and sprint performance during soccer matches: Beneficial effects of re-warm-up at half-time. *Scandinavian Journal of Medicine and Science in Sports, 14*, 156–162.

Murphy, J. R., Di Santo, M. C., Alkanani, T., & Behm, D. G. (2010). Aerobic activity before and following short-duration static stretching improves range of motion and performance vs. a traditional warm-up. *Applied Physiology, Nutrition and Metabolism, 35*, 679–690.

Nielsen, B., Hales, J. R., Strange, S., Christensen, N. J., Warberg, J., & Saltin, B. (1993). Human circulatory and thermoregulatory adaptations with heat acclimation and exercise in a hot, dry environment. *Journal of Physiology, 460*, 467–485.

Norlund, M. M., & Thorstensson, A. (2007). Strength training effects of whole-body vibration? *Scandinavian Journal of Medicine and Science in Sports, 17*, 12–17.

Nosaka, K., Sakamoto, K., Newton, M., & Sacco, P. (2004). Influence of pre-exercise muscle temperature on responses to eccentric exercise. *Journal of Athletic Training, 39*, 132–137.

Nybo, L. (2008). Hyperthermia and fatigue. *Journal of Applied Physiology, 104*, 871–878.

Parkin, J. M., Carey, M. F., Zhao, S., & Febbraio, M. A. (1999). Effects of ambient temperature on human skeletal muscle metabolism during fatiguing submaximal exercise. *Journal of Applied Physiology, 86*, 902–908.

Price, M. J., Boyd, C., & Goosey-Tolfrey, V. L. (2009). The physiological effects of pre-event and midevent cooling during intermittent running in the heat in elite female soccer players. *Applied Physiology, Nutrition and Metabolism, 34*, 942–949.

Racinais, S. (2010). Different effects of heat exposure upon exercise performance in the morning and afternoon. *Scandinavian Journal of Sports Medicine, 20*, S80–S89.

Racinais, S., & Oksa, J. (2010). Temperature and neuromuscular function. *Scandinavian Journal of Medicine and Science in Sports, 20*, S1–S18.

Robbins, D. W. (2005). Postactivation potentiation and its practical applicability: A brief review. *Journal of Strength and Conditioning Research, 19*, 453–458.

Ruben, R. M., Molinari, M. A., Bibbee, C. A., Childress, M. A., Harman, M. S., & Haff, G. G. (2010). The acute effects of an ascending squat protocol on performance during horizontal plyometric jumps. *Journal of Strength and Conditioning Research, 24*, 358–369.

Rubini, E. C., Costa, A. L. L., & Gomes, P. S. C. (2007). The effects of stretching on strength performance. *Sports Medicine, 37*, 213–224.

Safran, M. R., Garrett, W. E., Seaber, A. V., Glisson, R. R., & Ribbeck, B. M. (1988). The role of warmup in muscular injury prevention. *American Journal of Sports Medicine, 16*, 123–129.

Sale, D. G. (2002). Postactivation potentiation: Role in human performance. *Exercise and Sport Science Reviews, 30*, 138–143.

Saugen, E., & Vøllestad, N. K. (1995). Nonlinear relationship between heat production and force during voluntary contractions in humans. *Journal of Applied Physiology, 79*, 2043–2049.

Soligard, T., Nilstad, A., Steffen, K., Myklebust, G., Holme, I., Dvorak, J., . . . Andersen, T. E. (2010). Compliance with a comprehensive warm-up programme to prevent injuries in youth soccer. *British Journal of Sports Medicine, 44*, 787–793.

Starkie, R. L., Hargreaves, M., Lambert, D. L., Proietto, J., & Febbraio, M. A. (1999). Effect of temperature on muscle metabolism during submaximal exercise in humans. *Experimental Physiology, 84*, 775–784.

Steffen, K., Myklebust, G., Olsen, O. E., Holme, I., & Bahr, R. (2008). Preventing injuries in female youth football: A cluster-randomized controlled trial. *Scandinavian Journal of Medicine and Science in Sports, 18*, 605–614.

Steinen, G. J. M., Kiers, J. L., Bottinelli, R., & Reggiani, C. (1996). Myofibrillar ATPase activity in skinned human skeletal fibers: Fiber type and temperature dependence. *Journal of Physiology, 493*, 299–307.

Taylor, J., Weston, M., & Portas, M. D. (2013). The effect of a short, practical warm-up protocol on repeated-sprint performance. *Journal of Strength and Conditioning Research, 27*, 2034–2038.

Tillin, N. A., & Bishop, D. (2009). Factors modulating post-activation potentiation and its effect on performance of subsequent explosive activities. *Sports Medicine, 39*, 147–166.

Tucker, R., Marle, T., Lambert, E. V., & Noakes, T. D. (2006). The rate of heat storage mediates an anticipatory reduction in exercise intensity during cycling at a fixed rating of perceived exertion. *Journal of Physiology, 574*, 905–915.

Waldén, M., Atroshi, I., Magnusson, H., Wagner, P., & Hägglund, M. (2012). Prevention of acute knee injuries in adolescent female football players: Cluster randomized controlled trial. *British Medical Journal, 344*, e3042.

Weerapong, P., Hume, P. A., & Kolt, G. S. (2005). The mechanisms of massage and effects on performance, muscle recovery and injury prevention. *Sports Medicine, 35*, 235–256.

Wegmann, M., Faude, O., Poppendieck, W., Hecksteden, A., Frölich, M., & Meyer, T. (2012). Pre-cooling and sports performance: A meta-analytical review. *Sports Medicine, 42*, 545–564.

Woods, K., Bishop, P., & Jones, E. (2007). Warm-up and stretching in the prevention of muscular injury. *Sports Medicine, 37*, 1089–1099.

Young, W. B. (2007). The use of static stretching in warm-up for training and competition. *International Journal of Sports Physiology and Performance, 2*, 212–216.

Young, W. B., & Behm, D. G. (2003). Effects of running, static stretching and practice jumps on explosive force production and jumping performance. *Journal of Sports Medicine and Physical Fitness, 43*, 21–27.

Zois, J., Bishop, D., Fairweather, I., Ball, K., & Aughey, R. J. (2013). High-intensity re-warm-ups enhance soccer performance. *International Journal of Sports Medicine, 34*, 800–805.

CHAPTER 9

Performance Analysis in Sport

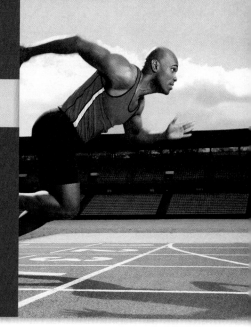

Chapter Objectives

At the end of this chapter, you will be able to:

- Explain the role of performance analysis in strength and conditioning

- Discuss the advantages and disadvantages of the different technologies used in notational and time–motion analyses

- Use time–motion analysis data to develop sport-specific workouts and tests

- Explain the use of different technologies to monitor workloads during training

- Discuss quantitative, predictive, and qualitative approaches to technique analysis

- Explain the use of the integrated model of qualitative analysis to observe and improve the techniques used in specific skills

- Discuss the role of biomechanical principles and deterministic models in the identification of critical features in technique analysis

Key Terms

Biomechanical principles

Closed motor skills

Continuous motor skills

Critical features

Deterministic model

Discrete motor skills

Fine motor skills

Gross motor skills

Model template

Motor skill

Movement

Movement phases

Needs analysis

Notational and time–motion analysis

Open motor skills

Performance

Performance indicators

Predictive approach

Qualitative approach

Quantitative approach

Skill

Technique

Technique analysis

Chapter Overview

Performance analysis methods can be used by strength and conditioning practitioners to gain insight into the physiological, mechanical, and technical demands of specific sports, and to assess the techniques used in the execution of sport-specific skills. The information derived from the various performance analysis methods can be used by practitioners to improve the performance of the athletes with whom they are working. Therefore, performance analysis methods constitute a first step for the strength and conditioning coach to consult when developing a sport-specific training program; however, continued use of performance analysis methods is essential for monitoring the progress of an athlete throughout the training process.

In this chapter, we introduce different methods of sports performance analysis that can be used by the strength and conditioning practitioner, focusing on those methods pertinent to biomechanical analyses and skill acquisition. We begin by introducing notational and time–motion analysis methods, which allow the identification of the movements required in successful sports performance. Next, we introduce the methods associated with technique analysis, which allow the practitioner to assess movements used by athletes during the execution of sport-specific skills and develop interventions to improve athletes' movements. We conclude by introducing an integrated model of qualitative technique analysis.

Methods of Performance Analysis

The different methods of performance analysis available to the strength and conditioning practitioner can be classified into two broad categories: **notational and time–motion analysis** and **technique analysis**. Notational and time–motion analysis methods are concerned with tracking the movements and technical actions of an athlete within his or her environment during competition and training. The data derived from such analyses can be used to guide the development of sport-specific training sessions and physical tests by identifying the categories of movements, selecting player-specific activities, and determining the effects of fatigue on performance (Carling, Bloomfield, Nelsen, & Reilly, 2008). Conversely, technique analysis methods are concerned with the analysis of specific sport skills and the way in which they are performed to provide a basis for improving future performance (Lees, 2002).

Performance analysis is concerned with the identification of **performance indicators** (Hughes & Bartlett, 2002). A performance indicator is an action variable that can define some or all aspects of performance of an individual athlete, a team, or an element of a team. The difference between notational and time–motion analyses and technique analyses is the scale at which the analysis takes place and the corresponding performance indicators that are produced. For example, a notational analysis of a soccer game might return performance indicators including the number of tackles won and lost, the number of successful passes completed, and the number of successful dribbles. A time–motion analysis of the same game might return information on the distances traveled by each player in different modes of locomotion (e.g., walking, running, sprinting), the total distance traveled, and the proportions of time spent in different locomotor modes. A technique analysis might focus on a specific technique used by an individual soccer player in an isolated skill such as a penalty kick, and would provide information including the placement of the support leg relative to the ball, the rotation of the trunk, and the timing of hip flexion and knee extension during the action phase of the skill.

The methods of performance analysis rely heavily on technology to provide information on performance indicators. Notational and time–motion analysis methods use either video- or satellite-based technology to record the movements and actions of the athletes, while technique analysis relies on video data to aid the coach in observing the specific skills performed by the athletes. The amount of data that can be gathered is enormous. For example, the analysis of elite soccer matches can result in approximately 4.5 million data points associated with player positions and more than 2000 touches of the ball (Carling et al., 2008). Similarly, technique analysis has the potential to generate large numbers of kinematic and kinetic variables that could be considered important determinants of successful execution of the specific skill. The requirement to analyze this wealth of data has implications for the time needed to provide feedback to the coaches and athletes. In recognition of this time demand, performance analysis methods utilize computer software to process and analyze the data, and automated systems have been developed for this purpose. Furthermore, more complex statistical techniques are being used to uncover patterns within the enormous amount of data generated (e.g., cluster analysis, artificial neural networks), and systematic approaches to the selection of appropriate variables to record during such analyses are being developed.

Notational and Time-Motion Analysis Methods

Notational and time–motion analysis methods provide data on physical efforts, movement patterns, and technical actions of the players and relate these data to the athletes' relative success. The activity profile of players in a given sport (e.g., work:rest ratios, distance, duration, and number of sprints) can be determined by continuously tracking the movements of players. These data can then inform the development of sport-specific training and testing protocols (Glaister, 2005). Furthermore, the data collected from notational analyses can be used to determine the importance of specific skills required during successful performance (Thomas, Fellingham, & Vehrs, 2009; Wheeler, Askew, & Sayers, 2010).

Early methods of notational analysis relied on direct observations, with the analyst taking written notes during this process. These methods have subsequently been replaced by more complex techniques relying on video-based technology, whereby key events are identified through computer-based coding software (e.g., Observer Pro). Player tracking systems are available that utilize video technology (both manual and automated technology) and Global Positioning System (GPS)–based methods. Some of these technologies allow for the collection of data in real time, thereby making information immediately available to the coach or athlete. With other technologies, the analysis is performed offline once the activities have been completed—an approach that can substantially delay the delivery of feedback. Table 9.1 shows examples of technologies used in notational and time–motion analyses. These technologies differ in terms of their cost, complexity, and reliability and validity.

Manual Video-Based Analysis Methods

Manual video-based methods of notational and time–motion analysis typically require the user to manually code videos of the activities with a specific computer-based software program (e.g., Observer Pro). The specific coding system can be developed by the user and can provide information on the frequency of specific actions and the

Table 9.1
Examples of Technologies Used in Notational and Time–Motion Analyses

System Name	Manufacturer	Technology	Description
Observer Pro	Noldus	Manual video-based	Videos of activities are recorded and analyzed offline. Requires the development of a specific coding protocol for the movements under observation, which the user must identify manually. Allows only single player analysis. Allows determination of frequency and duration of events.
Trak Performance	Sportstec	Manual video-based	The user tracks a single player using a computer pen and a commercially available tablet. The tablet area is scaled to the appropriate playing area. Allows determination of frequency and duration of events as well as distances covered. Allows only single player analysis. Analysis can be performed either online or offline.
Amisco Pro	Sport-Universal	Automatic video-based	Cameras are set permanently at stadia. Allows multiple players to be analyzed concurrently. Allows determination of the frequency and duration of events as well as the distances covered.
ProZone	Prozone Sports	Automatic video-based	Cameras are set permanently at stadia. Allows multiple players to be analyzed concurrently. Allows determination of the frequency and duration of events as well as the distances covered.
OptimEye	Catapult Sports	GPS-based	The player wears the unit in a vest. Multiple players can be analyzed concurrently, depending on the number of units purchased. Allows determination of the frequency and duration of events as well as the distances covered. Time spent at specific running speeds can be determined. GPS data are combined with heart rate (physiological load) and accelerometer data (e.g., number of tackles, jumps). Data can be viewed in real time. GPS devices are prohibited by most sports governing bodies during competitions.

Note: GPS = Global Positioning System.

duration of these activities. This information is then related to the effectiveness of the performance. Such techniques have been used to assess player movements and technical actions in a variety of sports, including rugby, soccer, basketball, volleyball, Australian Rules Football, badminton, and squash (Barris & Button, 2008). See Applied Research 9.1 and 9.2.

Manual notational and time–motion analysis methods have an advantage in that they do not require the athlete to wear any electronic devices; thus they are not likely to interfere with the performance in any way. These methods can be used with video data collected from a single commercially available camera that is either stationary or panning. They are also relatively inexpensive. However, manual methods are time consuming due to the requirement to analyze players separately, which delays feedback of information to the coach and athletes. Furthermore, the subjective interpretation of the activities of the athletes can result in poor inter-rater reliability and even intra-rater reliability (Barris & Button, 2008).

Applied Research 9.1
Manual notational analysis in Division I women's soccer

Thomas, Fellingham, and Vehrs (2009) developed a notational coding system that allowed scoring of the outcome associated with skills including passing, dribbling, first touch, and defensive tactics in soccer. The specific analysis system was derived from the previous literature, the expertise of the research team, and the testimony of expert coaches. The occurrence of the skills and the outcomes of the skills were manually coded in 10 Division I NCAA women's soccer games that were videotaped with a single digital camcorder. A statistical model was then used to determine the importance of each skill in creating goal-scoring opportunities. The authors reported that dribbling was the most important skill, followed by first touch, passing, and defensive tactics. This research has important consequences for the development of specific practices that are likely to influence the outcome of games in collegiate women's soccer.

Thomas, C., Fellingham, G., & Vehrs, P. (2009). Development of a notational analysis system for selected soccer skills of a women's college team. *Measurement in Physical Education and Exercise Science, 13*, 108–121.

Applied Research 9.2
Manual notational analysis in an elite rugby union

Duthie, Pyne, and Hooper (2005) developed a computer-based coding system that allowed the identification of nine specific activities—standing, walking, jogging, striding, sprinting, static exertion (e.g., scrums, rucks, mauls), jumping, lifting, and tackling—performed by rugby players. Video footage of 16 elite rugby matches recorded by commercial television stations and distributed on the public domain was analyzed. The manual coding system was used to quantify the total time spent in each activity, the total number of occurrences, the mean duration of each activity, and the durations of the work and rest periods. The players were categorized into positional groups to allow for comparison of activities between forwards and backs.

The authors reported that backs spent a greater amount of time standing, walking, and sprinting compared to forwards, while forwards performed fewer sprints (an average of 14 compared to 27 for backs). The duration of the sprint was also greater for the backs compared to the forwards (an average of 2.9 s compared to 2.2 s). The average work:rest ratio for the forwards was 6.2:39.8 s, while that for the backs was 4.1:75.8 s. These findings have significant implications for the development of training and testing methods for competitive rugby union players.

Duthie, G. M., Pyne, D. B., & Hooper, S. L. (2005). Time motion analysis of 2001 and 2002 Super 12 rugby. *Journal of Sports Sciences, 23*, 523–530.

Automatic Video-Based Analysis Methods

Automatic video-based player tracking technologies are used to track the locations of objects (e.g., players, ball) within a video field using mathematical algorithms to identify specific pixel configurations associated with the specific objects (see Performance Analysis Concept 9.1). The video data are gathered from multiple stationary high-quality video data recorders. Such systems have been used extensively in soccer (Carling et al., 2008) as well as in court sports such as handball and squash (Barris & Button, 2008).

The systems used to analyze elite soccer (e.g., Amisco Pro, ProZone) require multiple cameras installed within the stadia where the games are played. These cameras are calibrated to the specific dimensions of the field of play, which allows for determination of not only the duration of specific activities but also the distances covered by the players and associated derivatives such as speeds (Dellal et al., 2011). (See Applied Research 9.3.) However, the requirement for multiple cameras and an associated computer network within the location renders such systems expensive.

Performance Analysis Concept 9.1

Automated video-based player tracking technology

Automated video-based player tracking systems use a series of mathematical algorithms to identify and track an object of interest (e.g., a player, a ball). Once high-quality videos are collected from multiple cameras arranged around the field or court of play, a simple blob-tracking algorithm can be used in which the object of interest is identified by the collection of pixels (defined by their color and spatial similarity) associated with the object after the background images have been removed. Essentially, each frame of the video is compared to an image of the empty field or court, thereby allowing the blobs associated with the objects of interest to be identified. The central position of the pixelated blobs can then be used to determine the two-dimensional position of the object within a predetermined reference frame.

The automaticity of this technology is somewhat limited, however, and the systems require manual correction when the objects of interest become occluded, as is likely with the complexity of player movements in many sports or when the video quality is reduced. Although automated tracking systems usually rely on high-quality video data collected from multiple cameras, tracking algorithms have been developed that can be used on lower-quality videos shot from a single camera (Vučković, Perš, James, & Hughes, 2010; Yan, Christmas, & Kittler, 2005). These systems require that the user first identify the object of interest before it is tracked automatically; the analysis is performed offline once the video data have been collected. More complex tracking algorithms have been developed in tennis that can not only automatically track a player's movement but also determine the type of shot played (Bloom & Bradley, 2003).

Applied Research 9.3
Automated player tracking technology in elite men's soccer

Dellal et al. (2011) used an automated player tracking system (Amisco Pro) to characterize the physical and technical performance in 600 matches played in the top professional soccer leagues of England and Spain. The data were collected using eight stationary cameras located at specific stadia across the leagues. The outfield players were categorized based on their playing position; the variables analyzed were the physical activity of the players (total distance covered, distances covered at high intensities [running speed greater than 21 km/h] with and without the ball) and their technical actions (heading and ground duels, passing, time in possession, ball touches).

The authors reported that there was no difference in the total distance covered by the players in both leagues. However, the players in the English league tended to cover greater distances when sprinting, although the players in the Spanish league covered a greater total distance in sprinting when their team was in possession of the ball. Full backs in the Spanish league had smaller numbers and lower duration of ball possessions compared to the full backs in the English league; the reverse was true for the central attacking midfield players. The number of ground duels experienced by the players in the Spanish league was significantly smaller than that for the players in the English league, although there was no difference in the success rate of these ground duels. This information can be used to develop specific training and talent identification programs within the two countries.

Dellal, A., Chamari, K., Wong, D. P., Ahmaidi, S., Keller, D., Barros, R., . . . Carling, C. (2011). Comparison of physical and technical performance in European soccer match-play: FA Premier League and La Liga. *European Journal of Applied Sport Science, 11*, 51–59.

Moreover, their lack of portability allows these systems to be used only during competitions, and not in training. Furthermore, the data processing required means that the data are not immediately available to the coaches and players. As with the manual video-based technologies, the automated systems do not require the athletes to wear any associated device, so there is little chance of the technology interfering with their performance. In contrast to the manual technology, however, the automated systems provide an objective assessment of player movements. Unfortunately, there are few studies verifying the validity and reliability of these automated systems beyond manufacturer statements (Carling et al., 2008).

Global Positioning System–Based Methods

Global Positioning System (GPS) devices allow the online determination of distances covered by multiple athletes concurrently. This technology has been applied extensively in field sports such as soccer, rugby, field hockey, and Australian Rules Football to determine the activity profiles of players during training sessions and even competitions in some of these sports (Aughey, 2011). See Applied Research 9.4.

The GPS receivers are worn by the athlete in a vest placed on the upper body, which may preclude their use during competitions in certain sports. The positional and time data are telemetered to a computer, where they are analyzed by specific software. This approach allows other kinematic data, including velocity, to be calculated. The commercial receivers typically sample the position of the athlete at a frequency

Applied Research 9.4
Tracking of elite field hockey players during competitions

Jennings, Cormack, Coutts, and Aughey (2012) used GPS devices sampling at 5 Hz to record the total distance covered, distance of high-speed running (speeds greater than 4.17 m/s), and distance of low-speed activities (speeds of 0.10 to 4.17 m/s) in elite male field hockey players during six matches in a nine-day period of a world-class tournament. The players were from the same team and were categorized as defenders, midfielders, and strikers. Their values were compared to those recorded during the first match of the tournament and to the tournament averages for the team. Regardless of the comparison, all positional players were able to maintain or even increase the distances covered during high-speed running during the six tournament matches. This finding suggests that the players were able to resist fatigue across the six matches performed in the nine-day period.

Jennings, D., Cormack, S., Coutts, A. J., & Aughey, R. J. (2012). GPS analysis of an international field hockey tournament. *International Journal of Sports Physiology and Performance, 7,* 224–231.

of 1 or 5 Hz, although some devices record the data up to 10 Hz. The validity and reliability of the GPS devices are affected by the sampling frequency and the distance and speed of movement (Aughey, 2011). Specifically, a higher sampling frequency produces more valid and reliable distance measurements, while the devices are more valid and reliable over greater movement distances and lower movement speeds.

Each manufacturer of GPS receivers utilizes its own algorithms for signal acquisition and processing, resulting in differences in errors from different manufacturers (Witte & Wilson, 2004). Furthermore, even when devices from the same manufacturer are used, some evidence indicates the possibility of inter-unit differences in errors (Jennings, Cormack, Coutts, Boyd, & Aughey, 2010); thus it is recommended that the same unit be used for the same athlete throughout the monitoring process. Some GPS-based systems (e.g., OptimEye) include built-in heart rate monitors and accelerometers, which provide physiological data on the relative intensities of the actions performed by the player and allow the determination of the acceleration of the player and the frequency of events such as tackles and jumps executed. However, the accelerometer data derived from GPS devices has been shown to have relatively poor reliability (Waldron, Worsfold, Twist, & Lamb, 2011). Furthermore, not all sports governing bodies allow athletes to wear electronic devices such as GPS devices during competitions, limiting their use to training sessions.

In summary, the strength and conditioning coach can use a number of systems to track players, all of which rely on different technologies. Randers et al. (2010) reported large inter-device differences in the distances covered by soccer players during a test game recorded by manual and automated video-based and GPS tracking systems. Their work suggests that practitioners should exercise caution when comparing the results of player tracking studies performed with different technologies. All methods appear to have potential issues with validity and reliability, so other factors—such as system cost, portability, and analysis time—should be taken into consideration. The GPS systems are portable and allow online analysis of multiple athletes concurrently. Their validity and reliability can be enhanced by increasing the sampling frequency of the devices. Furthermore, GPS systems allow the determination of both physical (e.g., distance covered) and physiological (e.g., heart rate) loads. However, they will not provide information about tactical activities of the players. Moreover, they are not permitted during competitions in many sports and, therefore, can be used only in training and practice situations.

The behavior being analyzed using notational and time–motion analysis techniques is a complex pattern that takes place during the sporting event. The skills revealed as part of such analyses do not take place in isolation of each other; they do not occur as discrete skills, per se, but rather are linked together as part of a more complex overall pattern of movement (Vilar, Araújo, Davids, & Button, 2012). The discrete skills that emerge from such analyses are due to the framework associated with notational and time–motion analyses techniques; they should not be trained in isolation. An example of using time–motion analysis data to develop a sport-specific test is presented in **Worked Example 9.1**, while the use of time–motion analysis technology to develop and monitor training sessions is discussed in **Performance Analysis Concept 9.2**.

Worked Example 9.1
Using time–motion analysis data from basketball to develop a sport-specific test

A number of time–motion analysis studies have been performed on basketball (Abdelkrim, El Fazaa, & El Ati, 2007; Janeira & Maia, 1998; McInnes, Carlson, Jones, & McKenna, 1995). From these studies, it can be concluded that basketball is a repeated-sprint sport characterized by frequent bouts of short-duration, high-intensity movements (e.g., sprints, shuffling, jumping) interspersed with periods of low-intensity activity. **Table 9.2** shows the frequencies and durations of specific activities recorded during basketball matches collected from time–motion analysis studies. As well as the specific activities noted in this table, Janeira and Maia (1998) reported an average of 58 changes of direction during a game; McInnes et al. (1995) noted a change of movement activity every 2 s throughout a basketball game, with a high-intensity activity being performed every 21 s.

We can use this information to develop a basketball-specific repeated-sprint test. The high-intensity movements included in this test are forward sprinting, side shuffling, and jumping. The pattern of the test followed by the athlete is that of a T, with each section of the T comprising a distance of 5 m to ensure a change of direction every 2 s when the movement is performed at maximal intensity (**Figure 9.1**). Each trial begins with a countermovement vertical jump for maximal height performed on a contact mat, after which the player sprints forward 5 m and then side-shuffles 2.5 m to the right, placing the right foot in the marked square and touching a basketball placed at waist height with the right hand. From here, the player side-shuffles 5 m to the left, placing the left foot in the marked square and touching a waist-high basketball with the left hand before side-shuffling 2.5 m back to the right. When the player reaches the middle of the T pattern, he or she turns to sprint through the start line (this can be modified to backpedaling if required). Timing gates placed at the beginning of the T provide a measure of the time taken during each sprint, while the contact mat records the height of each jump.

Each trial has an estimated duration of 6 s and is repeated 5 times, with a 20-s recovery period between each iteration. Five repetitions are performed because evidence shows that athletes may pace themselves when they are requested to perform more than five

Table 9.2
Frequency and Average Duration of Specific Activities During Basketball Matches Derived from Time–Motion Analysis Studies

Activity	Frequency	Average Duration (s)	Percentage of Live Time
Sprint	55	1.7–2.1	5.3
Jump	44–46	1.0	2.1
High-intensity shuffle	63–94	2.0	8.8
Low-intensity activity	450	4.2	55.7

Note: Percentage of live time = duration of activity relative to the time when the game clock is running; low-intensity activities = jogging, walking, running.

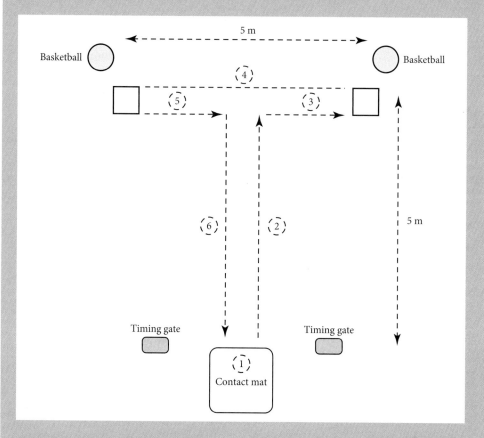

Figure 9.1 Schematic representation of the basketball-specific repeated-sprint test. (1) The player begins by jumping for maximum height on a contact mat. (2) The player then sprints forward. (3) The player changes direction and side-shuffles to the right. (4) The player places the right foot in the marked square and touches the basketball before side-shuffling to the left. (5) The player places the left foot in the marked square and touches the basketball before side-shuffling to the right. (6) The player reaches the middle of the pattern and turns to sprint through the start line.

(continues)

(continued)

Table 9.3
Frequency and Average Duration of Specific Activities During the Basketball-Specific Repeated-Sprint Test

Activity	Frequency	Average Duration (s)	Percentage of Test Time*
Forward sprint	10	1.5	12 (5.3)
Jump	5	1.0	4 (2.1)
High-intensity shuffle	15	1.0	12 (8.8)
Recovery	4	20	72 (55.7)

*Based upon a total test time of 110 s (5×6-s sprints; 4×20-s recovery). The numbers in parentheses denote the values derived from published time–motion analysis studies.

repetitions in a repeated-sprint test (Billaut, Bishop, Schaerz, & Noakes, 2011), which would violate the requirement of a maximal effort test. The recovery period between each sprint is taken from McInnes et al. (1995). Table 9.3 shows the frequency and duration of the different activities associated with the test. Note that this test is not designed to replicate the game, but rather seeks to assess the physical capacity of the players using activities that reflect the specific demands of the game.

This test can provide the coach with information about each player's maximum jump height and sprint time as well as the athlete's ability to resist fatigue, measured through such variables as the mean sprint values or the percent decrement in the sprint times (Bishop & Girard, 2011; Glaister, Stone, Stewart, Hughes, & Moir, 2004). Although the test's validity and reliability would have to be determined before it could be used with athletes, this example demonstrates how data gathered from time–motion analysis studies can be used to develop a sport-specific test.

A strength and conditioning coach would also need to consider the samples used in the studies from which the data were obtained. For example, the study conducted by McInnes et al. (1995) assessed players from the men's Australian National Basketball League during state-level competition or practice games, while the study of Abdelkrim et al. (2007) used data from elite Tunisian male under-19 players during competitions. Rule differences are also likely to influence the findings of time–motion analysis (i.e., time restrictions on possession, shot clocks), so careful interpretation of the results is warranted.

Performance Analysis Concept 9.2

Using GPS-based player tracking technology to design workouts and monitor training workloads

GPS-based tracking systems provide online recordings of the distance traveled by multiple athletes concurrently as well as the distance covered in different locomotor categories (e.g., walking, jogging, moderate running, fast running, sprinting). Furthermore, the addition of heart rate monitors in some GPS-based systems allows the synchronization of physiological data when the athletes are exercising. Taken collectively, these data allow coaches to monitor the physical (e.g., distance covered) and physiological (e.g., heart rate) workloads of athletes and to instigate changes in the workouts if required. In addition, accelerometers in the GPS receivers allow other activities to be logged (e.g., tackles, jumps).

GPS devices have been used to compare the workloads experienced by field athletes in competition to those experienced in training sessions. Gabbett (2010) reported that elite female field hockey players spent more time in low-intensity activities, but less time in moderate- and high-intensity activities, during training sessions compared to competitive matches. Hartwig, Naughton, and Searl (2011) found greater total distances covered in locomotor modes of jogging, striding, and sprinting as well as total distance covered during competitive matches compared to training sessions performed by adolescent rugby union players.

Loader, Montgomery, Williams, Lorenzen, and Kemp (2012) recorded the distance covered by professional Australian Rules Football players in seven velocity zones ranging from standing/walking (0–1.7 m/s) to maximal running (> 8.3 m/s) during different training drills. Heart rate data were also collected during the drills and categorized into one of eight zones, ranging from 0–80 beats/min to 201–220 beats/min. As the Australian Rules Football games rules permit the wearing of GPS and heart rate devices during competitions, these training data were then compared to those collected during competitive matches. Using a statistical procedure known as cluster analysis, the authors were able to categorize the distances covered in each of the seven velocity zones into three separate groups or clusters: (1) game-specific conditioning (including the data from the competitive matches), characterized by greater distances covered at high velocities; (2) skill refining/moderate-intensity dominant drills; and (3) skill refining/low-intensity dominant drills. The heart rate values expressed as the duration in the eight heart rate zones were significantly different between the training skills in the three groups. Loader et al. were able to identify a small number of drills that were generally prescribed as game-specific conditioning exercises but did not actually result in the same running velocity or heart rate characteristics as the competitive matches due to changes in the structure of the drills (e.g., playing area, number of players participating). The utility of this approach in other sports is limited by the prohibition of GPS devices in competition by many sports governing bodies, which would preclude the comparison of training data with data collected during competitive matches.

GPS systems have also been used to design small-sided games to be used by field-sport athletes. Casamichana and Castellano (2010) reported that reducing the playing area during small-sided soccer games (5 versus 5 plus a goalkeeper, for a duration of 8 minutes) from 275 m² to 75 m² reduced the total distance covered by each player, the maximum running speed, the work:rest ratio, and the frequency of sprints, while decreasing the physiological workload (time spent at more than 90% of the maximum heart rate). A concomitant reduction in the time that the ball was in play occurred as the playing area decreased, although certain activities (e.g., interceptions, control and dribble, control and shoot) were observed less frequently.

(continues)

(continued)

Other researchers have used GPS systems to assess the physical and physiological workloads experienced by athletes during different drills. Farrow, Pyne, and Gabbett (2008), for example, compared the responses to the closed and open practice drills commonly used in Australian Rules Football. Closed drills were performed without any opposition players, while the open drills mimicked the closed drills but added opponents. These researchers found that greater distances were covered and greater velocities were achieved in the open versus closed drills. Furthermore, greater heart rates were recorded during the open skills. Reid, Duffield, Dawson, Baker, and Crespo (2008) were able to record the distances covered and peak velocities achieved by well-trained tennis players during four common on-court drills (the Star, Suicide, Box, and Big X) performed under different work:rest ratios. These authors were then able to categorize the drills based on the physical workload for future use.

Finally, GPS systems can be used to provide an immediate measure of the physical and physiological workload experienced by athletes during specific practices. For example, DeMartini et al. (2011) monitored the distances covered and the velocity of activities during nine preseason practice sessions involving NCAA Division I football players. The starting players obtained higher velocities than the nonstarting players, while nonlinemen covered a greater distance at higher velocities than linemen, resulting in greater maximum heart rates for the former group.

In conclusion, GPS-based technology provides a very useful tool for strength and conditioning practitioners to monitor the training and practice sessions of their athletes.

Notational and time–motion analysis technologies can also be used to provide information regarding the movements executed by an athlete in specific situations encountered in both practice and competition, revealing the perceived affordances of the athlete. An *affordance* describes the opportunity for action provided by the environment, with an athlete determining whether an action is possible based on the athlete's attunement to task-relevant information and perception of his or her own capabilities (Fajen, Riley, & Turvey, 2008). For example, a rugby player might perceive a gap between two opposing defenders as traversable given the relative velocity between the players (task-relevant information) and the perception of the athlete's own sprinting capability, resulting in the rugby player sprinting between the two defenders to score a try. Another attacking player might perceive the exact same situation as affording the opportunity to pass the ball to a supporting player, given the perception of the athlete's own limited sprinting capability. In these two situations, sprinting speed represents an action-scaled affordance that results in different movements emerging from these player interactions to satisfy the goal of the task (scoring a try). The strength and conditioning practitioner can assess the perceived affordances through the use of notational and time–motion analysis technologies and then develop training methods and practices to allow athletes to explore their own unique affordances. Moreover, notational and time–motion analysis technologies can be used to guide the recalibration of action-scaled affordances following specific training blocks, allowing athletes to attune their altered action capabilities (e.g., sprinting speed) to the relevant task information (e.g., relative motion of the opposing players). As this discussion suggests, notational and time–motion analysis technologies should not be considered as merely methods to describe the performance of an athlete, but rather as tools to explain the behavior of the athlete during competition and training.

Technique Analysis Methods

Technique analysis includes analytical methods that are employed to understand the way in which sports skills are performed so as to provide a basis for improving performance (Lees, 2002). (See Performance Analysis Concept 9.3.) A **technique** is defined as a specific sequence or pattern of movements performed during a skill

Performance Analysis Concept 9.3

What are skills and movements?

A **skill** is defined as an action or task that has a specific goal to achieve, while a **motor skill** is defined as a skill that requires voluntary movements of the body, head, and/or limbs to achieve its goal (Magill, 2011). Specific to this definition is the notion that motor skills are goal-directed actions, such that the disclosure of the goal is important. Furthermore, the inclusion of *voluntary* in the definition means that reflexes are not considered skills.

Motor skills can be classified in a number of ways. For example, they can be categorized by the size of the musculature involved in the execution of the skill. **Gross motor skills** involve large muscle groups (e.g., running), whereas **fine motor skills** involve small muscle groups (e.g., writing). The specific beginning and ending points of the skills can be used to distinguish **continuous motor skills**, whose beginning and end are arbitrary (e.g., swimming), from **discrete motor skills**, whose beginning and ending can be specified (e.g., standing vertical jump). The stability of the environment in which the skills are performed can be used to categorize **open motor skills**, where the environment is relatively unstable and unpredictable due to objects and/or other participants being in motion that specify the beginning of the skill (e.g., hitting a live pitch in baseball), and **closed motor skills**, where the environment is both stable and predictable (e.g., hitting a baseball from a tee).

A **movement** is defined as the behavioral characteristics of the body, head, and/or limbs that are component parts of motor skills (Magill, 2011). A

(continues)

(continued)

movement is observable; thus and it is what is observed and recorded during a technique analysis. Categories of fundamental movements include walking, running, jumping, throwing, and kicking. The distinction between motor skills and movements is important because motor skills can be learned and improved upon to allow the individual to achieve the specific goal. However, the movements used to achieve the goal of the motor skill will be influenced by the constraints associated with the individual (e.g., muscular strength, limb length), the context in which the skill is performed (e.g., specific rules, implements used), and the physical and social aspects of the environment in which the skill is performed (e.g., ambient light, surface characteristics, societal expectations) (Davids, Button, & Bennett, 2008). *Constraints* are boundary conditions that channel and guide the motor system during movements, and that may rule out the appearance of certain elements of technique (Newell & Jordan, 2007). The interaction of these constraints means that the observable movements for a given motor skill will differ between athletes (e.g., novice versus elite), between different tasks (e.g., shot put versus javelin), and between different environments (e.g., outdoor versus indoor, practice versus competition) despite the goal of the motor skill remaining unchanged (i.e., maximize the horizontal distance covered by the projectile).

that results in an effective completion of the skill (Lees, 2002). It is distinct from **performance**, which is defined as the product or outcome of a sequence of movements (Lees, 2002). A technique is something that can be visually perceived and measured. The technique used in a specific skill can be measured by recording the spatial and temporal organization of body segments through the use of motion analysis systems and video-based technologies. Technique analysis usually focuses on closed motor skills, as these tend to produce more reliable data. However, the validity of such analyses can be questioned, as many of the skills observed in sport tend not to occur as discrete elements, but rather are linked together as part of a more complex overall pattern (Vilar et al., 2012).

Lees (2002) defined the goals of technique analysis as follows:

- Description of the movements used in a motor skill
- Determination of the effectiveness of the way movements are made
- Diagnosis or identification of faults in the performance of a motor skill
- Remediation or intervention to achieve the desired outcome

An assumption of technique analysis is that there are *good* and *poor* techniques for a given motor skill and that adopting a *good* technique will lead to superior performance. This reasoning, while difficult to demonstrate objectively, may hold only for certain tasks. For example, even a good running technique is unlikely to produce a world-class performance in a marathon race if the athlete is not endowed with appropriately high VO_{2max} and/or lactate threshold. However, improvements in the athlete's running technique could certainly contribute to an improved marathon performance, if not a world-class one. Some sports require the execution of multiple motor skills (e.g., soccer, rugby, tennis). The selection of which skills are important in these sports can be derived from notational and time–motion analysis studies, although the practitioner should remember that these skills are not executed in isolation during the respective sport. In other sports, technique makes a large contribution to the outcome (e.g., gymnastics, diving), and the athletes are actually scored directly on their technique.

Nevertheless, this line of thought leads us to contemplate what constitutes *good* technique for a specific motor skill. In sports such as gymnastics and diving, we can categorize *good* technique as determined in large part by the rules laid down by the sport. In other sports, it becomes more difficult to determine what constitutes a *good* technique compared to a *poor* technique (see Performance Analysis Concept 9.4). What can aid the practitioner in such instances is to determine the **critical features** of the skill (performance indicators) from biomechanical principles with reference to the constraints associated with the performance.

Performance Analysis Concept 9.4

Should athletes be driven by the attainment of good technique?

There has long been an interest in athletes' techniques, regardless of the sport. This interest is exemplified by the drill-based approach to coaching, whereby repetitious executions of drills that emphasize good/correct techniques are promoted. Recent advances in technology (e.g., digital cameras, smartphones) that allow the movements of athletes to be recorded and analyzed have undoubtedly increased the interest in technique. Even so, changing a technique is infinitely more difficult than recording and analyzing a technique. Furthermore, it is not always clear if an athlete should change his or her technique to improve performance.

There are a number of reasons for this lack of clarity. First, the techniques of athletes are usually recorded in situations that are not representative of their performance environment: Opposing players are absent, fatigue is avoided, and skills are executed in isolation. Such a scenario provides little useful information about an athlete's technique *in situ*. Second, there is rarely a single optimal technique for a given skill. Instead, the most appropriate technique to use in any given situation is determined by the confluence of organismic, task, and environmental constraints at that specific time. Rather than striving for a single, stable technique that fits a predetermined notion of what is "correct," it will be more effective for athletes to develop functionally variable movement solutions that they can adapt to satisfy the goals of the task in the face of the dynamic constraints associated with sporting performance.

(continues)

(continued)

Certainly, there are examples of poor or even wrong techniques in certain situations. For example, certain biomechanical factors predispose female athletes to noncontact injuries to the anterior cruciate ligament during landing tasks. Many of these biomechanical factors relate to the body postures adopted during the task. In turn, many of the interventions to reduce the risk of this injury are directed at changing athletes' specific movement patterns where the "correct" technique is specified (e.g., increased hip flexion, reduced knee abduction, increased knee flexion).

Latash (1996) noted that the brain does not seem to care about the specifics of the technique employed in a given movement task, so long as the goal of the task is satisfied. With their predilection for repetitious, drill-based training combined with a fondness of technology, it appears that many strength and conditioning coaches take the opposite view, concerning themselves with the specifics of the techniques used by their athletes, arguably to the detriment of the athletes' performance. What we should be doing as strength and conditioning practitioners is identifying the organismic, task, and environmental constraints that surround the performer and developing practices that allow the athlete to explore functional movements that support the achievement of task goals under the continually changing conditions associated with the sport. While this process can certainly be aided by appropriate methods of technique analysis, focusing solely on the attainment of a universally ideal technique will deter athletes from searching for and realizing their unique movement solutions to satisfy the goals of each specific movement task.

Approaches to Technique Analysis

Due to the nature of the goals defined for technique analysis, this mode of analysis is typically grounded in a biomechanical approach. Three general biomechanical approaches to technique analysis are quantitative, predictive, and qualitative (Lees, 2002). A **quantitative approach** to technique analysis involves the direct measurement of the mechanical aspects of a motor skill that are related to technique. Small details of the technique are recorded using biomechanical technologies and analyzed with the critical features revealed through statistical analyses (see Applied Research 9.5). This approach can be quite time consuming and typically involves the use of expensive technologies.

A **predictive approach** to technique analysis requires the development of computer-generated mathematical models of the human motor system. Through simulations of the techniques used in specific motor skills, predictive approaches can identify the most effective ways that movements are made, allowing the development of appropriate interventions that will affect the outcome of movements (see Applied Research 9.6). Despite the predictive approach's ability to study the effects of manipulating specific variables independently, such computer simulation models have been criticized because they ignore the multitude of constraints that surround the human motor system and that interact to determine the actual techniques used in a specific motor skill *in vivo* (Glazier & Davids, 2009).

A **qualitative approach** to technique analysis involves the application of biomechanical principles to guide observations of the athlete and the subjective interpretation and evaluation of the athlete's technique. Its evaluation of technique distinguishes the qualitative approach from the quantitative and predictive approaches to technique analysis. Introspective judgments are made by the observer in comparing the technique to the critical features derived from a representation of the technique based on either a model template, biomechanical principles of movements, or a deterministic model (see Applied Research 9.7). An advantage of the qualitative approach over the other approaches to technique analysis is that it requires relatively inexpensive equipment and can be used by a wide range of individuals in a wide range of environments.

Applied Research 9.5
A quantitative approach to analyzing technique during vertical jumps

Aragón-Vargas and Gross (1997) recorded various kinematic and kinetic variables from 52 participants performing countermovement vertical jumps for maximal height. A force plate and a motion analysis system were used to record 35 mechanical variables that were categorized as whole-body kinematic and kinetic variables, lower-body segmental kinematic and kinetic variables, and variables relating to the coordination of the body segments. A multiple regression analysis was performed to determine which combination of mechanical variables could predict jump height. The authors reported that a statistical model including whole-body peak and average mechanical power accounted for the greatest proportion of variation in jump height. The models including variables relating to the coordination of the jump (relative timing of lower-body joint reversals, timing of peak lower-body joint moments, timing of peak velocity difference between proximal and distal joints for each segment) were not strongly related to jump height.

Aragón-Vargas, L. F., & Gross, M. M. (1997). Kinesiological factors in vertical jump performance: Differences among individuals. *Journal of Applied Biomechanics, 13*, 24–44.

Applied Research 9.6
A predictive approach to analyzing technique during vertical jumps

Nagano and Gerritsen (2001) developed a two-dimensional computer model to investigate the effects of muscle strengthening on vertical jump performance. This model consisted of four rigid segments (head/arms/trunk, thighs, lower legs, feet) connected by three revolute joints representing the hip, knee, and ankle joints. Six muscles controlled the model, each of which consisted of a contractile element and a series elastic element. Standardized anthropometric (segmental masses, mass moments of inertia) and muscle (maximal isometric strength, optimal fiber length) parameters were used. The optimization criterion of the model was the muscle activation pattern that resulted in the greater jump height achieved.

The authors reported that a simultaneous increase in maximal isometric force, maximal muscle shortening velocity, and maximal activation amplitude resulted in an increase in jump height; the greatest improvements in jump height were attributed to the strengthening of the knee extensors. The authors also noted that an optimal muscle activation pattern was required to maximize the benefits in muscle strengthening. They concluded that a training program for improving jumping performance should include exercises to increase muscular force and jump-related exercises so that athletes can learn how to modify their technique appropriately to take advantage of the increased muscular strength.

Nagano, A., & Gerritsen, K. G. M. (2001). Effects of neuromuscular strength training on vertical jumping performance: A computer simulation study. *Journal of Applied Biomechanics, 17*, 113–128.

Applied Research 9.7
A qualitative approach to analyzing technique during vertical jumps

Ham, Knez, and Young (2007) modified an existing deterministic model of a standing vertical jump to identify the critical features of a running vertical jump. The critical features of the model were derived from research published in peer-reviewed journals in exercise science. The authors were able to categorize the determinants of jump height that can be altered into those relevant to a strength and conditioning intervention (e.g., run-up speed, reactive and concentric leg power, shoulder power) and those relevant to a skills training intervention (e.g., body position at takeoff, body position before takeoff, reach height). They then identified the training application of each of these determinants. The authors noted that the deterministic model should supplement the coaches' experience and direct the analysis of an athlete's performance in the motor skill in a systematic fashion, with all of these factors then being used to develop appropriate training strategies.

Ham, D. J., Knez, W. L., & Young, W. B. (2007). A deterministic model of the vertical jump: Implications for training. *Journal of Strength and Conditioning Research, 21*, 967–972.

The quantitative, predictive, and qualitative approaches to technique analysis are all interrelated to some extent. For example, the selection of variables to measure and manipulate in quantitative and predictive approaches may be derived from observations of motor skills. Conversely, the observation of those variables deemed the critical features of a given technique during a qualitative approach may be derived from studies employing quantitative or predictive methods. However, application of these approaches may lead to contrasting recommendations (see, for example, Applied Research 9.5 and 9.6); thus the strength and conditioning practitioner is required to gather information from a variety of sources to determine the important characteristics of a given technique. Obvious differences between the approaches to technique analysis include the use of equipment, the time required for the analysis, and the expertise of the analyst.

An Integrated Model of Qualitative Technique Analysis

This section outlines a systematic method of performing a qualitative analysis of technique, as this approach is most likely to be the one taken by a strength and conditioning coach. Knudson and Morrison (2002) provide a four-stage model that can be implemented to guide the qualitative analysis of technique during a given motor skill (**Figure 9.2**). The four stages of the model are depicted as circular to emphasize that this process is continually undergoing refinement and improvement. None of the stages in the model should be considered as any more important than any other. Indeed, a weakness in any one stage is likely to diminish the overall effectiveness of the analysis (Knudson & Morrison, 2002).

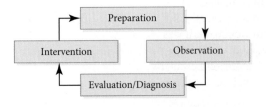

Figure 9.2 An integrated model to guide the qualitative analysis of technique.

Preparation Stage

The preparation stage of the integrated model of qualitative analysis begins with the analyst gathering information about the motor skill under observation. This information can come from a variety of sources (e.g., experiential knowledge, expert opinion, scientific research), but an "evidence-based" approach is strongly recommended (Bartlett, 2007; Knudson & Morrison,

2002). To synthesize the information drawn from different sources, the analyst must have an understanding of the anatomic terminology typically used to describe movements.

From the information gathered about the motor skill under observation, the analyst can then begin to identify the critical features and **movement phases**, both of which will aid the analyst in observation of the technique. The critical features of any technique can be identified through one of three methods:

- Use of a model template
- Use of a series of biomechanical principles
- Development of a deterministic model of the motor skill

A **model template** is an "ideal" representation of a technique used in a specific motor skill; this technique is often the one employed by an elite performer. While this approach of identifying the critical features of a technique is the simplest to adopt, it is not recommended because it ignores the fact that the actual technique will differ based on the constraints specific to the performer (see Performance Analysis Concept 9.5).

Performance Analysis Concept 9.5

Problems with using the best performers as the model template in technique analysis

It is perhaps logical to assume that those athletes who excel in a given sport must display the ideal technique—an assumption that is likely a result of the perceived relationship between good technique and superior performance. If this were the case, then technique analysis would simply involve having the athlete adopt the technique used by the best performer. This approach has been promoted somewhat with the advances in video-based technologies that have made it easy for a coach to display a video of an aspiring athlete next to that of a champion. In reality, this approach to technique analysis ignores the constraints surrounding the performer that influence the technique used in a specific motor skill. The interaction of the organismic task, and environmental constraints are unique to each performer; in turn, the technique displayed by the best performer is unlikely to be appropriate for all performers. Indeed, variations in technique have been noted even between elite performers in many sports (Ball, Best, & Wrigley, 2003; Bartlett, Wheat, & Robins, 2007; Brisson & Alain, 1996). Such variations may be functional, allowing the athletes to modify their movements to satisfy the demands of a given task in the dynamic environments typically experienced in sport (Davids et al., 2008). This is not to say that coaches should not observe and analyze the technique of the elite performers; rather, practitioners should not assume a generic "ideal" technique for any motor skill. Each performer will have an "optimal" technique determined by the interaction of the organismic task, and environmental constraints. The role of the coach is to aid the athlete in developing functional techniques that allow the adaptation of the technique to the constraints that surround the performer.

Table 9.4

Biomechanical Principles Used in a Qualitative Analysis of Technique

Principle	Explanation
Use of the stretch–shortening cycle	An initial movement of a body segment in the opposite direction to that intended will stretch the musculotendinous units. This principle is universal for movements requiring force or speed, or to minimize metabolic energy cost.
Minimization of energy	Minimizing unnecessary movements of body segments during the execution of a motor skill will reduce the energy expenditure.
Number of body segments	A greater number of body segments will tend to increase the force generated, given $F = ma$. However, the more segments involved in a technique, the more complex the control of the technique for novice performers.
Coordination of body segments	Any movements of the body require rotation of body segments. The mass moment of inertia and the muscle mass are reduced from the proximal to the distal body segments. During motor skills requiring high velocities (e.g., striking, throwing), the rotations should be coordinated in a proximal-to-distal pattern. During motor skills that require high force generation (e.g., bench press) or accuracy (e.g., basketball free throw), the rotations should occur in a simultaneous manner.
Maximization of the acceleration path	As per the work–energy theorem, a large change in energy requires the application of a large average force and a large displacement undergone by the force being applied to a body. This relationship is important in motor skills involving force or speed generation.
Stability	A large base of support increases the stability of a body.
Path of projection	Where an implement or the human body is projected (e.g., javelin, long jump), consideration should be given to the speed, angle, and height of the projectile at release.

Another method of identifying the critical features of a technique is to refer to a list of **biomechanical principles**, such as those shown in Table 9.4 (Bartlett, 2007; Hudson, 1995; Knudson, 2007). Whichever biomechanical principles are selected, they should be observable to facilitate a qualitative analysis of technique. The seven biomechanical principles in Table 9.4 have been proposed to provide a theoretical structure to facilitate the evaluation and teaching of motor skills (Knudson, 2007), although such principles appear to be useful only when evaluating low-skilled performers (Bartlett, 2007).

A final method of identifying the critical features of a motor skill is to develop a **deterministic model** (Bartlett, 2007; Hay & Reid, 1988). These models require that the analyst first establish the outcome of the motor skill. Next, the factors that determine the outcome are identified and placed in a hierarchy, where each factor is

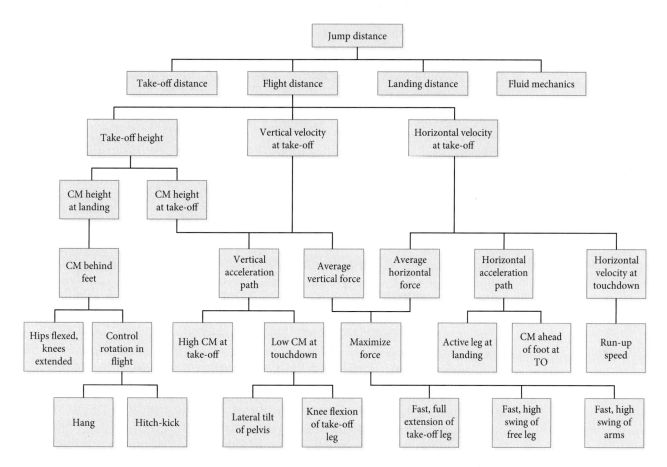

Figure 9.3 A deterministic model of long jump performance.

Data from Bartlett, R. (2007). *Introduction to sports biomechanics: Analysing human movement patterns.* London, UK: Routledge.

determined by those factors appearing immediately below it either by addition or by a biomechanical principle (Figure 9.3). Such models require knowledge of the biomechanical principles shown in Table 9.4.

Deterministic models have been criticized as being models of performance as opposed to models of technique, informing the analyst only of which performance parameters are important and not how these performance parameters are generated (Glazier & Robins, 2012). This may certainly be true, although these models were never developed as models of technique (Hay & Reid, 1988). Nevertheless, they provide a valuable framework for analyzing technique (Lees, 2002). The development of a deterministic model for the technique during a long jump is presented in **Worked Example 9.2**

In the preparation stage the analyst should consider breaking the motor skills down into different movement phases that are linked. (Note that the reduction of movements into phases forms an analysis technique and is not part of a strategy used to practice the motor skills.) The division of each phase should be based on

Worked Example 9.2
Developing a deterministic model of the long jump

This example comes from Bartlett (2007).

Step 1. Determine the goal of the motor skill. The goal of the motor skill is to maximize the distance jumped. This variable is placed at the top of the model.

Step 2. Identify the important phases of the motor skill. The distance jumped by the athlete can be reduced to three phases: the takeoff phase, the flight phase, and the landing phase (Figure 9.4).

The identification of the three phases can be added to the goal of the motor skill to provide the first two levels of the model, to which we add fluid mechanical factors (e.g., drag forces) as variables that act to reduce jump distance (Figure 9.5). For the sake of clarity, we will focus on the flight distance here.

Step 3. Identify the factors that determine flight distance. Here we can use the biomechanical principle of projectile motion—namely, that the distance traveled by a projectile is determined by the speed, angle, and height of the projectile at takeoff. As the speed and angle at takeoff will be determined by the interaction of the vertical and horizontal components of the athlete's velocity, we use these variables in the model (Figure 9.6).

Step 4. Identify the factors that determine takeoff height. Takeoff height is defined as the difference between the height of the center of mass (CM) at takeoff and the CM height at landing (Figure 9.4). The CM height at takeoff is determined by the change in gravitational potential energy (E_{GP}) during takeoff, as determined by the work–energy theorem, and the athlete's mass (as mass is unlikely to have a large effect on the performance, we exclude this from the model). The work performed to change E_{GP} is simply the product of the average vertical force and the vertical displacement undergone by the force (vertical acceleration path). From the biomechanical principles, we know that the involvement of other body segments can influence the magnitude of the vertical force applied during takeoff, so we include the swing

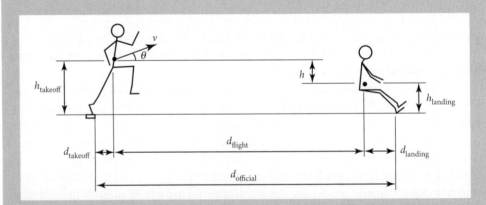

Figure 9.4 The takeoff, flight, and landing phases of the long jump. The three phases are determined by the takeoff distance, flight distance, and landing distance.

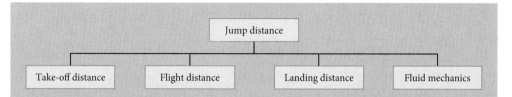

Figure 9.5 The first two levels of the deterministic model of the long jump.

Data from Bartlett, R. (2007). *Introduction to sports biomechanics: Analysing human movement patterns.* London, UK: Routledge.

of the contralateral leg and the arms at takeoff to the extension of the takeoff leg in determining the magnitude of the vertical force. The length of the vertical path undergone by the athlete's CM is determined by the lowest position of the CM. The lowest position of the CM is determined by the amount of knee flexion (although a large knee flexion is likely to minimize takeoff speed and so should be avoided) and the lateral tilt of the pelvis.

The height of the CM at landing will be determined by the body position of the athlete upon landing. The CM is behind the feet upon landing, and the athlete is required to flex the hips and extend the knees. Furthermore, the athlete is required to control the forward rotation during flight, as this rotation would naturally result in the feet touching down prematurely. The forward rotation is induced because the ground reaction force acts behind the CM at takeoff, increasing the angular momentum of the body. Given the conservation of angular momentum, this angular momentum cannot be reduced during flight. However, it can be transferred from the trunk to the limbs if they are rotated during flight—a technique known as the hitch-kick. Alternatively, the rate of forward rotation during flight can be reduced by increasing the mass moment of inertia of the body—the so-called hang technique.

We add all of these factors to our model under the variable of takeoff height (Figure 9.7).

Step 5. Identify the factors that determine the vertical velocity at takeoff. From the work–energy theorem, the work done during takeoff will determine the takeoff velocity. We therefore add vertical acceleration path and average vertical force to the model to represent the work done. These variables are determined by the same

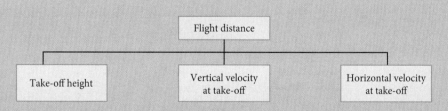

Figure 9.6 The factors that determine flight distance.

Data from Bartlett, R. (2007). *Introduction to sports biomechanics: Analysing human movement patterns.* London, UK: Routledge.

(continues)

(continued)

factors included in Step 4 for the CM height at takeoff (high CM at takeoff, low CM at touchdown, maximize force) and are added to this portion of the model (Figure 9.8).

Step 6. Identify the factors that determine the horizontal velocity at takeoff. We can apply the same procedures used in Step 5 to identify the factors determining the horizontal velocity of the athlete. The length of horizontal acceleration path is determined by the horizontal location of the CM relative to the takeoff foot. At touchdown, the foot should not be so far in front of the CM that it increases the braking force, as this could reduce the horizontal velocity at takeoff. We may want the athlete to actively pull the foot backward prior to touchdown to minimize this braking force. However, the CM should be in front of the foot at takeoff to increase the length of the horizontal acceleration path. (Note that this posture would increase the takeoff distance, but reduce the takeoff height.) The run-up speed is also added at this stage of the model development, as it determines the horizontal velocity of the athlete at touchdown (Figure 9.9).

Step 7. Combine the elements of the model. We can now combine the elements of the model (Figures 9.5 through 9.9) to reveal our final deterministic model of the long jump (Figure 9.10).

Although this model does not specify the technique that should be used during the motor skill, it does highlight the important critical features, all of which are observable (shown as the shaded boxes in Figure 9.10). This model and the critical features can be used to guide the observation of the motor skill. For example, the observer requires a sagittal view of the jump to identify most of the features, but a frontal view is also required to observe the lateral pelvic tilt. Furthermore, the observations could be supplemented with data recorded from timing gates to provide a measure of the run-up speed of the athlete.

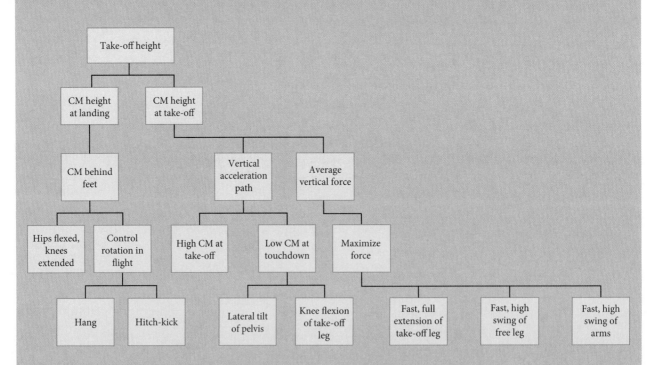

Figure 9.7 The factors that determine takeoff height.

Data from Bartlett, R. (2007). *Introduction to sports biomechanics: Analysing human movement patterns.* London, UK: Routledge.

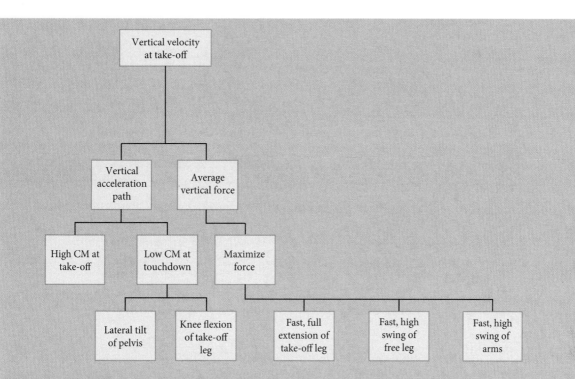

Figure 9.8 The factors that determine vertical velocity at takeoff.

Data from Bartlett, R. (2007). *Introduction to sports biomechanics: Analysing human movement patterns.* London, UK: Routledge.

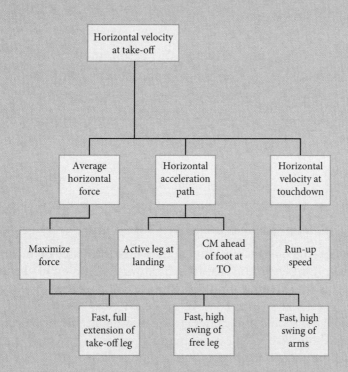

Figure 9.9 The factors that determine horizontal velocity at takeoff.

Data from Bartlett, R. (2007). *Introduction to sports biomechanics: Analysing human movement patterns.* London, UK: Routledge.

(continues)

(continued)

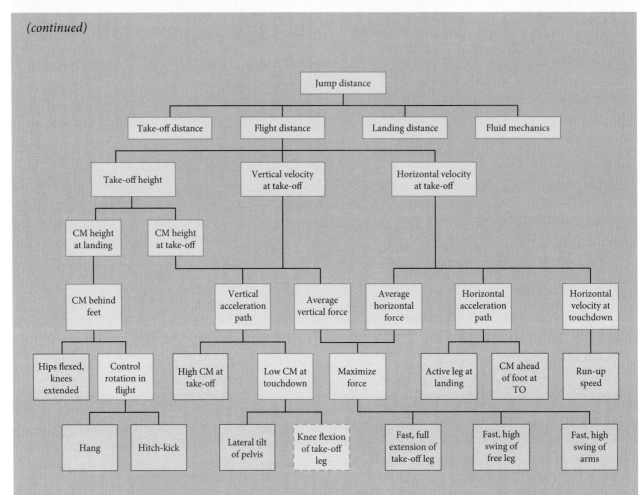

Figure 9.10 The deterministic model of the long jump. The observable critical features are shaded. The dashed box shows a misleading feature of the motor skill.

Data from Bartlett, R. (2007). *Introduction to sports biomechanics: Analysing human movement patterns*. London, UK: Routledge.

clearly defined biomechanical functions, with identifiable boundaries separating each phase (Bartlett, 2007). Table 9.5 shows the division of phases used in specific motor skills. The identification of the movement phases can greatly simplify the analysis.

The analyst should also gather information about the performer including his or her age (both chronological and training), sex, standard of performance, physical abilities, injury status and history, and cognitive development (Bartlett, 2007). This information will be crucial not only for identifying critical features of the technique, but also in developing the intervention to improve the technique; it can be garnered from an appropriate **needs analysis**.

Table 9.5
Division of Ballistic Motor Skills Such as Throwing, Kicking, and Striking into Movement Phases

Movement Phase	Function	Determination of Beginning
Preparation/Windup	Maximizes range of movement	Initiation of ball toss (tennis serve)
	Allows large segments to initiate movement	Rearward movement of ball (overarm throw)
	Involvement of the stretch–shortening cycle	Planting the contralateral leg (kicking)
Action/Propulsion	Large proximal segments initiate movement	Racket at lowest point behind performer (tennis serve)
	Movement proceeds with a proximal-to-distal coordination of segments	Forward movement of the ball (overarm throw)
	Segmental forces applied in the direction of movement	Hip flexion of kicking leg (kicking)
Recovery Follow-through	Controlled deceleration of segments	Impact of the ball (tennis serve, kicking)
	Achievement of a position of temporary stability	Release of the ball (overarm throw)

Data from Bartlett, R. (2007). *Introduction to sports biomechanics: Analysing human movement patterns*. London, UK: Routledge; Flanagan, S.P. (2014). *Biomechanics. A case-based approach*. Burlington, MA: Jones & Bartlett Learning; Knudson, D. V., & Morrison, C. S. (2002). *Qualitative analysis of human movement*. Champaign, IL: Human Kinetics.

The analyst should develop a systematic observation strategy during the preparation phase. This strategy should include how to observe, where to observe from, and how many observations are required (Bartlett, 2007).

Observation Stage

During this stage, the analyst implements the observation strategy developed previously. Although an observer should use all senses during the observation (Knudson & Morrison, 2002), vision is the most important sense in this phase. Analysts should place themselves where they are able to receive information pertinent to the critical features associated with the technique. This information can be gathered from the deterministic model of the technique.

One issue that arises in observing live performances is that the human visual system is often unreliable, particularly when the movements are fast, such as occurs in many sports. Video-based technology can provide slow-motion play-back facilities that can improve the evaluation of the critical features of the motor skill by the observer; indeed, it has been shown to improve the reliability of qualitative analyses

(Borel, Schneider, & Newman, 2011; Schultz et al., 2011). Furthermore, videos can be used as a means of augmenting the feedback provided to the performer when attempting to modify technique (Davids et al., 2008). Video footage also serves as a permanent record of the athlete's technique over time and, in this capacity, can be used to demonstrate improvement. As with live observation, questions may occur regarding where to place the camera as well as how many cameras to use. It is important to remain consistent when identifying the location and number of cameras, as this will contribute to the reliability of the observations and, therefore, to the ability of the analyst to track the change in technique over time.

The number of trials to be observed should be considered when developing the observation strategy. If the observation takes place during competition, then the number of trials will be out of the analyst's control. However, even in a controlled environment such as a practice session, the number of trials to be observed is affected by the inherent variability of the human motor system (see Performance Analysis Concept 9.6). This variability precludes a single trial as being representative of an athlete's technique.

Performance Analysis Concept 9.6

Variability in technique

The human motor system is a complex system that comprises a huge number of interacting components (e.g., joints, muscles, cell types, neurons and neuronal connections). Given the overwhelming number of components that interact to negotiate the dynamic environments associated with sport, variations in technique between repetitions of the same motor skills are to be expected. Indeed, Hatze (1986) noted that the exact reproduction of any given motor skill is statistically improbable. This assertion has subsequently been confirmed empirically, even with elite athletes (Bartlett et al., 2007). Variability in technique during repeated executions of specific motor skills is proposed to serve a functional purpose by allowing the performer to adapt to changing task and environmental constraints (Davids et al., 2008). Furthermore, variations in technique parameters have been proposed to prevent injuries in repetitive cyclical movements such as running (Hamill, Haddad, Heiderscheit, van Emmerik, & Li, 2006).

The issue of variability in technique does raise some important issues for the observer performing a technique analysis. For example, the observer needs to consider the number of trials that are required for a reliable measure of performance. Moreover, the observer needs to be aware that deviations from the critical features associated with the technique may not represent errors in the execution of the movement, but rather serve as a functional aspect of the technique that allows the athlete to attune his or her movements to a dynamic environment (Davids et al., 2008). It therefore falls to the observer to resolve these issues based on an understanding of the specific constraints surrounding the athlete during the performance.

There are no objective methods for determining the number of trials to observe in a qualitative analysis. While some evidence suggests that a large number of trials (12 or more) may be required to establish a reliable measure of discrete kinetic variables during specific motor skills (Rodano & Squadrone, 2002), there is currently no information regarding the appropriate number of trials necessary to ensure reliable measures of technique variables. As such, the determination of the number of trials to observe is subjective. For example, some authors recommend 10 trials be observed (Bartlett, 2007), although issues of fatigue and performer motivation should be considered when determining the number of trials to observe.

The final element to be considered in the development of a systematic observation strategy is the instructions provided to the performer prior to the execution of each trial. Such instructions represent an important constraint that can affect the technique executed in a given motor skill (Davids et al., 2008).

Evaluation/Diagnosis Stage

The third stage of the integrated model of qualitative analysis is that of evaluation/diagnosis. The analyst is tasked with evaluating the technique and identifying the strengths and weaknesses of the performer relative to the critical features identified in the preparation stage by making a judgment about the quality of the technique. The evaluation process can be aided through the use of video analysis software (e.g., Dartfish, siliconCOACH, Quintic). These software packages allow for digital video recorded from multiple cameras to be analyzed concurrently and annotated. In addition, they allow the determination of kinematic variables associated with the specific technique being analyzed, including linear and angular displacements, and have been shown to be reliable (Cronin, Nash, & Whatman, 2006). Unfortunately, these software packages lack appropriate signal processing features (e.g., filtering algorithms) that would enhance the reliability of the kinematic variables derived (Melton, Mullineaux, Mattacola, Mair, & Uhl, 2011). Thus these software packages are very useful in supporting the qualitative analysis of technique, but they should not be considered replacements for more comprehensive opto-reflective motion analysis systems if a quantitative approach to technique analysis is required.

A further task of the analyst is the diagnosis of which of the identified weaknesses to tackle and how to prioritize the correction of these weaknesses. Bartlett (2007) provides the following methods for prioritizing the correction of identified weaknesses:

- Look at the sequence of features as per phases of movement.
- Prioritize critical features that maximize performance improvements.
- Prioritize critical features based on which will be easiest to improve.

Intervention Stage

The final stage of the integrated model of qualitative analysis involves the development of an appropriate intervention to correct the weaknesses in technique identified in the evaluation/diagnosis stage. Typically, the interventions revolve

Table 9.6

Summary of the Stages of the Integrated Model Used for the Qualitative Analysis of Technique

Stage	Tasks Within Each Stage
Preparation	Gather knowledge of activity and performer
	Identify critical features of the activity
	Develop systematic observation strategy
	Present data
	Obtain knowledge of effective instruction
Observation	Implement the observation strategy
Evaluation/diagnosis	Evaluate critical features
	Prioritize critical features
Intervention	Develop an appropriate practice regimen

around the development of physical practices, accompanied by feedback to the performer that guides the required changes in technique (Bartlett, 2007; Knudson & Morrison, 2002).

Table 9.6 shows the sequencing of the stages associated with the integrated model of qualitative analysis and the general tasks within each of those stages.

Chapter Summary

Performance analysis methods can be used by strength and conditioning practitioners to gain insight into the physiological, mechanical, and technical demands of specific sports, and to assess the techniques used in the execution of sport-specific skills. Notational and time–motion analysis methods provide data on physical efforts, movement patterns, and technical actions of the players and relate these data to the athletes' relative success. The technologies used include manual video-based analysis methods, automatic video-based analysis methods, and Global Positioning System–based methods.

Technique analysis relies on analytical methods that seek to understand the way in which sports skills are performed so as to provide a basis for improving performance. A quantitative approach to technique analysis involves the direct measurement of the mechanical aspects of a motor skill that are related to technique. A predictive approach to technique analysis requires the development of computer-generated mathematical models of the human motor system. A qualitative approach to technique analysis involves the application of biomechanical principles to guide observations of movements and the subjective interpretation and evaluation of the technique. An integrated model of qualitative technique analysis involves the stages of preparation, observation, evaluation/diagnosis, and intervention.

Review Questions and Projects

1. List the advantages and disadvantages of the different technologies that can be used to track players in field sports.

2. A group of soccer players is participating in a small-sided game format (5 versus 5 players) in an area where each player covers an approximate area of 50 m². You are monitoring the physical (distances covered) and physiological (heart rate) workloads of the session with a GPS system. During a scheduled break in the workout, you notice that the number of sprints performed by each player and their heart rates are lower than you had planned. Explain how you can change the session to increase the demands of the workout.

3. A strength and conditioning practitioner working with a basketball team reviews the extant time–motion analysis data and finds that basketball players typically execute between 44 and 46 vertical jumps during a game. What other factors should the practitioner consider before simply having her athletes practice isolated vertical jumps in training?

4. What are the goals of technique analysis?

5. What is the difference between a movement and a skill?

6. Highlight the problems with using the techniques demonstrated by elite performers to identify the critical features in a specific motor skill.

7. What are the main differences between the quantitative, predictive, and qualitative approaches to technique analysis?

8. Explain the advantages of using video footage in the qualitative analysis of an athlete's technique in a given motor skill.

9. Explain why multiple observations are more beneficial in determining an athlete's movement capabilities than a single observation.

10. Explain the functional role of movement variability for an athlete.

References

Abdelkrim, N. B., El Fazaa, S., & El Ati, J. (2007). Time–motion analysis and physiological data for elite under-19-year-old basketball players during competition. *British Journal Sports Medicine*, *41*, 69–75.

Aughey, R. J. (2011). Applications of GPS technologies to field sports. *International Journal of Sports Physiology and Performance*, *6*, 295–310.

Ball, K. A., Best, R. J., & Wrigley, T. V. (2003). Body sway, aim point fluctuation and performance in rifle shooters: Inter- and intra-individual analysis. *Journal of Sports Sciences*, *21*, 559–566.

Barris, S., & Button, C. (2008). A review of vision-based motion analysis in sport. *Sports Medicine, 38*, 1025–1043.

Bartlett, R. (2007). *Introduction to sports biomechanics: Analysing human movement patterns.* London, UK: Routledge.

Bartlett, R., Wheat, J., & Robins, M. (2007). Is movement variability important for sports performance? *Sports Biomechanics, 6*, 234–245.

Billaut, F., Bishop, D. J., Schaerz, S., & Noakes, T. D. (2011). Influence of knowledge of sprint number on pacing during repeated-sprint exercise. *Medicine and Science in Sports and Exercise, 43*, 665–672.

Bishop, D., & Girard, O. (2011). Repeated-sprint ability (RSA). In M. Cardinale, R. Newton, & K. Nosaka (Eds.), *Strength and conditioning: Biological principles and practical applications* (pp. 223–241). West Sussex, UK: Wiley-Blackwell.

Bloom, T., & Bradley, A. P. (2003, February 7). Player tracking and stroke recognition in tennis video. In B. Lovell & A. Maeder (Eds.), *Proceedings of the APRS Workshop on Digital Image Computing* (pp. 93–97.). Brisbane.

Borel, S., Schneider, P., & Newman, C. J. (2011). Video analysis software increases the interrater reliability of video gait assessments in children with cerebral palsy. *Gait and Posture, 33*, 727–729.

Brisson, T. A., & Alain, C. (1996). Should common optimal movement patterns be identified as the criterion to be achieved? *Journal of Motor Behavior, 28*, 211–223.

Carling, C., Bloomfield, J., Nelsen, L., & Reilly, T. (2008). The role of motion analysis in elite soccer: Contemporary performance measurement techniques and work rate data. *Sports Medicine, 38*, 839–862.

Casamichana, D., & Castellano, J. (2010). Time–motion, heart rate, perceptual and motor behaviour demands in small-sided soccer games: Effects of pitch size. *Journal of Sports Science, 28*, 1615–1623.

Cronin, J., Nash, M., & Whatman, C. (2006). Assessing dynamic knee joint range of motion using Siliconcoach. *Physical Therapy in Sport, 7*, 191–194.

Davids, K., Button, C., & Bennett, S. (2008). *Dynamics of skills acquisition: A constraints-led approach.* Champaign, IL: Human Kinetics.

Dellal, A., Chamari, K., Wong, D. P., Ahmaidi, S., Keller, D., Barros, R., . . . Carling, C. (2011). Comparison of physical and technical performance in European soccer match-play: FA Premier League and La Liga. *European Journal of Applied Sport Science, 11*, 51–59.

DeMartini, J. K., Martschinske, J. L., Casa, D. J., Lopez, R. M., Ganio, M. S., Walz, S. M., & Coris, E. E. (2011). Physical demands of National Collegiate Athletic Association Division I football players during preseason training in the heat. *Journal of Strength and Conditioning Research, 25*, 2935–2943.

Fajen, B. R., Riley, M. A., & Turvey, M. T. (2008). Information, affordances, and the control of action in sport. *International Journal of Sport Psychology, 40*, 79–107.

Farrow, D., Pyne, D., & Gabbett, T. (2008). Skill and physiological demands of open and closed training drills in Australian Football. *International Journal of Sports Science and Coaching, 3*, 489–499.

Gabbett, T. J. (2010). GPS analysis of elite women's field hockey training and competition. *Journal of Strength and Conditioning Research, 24*, 1321–1324.

Glaister, M. (2005). Multiple sprint work: Physiological responses, mechanisms of fatigue and the influence of aerobic fitness. *Sports Medicine, 35*, 757–767.

Glaister, M., Stone, M. H., Stewart, A. M., Hughes, M., & Moir, G. L. (2004). Reliability and validity of fatigue measures during short-duration maximal intensity intermittent cycling. *Journal of Strength and Conditioning Research, 18*, 459–462.

Glazier, P. S., & Davids, K. (2009). Constraints on the complete optimization of human motion. *Sports Medicine, 39*, 15–28.

Glazier, P. S., & Robins, M. T. (2012). Comment on "Use of deterministic models in sports and exercise biomechanics research" by Chow and Knudson (2011). *Sports Biomechanics, 11*, 120–122.

Hamill, J., Haddad, J. M., Heiderscheit, B. C., van Emmerik, R. E. A., & Li, L. (2006). Clinical relevance of variability in coordination. In K. Davids, S. Bennett, & K. Newell (Eds.), *Movement system variability* (pp. 133–152). Champaign, IL: Human Kinetics.

Hartwig, T. B., Naughton, G., & Searl, J. (2011). Motion analyses of adolescent rugby union players: A comparison of training and game demands. *Journal of Strength and Conditioning Research, 25,* 966–972.

Hatze, H. (1986). Motion variability: Its definition, quantification, and origin. *Journal of Motor Behavior, 18,* 5–16.

Hay, J. G., & Reid, J. G. (1988). *Anatomy, mechanics and human motion.* Englewood Cliffs, NJ: Prentice Hall.

Hudson, J. L. (1995). Core concepts of kinesiology. *Journal of Physical Education, Recreation and Dance, 66,* 54–55, 59–60.

Hughes, M. D., & Bartlett, R. M. (2002). The use of performance indicators in performance analysis. *Journal of Sports Sciences, 20,* 739–754.

Janeira, M. A., & Maia, J. (1998). Game intensity in basketball: An interactionist view linking time–motion analysis, lactate concentration and heart rate. *Coaching and Sport Science Journal, 3,* 26–30.

Jennings, D., Cormack, S., Coutts, A. J., Boyd, L., & Aughey, R. J. (2010). Variability of GPS units for measuring distance in team sport movements. *International Journal of Sports Physiology and Performance, 5,* 565–569.

Knudson, D. V. (2007). Qualitative biomechanical principles for application in coaching. *Sports Biomechanics, 6,* 109–118.

Knudson, D. V., & Morrison, C. S. (2002). *Qualitative analysis of human movement.* Champaign, IL: Human Kinetics.

Latash, M. L. (1996). The Bernstein problem: How does the central nervous system make its choices? In M. L. Latash & M. J. Turvey (Eds.), *Dexterity and its development* (pp. 277–304). Mahwah, NJ: Erlbaum.

Lees, A. (2002). Technique analysis in sports: A critical review. *Journal of Sports Sciences, 20,* 813–828.

Loader, J., Montgomery, P. G., Williams, M. D., Lorenzen, C., & Kemp, J. G. (2012). Classifying training drills based upon movement demands in Australian Football. *International Journal of Sports Science and Coaching, 7,* 57–67.

Magill, R. A. (2011). *Motor learning and control: Concepts and applications.* New York, NY: McGraw-Hill.

McInnes, S. E., Carlson, J. S., Jones, C. J., & McKenna, M. J. (1995). The physiological load imposed on basketball players during competition. *Journal of Sports Sciences, 13,* 387–397.

Melton, C., Mullineaux, D. R., Mattacola, C. G., Mair, S. D., & Uhl, T. L. (2011). Reliability of video motion-analysis systems to measure amplitude and velocity of shoulder elevation. *Journal of Sport Rehabilitation, 20,* 393–405.

Newell, K. M., & Jordan, K. (2007). Task constraints and movement organization: A common language. In W. E. Davis & G. D. Broadhead (Eds.), *Ecological task analysis and movement* (pp. 5–23). Champaign, IL: Human Kinetics.

Randers, M. B., Mujika, I., Hewitt, A., Santisteban, J., Bischoff, R., Solano, R., . . . Mohr, M. (2010). Application of four different football match analysis systems: A comparative study. *Journal of Sports Sciences, 28,* 171–182.

Reid, M., Duffield, R., Dawson, B., Baker, J., & Crespo, M. (2008). Quantification of the physiological and performance characteristics of on-court tennis drills. *British Journal of Sports Medicine, 42,* 146–151.

Rodano, R., & Squadrone, R. (2002). Stability of selected lower limb joint kinetic parameters during vertical jump. *Journal of Applied Biomechanics, 18,* 83–89.

Schultz, R., Mooney, K., Anderson, S., Marcello, B., Matheson, G. O., & Besier, T. (2011). Functional movement screen: Inter-rater and subject reliability. *British Journal of Sports Medicine, 45,* 374–375.

Thomas, C., Fellingham, G., & Vehrs, P. (2009). Development of a notational analysis system for selected soccer skills of a women's college team. *Measurement in Physical Education and Exercise Science, 13,* 108–121.

Vilar, L., Araújo, D., Davids, K., & Button, C. (2012). The role of ecological dynamics in analyzing performance in team sports. *Sports Medicine, 42*, 1–10.

Vučković, G., Perš, J., James, N., & Hughes, M. (2010). Measurement error associated with the SAGIT/Squash computer tracking software. *European Journal of Sport Sciences, 10*, 129–140.

Waldron, M., Worsfold, P., Twist, C., & Lamb, K. (2011). Concurrent validity and test–retest reliability of a Global Positioning System (GPS) and timing gates to assess sprint performance variables. *Journal of Sports Sciences, 29*, 1613–1620.

Wheeler, K. W., Askew, C. D., & Sayers, M. G. (2010). Effective attacking strategies in rugby union. *European Journal of Sports Sciences, 10*, 237–242.

Witte, T. H., & Wilson, A. M. (2004). Accuracy of non-differential GPS for the determination of speed over ground. *Journal of Biomechanics, 37*, 1891–1898.

Yan, F., Christmas, W., & Kittler, J. (2005, September). A tennis ball tracking algorithm for automatic annotation of tennis match. In W. F. Clocksin, A. W. Fitzgibbon, & P. H. S. Torr (Eds.), *Proceedings of the British Machine Vision Conference* (pp. 619–628). Oxford, UK.

CHAPTER 10

Skill Acquisition

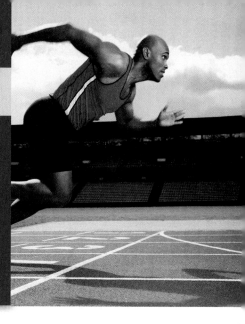

Chapter Objectives

At the end of this chapter, you should be able to:

- Explain the processes by which motor skills are acquired
- Describe the major tenets of different theoretical approaches to the coordination and control of motor skills
- Understand which factors influence the processes of skill acquisition and adaptations in coordination during the execution of motor skills
- Identify organismic, environmental, and task constraints that influence the emergence of the coordination and control of movements during the execution of specific motor skills
- Explain how organismic, environmental, and task constraints influence the acquisition of motor skills
- Explain how the variables of practice structure and attentional focus influence the acquisition of motor skills
- Identify the ways in which the variables of practice structure and attentional focus can be manipulated by a coach to ensure the effective acquisition of motor skills

Key Terms

Action-scaled affordances

Affordance

Angle–angle diagram

Attractor state

Blocked practice

Body-scaled affordances

Challenge-point framework

Complex system

Contextual interference

Continuous relative phase

Control parameter

Control space

Coordination

Coordinative structures

Degeneracy

Degree of freedom

Degrees of freedom problem

Differential learning

Direct perception

Environmental constraints

Event space

Explicit learning

External attentional focus

Faded feedback

General motor programs

Guided discovery

Implicit learning

Internal attentional focus

Knowledge of performance

Knowledge of results

Learning

Motor program

Order parameter

Organismic constraints

Part-task practice

Perceptual attunement

Perceptual-motor
recalibration

Perceptual-motor workspace

Phase portraits

Random practice

Rate-limiter

Retention test

Schema

Self-organization

Serial practice

Simplification

State space

Task constraints

Transfer test

Chapter Overview

A core concept of sport is that optimization of athletic performance requires practice. Ericsson (2007) proposed that achieving expertise in a range of different domains, including sport, requires the engagement of deliberate practice on behalf of the performer—specifically, 10,000 hours of practice. While it is typically accepted that the engagement in many hours of practice is necessary for expertise, it is unlikely that time spent in practice will be sufficient to produce expert performance. For example, there is a potent genetic component to expertise (Baker & Young, 2014; Tucker & Collins, 2012). Moreover, the assumption that amassing a greater number of practice hours leads to expertise ignores the importance of the content and structure of the practices. In fact, it is the content and structure of practices that the strength and conditioning practitioner is readily able to manipulate—and hence the focus of the chapter.

In this chapter, we discuss skill acquisition as a process and its theoretical underpinnings to understand how we acquire new skills, improve existing patterns of coordination to enhance performance, and develop new coordination patterns to meet changing demands associated with the training tasks and those associated with sports performance. Based on our understanding of the processes involved in skill acquisition, we can develop effective practices.

Defining Skill Acquisition

A skill is an action or task directed toward achieving a specific goal. A motor skill is a skill that requires voluntary movements of the body, head, and/or limbs to achieve the task goal, with these movements being component parts of motor skills (Magill, 2011). Motor skills can be classified in a number of ways. For example, they can be categorized by the size of the musculature involved in the execution of the skill, where *gross motor skills* involve large muscle groups (e.g., running) and *fine motor skills* involve small muscle groups (e.g., writing). The specific beginning and ending points of the skills can be used to distinguish *continuous motor skills*, whose beginning and end are arbitrary (e.g., swimming stroke), from *discrete motor skills*, whose beginning and ending can be specified (e.g., standing vertical jump). The stability of the environment in which the skills are performed can be used to distinguish *open motor skills*, where the environment is relatively unstable and unpredictable due to objects and/or other participants being in motion that specify the beginning of the skill (e.g., hitting a live pitch in baseball), from *closed motor skills*, where the environment is both stable and predictable (e.g., hitting a baseball from a tee). Skill acquisition then becomes the ongoing process of attaining functional movement task solutions to satisfy the goal of motor skills (Davids, Button, & Bennett, 2008).

The human motor system can be viewed as a **complex system**, composed of many independent components operating at different structural and functional levels (e.g., limb segments, joints, muscles, motor units); the actions of these components need to be coordinated and controlled to successfully execute the movements required to accomplish the goal of a motor skill. Each independent component of the human motor system represents a **degree of freedom** (DOF) that can be organized in many different ways during goal-directed movements. The organization of the DOF during the execution of a given movement represents the **coordination** of the motor system, which is revealed in the topological characteristics of the relative motion of the limb segments (see **Worked Example 10.1**). (Notice that the individual players can

Worked Example 10.1
Measuring intra-limb coordination during motor skills using the topological characteristics of relative motion

Coordination in a specific motor skill can be measured by recording the spatial and temporal organization of body segments. In turn, kinematic variables can be used to describe the coordination pattern. Topological characteristics of movements are revealed in the form and shape of the relative motion of the limbs recorded during movements, allowing the coordination of the degrees of freedom during the execution of a motor skill to be evaluated. A topological framework of the assessment of movements is based on the assumption that only one single point of the body (joint, segment, or specific point) can occupy a position in space at any given instant in time—a notion called the concept of impenetrability (McGinnis & Newell, 1982). The concept of impenetrability asserts that motions of a number of constituent parts of a particular movement system can be represented within certain action boundaries, known as a **control space** (McGinnis & Newell, 1982). A control space represents a three-dimensional reference frame in which a body segment is located during a motor skill.

Two control spaces are important in describing coordination used in motor skills: the **event space** and the **state space**. The event space allows the position of a body segment or joint angle to be specified at any given time during the activity and is important during tasks where time becomes a constraint to the movement (Figure 10.1). Plotting the angles of two joints on the same graph produces an **angle–angle diagram** (Figure 10.2). Two general coordination patterns can be derived from the topological characteristics of angle–angle diagrams: (1) in-phase patterns, where both joints extend or flex concurrently, and (2) antiphase patterns

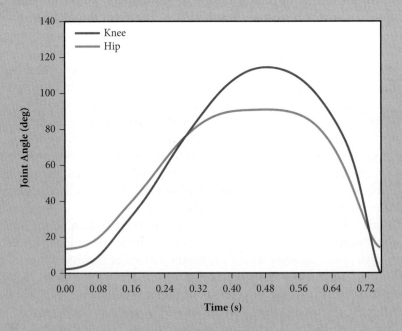

Figure 10.1 Hip and knee joint angles recorded in the sagittal plane from one athlete during a countermovement vertical jump.

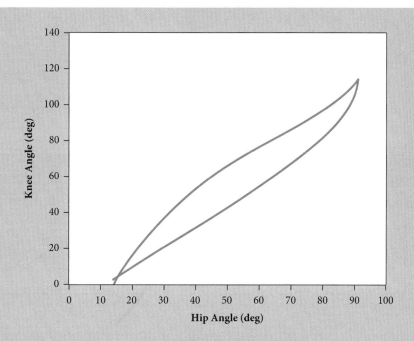

Figure 10.2 Hip–knee angle–angle diagram recorded in the sagittal plane from one athlete during a countermovement vertical jump. The angle–angle diagram reveals the coordination of the degrees of freedom in event space.

where each joint performs the opposite action concurrently (**Figure 10.3**). From Figure 10.2, it can be seen that the hip and knee joints tend to operate in phase during a countermovement vertical jump when they are described in event space.

Kilding et al. (2007) used angle–angle diagrams to investigate the coordination of lower-body segments during over-ground and deep-water running. These authors recorded two-dimensional lower-body joint angles in the sagittal plane of endurance runners completing five running trials through a 50-m over-ground course and running in deep water with the aid of a flotation device. Angle–angle diagrams of the hip–knee coordination patterns were constructed and analyzed using cross-correlations to quantify the coordination between the two joints. Kilding et al. reported that the hip–knee coordination pattern during over-ground running was characterized by the hip joint moving before the knee joint, whereas during deep-water running the joints tended to move in a more in-phase pattern. These differences could arise from the lack of a stance phase during deep-water running and have implications for the specificity of adaptations that are likely when using this mode of exercise.

Plotting the joint angle during a motor skill against the angular velocity of the joint allows elements of the coordination to be described in the state space, which is important for tasks where velocity is considered a constraint (**Figure 10.4**). Such plots of joint angle against joint angular velocity are known as **phase portraits**.

The coordination between two joints can also be derived from their phase portraits by calculating the **continuous relative phase** (CRP) variable. To do so, the phase angle of each data point is calculated for each phase portrait following normalization of the joint angle

(continues)

(continued)

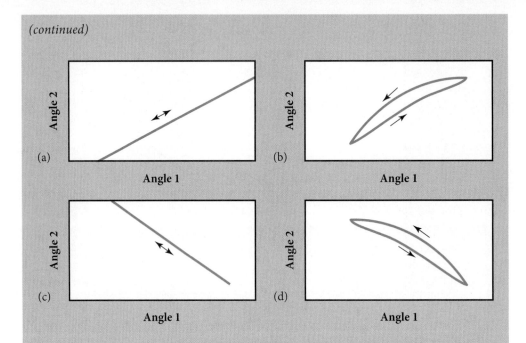

Figure 10.3 Trajectories of angle–angle diagrams representing in-phase (a and b) and anti-phase (c and d) coordination of joints.

Reproduced from Bartlett, R. (2007). *Introduction to sports biomechanics: Analysing human movement patterns.* London: Routledge.

and joint angular velocity data (**Figure 10.5**). The phase angle is then defined as the angle between the right horizontal and a line drawn from the origin of the phase portrait to each data point in the portrait (Hamill, van Emmerick, Heiderscheit, & Li, 1999) and is calculated as follows:

$$\phi = \tan^{-1}\frac{\omega}{\theta}$$

where ϕ is the phase angle for the data point, ω is the angular velocity of the data point, and θ is the angular displacement of the data point. The CRP is then calculated as the difference between the phase angle associated with the proximal joint and that associated with the distal joint:

$$\text{CRP} = \phi_{\text{promixal}} - \phi_{\text{distal}}$$

where CRP is the continuous relative phase, ϕ_{proximal} is the phase angle of the proximal joint, and ϕ_{distal} is the phase angle of the distal joint. General patterns of coordination are determined by the magnitude of CRP, with 0° representing an in-phase pattern between the joints and 180° representing an antiphase pattern (**Figure 10.6**).

Figure 10.6 shows that the hip and knee tend to operate in-phase during the propulsive phase of the countermovement vertical jump, as was revealed in the angle–angle diagram.

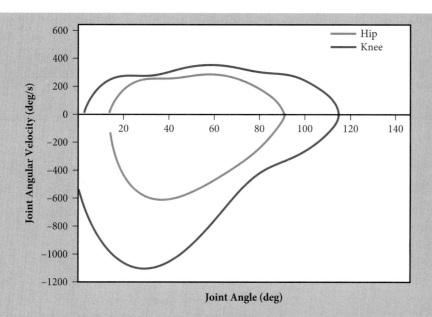

Figure 10.4 Phase portraits for the hip and knee joints recorded in the sagittal plane from one athlete during a countermovement vertical jump. The data reveal the coordination of degrees of freedom in state space.

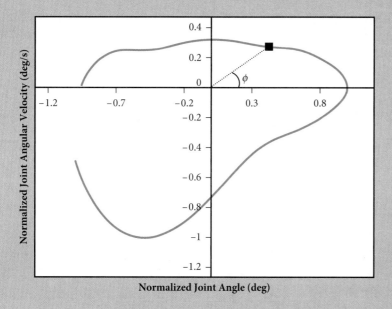

Figure 10.5 The phase portrait for the knee joint recorded in the sagittal plane from one athlete during a countermovement vertical jump. The joint angle and joint angular velocity data have been normalized. The phase angle (ϕ) is defined as the angle between the right horizontal and a line drawn from the origin of the phase portrait to each data point in the portrait.

(continues)

(continued)

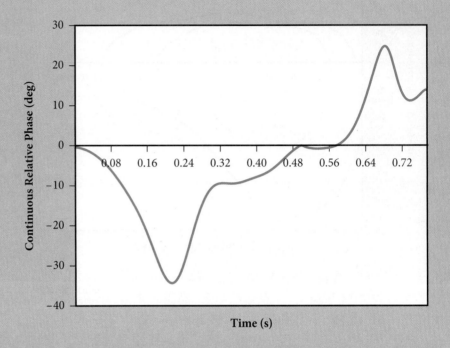

Figure 10.6 The continuous relative phase between the hip and knee joints recorded in the sagittal plane from one athlete during a countermovement vertical jump. The continuous relative phase plot reveals the coordination pattern of the degrees of freedom in state space.

Kurz, Stergiou, Buzzi, and Georgoulis (2005) investigated the differences in CRP measures for the interaction of two pairs of lower-body segments (thigh–leg and leg–foot) between a group of healthy participants and a group of individuals who were 10 months post anterior cruciate ligament (ACL) reconstruction. Kinematic data of the lower-body segments were recorded in the sagittal plane during trials of walking and running at the individuals' preferred speeds. The CRP data for both segment couplings were averaged across strides to provide mean CRP values. The researchers found that the patients who were post ACL surgery walked with a more antiphase leg–foot coupling, but ran with a more in-phase coupling compared to the healthy participants. The authors concluded that the differences between the two groups could arise from a loss of somatosensory information in the patients who underwent reconstructive surgery combined with an adaptive response from the early stages of postsurgery rehabilitation to avoid pain during gait.

The topological characteristics of the plots derived from the methods outlined in these examples can be interpreted either qualitatively or quantitatively to allow the coordination to be assessed during the execution of motor skills. These methods, however, rely on the accurate and reliable recording of kinematic data. While some basic video analysis systems allow the determination of kinematic data, including joint angles, at specific time instances during a motor skill, previous researchers have reported that time-continuous data provide more information than time-discrete data for the analysis of coordination patterns (Schöllhorn, Nigg, Stefanyshyn, & Liu, 2002).

represent DOF in a macroscopic analysis of team sports such that the relative motion of each player provides a measure of the coordination of the complex system. This type of analysis can reveal important information about the movements of individual players that result in successful outcomes.)

The human motor system actually has a greater number of DOF than the dimensions of the workspace (defined as the region of space within which the motor system operates). For example, any rigid body, such as a limb segment, requires six spatial coordinates to specify its position and orientation in three-dimensional space (three translational and three rotational coordinates), yet the shoulder, elbow, and wrist joints constitute at least seven anatomic DOF that need to be controlled to position the arm appropriately.

Furthermore, the coordination of different independent components of the motor system can result in the same movements being produced, encapsulating the **degeneracy** of the human motor system (Edelman & Gally, 2001). Degeneracy is associated with complex systems and confers adaptability and flexibility on the human motor system, allowing the goal of movement tasks to be achieved in the face of changing environmental conditions or characteristics of the performer. However, it would appear that the degeneracy of the motor system presents a problem for the coordination and control of movements (an issue addressed elsewhere in the chapter).

Appropriate movement solutions to satisfy the goal of motor skills are attained through experience and exposure to motor tasks, including formal practice, game play, free play, and even observation of others performing the tasks. It is through this experience and exposure that the motor skills are learned. **Learning** is defined as a relatively permanent improvement in performance and is assessed through the use of retention and transfer tests (Magill, 2011). A **retention test** entails the administration of a test after a period of time during which the performer has not been practicing the skill. The period of abstinence from practice allows for the dissipation of other factors that could influence performance of the motor skill, thereby enabling the degree of permanence of performance level to be determined (Magill, 2011). A **transfer test** requires that the performance of the skill be assessed in a different context from that of the practice trials or that a novel variation of the practiced skill be assessed (Magill, 2011). Such a test assesses the adaptability of the learned skill.

The use of retention and transfer tests to assess learning is important, as inferring learning from the performance of athletes during practice can be misleading (see Skill Acquisition Concept 10.1). With the use of such tests, the outcome in motor tasks is the determining factor in establishing that learning has occurred. However, learning may be accompanied by the acquisition of a new coordination pattern or the modification of an existing coordination pattern. These changes can be determined through the assessment of angle–angle diagrams and phase portraits.

Skill acquisition is defined as the process of attaining functional movement task solutions. How this process unfolds and how it is affected by the experience of the learner and exposure to movements requires knowledge of the different approaches to the coordination and control of movement.

Different Approaches to the Coordination and Control of Movement

A problem faced by the human motor system when learning motor skills is the coordination and control of the many DOF during goal-directed movements (Bernstein, 1967).

Skill Acquisition Concept 10.1

How is learning assessed?

The learning of motor skills is assessed by examining the learner's performance on retention and transfer tasks. Learning is not assessed during practice, as the performance of a learner during such sessions is not always indicative of how the learner will perform during retention and transfer tasks. For example, performance is largely improved at the end of practices that follow a blocked structure (i.e., only one skill is practiced) compared to when a random structure is followed (i.e., multiple motor skills are practiced in a random order). However, the blocked practice structure tends to elicit reductions in performance when the skills are retested following a period of no practice (retention test) and when the skill is assessed in a different context (transfer test); in contrast, performance in retention and transfer tests is improved following a random practice structure. For this reason, learning should not be assessed at the end of a practice session. Traditional approaches to acquiring motor skills that emphasize the execution of multiple repetitions of drills with the "correct" movements as prescribed a priori by the coach would be deemed successful if learning were assessed at the end of a practice session; however, such outcomes simply demonstrate that the athlete can "perform" and do not confirm that the athlete has "learned."

In contrast to retention tasks, transfer tasks are rarely included in motor learning studies. Therefore, we cannot always determine how adaptable and robust the learning is.

Many theoretical approaches have been forwarded in an attempt to explain this **degrees of freedom problem**. In this section, we discuss two opposing approaches: the information processing approach and the constraints-led approach. Although the constraints-led approach is favored here, a discussion of these two disparate approaches provides an informative foundation for the strength and conditioning coach to understand the implications of the constraints-led approach.

Information Processing Approach

Information processing approaches to the coordination and control of movement emphasize cognitive processes—particularly memory processes—and involve model structures that are analogous to a computer, with the storage and execution of "programs" for specific movement tasks based on sensory information (Schmidt & Wrisberg, 2008). For example, early information processing approaches promoted a form of memory representation (a motor program) that contained a set of movement commands to produce movements under specific circumstances (Keele, 1968). The concept of the **motor program** emanated from the notion that the sequencing of movements observed in motor skills were preplanned prior to their execution. According to this model, the execution of a specific motor program resulted from processes including perception, decision making, and response execution. However, feedback was not required and the models developed relied on open-loop control systems.

Subsequent theories incorporated feedback by including a comparator function that regulated the ongoing movement; it did so by comparing the sensory information generated during the movement with the sensory information from the execution of successful movements that was stored in memory (Adams, 1971). These stored representations of the expected movement were generated by using outcome-related feedback (knowledge of results) to guide successful movements. The inclusion of feedback in the models provided a closed-loop control system.

One notable problem associated with motor programs was that of storage. With each program representing a specific movement, the storage capacity of the central nervous system was called into question. This issue was circumvented by the development of **general motor programs** (Schmidt, 1975). A general motor program contains invariant features (e.g., sequencing, relative timing, relative force) that are common to movements within a given movement class, such that the one-to-one memory construct is replaced by a one-to-many relationship. With this model, motor programs could be executed in myriad ways so as to account for different variations of the same movement.

Schmidt (1975) also added another concept to the model of coordination and control: a **schema**, defined as a rule that describes the relationship between the outcomes of previous motor programs and the parameters of the programs associated with those attempts. A recall schema describes the relationship between the parameters associated with a program and the outcome of the movement, whereas a recognition schema describes the relationship between the past sensory consequences of the program and the outcome of the program (Schmidt, 2003). These schemata are developed through practice and experiences.

Criticisms of the information processing approaches to the coordination and control of movement focus on the prescriptive nature of the proposed models, with each requiring a representational scheme of the movement that prescribes the movement sequence to be stored (Newell, 1991). With such models, the process of skill acquisition is regarded as the process of attaining more appropriate prescriptions for movements to satisfy the goal of a motor skill. The information processing approach does not provide a mechanism by which the DOF are coordinated and controlled during the acquisition of new motor skills. Moreover, the ability of the motor system to compensate for perturbations to an ongoing movement sequence is not addressed, as it would require a representation of the "correct" movement sequence (Newell, 1991). It is also not clear what form the motor program takes—that is, what is represented in a motor program? Typically, the notion of a motor program relates to a set of muscle commands, although this definition is subject to disagreement (Summers & Anson, 2009). Certainly, at least some evidence points to strengthening of activity in certain areas of the brain as motor skills are learned (Nielsen & Cohen, 2007), but this evidence falls short of elucidating "programs" that store representations of the movement. Furthermore, the acquisition of these programs has not been explained adequately.

The computer analogy that forms the foundation of the information processing approaches to the coordination and control of movement assumes variability in the movements represents an error in one of the processes associated with the selection and execution of a motor program, promoting the minimization of variability as one of the goals of practice. This perspective stands in contrast to the evidence that even skilled athletes demonstrate considerable variability, oftentimes greater than that associated with the novice performer (Davids, Bennett, & Newell, 2006). The notion of skilled behavior residing in an internal structure that is prominent in the information processing approach downplays the influence of the task and the environment in shaping skilled behavior. In turn, information processing approaches to the coordination and control of movement have been criticized for promoting "organismic asymmetry" (Davids & Araújo, 2010). Yet despite the organismic asymmetry promoted by these approaches, little consideration is given to the characteristics of the performer's motor system (e.g., biomechanical, physiological, neural processes) and the means by which they influence the execution of movements and the learning of motor skills.

Finally, the information processing approaches have little to offer regarding the coordination and control of movements between individual athletes such as are observed during subphases of play in invasion sports such as basketball, rugby, and soccer. While this shortcoming is not surprising given that the information processing approaches were never developed to address such situations, it severely limits the utility of the approaches for the strength and conditioning practitioner.

Collectively, these criticisms of the information processing approach to the coordination and control of movements have led to a search for alternative approaches that better explain the performance in motor skills and the acquisition of these skills.

Constraints-Led Approach

At the heart of the constraints-led approach is the simple proposition that the coordination and control of movements emerge from the confluence of constraints associated with the organism, the environment, and the task (Davids et al., 2008). A constraint is a variable that limits the configuration of the motor system, guiding the movements of the performer as he or she executes a motor skill (Newell, 1986).

Organismic constraints are associated with the performer and include the physical properties of the motor system (e.g., height, mass, limb lengths) as well as biomechanical/physiological variables (e.g., heart rate, fatigue, muscle strength, flexibility) and psychological variables (e.g., motivation, attentional focus). These constraints operate across different time scales. For example, a change in height, limb length, or muscular strength will take longer to become fully realized than a change in heart rate or motivation. Although evidence of the influence of organismic constraints on performance of motor skills is readily apparent, fewer data have been published that demonstrate the influence of organismic constraints on the coordination and control of movements.

Investigations of the kinematics of locomotion following anterior cruciate ligament (ACL) injury, however, reveal the influence of organismic constraints. Following an ACL rupture, patients typically experience a loss of proprioception and/or reduced strength of the muscles around the knee joint that can lead to instability and episodes of "giving way" during weight acceptance (Buss et al., 1995; Daniel et al., 1994). To compensate for these changes in organismic constraints, ACL-deficient patients reduce knee flexor and knee extensor moments during the stance phases of walking (Berchuck, Andriacchi, Bach, & Reider, 1990; Rudolph, Eastlack, Axe, & Snyder-Mackler, 1998). Furthermore, a comparison of ACL-deficient patients and healthy controls revealed that both groups walked and jogged at the same self-selected speeds; however, the ACL-deficient patients achieved these speeds with reduced knee flexion moments (Lewek, Rudolph, Axe, & Snyder-Mackler, 2002).

Aging is associated with a number of adaptations within the motor system, including a decrease in muscular strength, a loss of motor units, a shift toward a higher percentage of type I muscle fibers, and a decrease in the extensibility of soft tissue (Luff, 1998; Maharam, Bauman, Kalman, Skolnik, & Perle, 1999; Porter, Myint, Kramer, & Vandervoort, 1995). These changes in organismic constraints are likely to result in alterations in the coordination and control of movements. In an analysis of sprint running,

Roberts, Cheung, Abdel Hafez, and Hong (1997) reported that elderly runners achieved lower sprinting speeds than their younger counterparts. However, an analysis of the kinematic and kinetic variables of the lower-body joints during each running stride revealed a similar pattern between the two groups: The elderly group simply produced lower joint angular velocities and lower joint moments. The authors suggested that the elderly runners preserved the overall coordination pattern by reducing the range of motion at the joints through reductions in the joint moments, ensuring the timing of the swing leg corresponded to the timing of the stance leg. Furthermore, the reduced muscular force of the elderly runners resulted in an increased stance duration, requiring an adaptation of the joint moments of the swing leg to maintain the overall coordination pattern. Transient changes in the mechanical characteristics of muscles caused by fatigue have also been shown to elicit changes in coordination during sprint running (Pinniger, Steele, & Groeller, 2000; Sprague & Mann, 1983). From such studies, it is apparent that organismic constraints influence the coordination patterns observed during the execution of motor skills.

Environmental constraints are associated with the physical properties of the environment in which the athlete is performing. Environmental constraints readily influence performance in motor skills. For example, high ambient temperatures and altitude can result in reduced distance-running performance (El Helou et al., 2012; Wehrlin & Hallen, 2006), while sprinting speeds are lower when an individual is sprinting up a hill or around a curve (Paradisis & Cooke, 2001; Usherwood & Wilson, 2006). Evidence also indicates that environmental constraints influence the coordination and control of movements. For example, sprinting on sand results in a lower center of mass during stance, greater forward lean of the trunk, and reduced hip extension at takeoff compared to when the motor skill is performed on an athletic track (Alcaraz, Palao, Elvira, & Linthorne, 2011). A shorter touchdown distance, a greater takeoff distance, and a greater forward lean of the trunk at touchdown and takeoff have been reported when sprinting uphill compared to horizontal sprinting (Paradisis & Cooke, 2001; Slawinski et al., 2008). Interestingly, a reduction in gravitational force has been shown to reduce the speed at which individuals transition from a walking coordination pattern to a running coordination pattern (Kram, Domingo, & Ferris, 1997).

Notice that these environmental constraints operate over very short time scales to exert their influence on the coordination and control of movement. In addition to the physical characteristics of the performance environment, societal expectations can be considered to represent environmental constraints.

Task constraints include the goal of the task. Such constraints have been shown to affect the outcome of motor skills. For example, the use of an overhead goal that the athlete has to aim for has been shown to increase jump height (Ford et al., 2005), while sprinting speed is reduced when the task is modified by the athlete carrying a hockey stick (Wdowski & Gittoes, 2013) or carrying a rugby ball (Walsh, Young, Hill, Kittredge, & Horn, 2007).

Task constraints can also be altered by the coach giving specific instructions to the athlete. For example, providing the explicit instruction of "jumping for maximal height" as opposed to the instruction of "jumping while extending the legs as fast as possible to maximize explosive force" results in different kinematic outcomes during vertical jumps (Talpey, Young, & Beseler, 2014). Instructing female athletes to "land softly" during a landing task results in changes in lower-body coordination during the absorption phase of the task that lowers the vertical ground reaction force acting on the athlete (Milner, Fairbrother, Srivatsan, & Zhang, 2012; Walsh, Waters, & Kersting, 2007). The use of instructions prior to the execution of a motor skill acts to change the coordination and control of the movements by altering the intention of the athlete; thus such instructions represent a form of informational constraint on movements. However, the goal of the task may not be explicitly stated prior to the execution of the movement, being biomechanical in nature. For example, accelerative sprinting requires the athlete to employ a "rotation–extension" strategy to satisfy the goal of the task, whereby the forceful extension of the lower-body joints is delayed until the center of mass is rotated ahead of the ground reaction force by the reciprocal activation of the biarticular muscles crossing the hip and knee joints (Jacobs & van Ingen Schenau, 1992). It is unlikely that this task goal is apparent to the athlete prior to executing an accelerative sprint, but it acts to constrain the movement of the athlete.

Finally, task constraints can include any rules specifying the movements used to achieve the goal (e.g., swimming strokes, race walking).

The constraints-led approach to the coordination and control of movement places the coach in the role of guiding the athlete during practice while searching for functional movement task solutions that satisfy the goal of the motor skill (Davids et al., 2008). The guidance provided by the coach comes in the form of manipulating the constraints surrounding the athlete because functional movement solutions emerge from the confluence of constraints. Therefore, the coach needs to consider the specific constraints before attempting to enhance the performance of the athlete; failure to consider the interaction of constraints may lead to the development of ineffective practices (see Skill Acquisition Concept 10.2).

The role of the coach in guiding the athlete in his or her search for a functional movement solution reflects the principle of **guided discovery**, which is exemplified by the constraints-led approach to the coordination and control of movement, and which promotes **implicit learning**. Implicit learning occurs when the athlete accumulates task-relevant information without conscious awareness of what has been learned. Such learning has been shown to be resistant to factors including anxiety, emotions, and changes in environmental constraints that act to perturb the learned movements (Masters & Poolton, 2012). In contrast, **explicit learning** occurs when the athlete is consciously aware of the elements of the movement that are to be learned, resulting in conscious control of movement that can be easily perturbed (Masters & Poolton, 2012). Explicit learning is likely to occur when the coach prescribes the to-be-learned movement pattern through instructions and feedback rather than allowing a functional movement pattern to emerge naturally through the manipulation of constraints during learning.

To explain how functional movement patterns emerge, we need to discuss dynamical systems theory and ecological psychology upon which the constraints-led approach is founded.

Dynamical Systems Theory

Dynamical systems theory is an interdisciplinary framework used to describe and examine different types of systems (i.e., biological, ecological, social) that are in a constant state of flux, changing and evolving over time (Davids, Glazier, Araújo, & Bartlett, 2003). Recall that the motor system is regarded as a complex system, being characterized by an enormous number of DOF that interact across many different levels. From a dynamical systems perspective, the coordination and control of the DOF is achieved through the formation of **coordinative structures** (Turvey, Fitch, &

Skill Acquisition Concept 10.2

Constraints during maximal speed sprinting

An athlete is required to generate a vertical impulse during each stance phase when sprinting so as to support body weight and prevent the center of mass (CM) from falling. While there is little difference in the magnitude of the vertical impulse generated during the acceleration and maximal speed phases of sprinting, the duration of the stance phases is much shorter when the athlete attains maximal speed (Girard, Miscallef, & Millet, 2011). In turn, the requirement to exert a sufficient vertical impulse to support body weight and project the CM into the subsequent aerial phase in short stance times has been identified as a substantial biomechanical limitation to the attainment of maximal running speed (Weyand, Sandell, Prime, & Bundle, 2010; Weyand, Sternlight, Bellizzi, & Wright, 2000). To exert a sufficient impulse, the athlete must generate force rapidly and, therefore, must possess sufficiently high levels of explosive strength.

Goodwin (2011) noted that an athlete who possesses insufficient muscular strength (explosive strength) to generate the required vertical impulse during the short stance phases associated with maximal speed sprinting will likely compensate by over-striding, placing the stance leg far ahead of the CM at touchdown. This compensatory alteration in coordination increases the duration of the stance phase, providing the athlete with sufficient time to exert the necessary vertical impulse. However, the compensatory change in coordination also increases the braking force acting on the athlete, further increasing the requirement for a propulsive impulse during stance.

A coach may observe the over-striding and attempt to rectify the problem by changing the athlete's movements through instruction, feedback, and possibly repetitious sprint drills promoting the appropriate sprinting technique. This approach is unlikely to be successful, as over-striding will emerge once again when the athlete attains a sufficiently high speed. In contrast, couching the problem within the constraints-led framework can allow the coach to develop a different, more effective approach to the problem.

To do so, we can define the requirement to exert sufficient vertical impulse during the stance phases associated with maximal speed sprinting as a task constraint. Explosive strength is an organismic constraint. Altering the organismic constraint through resistance training methods will allow the athlete to select a more appropriate coordination pattern to satisfy the goal of the task given the specific task constraint; the athlete will no longer need to over-stride to provide sufficient time to produce the required vertical impulse. Within this model, the over-striding problem is not viewed as a technical flaw to be remedied through repeated drilling; rather, it is seen as a technical adaptation to compensate for insufficient muscular strength. Successful application of the constraints-led approach, however, is possible only when the coach has a biomechanical understanding of the motor skill obtained through quantitative and qualitative approaches.

Tuller, 1982). A coordinative structure is a temporary organization of DOF that emerges through the process of self-organization under constraint.

The process of **self-organization** associated with complex systems was a well-documented phenomenon in physical and chemical systems long before any attempts were made to empirically verify its presence in a system of human movement coordination (Schöner & Kelso, 1988). In this context, self-organization implies spontaneous pattern generation as a consequence of the interaction of a very large collection of DOF that may adapt in response to changing internal and external conditions, by adopting coordination patterns without any explicit prescription of the emergent pattern (Beek, Schmidt, Morris, Sim, & Turvey, 1995; Schöner & Kelso, 1988). This process stands in stark contrast to the prescriptive representations of the coordination patterns promoted in the information processing approach.

The coordinative structures that emerge under constraint are intentional, being influenced by the goal of the specific motor skill, and they are soft-assembled, existing only until the goal of the motor skill is achieved. Furthermore, coordinative structures are autonomous, emerging from the intrinsic dynamics of an athlete's motor system and the constraints imposed on the athlete. If the constraints under which the motor system is operating during a motor skill do not change, then the coordinative structure will remain in place and a stable coordination pattern will develop. Stability within the framework of dynamical systems refers not to a persistent, stereotypic repetition of a coordination pattern, but rather to the capacity of a system to quickly return to a coordination pattern after perturbation (Nourrit, Deschamps, Lauriot, Caillou, & Delignieres, 2000). Stability in this sense enables performers to maintain "stable" task-related coordinative structures while simultaneously possessing a degree of flexibility and adaptability that enables them to modify coordination patterns as a consequence of perturbations (e.g., changes in constraints). Changing the constraints will lead to instabilities in the coordination pattern and the formation of different coordinative structures to satisfy the goal of the task. This notion is important because instabilities can force the search for a new, more functional coordination pattern.

According to Schöner and Kelso (1988), the many possible coordination patterns of a movement system (irrespective of the system's initial conditions) will eventually converge around a limited set of stable coordination patterns, otherwise referred to as an **attractor state**. Attractor states may be characterized as wells within the **perceptual-motor workspace** (Figure 10.7). Glazier, Davids, and Bartlett (2003) propose that functionally preferred, highly stable coordination or attractor states evolve and develop through experience and practice to enable and sustain goal-directed actions. Therefore, the goal of coaches is not to guide performers toward a to-be-learned movement pattern that is specified a priori, but rather to facilitate a shift in coordination away from the initial attractor state and thus enable a search for an optimal solution to the task (Delignières et al., 1998). This may require the acquisition of a new movement pattern or the modification of an existing movement pattern by enabling performers to search their perceptual-motor workspace. Performers will have natural coordination tendencies or attractor states due to the intrinsic dynamics of their motor system. These attractor states may compete or cooperate with the to-be-learned coordination pattern to satisfy the goal of a movement task, providing an explanation as to why some individuals may learn at a different rate than others (Kelso, 1995).

Central to the dynamical systems approach to movement coordination and control is the identification of a system's attractor state or states, and the transitions between

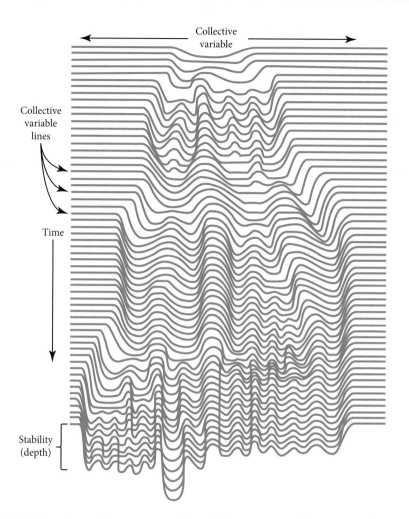

Figure 10.7 A schematic representation of the perceptual-motor workspace as a dynamic landscape. The perceptual-motor landscape contains the perceptual information associated with the to-be-learned motor skill, the constraints of the to-be-learned motor skill, and the intrinsic dynamics of the performer. It represents the context in which an athlete learns a motor skill through experience and practice. The deep regions within the topological landscape correspond to attractor states. The journey of the motor system around this theoretical landscape is driven by the change in control parameters.

Reproduced from Handford, C., Davids, K., Bennett, S., & Button, C. (1997). Skill acquisition in sport: Some applications of an evolving practice ecology. *Journal of Sports Sciences, 15,* 621–640. Reprinted by permission of the publisher (Taylor & Francis Ltd, http://www.tandfonline.com).

states as a consequence of a variation in a specific control parameter (Beek et al., 1995). A **control parameter** is a variable that moves the system through different states of coordination, although it does not contain any specific (prescribed) information regarding the organization of the system (Kelso, 1995). Control parameters can be thought of as constraints surrounding the motor system. An **order parameter**, or a collective variable, is a variable that describes the "state" of a system at any given time, identifying both the macroscopic aspects of a system and the "collective behavior" of the component subsystems involved (Van Emmerik, Rosenstein, McDermott, & Hamill, 2004); an order parameter, therefore, describes the coordination pattern during a motor skill. Returning to the example of maximal sprinting speed highlighted in Skill Acquisition Concept 10.2, we can consider speed to be the control parameter, as scaling up speed (as the athlete sprints faster) results in a change in the order parameter (the adoption of a coordination pattern exemplified by over-striding). Furthermore, explosive strength can be considered as a **rate-limiter** in this example because it precludes the attainment of the more task-relevant coordination pattern (Thelen, 1986).

The dynamical systems approach promotes the functional role of variability in movements. The variability inherent in the movements of even skilled performers arises from the vast number of DOF, facilitating more flexible control of the system (multiple states of coordination can be brought into play to solve a specific task). Having an abundant number of DOF allows various combinations of these DOF to be formed into temporally available task-dependent coordinative structures (Kugler & Turvey, 1987; Turvey, 1990). (See Skill Acquisition Concept 10.3.) The importance of the dynamical systems concepts of control and order parameters, stability, variability, and transitions between attractor states, along with an understanding of how they relate to the coordination and control of movements, can be derived from a discussion of a simple experiment (see Worked Example 10.2).

The concepts from dynamical systems theory that have been applied to the coordination and control of the movements performed by individual athletes during the execution of motor skills have also been applied to team sports. For example, the movements of an attacker and a defender in invasion sports such as basketball, rugby, or soccer can be viewed as a dynamical system, whereby the coordination between the two players emerges from the dynamics of the component parts (i.e., the position and motion of other players, the ball, boundaries of the playing area) (Balague, Torrents, Hristovski, Davids, & Araújo, 2013). The movements of the two players may be synchronous (i.e., as the attacker moves in one direction, the defender counters by moving in the same direction) or asynchronous. Such coordination patterns can be revealed in the relative phase of the positioning and running speeds of the two players in the dyad. The stability of these coordination patterns is influenced by the interpersonal distance between the attacker and the defender (Duarte et al., 2010). Specifically, when the players approach each other and the interpersonal distance decreases, they enter a critical region where an increase in the running speed of the attacker relative to the defender destabilizes the coordination of the dyad, providing an opportunity for the attacker to pass the defender and maintain the attack. Conversely, the defender is tasked with maintaining the interpersonal distance beyond the critical region so as to maintain the stability of the coordination pattern. In such situations, both interpersonal distance and relative speed can be considered control parameters that move the dyad through different states of coordination (Duarte et al., 2010; Esteves, de Oliveira, & Araújo, 2011; Passos et al., 2009). From the dynamical systems perspective, both the attacker and the defender are required to recognize the appropriate moment when the interpersonal distance enters the critical region so that they can execute their appropriate movements to satisfy the specific goal of the task. The coach can promote their awareness of these critical regions by manipulating the task constraints during practices to expose the players to these one-versus-one subphases of the game and allow the development of functional movement task solutions (Passos, Araújo, Davids, & Shuttleworth, 2008).

Skill Acquisition Concept 10.3

Are more skilled performers less variable?

The human motor system comprises an enormous number of degrees of freedom (e.g., joints, muscles, cell types, neurons and neuronal connections), so variation in performance is inevitable. However, the definition of skilled behavior typically incorporates the notion of a certainty in the outcome of a motor task (Guthrie, 1952), implying that the performance of a skilled athlete will be less variable than that of a less skilled athlete. In reality, this is not the case: Elite performers actually show greater variability in their performances than less skilled athletes (Woo & Zatsiorsky, 2006). Furthermore, the movement patterns of elite performers have been shown to be highly variable (Bartlett, Wheat, & Robins, 2007)—perhaps not surprising given the enormous number of DOF. At the same time, evidence suggests that skilled performers display greater variation in coordination patterns than less skilled athletes (Davids et al., 2006). The question then becomes, What purpose could this increased variability serve?

Variability in coordination during repeated executions of specific motor skills is proposed to serve a functional purpose by allowing the performer to adapt to changing task and environmental constraints (Davids et al., 2008). Variations in coordination patterns may also prevent injuries in repetitive cyclical movements such as running (Hamill, Haddad, Heiderscheit, van Emmerik, & Li, 2006). Finally, the acquisition of new attractor states may be facilitated if variability is enhanced during practice. Therefore, variability in coordination is not a characteristic particular to novice athletes and something that should be eliminated through practice; rather, variability should be embraced as a functional characteristic of an adaptable athlete.

Worked Example 10.2
The dynamical systems approach to coordination and control of movement in a finger waggling experiment

Try the following simple experiment:

1. Sit with your hands on a table in front of you, palms facing down.
2. Extend the index finger on each hand while clenching the other fingers.
3. Move the right index finger toward the midline of the body while simultaneously moving the left index finger away from the midline of the body before reversing the motion of the fingers. Continue this slow rhythmical motion.
4. Begin to slowly increase the frequency of the motion of the fingers until you are moving them as fast as possible.
5. What should become apparent is that the fingers are now moving toward and away from the midline of the body at the same time rather than one moving toward the midline while the other moves away from it. The coordination pattern of the fingers has changed.

This seemingly simple experiment was initially performed by Kelso (1984) to investigate the processes involved in the coordination and control of movements from the dynamical

(continues)

(continued)

systems perspective. The experiment required participants to time the motion of the fingers to a metronome. The initial motion of the fingers was antiphase (as the right index finger moves toward the midline, the left index finger moves away from the midline). This phase relationship between the fingers represents the order parameter that describes the coordination of the component parts of the system. The frequency of the metronome was then increased from 1.25 Hz to 3.50 Hz, and the participants were asked to maintain the original coordination pattern (antiphase). The researchers observed that a spontaneous change in the coordination pattern occurred as the frequency increased: The relative phase between the fingers changed from antiphase (one finger moves toward the midline as the other moves away from the midline) to in-phase (both fingers move toward and away from the midline simultaneously). Expressing this finding in the language of dynamical systems theory, a transition occurred in the order parameter (antiphase to in-phase coordination pattern) as the control parameter (frequency) was scaled, such that a more stable attractor state was realized (the antiphase pattern was unable to be maintained in the face of a perturbation caused by scaling the control parameter). Furthermore, as the transition between the attractor states (antiphase and in-phase coordination patterns) was approached, the variability of the order parameter increased, as evidenced by the standard deviation of the relative phase between the fingers.

What are the implications of these findings when we are looking to understand the processes of coordination and control of movements? It should be acknowledged that the experimental protocol over-constrained the participants by allowing them only two degrees of freedom (Newell & Jordan, 2007). However, the results reveal a number of interesting characteristics of coordination and control. First, abrupt changes in coordination occur when a control parameter is scaled. In the original experiment, the control parameter was movement frequency. A similarly abrupt change in coordination has been shown when the speed of locomotion is increased and the participant transitions from a walking coordination pattern to a running coordination pattern (Diedrich & Warren, 1995). This implies that the search for a more appropriate coordination pattern to satisfy the goal of a motor skill can be facilitated by scaling a control parameter. The scaling of the control parameter creates a perturbation that increases the instability of the system and triggers a search for a new coordination pattern. Strength and conditioning coaches should consider the control parameters for their athletes in different motor skills when seeking to improve their performance.

Another implication of the finger waggling experiment relates to the role of variability in signifying a transition between coordination patterns. An increase in the variability observed in the order parameter as it deviates away from an attractor state around a transition point is known as a critical fluctuation (Kelso, Scholz, & Schöner, 1986; Schöner, Haken, & Kelso, 1986). The walk–run transition is also preceded by a critical fluctuation in coordination pattern (Diedrich & Warren, 1995). Furthermore, the movement patterns of novice performers are characterized by greater variability than those of intermediate-level performers (Wilson, Simpson, van Emmerik, & Hamill, 2008), implying a search for a more appropriate coordination pattern by the novices. This highlights the functional role of variability that is inherent in the motor system and suggests that the measurement of variability in coordination patterns might provide information about an impending change in coordination pattern (Davids et al., 2006; Van Emmerik, 2007).

Finally, the finger waggling experiment reveals the natural coordination tendencies of the human motor system. Specifically, the finger waggling task was characterized by two stable coordination patterns: in-phase and antiphase. These stable coordination patterns were not specified by a representation stored in the central nervous system, and control was not given to a central executive. Rather, these coordination patterns emerged as the system self-organized under constraint.

Ecological Psychology

A major tenet of ecological psychology is that of **direct perception**, whereby patterns of ambient energy found in the environment (e.g., light, sound) are attended to directly by the performer to provide information that can guide movement (Jacobs & Michaels, 2007). This perspective contrasts with the information processing approaches that require the stimuli found in the environment to be ambiguous and the performer to interpret the information through processes of inference and memories (Jacobs & Michaels, 2007). Ecological approaches to the coordination and control of movement promote reciprocity between movements and the information found within the environment, such that the information constrains the observed movements while the movement reveals further information within the environment (Jacobs & Michaels, 2007). Therefore, one cannot understand movements without reference to the environment in which the performer operates.

Central to the notion of the coupling between the direct perception of environmental information and the subsequent movement promoted by the ecological approach (perception–action coupling) is the concept of affordances. An **affordance** can be described as an opportunity for movement provided by the environment as perceived by the performer (Fajen, Riley, & Turvey, 2008). For example, the ambient light energy may present a surface that the athlete can walk or run upon; alternatively, it may reveal the location of a teammate who is in a position to receive a pass in soccer. Athletes need to detect affordances so that they can select an appropriate movement solution to achieve the goal of the task. The detection of specifying information (task-relevant environmental information that acts to constrain the movements) is a skill that can be learned through the process of **perceptual attunement** (Fajen et al., 2008). The ecological approach, therefore, promotes motor learning as the process of the attunement to task-relevant environmental information, with the differences between experts and novices then reflecting differences between the specifying information upon which the athletes rely (Fajen et al., 2008). For example, expert soccer goalkeepers who were successful in saving a penalty kick have been shown to demonstrate a different visual search strategy compared to those who were unsuccessful and attended to different body parts of the kicker (Savelsbergh, Van Der Kamp, Williams, & Ward, 2005). An important corollary for the strength and conditioning practitioner is the notion of representative learning practices (Pinder, Davids, Renshaw, & Araújo, 2011). (See Skill Acquisition Concept 10.4.)

Instructions presented to the athlete by the coach can be used to expedite the process of perceptual attunement by directing the attention of the athlete toward "information-rich" areas of the practice environment (Magill, 1998). However, if the specific to-be-learned movements are prescribed by the coach with explicit instructions, the athlete does not learn to detect the specifying information and, therefore, does not achieve skill acquisition. Perceptual attunement can also be expedited by the coach posing questions to the athlete between executions of the motor skills. As another example of the principle of guided discovery, this questioning strategy would appear to be appropriate given the rest periods that will be scheduled during any practice session.

Body-scaled affordances represent the relation between a measurable dimension of an athlete's body and a property of the environment that determines whether a movement is possible (Fajen et al., 2008). For example, the arm length of a basketball player may be perceived as allowing for the interception of a pass from the athlete's current position or the requirement to move so as to intercept the ball. In contrast,

Skill Acquisition Concept 10.4

Representative learning practices

Representative learning design refers to the generalization of task constraints in practice to the constraints encountered in the specific sporting environments in which athletes operate (Pinder, Davids, et al., 2011). A congruency between the two would promote perception–action coupling, which in turn is an important element of the ecological approach to the coordination and control of movements. The process of perceptual attunement requires that the environmental information presented in practice match the information encountered during actual sports performance. For example, expert baseball batters use the information associated with the movement of pitchers to constrain their swing (Ranganathan & Carlton, 2007). The use of pitching machines would, therefore, violate the assumption of representative learning practices, because it removes task-relevant information from the movement (Pinder, Renshaw, Davids, & Kerhervé, 2011). Similarly, the use of cone drills for the promotion of agility performance violates the principle of representative learning practices. Indeed, Young and Rogers (2014) have reported that the use of cone drills during training is ineffective in improving agility performance. In contrast, the use of small-sided games was found to be effective. This difference likely reflects the attunement of the athletes to task-relevant information through the use of practices that were representative of the task constraints associated with agility performance. To assist athletes in improving their performance, the strength and conditioning practitioner should be aware of the importance of developing representative learning practices.

action-scaled affordances represent the relation between the perception of an athlete's physical capabilities and the possibility for movement (Fajen et al., 2008). For example, a gap between two opposing players may be identified as traversable by one athlete who perceives his or her sprinting speed as being sufficient to achieve this goal, whereas another athlete may determine that a pass to a teammate is the more appropriate action under the same circumstances. What is important here is that both types of affordances can be learned through training. Furthermore, an alteration in body dimensions or physical capabilities through either natural growth processes or specific training will require **perceptual-motor recalibration** to allow the athlete to become attuned to these affordances. Thus the process of perceptual-motor recalibration is likely to be important as an athlete progresses through his or her training program and requires consideration on the part of the coach.

In summary, the constraints-led approach promotes the emergence of coordination and control of movement from the confluence of constraints associated with the athlete, the environment, and the task. It immediately precludes the "organismic asymmetry" that is inherent in the information processing approaches (Davids & Araújo, 2010). Indeed, the athlete–environment system becomes the unit of study during skill acquisition rather than solely the athlete. This approach highlights the potential for individual differences in coordination to emerge during the execution of the same motor skills, precluding the notion of an optimal movement pattern. Moreover, the constraints-led approach rules out a prescriptive approach to the acquisition of motor skills, promoting instead the principle of guided discovery and the emergence of functional movement task solutions. It also suggests the use of an interdisciplinary approach to movement coordination, which in turn requires the coach to understand the biomechanical characteristics of the motor system and the task. The approach emphasizes the functional role of variability in movements and suggests that representative learning practices should be employed in which the task constraints experienced in practice reflect those found in the performance environment. Finally, the constraints-led approach can explain the interpersonal coordination between players in team sports, something that the information processing approach is unable to do.

Using the constraints-led framework, we can now provide more informative definitions of the terms of *coordination*, *control*, and *skill*. Any definition of coordination must acknowledge the mutuality of the movements of athletes and the environment in which they are performing, such that coordination is viewed as the "patterning of body and limb motions relative to the patterning of environmental objects and events" (Turvey, 1990, p. 938). Control represents the ability of athletes to vary the parameters of their coordination patterns in relation to the specific task constraints, while skill refers to the optimization of the control process (Newell, 1985). The optimization criteria may comprise the minimization of energy expenditure during the execution of the motor skill or the minimization of the time to complete the motor skill. Alternatively, the optimization criteria may involve a variable being maximized, such as jump height or sprinting speed. However, performance in a motor skill does not always have to be maximized. Rather, skilled behavior should be regarded as an improved fit between the athlete and the environment (Jacobs & Michaels, 2007); that is, skilled behavior is characterized by flexible coordination patterns that the athlete is able to adapt to changing constraints so as to achieve the goal of the motor task.

Stages of Learning

The process of learning involves a search for and stabilization of specific, functional movement patterns across the perceptual-motor workspace as each individual adapts to a new set of changing constraints (Davids et al., 2008). Newell (1991) proposed that learning is a discontinuous process, characterized by nonlinear changes in motor behavior in response to the interacting constraints on the system and the continual search of the perceptual-motor workspace. Table 10.1 describes the three general stages as the learner progresses from novice to skilled performer (Newell, 1985).

Vereijken et al. (1997) provided some evidence to support the validity of these stages of learning. Having participants learn a novel ski simulator task, the authors reported low variability and high correlations between joint angles early in learning, characteristics of the participants freezing the available DOF. Later in learning, the participants were observed to free the DOF with increased variability and low correlations between joint angles. The research of Nourrit, Delignières, Caillou, Deschamps, and Lauriot (2003) also supported these three stages of learning, demonstrating the manner in which the motor system searches the state space (which

Table 10.1
Three General Stages of Learning

Stage	Characteristics
1. Coordination	The learner establishes the coordination pattern
	Freezing of the degrees of freedom
	Successful coordination pattern appears regularly during practice
	High movement and outcome variability
2. Control	Gaining control of coordinative structures
	Exploration to attune movements to environmental demands
	Adoption of an external attentional focus
	Freeing of the degrees of freedom
	Formation of strong information–movement coupling
3. Skill	Optimization of control
	Flexible coordination to exploit environmental information
	High (functional) movement variability

manifests as high variability), stabilizes around particular patterns of coordination as learning progresses (reduced variability), and then increases variability as the system searches for even more efficient and effective coordination patterns. An increase in variability occurs as practice of a particular task continues, and as the learner becomes more able to control, "unfreeze," or release the DOF (Van Emmerik et al., 2004). The concomitant increase in variability represents the learner searching and adjusting to the environment so as to discover more appropriate and/or successful coordination patterns in light of the changes occurring as a consequence of the release of DOF. As learning continues, reductions in the variability of coordination occur, perpetuating the search process.

Wilson et al. (2008) reported high levels of movement variability for both novice and expert triple-jumpers, with relatively low movement variability observed in the intermediate-level athletes. These authors suggested that the high variability in the novice athletes represented the assimilation of the coordination pattern, while that in the elite performers represented a flexible motor system that could adapt to perturbations. This view is commensurate with the stages of learning presented by Newell (1985).

According to Chow, Davids, Button, and Koh (2008), progression through the stages of learning may not be sequential; that is, learners may be able to shift between states. For example, an expert golfer trying a new grip may exhibit characteristics associated with a stage 1 or 2 learner.

Implications for Practice Design

The constraints-led approach to skill acquisition and the three stages of learning have significant implications for the design of effective practices to enhance learning. Practice is characterized as the search for the optimal movement solution given the specific task goal. Through experience and exposure to motor skills, it is seen as repeating the *solving* of the movement problem rather than simply repeating the *solution* to the problem (Newell, 1991). This is in sharp contrast to traditional approaches to practice, which promote the repetitions of drills to guide the athlete toward a movement pattern that reflects the "correct" technique. Furthermore, practice is a process of manipulating specific task constraints for each individual learner (Handford, Davids, Bennett, & Button, 1997). By modifying these constraints, the coach can induce instabilities that result in the emergence of functional movement task solutions. The task constraints that can be manipulated by the coach include the structure of the practices (e.g., blocked, serial, random regimes) and the provision of instructions and feedback (which influence the attentional focus of the athlete).

Practice Structure

There are a number of ways in which the motor skills executed in a practice can be performed:

- In a **blocked practice** structure, a single motor skill is executed.
- In a **serial practice** structure, a number of motor skills are executed successively.
- In a **random practice** structure, multiple motor skills are executed in a random order.

Table 10.2 shows the structure of practices using these three regimens for learning three resistance training exercises across three days. Notice that the total time spent practicing each exercise across the three days is the same under each regimen

Table 10.2

Structure of Practices Using Blocked, Serial, and Random Regimens for Learning Deadlift, Back Squat, and Bench Press Exercises

Practice Regimen	Practice Time	Day 1	Day 2	Day 3
Blocked	30 min	All deadlift	All back squat	All bench press
Serial	5 min	Deadlift	Deadlift	Deadlift
	5 min	Back squat	Back squat	Back squat
	5 min	Bench press	Bench press	Bench press
	5 min	Deadlift	Deadlift	Deadlift
	5 min	Back squat	Back squat	Back squat
	5 min	Bench press	Bench press	Bench press
Random	5 min	Bench press	Deadlift	Back squat
	5 min	Deadlift	Back squat	Deadlift
	5 min	Bench press	Back squat	Back squat
	5 min	Back squat	Bench press	Bench press
	5 min	Bench press	Deadlift	Bench press
	5 min	Deadlift	Deadlift	Back squat

(30 min). The difference between the regimens is the amount of variability experienced by the athlete due to the different practice structures: There is very limited variation experienced during blocked practice, whereas large variations are experienced during random practice. The amount of variation can influence the degree of learning achieved through practice.

Contextual interference (CI) refers to a performance disruption that results from performing multiple motor skills or variations of a motor skill within the context of practice (Magill, 2011). In the contextual interference effect, the learning benefit results from performing multiple motor skills in a high-CI practice structure (random practice) rather than from performing motor skills in a low-CI structure (blocked practice) (Magill, 2011). The benefits of random practice are believed to derive from learners having to frequently explore their perceptual-motor workspace and reorganize the DOF; this behavior produces instabilities that can aid the acquisition of appropriate movement solutions while providing learners with a more comprehensive realization of their movement capabilities (Davids et al., 2008; Newell & McDonald, 1991). Note that increased variability in the structure of a practice will produce poorer performance of the motor skills during practice but better performance on retention and transfer tests. Given this factor, it is inappropriate to assess learning at the end of a practice session (see Skill Acquisition Concept 10.1).

A number of variables influence the effectiveness of variability in practice. In general, less difficult tasks benefit more from high practice variability than more difficult tasks (Magill, 2011). This effect is likely due to the greater complexity of the more difficult tasks, which by itself produces sufficient variability during task execution. Early learners tend to benefit from reduced variability in practice, whereas advanced learners benefit more from increased variability in practice (Magill, 2011). The reduced variability in practice allows the early learner to assemble the coordination pattern, while the increased variability allows the advanced learner to explore the perceptual-motor workspace while searching for appropriate movement solutions as task constraints are manipulated and to attune their affordances. Thus it appears that the variability in practice should be systematically increased as the learner progresses (Porter & Magill, 2010).

Recently, **differential learning** has been proposed as an effective method for motor learning (Schöllhorn, Hegen, & Davids, 2012). Differential learning emphasizes the variability in an athlete's natural movements by deliberately precluding repetitions of the same movements during practice. For example, when learning to control and pass a soccer ball, the coach ensures that the athlete executes each trial from a different starting posture and requires different movements during the execution of the same skill. Such increased variability in coordination during the acquisition of skilled movements provides greater information to the learner about his or her capabilities by forcing the athlete to explore a larger region of the perceptual-motor workspace. Differential learning has been shown to be more effective than the traditional repetition-based approaches to motor learning in which learners are required to adopt an ideal starting position prior to movement execution and the "correct" technique is emphasized (Schöllhorn et al., 2012). See Applied Research 10.1.

Practices can also be structured around the decomposition of motor skills. For example, rather than executing the entire movement when learning a clean and jerk, decomposing the skill into component parts is often promoted (e.g., first pull, scoop, second pull, catch, and recovery), with some of the components

Applied Research 10.1
Differential learning promotes enhanced learning compared to traditional repetition- and correction-based approaches

Schöllhorn, Hegen, and Davids (2012) compared the effects of traditional repetition- and correction-based learning methods to differential learning methods in the soccer skills of shooting and ball control. Competitive soccer players from the lower leagues in Germany were randomly assigned to a traditional practice group, a differential blocked practice group, or a differential random practice group. The traditional practice group performed drills that emphasized the "correct" technique for each skill, with the emphasis placed on performance criteria including position of the standing leg, orientation of the head, amplitude of the kicking leg for the shooting skill, fixation on the approaching ball, and soft first ball contact for the ball control skill. The drills were completed in a blocked order within each practice, with the shooting drills being done first. The two differential learning groups completed drills that deliberately altered the starting posture and the motion of specific body parts during the execution of the drills such that a single movement was never repeated during a practice session. The differential blocked practice group performed the drills in a blocked order, beginning with the ball control drills, while the differential random practice group completed the drills in a random order. As the result of this design, the two differential groups experienced different degrees of variation during practice, with the greatest variation being associated with the differential random practice group.

The training intervention lasted four weeks, with two practice sessions completed each week, resulting in a total of 160 performances of the shooting and control exercises being completed by each participant. The authors reported greater improvements in both the shooting skills and the ball control skills resulting from the differential learning practices compared to the traditional learning group. Although there were no significant differences between the two differential learning groups in terms of improvements in their ball control skills, the differential random practice group demonstrated greater improvements in their shooting skills.

Schöllhorn, W. I., Hegen, P., & Davids, K. (2012). The nonlinear nature of learning: A differential learning approach. *Open Sports Sciences Journal, 5,* 100–112.

being practiced in isolation before the movement is executed in its entirety (Judge, Wang, Craig, & Bellar, 2012). This **part-task practice** structure is intended to avoid the attentional overload often associated with learning a complex motor skill (Magill, 2011). The principle of component interdependence can allow the coach to determine which motor skills to decompose during practice; specifically, motor skills that involve high task interdependence and low complexity may not require decomposition.

Although part-task practice leads to a greater degree of learning than no practice (Lee, Chamberlin, & Hodges, 2001), the decomposition of skills reduces or eliminates important perceptual information that would normally be available to the learner, removing the reciprocity between the movements and the environment (Davids et al., 2008). For example, information about the transition between the first pull and the scoop during the clean is eliminated when these elements of the clean and jerk are practiced in isolation.

Rather than decomposing skills into component parts, Davids et al. (2008) recommend simplifying the skill so that the perception–action couplings are preserved. The **simplification** process involves reducing key performance variables such as the velocities of objects and other performers, the distances between surfaces and objects, and the forces of objects and other performers, while maintaining the natural performance conditions. In the case of learning the clean, simply reducing the load on the barbell and having the athlete execute the entire movement with reduced velocity would reflect the principle of simplification. The load on the barbell can be gradually increased as the athlete becomes more skilled.

Another example of simplification (rather than decomposition) comes from the long jump. In the long jump event, the coupling of visual information to establish the location of the takeoff board with the physical task of placing the takeoff leg on the board is important in increasing the distance jumped. As such, athletes are often encouraged to perform "run-throughs," whereby they run and contact the board without physically jumping from the takeoff board to increase the precision of their run-up. The athlete may even practice the run-up without a board present. However, researchers have determined that the visual regulation of a run-through drill is different from that observed when a jump is executed following the run-up, limiting the utility of such drills (Bradshaw & Aisbett, 2006). Such drills remove the perception–action coupling required by the athlete; simplifying the task by having the athlete perform the run-up from a reduced distance but still complete the jump would represent an appropriate practice (Davids et al., 2008).

Attentional Focus

The attentional focus of an athlete refers to the location of the sources of information to which the athlete attends when executing a motor skill. With an **external attentional focus**, athletes focus on variables external to their body and in particular to the outcome of the movements that they are performing (Wulf, 2013). Conversely, with an **internal attentional focus**, athletes focus on variables associated with their body and the movement itself (Wulf, 2013).

The adoption of an external attentional focus has been shown to improve performance in a variety of motor tasks (Marchant, Greig, Bullogh, & Hitchen, 2011; Schücker, Hagemann, Strauss, & Völker, 2009). In particular, adopting an external attentional focus is more effective during learning than adopting an internal focus where attention is focused on the movement itself (Wulf, 2013). An external attentional focus likely rules out the constraint imposed on the movement by an internal attentional focus; an internal focus might potentially interfere with the natural self-organizing properties associated with the motor system that hinder the acquisition of a functional movement task solution (Southard, 2011). An external attentional focus leads to implicit learning, which has been shown to be more robust and resist deterioration under conditions characterized by high pressure compared to explicit learning (Masters & Poolton, 2012).

Others have suggested that during the early stages of learning, when the athlete is attempting to develop a basic coordination pattern, an internal attentional focus may be effective (Peh, Chow, & Davids, 2011). Indeed, both internal and external foci appear to be equally effective at improving both the outcome and the coordination pattern when novices learn a multijoint motor skill (Uehara, Button, & Davids, 2008). The attentional focus adopted by an athlete during the acquisition of motor skills is influenced by the instructions and feedback presented to the athlete by a coach.

Instructions

Instructions are provided to the learner before the execution of a movement and, therefore, are considered prescriptive. Instructions include verbal information provided by the coach as well as a demonstration provided by a model that is live or shown on video. Instructions provide task-relevant information to learners that can alter their intention and channel their search for an appropriate movement solution (Newell & Ranganathan, 2010). Therefore, instructions represent a form of informational constraint.

Verbal Instructions

A multitude of evidence confirms that the verbal instructions presented to the athlete prior to the execution of a movement task influence the subsequent performance. For example, greater jump heights are achieved when athletes are instructed to "jump for maximum height" as opposed to "extend the legs as fast as possible" (Talpey et al., 2014), while the instruction to "land softly" alters the coordination pattern and force experienced during landing tasks (Milner et al., 2012; Walsh, Waters, et al., 2007). Furthermore, instructions can influence the movements observed during team sports such as soccer. For example, the presentation of instructions to the attacker that his or her team was losing and that the game would soon end, necessitating a goal to be scored quickly, resulted in greater speeds being achieved by the players in a one-versus-one subphase of a game compared to when the attacker was instructed to attack whenever a scoring opportunity was presented (Clemente, Couceiro, Martins, Dias, & Mendes, 2013).

The verbal instructions presented to an athlete can promote either an external or an internal attentional focus, influencing the acquisition of motor skills. In general, verbal instructions that promote an external attentional focus have been shown to be more effective in promoting learning (as determined by retention and transfer tests) (Wulf, 2013). These instructions contain terms relating to the outcome of the movement rather than referencing specific body parts. Other researchers have supported the use of analogies in the verbal instructions presented to athletes (Lam, Maxwell, & Masters, 2009). Effective analogies allow athletes to make inferences about the appropriate movements without requiring them to consider the specifics of the coordination pattern by using biomechanical metaphors (Masters & Poolton, 2012). Such analogies reduce the prescriptive nature of the instructions and allow the natural self-organizing tendencies of the motor system to emerge. Examples of instructions to promote an external attentional focus and the use of analogies are shown in Table 10.3.

Observation of a Model

Prior to the execution of a movement, the coach may demonstrate the movement or have another athlete demonstrate the movement for the learner. Alternatively, the learner may view a video of a model performing the movement. These modes of observing a model perform the movement represent a form of visual instruction.

Table 10.3

Examples of Instructions Promoting an External Attentional Focus and Using Analogies

Scenario	Instruction	Explanation
Learning a golf shot	"Focus on the path of the club head as you swing."	External attentional focus
Learning the bench press	"At the bottom of the movement, push the barbell upward and back toward the spotter."	External attentional focus
Learning swimming strokes	"Pull through the water."	External attentional focus
Learning a soccer chip	"Stay behind the ball and kick underneath it."	External attentional focus
Learning a golf shot	"Swing the club like a long pendulum."	External attentional focus using an analogy
Learning a tennis shot	"Move the racket up the slope when you hit the ball."	External attentional focus using an analogy
Learning the volleyball spike	"Hit the ball like you're cracking a whip."	External attentional focus using an analogy

The observation of a model will provide relative motion information to the learner that would not necessarily be present in verbal forms of instructions. This is important in the early stages of learning when the learner is assembling his or her coordination pattern and has been shown to result in a more rapid acquisition of an appropriate coordination pattern (Sakadjian, Panchuk, & Pearce, 2014). (See Applied Research 10.2.) An important consideration when using observational

Applied Research 10.2
Observing a skilled video model facilitates learning of a power clean

Sakadjian, Panchuk, and Pearce (2014) compared the effects of traditional coaching methods with the addition of observational learning on the technique and performance of a power clean exercise. Australian football players with no previous experience of performing the power clean exercise were organized into either a traditional group, who received verbal cues from a coach combined with physical practice, or an observation group, who received the same practices as the traditional group but were able to observe a video of a skilled model performing the movement before they completed each practice set. The practices were completed during a four-week general preparation phase of an annual periodized training program, with 12 sessions completed by both groups.

Alterations in the power clean technique were assessed by recording two-dimensional kinematic data in the sagittal plane (joint and segment angles); power clean performance was assessed by recording the mean peak power output recorded from a linear position transducer. These measures were assessed at the end of weeks 2, 3, and 4. The authors reported that both groups demonstrated significant performance and technical improvements across the four weeks of the intervention, but the observation group produced faster technical improvements than the traditional group.

Sakadjian, A., Panchuk, D., & Pearce, A. J. (2014). Kinematic and kinetic improvements associated with action observation facilitated learning of the power clean in Australian footballers. *Journal of Strength and Conditioning Research, 28*, 1613–1625.

methods of instruction is the characteristics of the model relative to those of the learner. Because the learner may attempt to assimilate and adopt/replicate the movements of the model, the organismic constraints may need to be matched between learner and model. For example, it may not be appropriate to present an adult model to an adolescent athlete. Observing other novices may help novice learners, however, as they are able to identify errors in the execution of the movements (Hodges & Franks, 2002).

Feedback

Feedback is information provided to the learner after the performance of a motor skill in relation to the task goal. Each execution of a movement represents a performance of the motor skill. The outcome of the movement relative to the goal of the motor skill, known as **knowledge of results**, provides feedback to the performer. This type of feedback can take the form of mechanical information relating to the movement (e.g., power output, acceleration) using various devices (see Applied Research 10.3). It may be employed to modify the intentions of the performer prior to the next performance, thereby promoting the search for an appropriate movement solution.

Other types of feedback can also be provided to performers that they would not normally receive simply by completing the motor skill. For example, the coach can provide verbal feedback about the movement or performers can watch a video of their movements following the completion of the motor skill, both of which provide **knowledge of performance**.

Feedback provides a temporary constraint, directing the search for movement solutions (Davids et al., 2008). It also has a motivational effect. While this is important, the learner should not become reliant on the feedback. Thus methods of systematically removing the provision of feedback by the coach should be employed. In **faded feedback** regimens, for example, the feedback provided to athletes is systematically withdrawn as they progress through a period of practice (Crowell & Davis, 2011; Davis, 2005; Willy, Scholtz, & Davis, 2012).

Applied Research 10.3
Using feedback to enhance power output during resistance training

Staub et al. (2013) compared the effects of presenting feedback in the form of peak power output following countermovement vertical jumps with the effects of withholding that same information from a group of Division I track and field and crew athletes. In a study using a crossover design, the athletes performed two plyometric workouts where they completed three sets of five countermovement vertical jumps for maximal height. In one session, the athletes received the peak power output information following each jump; this information was derived from force plate data. In the other session, this information was withheld from the athletes. The authors reported that the mean power output and the peak power outputs were greater in the session where the kinetic information was presented as feedback to the athletes.

Staub, J. N., Kraemer, W. J., Pandit, A. L., Haug, W. B., Comstock, B. A., Dunn-Lewis, C., ... Häkkinen, K. (2013). Positive effects of augmented verbal feedback on power production in NCAA Division I collegiate athletes. *Journal of Strength and Conditioning Research, 27*, 2067–2072.

When providing verbal feedback, the coach should consider the content of the feedback and assess whether it is meaningful to the athlete. Given that verbal feedback can influence the intention of the learner and his or her attentional focus, feedback related to the task-goal, rather than movement of limbs, has been recommended, as such information will promote an external attentional focus (Hodges & Franks, 2002). In contrast, the use of verbal feedback directing the athlete's attention to his or her body parts (internal attentional focus) may be effective when the performer is attempting to establish a coordination pattern to satisfy the goal of the motor task (Peh et al., 2011).

The advent of affordable video technologies allows the coach to use video footage as a form of feedback. This footage can be shown concurrently with the execution of the movement (Eriksson, Halvorsen, & Gullstrand, 2011), or it can be shown following the completion of the movements (Janelle, Barba, Frehlich, Tennant, & Cauraugh, 1997). The effectiveness of video feedback as a means of enhancing performance depends on the skill level of the learner. For example, novices have been shown to benefit more from verbal feedback as opposed to video feedback, while advanced learners benefit more from a combination of the two (Bertram, Marteniuk, & Guadagnoli, 2007). The coach also needs to guard against comparing the video footage of the athlete to "correct models." The constraints-led approach precludes the notion of a single "correct" coordination pattern in any motor skill; thus video feedback should be used to enhance the learner's awareness of the biomechanical principles that underpin the motor skill.

The timing of the presentation of feedback is an important consideration. Feedback that is presented after every trial is likely to be detrimental to learning, as the learner will not engage in the problem-solving process and is likely to ignore other important sources of information that can be used to select an appropriate movement solution to satisfy the goal of the task. The learner is also likely to become dependent upon the provision of feedback. Providing feedback after successful performances, however, may enhance the motivation of the learner. When the coach is seeking to determine the frequency of feedback, he or she should consider that a reduced frequency (after 33% versus 100% of repetitions) has been shown to be more effective in certain tasks (Wulf, McConnel, Gärtner, & Schwarz, 2002). Researchers have reported that providing feedback when the learner requests it is actually the most effective schedule for both verbal and video-based feedback (Aiken, Fairbrother, & Post, 2012; Janelle et al., 1997), but coaches should appreciate that novice or young learners may be intimidated and not ask for feedback.

Finally, the **challenge-point framework** is an important concept when considering the design of practices for athletes. This framework holds that learning is optimized when the learner is appropriately challenged (Guadagnoli & Lee, 2004). Too much difficulty in the practice tasks or too little difficulty can hinder the learning process. The optimal challenge point depends on the skill level of the learner and the difficulty of the task, implying that the optimal challenge point will change as the athlete becomes more skilled. Furthermore, manipulation of the practice structure, instructions, and feedback can be used to alter the challenge faced by the learner.

We now present two scenarios relevant for the strength and conditioning practitioner that bring together all of the concepts used to promote motor learning in athletes. The first scenario involves learning the Olympic lifts (see Skill Acquisition Concept 10.5), while the second scenario involves gait retraining in distance runners to reduce the risk of musculoskeletal injury (see Skill Acquisition Concept 10.6).

Skill Acquisition Concept 10.5

Learning the Olympic lifts

- **Assess intrinsic dynamics:** Have the athlete perform the lift without instructions and assess the intrinsic coordination dynamics.

- **Develop cooperative coordination dynamics:** Develop competency with the deadlift, front squat, and push jerk exercises before beginning to learn the Olympic lifts.

- **Practice structure:** Blocked practice for novice athletes; increase the variability of the practice for a more advanced athlete.

- **Instructions:** Internal attentional focus if the athlete is unable to demonstrate the basic coordination pattern (position and orientation of specific body parts); external focus if the athlete exhibits the basic coordination pattern (motion of the barbell). Emphasize control parameter (barbell velocity). Present video of a skilled model performing the lift.

- **Simplification of the task:** Lighter loads allow the execution of the full lift to ensure the appropriate movement information.

- **Alter task constraints:** Introduce instabilities in the coordination pattern during the skill to promote a search for a more appropriate movement solution. Increase the load of the barbell; load the barbell asymmetrically; attach chains or elastic bands to the barbell.

- **Feedback:** Barbell velocity through linear position transducer; video feedback; verbal feedback. Ensure a performer-scheduled feedback regimen.

Skill Acquisition Concept 10.6

Gait retraining to reduce the risk of musculoskeletal injuries in distance runners

Gait retraining strategies aim to change the movements of distance runners so as to either improve performance or reduce the risk of injuries. The focus here is on using gait retraining strategies to reduce the risk of tibial stress fractures and patellofemoral pain, as these are the topics addressed by most of the extant research (Davis, 2005; Heiderscheit, 2011). The long distances covered during training undertaken by distance runners results in a large number of loading cycles for these athletes. For example, assuming an average running speed of 3.80 m/s and an average step length of 1.30 m, an athlete would experience 385 steps per foot per kilometer during a marathon (Cavanagh & Williams, 1982). This equates to approximately 16,170 loading cycles per leg during the event. Evidence indicates that the training distance covered each week is a risk factor for incurring lower-extremity musculoskeletal injuries (van Gent et al., 2007).

(continues)

(continued)

Tibial Stress Fracture

A stress fracture in bone is a focal structural weakness resulting from repeated application of sub-fracture threshold stresses (Beck, 1998). Tibial stress fractures are often incurred by distance runners (Taunton et al., 2002), with the middle and distal thirds of the medial border of the bone being the most common sites of injury (Beck, 1998). Researchers have implicated large vertical loading rates, large passive peaks, and large tibial accelerations in the etiology of tibial stress fractures (Milner, Ferber, Pollard, Hamill, & Davis, 2006).

Footwear has been shown to affect the magnitude of the loading rate associated with the initial passive peak of the vertical ground reaction force (GRF), with greater loading rates being observed when men run at a given speed in racing flats and spikes compared to running shoes (Logan, Hunter, Hopkins, Feland, & Parcell, 2010). Furthermore, the strike pattern at touchdown has been shown to influence the initial vertical loading rate. For example, Hennig et al. (1993) demonstrated that a rearfoot strike pattern during stance is associated with a greater vertical loading rate and greater tibial acceleration as compared to a forefoot striking pattern.

Lieberman et al. (2010) observed that the initial passive peak was absent from the GRF of habitually barefoot distance runners. These runners present a forefoot or midfoot strike pattern as opposed to a rearfoot strike pattern. This finding has led to recent interest in the use of minimalist shoes or barefoot running. In a recent systematic review of the literature, Hall, Barton, Jones, and Morrissey (2013) concluded that some evidence supports an association of barefoot running with biomechanical changes that may reduce overuse injuries associated with running such as stress fractures. However, Willy and Davis (2014) have reported that running in minimalist shoes when unaccustomed to them can increase the loading of the leg during stance, possibly predisposing the athlete to a stress fracture. Therefore, if the athlete plans to change to minimalist footwear, he or she should instigate this change over a long period of time to allow for sufficient adaptation.

Athletes' stride length has a significant influence on the dynamics of the vertical ground reaction force, with longer strides being associated with a greater passive peak and tibial accelerations (Clarke, Cooper, Clark, & Hamill, 1985; Derrick, Cladwell, & Hamill, 2000). Indeed, reducing stride length has been suggested as a method to reduce the risk of incurring a stress fracture despite the concomitant increase in the number of loading cycles that would accompany this strategy (Edwards, Taylor, Rudolphi, Gillette, & Derrick, 2009). Runners who have previously incurred a tibial stress fracture have been shown to exhibit greater peak hip adduction and rearfoot eversion angles during stance (Milner, Hamill, & Davis, 2010), highlighting these kinematic variables as potential risk factors for tibial stress fractures.

Researchers have begun to explore the effects of gait retraining strategies using specific forms of feedback presented to the athlete in combination with practice to modify the runner's running movement and thereby reduce the loading experienced during the stance phases (Crowell & Davis, 2011; Davis, 2005).

Practices to Reduce the Risk of Tibial Stress Fracture (Crowell & Davis, 2011; Davis, 2005)

- The runners (men and women with tibial acceleration greater than 8 g) attended eight sessions over a two-week period.

- The runners were instructed to "run softer" and to make their footfalls quieter during each session.

- Participants ran at a self-selected pace for 15 min during week 1, with the duration increased to 30 min by week 8.

- The runners were provided with online visual feedback (concurrent feedback) from an accelerometer placed on the distal tibia. They were instructed to reduce the peak acceleration and keep it at less than 50% of the peak during their first session.

- Feedback was provided continuously for the first four sessions, but was progressively reduced such that during the last four sessions, one-third of the feedback was provided at the beginning of the session, one-third in the middle of the session, and one-third at the end of the session (faded feedback). By the final session, the runners were provided with 1 min of feedback at the beginning, middle, and end of the session.

- The runners decreased the peak loading rate and the magnitude of the passive peak in the vertical GRF by 30% and 20%, respectively, as a result of the intervention. These mechanical improvements were maintained at a one-month follow-up.

Patellofemoral Pain

The knee is the most common lower-extremity site of injuries in distance runners (van Gent et al., 2007), and patellofemoral pain (PFP) is the most prevalent complaint reported by runners (Taunton et al., 2002). PFP is characterized by diffuse pain over the anterior knee that is aggravated by any activities that increase the compressive forces at the patellofemoral joint, including running (Witvrouw et al., 2014). The pain associated with this complaint interferes with the activities of these athletes, limiting their ability to train for their sport. There is evidence that females may be more likely to develop PFP than males (Boling et al., 2010).

Structural factors have been implicated in PFP. For example, factors including a high Q-angle, a high congruence angle, and osseous sclerosis of the lateral facet may cause malalignment of the patella that results in pain in the knee, although these factors are not always present in patients with PFP (Dye, 2001). More recently, biomechanical factors associated with PFP have been investigated— these factors have particular relevance for distance runners. The biomechanical factors implicated in PFP include trunk and hip mechanics (e.g., excessive hip adduction and internal rotation during stance, contralateral pelvic drop during stance) and knee and foot mechanics (e.g., increased tibial internal rotation during stance, greater rearfoot eversion) (Witvrouw et al., 2014). Increasing stride frequency has been shown to decrease the patellofemoral joint forces during

(continues)

(continued)

distance running performance, potentially reducing the risk for PFP (Lenhart, Thelen, Wille, Chumanov, & Heiderscheit, 2014). Although the exact mechanisms underlying PFP remain to be determined, it is likely that structural and biomechanical factors interact to elicit PFP (Witvrouw et al., 2014).

Modifications of the structural factors associated with PFP are beyond the capabilities of the strength and conditioning practitioner, but the modification of the biomechanical factors is not. Gait retraining strategies have been proposed as a means of modifying the biomechanical factors implicated in PFP during distance running by using specific forms of feedback presented to the athlete (Davis, 2005; Willy et al., 2012).

Practices to Reduce the Risk of Patellofemoral Pain (Davis, 2005; Willy et al., 2012)

- Ten female runners with PFP attended eight sessions across a two-week period.
- The runners ran at a self-selected pace for between 15 min (session 1) and 30 min (session 8).
- Runners received instructions ("run with your knees apart, with your kneecaps pointing straight ahead," "squeeze your buttocks") and visual feedback of their running technique via a mirror placed in front of them as they ran on a treadmill.
- The visual feedback was provided continuously during the trials over the first four weeks and was progressively reduced during the final four sessions (faded feedback).
- The intervention resulted in reduced peak hip adduction angles, reduced contralateral pelvic drop, and hip abduction moments during stance when running. The runners also reported improvements in pain. These improvements were maintained at a three-month follow-up.

It is important to consider whether the improvements in running mechanics observed from these interventions occur simply because the athlete is asked to adopt the modified running mechanics in the laboratory in front of the experimenters or whether the athlete continues to produce the modified running mechanics in his or her unobserved training runs (Heiderscheit, 2011). This issue could be tested by administering transfer tests in addition to the retention tests that are performed in the gait retraining studies.

Chapter Summary

Skill acquisition is the ongoing process of attaining functional movement task solutions to satisfy the goal of motor skills. Learning is a relatively permanent improvement in performance and is assessed through the use of retention and transfer tests. The human motor system can be viewed as a complex system, encompassing many degrees of freedom that need to be coordinated and controlled to successfully execute the movements required to accomplish the goal of a motor skill. The information processing approach to the coordination and control of movements emphasizes cognitive processes, particularly memory processes, and involves models that are analogous to a computer (i.e., the storage and execution of "programs" for specific movement tasks based upon sensory information).

The constraints-led approach proposes that the coordination and control of movements emerge from the confluence of constraints associated with the organism, the environment, and the task; these factors collectively guide the movements of the performer as he or she executes a motor skill. This approach precludes "organismic asymmetry" in skill acquisition processes and avoids the prescriptive approach to the acquisition of motor skills, instead emphasizing the principle of guided discovery and the emergence of functional movement task solutions. The constraints-led approach also promotes an interdisciplinary approach to movement coordination, requiring the coach to understand biomechanical characteristics of the motor system and the task to support the athlete's acquisition of motor skills. Learning is regarded as a discontinuous process, characterized by nonlinear changes in motor behavior in response to the interacting constraints on the system and the continual search of the perceptual-motor workspace. It is characterized by three general stages as the learner progresses from novice to skilled performer. Practice is a process of manipulating specific task constraints for each individual learner so as to induce instabilities that result in the emergence of functional movement task solutions. The task constraints that can be manipulated by the coach include the structure of the practices and the provision of instructions and feedback, both of which influence the attentional focus of the athlete.

Review Questions and Projects

1. What is a motor skill?

2. Provide a basic classification of motor skills.

3. When describing the human motor system, what are degrees of freedom?

4. What is degeneracy of the motor system, and why might it be important in the performance of motor skills?

5. What is a retention test?

6. What is a transfer test?

7. Why is the use of retention and transfer tests important when assessing motor learning?

8. Explain some of the criticisms leveled at the information processing approach to the coordination and control of movements.

9. From the perspective of dynamical systems theory, explain how the enormous number of degrees of freedom associated with the human motor system are controlled.

10. What is an attractor state in the perceptual-motor workspace?

11. Explain the relations between control and order parameters.

12. What are affordances, and why are they important in coordination?

13. What is knowledge of results, and how does it represent an informational constraint on the performer?

14. What is the contextual interference effect, and why is it useful for motor learning?

15. What are some problems associated with part-task practice that may reduce its effectiveness?

16. How do verbal instructions provided by the coach influence movement coordination?

17. Which characteristics of the model are important to consider when using observational learning?

18. Define augmented feedback, and provide examples of this form of feedback.

19. Which schedule appears to be appropriate for the provision of augmented feedback?

20. What is the challenge-point hypothesis, and what does it tell the strength and conditioning practitioner about the manipulation of task constraints during practice?

References

Adams, J. A. (1971). A closed-loop theory of motor learning. *Journal of Motor Behavior, 3*, 111–150.

Aiken, C. A., Fairbrother, J. T., & Post, P. G. (2012). The effects of self-controlled video feedback on the learning of the basketball set shot. *Frontiers in Psychology, 3*, Article 338, 1–8.

Alcaraz, P. E., Palao, J. M., Elvira, J. L. L., & Linthorne, N. P. (2011). Effects of a sand running surface on the kinematics of sprinting at maximum velocity. *Biology of Sport, 28*, 95–100.

Baker, J., & Young, B. (2014). 20 years later: Deliberate practice and the development of expertise in sport. *International Review of Sport and Exercise Psychology, 7*, 135–157.

Balague, N., Torrents, C., Hristovski, R., Davids, K., & Araújo, D. (2013). Overview of complex systems in sport. *Journal of Systems Science and Complexity, 26*, 4–13.

Bartlett, R., Wheat, J., & Robins, M. (2007). Is movement variability important for sports performance? *Sports Biomechanics, 6*, 234–245.

Beck, B. R. (1998). Tibial stress injuries: An aetiological review for the purposes of guiding management. *Sports Medicine, 26*, 265–279.

Beek, P. J., Schmidt, R. C., Morris, A. W., Sim, M. Y., & Turvey, M. T. (1995). Linear and nonlinear stiffness and friction in biological rhythmic movements. *Biological Cybernetics, 73*, 449–507.

Berchuck, M., Andriacchi, T. P., Bach, B. R., & Reider, B. (1990). Gait adaptations by patients who have a deficient anterior cruciate ligament. *Journal of Bone and Joint Surgery, 72*, 871–877.

Bernstein, N. A. (1967). *The control and regulation of movements*. London, UK: Pergamon Press.

Bertram, C. P., Marteniuk, R. G., & Guadagnoli, M. A. (2007). On the use and misuse of video analysis. *International Journal of Sports Science and Coaching, 2*, 37–46.

Boling, M., Padua, D., Marshall, S., Guskiewicz, K., Pyne, S., & Beutler, A. (2010). Gender differences in the incidence and prevalence of patellofemoral pain syndrome. *Scandinavian Journal of Medicine and Science in Sports, 20*, 725–730.

Bradshaw, E. J., & Aisbett, B. (2006). Visual guidance during competition performance and run-through training in long jumping. *Sports Biomechanics, 6*, 1–14.

Buss, D. D., Min, R., Skyhar, M., Galinat, B., Warren, R., & Wickiewicz, T. L. (1995). Nonoperative treatment of acute anterior cruciate ligament injuries in a selected group of patients. *American Journal of Sports Medicine, 23*, 160–165.

Cavanagh, P. R., & Williams, K. R. (1982). The effect of stride length variation on oxygen uptake during distance running. *Medicine and Science in Sports and Exercise, 14*, 30–35.

Chow, J. Y., Davids, K., Button, C., & Koh, M. (2008). Coordination changes in a discrete multi-articular action as a function of practice. *Acta Psychologica, 127*, 163–176.

Clarke, T. E., Cooper, L., Clark, D. E., & Hamill, C. L. (1985). The effects of increased running speed upon peak shank deceleration during ground contact. In D. A. Winter, R. W. Norman, R. P. Wells, K. C. Hayes, & A. E. Patla (Eds.), *Biomechanics IX-B* (pp. 101–105). Champaign, IL: Human Kinetics.

Clemente, F. M., Couceiro, M. S., Martins, F. M. L., Dias, G., & Mendes, R. (2013). Interpersonal dynamics: 1v1 sub-phases at sub-18 football players. *Journal of Human Kinetics, 36*, 181–191.

Crowell, H. P., & Davis, I. S. (2011). Gait retraining to reduce lower extremity loading in runners. *Clinical Biomechanics, 26*, 78–83.

Daniel, D. M., Stone, M. L., Dobson, B. E., Fithian, D. C., Rossman, D. J., & Kaufman, K. R. (1994). Fate of the ACL injured patient: A prospective outcome study. *American Journal of Sports Medicine, 22*, 632–644.

Davids, K., & Araújo, D. (2010). The concept of "organismic asymmetry" in sport science. *Journal of Science and Medicine in Sport, 13*, 633–640.

Davids, K., Bennett, S. J., & Newell, K. (2006). *Movement system variability*. Champaign, IL: Human Kinetics.

Davids, K., Button, C., & Bennett, S. (2008). *Dynamics of skills acquisition: A constraints-led approach*. Champaign, IL: Human Kinetics.

Davids, K., Glazier, P., Araújo, D., & Bartlett, R. (2003). Movement systems as dynamical systems. *Sports Medicine, 33*, 245–260.

Davis, I. S. (2005). Gait retraining in runners. *Orthopaedic and Physical Therapy Practice, 17*, 8–13.

Delignières, D., Nourrit, D., Sioud, R., Leroyer, P., Zattara, M., & Micaleff, J. P. (1998). Preferred coordination modes in the first steps of the learning of a complex gymnastics skill. *Human Movement Science, 17*, 221–241.

Derrick, T. R., Cladwell, G. E., & Hamill, J. (2000). Modeling the stiffness characteristics of the human body while running with various stride lengths. *Journal of Applied Biomechanics, 16*, 36–51.

Diedrich, F. J., & Warren, W. H. (1995). Why change gaits? Dynamics of the walk to run transition. *Journal of Experimental Psychology, 21*, 183–201.

Duarte, R., Araújo, D., Gazimba, V., Fernandes, O., Folgado, H., Marmeleira, J., & Davids, K. (2010). The ecological dynamics of 1 vs 1 sub-phases in Association Football. *Open Sports Sciences Journal, 3*, 16–18.

Dye, S. F. (2001). Patellofemoral pain current concepts: An overview. *Sports Medicine and Arthroscopy Review, 9*, 264–272.

Edelman, G. M., & Gally, J. A. (2001). Degeneracy and complexity in biological systems. *Proceedings of the National Academy of Sciences, 98*, 13763–13768.

Edwards, W. B., Taylor, D., Rudolphi, T. J., Gillette, J. C., & Derrick, T. R. (2009). Effects of stride length and running mileage on a probabilistic stress fracture model. *Medicine and Science in Sports and Exercise, 41*, 2177–2184.

El Helou, N., Tafflet, M., Berthelot, G., Tolaini, J., Marc, A., Guillaume, M., . . . Toussaint, J.-F. (2012). Impact of environmental parameters on marathon running performance. *PLoS One, 7*, e37407.

Ericsson, K. A. (2007). Deliberate practice and the modifiability of body and mind: Toward a science of the structure and acquisition of expert and elite performance. *International Journal of Sport Psychology, 38*, 4–34.

Eriksson, M., Halvorsen, K. A., & Gullstrand, L. (2011). Immediate effect of visual and auditory feedback to control the running mechanics of well-trained athletes. *Journal of Sports Sciences, 29*, 253–262.

Esteves, P. T., de Oliveira, R. F., & Araújo, D. (2011). Posture-related affordances guide attacks in basketball. *Psychology of Sport and Exercise, 12*, 639–644.

Fajen, B., Riley, M. A., & Turvey, M. T. (2008). Information, affordances, and the control of action in sport. *International Journal of Sport Psychology, 40*, 79–107.

Ford, K. R., Myer, G. D., Smith, R. L., Byrnes, R. N., Dopirak, S. E., & Hewett, T. E. (2005). Use of an overhead goal alters vertical jump performance and biomechanics. *Journal of Strength and Conditioning Research, 19*, 394–399.

Girard, O., Miscallef, J.-P., & Millet, G. P. (2011). Changes in spring-mass model characteristics during repeated running sprints. *European Journal of Applied Physiology, 111,* 125–134.

Glazier, P. S., Davids, K., & Bartlett, R. M. (2003). Dynamical systems theory: A relevant framework for performance-oriented sports biomechanics research. *Sportscience, 7.* http://www.sportsci.org/

Goodwin, J. (2011). Maximum velocity is when we can no longer accelerate: Using biomechanics to inform speed development. *UK Strength and Conditioning Association, 21,* 3–9.

Guadagnoli, M. A., & Lee, T. D. (2004). Challenge point: A framework for conceptualizing the effects of various practice conditions in motor learning. *Journal of Motor Behavior, 36,* 212–224.

Guthrie, E. R. (1952). *The psychology of learning.* New York: Harper & Row.

Hall, J. P., Barton, C., Jones, P. R., & Morrissey, D. (2013). The biomechanical differences between barefoot and shod distance running: A systematic review and preliminary meta-analysis. *Sports Medicine, 43,* 1335–1353.

Hamill, J., Haddad, J. M., Heiderscheit, B. C., van Emmerik, R. E. A., & Li, L. (2006). Clinical relevance of variability in coordination. In K. Davids, S. Bennett, & K. Newell (Eds.), *Movement system variability* (pp. 133–152). Champaign, IL: Human Kinetics.

Hamill, J., van Emmerick, R. E. A., Heiderscheit, B. C., & Li, L. (1999). A dynamical systems approach to lower extremity running injuries. *Clinical Biomechanics, 14,* 297–308.

Handford, C., Davids, K., Bennett, S., & Button, C. (1997). Skill acquisition in sport: Some applications of an evolving practice ecology. *Journal of Sports Sciences, 15,* 621–640.

Heiderscheit, B. (2011). Gait retraining for runners: In search of the ideal. *Journal of Orthopaedic and Sports Physical Therapy, 41,* 909–910.

Hennig, E., Milani, T., & Lafortune, M. (1993). Use of ground reaction force parameters in predicting peak tibial accelerations in running. *Journal of Applied Biomechanics, 9,* 306–314.

Hodges, N. J., & Franks, I. M. (2002). Modelling coaching practice: The role of instruction and demonstration. *Journal of Sports Science, 20,* 739–811.

Jacobs, D. M., & Michaels, C. F. (2007). Direct learning. *Ecological Psychology, 19,* 321–349.

Jacobs, R., & van Ingen Schenau, G. J. (1992). Intermuscular coordination in a sprint push-off. *Journal of Biomechanics, 25,* 953–965.

Janelle, C. M., Barba, D. A., Frehlich, S. G., Tennant, L. K., & Cauraugh, J. H. (1997). Maximizing performance effectiveness through videotape replay and a self controlled learning environment. *Research Quarterly for Exercise and Sport, 68,* 269–279.

Judge, L. W., Wang, L., Craig, B., & Bellar, D. (2012). Teaching rhythm: A key to learning proper technique in the power clean. *Strength and Conditioning Journal, 34,* 22–26.

Keele, S. W. (1968). Movement control in skilled motor performance. *Psychological Bulletin, 70,* 387–403.

Kelso, J. A. S. (1984). Phase transitions and critical behavior in human bimanual coordination. *American Journal of Physiology, 15,* R1000–R1004.

Kelso, J. A. S. (1995). *Dynamic patterns: The self-organization of brain and behavior.* Cambridge, MA: MIT Press.

Kelso, J. A. S., Scholz, J. P., & Schöner, G. (1986). Nonequilibrium phase transitions in coordinated biological motion: Critical fluctuations. *Physics Letters A, 118,* 279–284.

Kilding, A. E., Scott, M. A., & Mullineaux, D. R. (2007). A kinematic comparison of deep water running and overground running in endurance runners. *Journal of Strength and Conditioning Research, 21,* 476–480.

Kram, R., Domingo, A., & Ferris, D. P. (1997). Effect of reduced gravity on the preferred walk–run transition speed. *Journal of Experimental Biology, 200,* 821–826.

Kugler, P. N., & Turvey, M. T. (1987). *Information, natural law, and the self-assembly of rhythmic movement: Theoretical and experimental investigations.* Hillsdale, NJ: Erlbaum.

Kurz, M. J., Stergiou, N., Buzzi, U. H., & Georgoulis, A. D. (2005). The effect of anterior cruciate ligament reconstruction on lower extremity relative phase dynamics during walking and running. *Knee Surgery and Sports Traumatology and Arthroscopy, 13,* 107–115.

Lam, W. K., Maxwell, J. P., & Masters, R. (2009). Analogy learning and the performance of motor skills under pressure. *Journal of Sport and Exercise Psychology, 31,* 337–357.

Lee, T. D., Chamberlin, C. J., & Hodges, N. J. (2001). Practice. In B. Singer, H. Hausenblas, & C. Jannelle (Eds.), *Handbook of sport psychology* (pp. 115–143). New York, NY: Wiley.

Lenhart, R. L., Thelen, D. G., Wille, C. M., Chumanov, E. S., & Heiderscheit, B. C. (2014). Increasing running step rate reduces patellofemoral joint forces. *Medicine and Science in Sports and Exercise, 46,* 557–564.

Lewek, M., Rudolph, K., Axe, M., & Snyder-Mackler, L. (2002). The effect of insufficient quadriceps strength on gait after anterior cruciate ligament reconstruction. *Clinical Biomechanics, 17,* 56–63.

Lieberman, D. E., Venkadesan, M., Werbel, W. A., Daoud, A. I., D'Andrea, S., Davis, I. S., . . . Pitsiladis, Y. (2010). Foot strike patterns and collision forces in habitually barefoot versus shod runners. *Nature, 463,* 531–535.

Logan, S., Hunter, I., Hopkins, J. T., Feland, J. B., & Parcell, A. C. (2010). Ground reaction force differences between running shoes, racing flats, and distance spikes in runners. *Journal of Sports Science and Medicine, 9,* 147–153.

Luff, A. R. (1998). Age-associated changes in the innervation of muscle fibers and changes in the mechanical properties of motor units. *Annals of the New York Academy of Sciences, 854,* 92–101.

Magill, R. A. (1998). Knowledge is more than we can talk about: Implicit learning in motor skill acquisition. *Research Quarterly for Exercise and Sport, 69,* 104–110.

Magill, R. A. (2011). *Motor learning and control: Concepts and applications.* New York, NY: McGraw-Hill.

Maharam, L. G., Bauman, P. A., Kalman, D., Skolnik, H., & Perle, S. M. (1999). Masters athletes: Factors affecting performance. *Sports Medicine, 28,* 273–285.

Marchant, D. C., Greig, M., Bullogh, J., & Hitchen, D. (2011). Instructions to adopt an external focus enhance muscular endurance. *Research Quarterly for Exercise and Sport, 82,* 466–473.

Masters, R. S., & Poolton, J. M. (2012). Advances in implicit motor learning. In N. J. Hodges & A. M. Williams (Eds.), *Skill acquisition in sport: Research, theory and practice* (pp. 59–75). Oxford, UK: Routledge.

McGinnis, P. M., & Newell, K. M. (1982). Topological dynamics: A framework for describing movements and its constraints. *Human Movement Science, 1,* 289–305.

Milner, C. E., Fairbrother, J. T., Srivatsan, A., & Zhang, S. (2012). Simple verbal instruction improves knee biomechanics during landing in female athletes. *The Knee, 19,* 399–403.

Milner, C. E., Ferber, R., Pollard, C. D., Hamill, J., & Davis, I. S. (2006). Biomechanical factors associated with tibial stress fracture in female runners. *Medicine and Science in Sports and Exercise, 38,* 323–328.

Milner, C. E., Hamill, J., & Davis, I. S. (2010). Distinct hip and rearfoot kinematics in female runners with a history of tibial stress fracture. *Journal of Orthopaedic and Sports Therapy, 40,* 59–66.

Newell, K. M. (1985). Coordination, control and skill. In D. Goodman, R. B. Wilberg, & I. M. Franks (Eds.), *Differing perspectives in motor learning, memory, and control* (pp. 295–317). Amsterdam, Netherlands: Elsevier.

Newell, K. M. (1986). Constraints on the development of coordination. In M. G. Wade, & H. T. A. Whiting (Eds.). *Motor development in children: Aspects of coordination and control* (pp. 341–360). Boston, MA: Martinus Nijhoff.

Newell, K. M. (1991). Motor skill acquisition. *Annual Review of Psychology, 42,* 213–237.

Newell, K. M., & Jordan, K. (2007). Task constraints and movement organization: A common language. In W. E. Davis & G. D. Broadbent (Eds.), *Ecological task analysis and movement* (pp. 5–23). Champaign, IL: Human Kinetics.

Newell, K. M., & McDonald, P. V. (1991). Practice: A search for task solutions. In R. Christina & H. M. Eckert (Eds.), *American Academy of Physical Education papers: Enhancing human performance in sport: New concepts and developments* (pp. 51–60). Champaign, IL: Human Kinetics.

Newell, K. M., & Ranganathan, R. (2010). Instructions as constraints in motor skill acquisition. In I. Renshaw, K. Davids, & G. J. P. Savelsbergh (Eds.), *Motor learning in practice: A constraints-led approach* (pp. 17–32). London, UK: Routledge.

Nielsen, J. B., & Cohen, L. G. (2007). The Olympic brain: Does corticospinal plasticity play a role in acquisition of skills required for high-performance sports? *Journal of Physiology, 586,* 66–70.

Nourrit, D., Delignières, D., Caillou, N., Deschamps, T., & Lauriot. B. (2003). On discontinuities in motor learning: A longitudinal study of complex skill acquisition on a ski-simulator. *Journal of Motor Behavior, 35,* 151–170.

Nourrit, D., Deschamps, T., Lauriot, B., Caillou, N., & Delignieres, D. (2000). The effects of required amplitude and practice on frequency stability and efficiency in a cyclical task. *Journal of Sports Sciences, 18,* 201–212.

Paradisis, G. P., & Cooke, C. B. (2001). Kinematic and postural characteristics of sprint running on sloping surfaces. *Journal of Sports Sciences, 19,* 149–159.

Passos, P., Araújo, D., Davids, K., Gouveia, L., Serpa, S., Milho, J., & Fonseca, S. (2009). Interpersonal pattern dynamics and adaptive behavior in multi-agent neurobiological systems: A conceptual model and data. *Journal of Motor Behavior, 41,* 445–459.

Passos, P., Araújo, D., Davids, K., & Shuttleworth, R. (2008). Manipulating constraints to train decision making in rugby union. *International Journal of Sports Science and Coaching, 3,* 125–140.

Peh, S. Y.-C., Chow, J. Y., & Davids, K. (2011). Focus of attention and its impact on movement behavior. *Journal of Science and Medicine in Sport, 14,* 70–78.

Pinder, R. A., Davids, K., Renshaw, I., & Araújo, D. (2011). Representative learning design and functionality of research and practice in sport. *Journal of Sport and Exercise Psychology, 33,* 146–155.

Pinder, R. A., Renshaw, I., Davids, K., & Kerhervé, H. (2011). Principles for use of ball projection machines in elite developmental sport programmes. *Sports Medicine, 41,* 793–800.

Pinniger, G. J., Steele, J. R., & Groeller, H. (2000). Does fatigue induced by repeated dynamic efforts affect hamstring muscle function? *Medicine and Science in Sports and Exercise, 32,* 647–653.

Porter, J. M., & Magill, R. A. (2010). Systematically increasing contextual interference is beneficial for learning sport skills. *Journal of Sports Sciences, 28,* 1277–1285.

Porter, M. M., Myint, A., Kramer, J. F., & Vandervoort, A. A. (1995). Concentric and eccentric knee extension strength in older and younger men and women. *Canadian Journal of Applied Physiology, 20,* 429–439.

Ranganathan, R., & Carlton, L. G. (2007). Perception–action coupling and anticipatory performance in baseball batting. *Journal of Motor Behavior, 39,* 369–380.

Roberts, E. M., Cheung, T. K., Abdel Hafez, A. M., & Hong, D.-A. (1997). Swing limb biomechanics of 60- to 65-year-old male runners. *Gait and Posture, 5,* 42–53.

Rudolph, K. S., Eastlack, M. E., Axe, M. J., & Snyder-Mackler, L. (1998). Movement patterns after anterior cruciate ligament injury: A comparison of patients who compensate well for the injury and those who require operative stabilization. *Journal of Electromyography and Kinesiology, 8,* 349–362.

Sakadjian, A., Panchuk, D., & Pearce, A. J. (2014). Kinematic and kinetic improvements associated with action observation facilitated learning of the power clean in Australian footballers. *Journal of Strength and Conditioning Research, 28,* 1613–1625.

Savelsbergh, G. J. P., Van Der Kamp, J., Williams, A. M., & Ward, P. (2005). Anticipation and visual search behavior in expert soccer goalkeepers. *Ergonomics, 48,* 1686–1697.

Schmidt, R. A. (1975). A schema theory of discrete motor skill learning. *Psychological Reviews, 82,* 225–260.

Schmidt, R. A. (2003). Motor schema theory after 27 years: Reflections and implications for a new theory. *Research Quarterly for Exercise and Sport, 74,* 366–375.

Schmidt, R. A., & Wrisberg, C. A (2008). *Motor learning and performance: A situation-based learning approach.* Champaign, IL: Human Kinetics.

Schöllhorn, W. I., Hegen, P., & Davids, K. (2012). The nonlinear nature of learning: A differential learning approach. *Open Sports Sciences Journal, 5,* 100–112.

Schöllhorn, W. I., Nigg, B. M., Stefanyshyn, D. J., & Liu, W. (2002). Identification of individual walking patterns using time discrete and time continuous data sets. *Gait and Posture, 15,* 180–186.

Schöner, G., Haken, H., & Kelso, J. A. S. (1986). A stochastic theory of phase transitions in human hand movement. *Biological Cybernetics, 53,* 247–257.

Schöner, G., & Kelso, J. A. S. (1988). Dynamic pattern generation in behavioral and neural systems. *Science, 239,* 1513–1520.

Schücker, L., Hagemann, N., Strauss, B., & Völker, K. (2009). The effect of attentional focus on running economy. *Journal of Sports Sciences, 27,* 1241–1248.

Slawinski, J., Dorel, S., Hug, F., Couturier, A., Fournel, V., Morin, J.-B., & Hanon, C. (2008). Elite long sprint running: A comparison between incline and level training sessions. *Medicine and Science in Sports and Exercise, 40*, 1155–1162.

Southard, D. (2011). Attentional focus and control parameter: Effect on throwing pattern and performance. *Research Quarterly for Exercise and Sport, 82*, 652–666.

Sprague, P., & Mann, R. V. (1983). The effects on muscular fatigue on the kinetic of sprint running. *Research Quarterly for Exercise and Sport, 54*, 60–66.

Summers, J. J., & Anson, J. G. (2009). Current status of the motor program: Revisited. *Human Movement Science, 28*, 566–577.

Talpey, S., Young, W., & Beseler, B. (2014). Effects of instructions on selected jump squat variables. *Journal of Strength and Conditioning*, Epub ahead of print.

Taunton, J. E., Ryan, M. B., Clement, D. B., McKenzie, D. C., Lloyd-Smith, D. R., & Zumbo, B. D. (2002). A retrospective case-control analysis of 2002 running injuries. *British Journal of Sports Medicine, 36*, 95–101.

Thelen, E. (1985). Developmental origins of motor coordination: Leg movements in human infants. *Developmental Psychobiology, 18*, 1–22.

Tucker, R., & Collins, M. (2012). What makes a champion? A review of the relative contribution of genes and training to sporting success. *British Journal of Sports Medicine, 46*, 555–561.

Turvey, M. T. (1990). Coordination. *American Psychologist, 45*, 938–953.

Turvey, M. T., Fitch, H. L., & Tuller, B. (1982). The Bernstein perspective I: The problem of degrees of freedom and context conditioned variability. In J. A. S. Kelso (Ed.), *Human motor behavior: An introduction* (pp. 239–252). Hillsdale, NJ: Erlbaum.

Uehara, L. A., Button, C., & Davids, K. (2008). The effects of focus of attention instructions on novices learning soccer chip. *Brazilian Journal of Biometricity, 2*, 63–77.

Usherwood, J. R., & Wilson, A. M. (2006). Accounting for elite indoor 200 m sprint results. *Biology Letters, 2*, 47–50.

Van Emmerik, R. E. A. (2007). Functional role of variability in movement coordination and disability. In W. E. Davis & G. D. Broadbent (Eds.), *Ecological task analysis and movement* (pp. 25–52). Champaign, IL: Human Kinetics.

Van Emmerik, R. E. A., Rosenstein, M. T., McDermott, W. J., & Hamill, J. (2004). A nonlinear dynamics approach to human movement. *Journal of Applied Biomechanics, 20*, 396–420.

van Gent, R. N., Siem, D., van Middelkoop, M., van Os, A. G., Bierma-Zeinstra, S. M., & Koes, B. W. (2007). Incidence and determinants of lower extremity running injuries in long distance runners: A systematic review. *British Journal of Sports Medicine, 41*, 469–480.

Vereijken, B., van Emmerik, R. E. A., Bongaardt, R., Beek, W. J., & Newell, K. M. (1997). Changing coordinative structures in complex skill learning acquisition. *Human Movement Science, 16*, 823–844.

Walsh, M. S., Waters, J., & Kersting, U. G. (2007). Gender bias on the effects of instruction on kinematic and kinetic jump parameters of high-level athletes. *Research in Sports Medicine, 15*, 283–295.

Walsh, M., Young, B., Hill, B., Kittredge, K., & Horn, T. (2007). The effect of ball-carrying technique and experience on sprinting in rugby union. *Journal of Sports Sciences, 25*, 185–192.

Wdowski, M. M., & Gittoes, M. J. R. (2013). Kinematic adaptations in sprint acceleration performance without and with the constraint of holding a field hockey stick. *Sports Biomechanics, 12*, 143–153.

Wehrlin, J. P., & Hallen, J. (2006). Linear decrease in VO_{2max} and performance with increasing altitude in endurance athletes. *European Journal of Applied Physiology, 96*, 404–412.

Weyand, P. G., Sandell, R. F., Prime, D. N. L., & Bundle, M. W. (2010). The biological limits to running speed are imposed from the ground up. *Journal of Applied Physiology, 108*, 950–961.

Weyand, P. G., Sternlight, D. B., Bellizzi, M. J., & Wright, S. (2000). Faster top running speeds are achieved with greater ground forces not more rapid leg movements. *Journal of Applied Physiology, 81*, 1991–1999.

Willy, R. W., & Davis, I. S. (2014). Kinematic and kinetic comparison of running in standard and minimalist shoes. *Medicine and Science in Sports and Exercise, 46*, 318–323.

Willy, R. W., Scholtz, J. P., & Davis, I. S. (2012). Mirror gait retraining for the treatment of patellofemoral pain in female runners. *Clinical Biomechanics, 27*, 1045–1051.

Wilson, C., Simpson, S. E., van Emmerik, R. E. A., & Hamill, J. (2008). Coordination variability and skill development in expert triple jumpers. *Sports Biomechanics, 7*, 2–9.

Witvrouw, E., Callaghan, M. J., Stefanik, J. J., Noehren, B., Bazett-Jones, D. M., Willson, J. D., . . . Crossley, K. M. (2014). Patellofemoral pain: Consensus statement from the 3rd International Patellofemoral Pain Research Retreat held in Vancouver, September 2013. *British Journal of Sports Medicine, 48*, 411–414.

Woo, B. H., & Zatsiorsky, V. M. (2006). Variability of competition performance in throwing and jumping events in elite athletes. *Human Movement, 7*, 5–13.

Wulf, G. (2013). Attentional focus and motor learning: A review of 15 years. *International Review of Sport and Exercise Psychology, 6*, 77–104.

Wulf, G., McConnel, N., Gärtner, M., & Schwarz, A. (2002). Enhancing the learning of sport skills through external-focus feedback. *Journal of Motor Behavior, 34*, 171–182.

Young, W., & Rogers, N. (2014). Effects of small-sided game and change-of-direction training on reactive agility and change-of-direction speed. *Journal of Sports Sciences, 32*, 307–314.

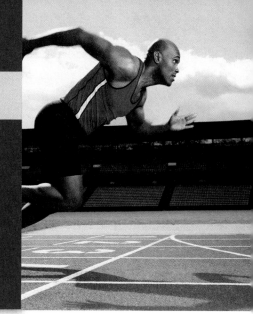

CHAPTER 11

Biomechanics of Fundamental Movements: Jumping

Chapter Objectives

At the end of this chapter, you will be able to:

- Explain the mechanical factors that determine performance when jumping for vertical and horizontal distance

- Explain the biomechanical aspects of jumping tasks

- Explain modifications to jumping movements that can enhance performance

- Explain modifications to task and informational constraints that a coach can implement to enhance jumping performance

- Perform a qualitative analysis of jumping

- Develop specific workouts targeting muscular strength commensurate with the biomechanical aspects of jumping tasks to enhance jumping performance

- Develop specific workouts based on representative learning to enhance the attunement of the athletes' jumping movements to environmental information

Key Terms

Assisted jump training	Flight phase	Predictive approach	Takeoff angle
Braking phase	Informational constraints	Propulsive phase	Takeoff distance
Countermovement	Instructions	Relative projection height	Takeoff height
Countermovement vertical jump	Knowledge of results	Standing long jump	Task constraints
Drop jump	Landing distance	Standing vertical jump	Tendon function
Eccentric utilization ratio	Leg stiffness	Static vertical jump	Whole-body vibration
	Pivot mechanism	Stretch–shortening cycle	

Chapter Overview

The execution of jumps is a requirement in many sports. In some athletic events, the jumping task represents a goal in itself, with performance being judged solely on the horizontal distance or vertical height achieved by the athlete during the jump, as with the long jump and high jump events in track and field, respectively. In other sports, the athlete is required to execute jumps to satisfy the strategic/tactical elements, such as jumping to intercept a ball in basketball or to avoid an attempted tackle by an opponent in soccer. Furthermore, the athlete may have to perform multiple jumps during the sport. For example, time–motion analysis data reveal that basketball players may perform as many as 49 jumps during a game (Abdelkrim, El Fazaa, & El Ati, 2007), while soccer players have been reported to perform as many as 36 jumps during competitive matches (Bangsbo, Mohr, & Krustrup, 2006). Sheppard et al. (2007) have reported that elite volleyball players perform as many as 75 jumps of different types (e.g., block jumps, jump sets, spike jumps) during games. It is unlikely that all of these jumps will be maximal, as the required height of the jump is determined by the location of the ball to be intercepted or the location of the opponent to be avoided. These interceptive and avoidance requirements represent considerable constraints on the jumping tasks and necessitate that the athlete effectively couple his or her movements to the environmental information available during the sport to be successful. Furthermore, it is unlikely that each jump will be performed under optimal mechanical conditions, with alterations in the posture of the athlete likely precluding maximal performance in each jump. These constraints have considerable implications for training and practice regimens that can be developed by the strength and conditioning practitioner to improve athletes' jumping ability.

The performance in jumping tasks also constitutes a common assessment tool used to monitor the ability of athletes (Markovic & Jaric, 2007). In many sports, the better athletes tend to jump higher than their lesser counterparts, while jumping performance distinguishes various player positions (Haugen, Tønnessen, & Seiler, 2013). Jumps are also recommended as training exercises for athletes in many different sports, forming the basis of many plyometric exercises (Radcliffe & Farentinos, 1999). It is clear, then, that improving performance in jumping tasks will be beneficial for athletes involved in numerous sports.

This chapter introduces the mechanical aspects of jumping that influence the distance achieved by the athlete. It discusses the biomechanical variables that determine the mechanical output during jumping tasks. Enhancements to jumping performance are highlighted, including modifications in the movement as well as the manipulation of task and informational constraints that can be implemented by the coach. Finally, the role of specific training methods to improve muscular strength and their application to the enhancement of jumping performance are discussed, as is the requirement for representative learning practices to enhance sport-specific jumping tasks.

Mechanics of Jumping

A jump is a ballistic movement that requires the athlete to project himself or herself into a **flight phase** so as to displace the center of mass (CM) vertically or horizontally. The flight phase begins at the point of takeoff when the athlete loses contact with the ground, and ends when the athlete makes contact with the ground upon landing. The displacement of the CM during the flight phase is determined by the kinematics of the CM at the point of takeoff. Accordingly, the peak vertical displacement of the CM during flight can be determined from the following equation of motion:

$$s = \frac{(v^2 \times \sin\theta)}{2g}$$

Eq. (11.1)

where s is the peak vertical displacement during flight, v is the resultant velocity of the CM at takeoff, θ is the angle of the resultant velocity with respect to the horizontal axis of the reference frame (known as the **takeoff angle**), and g is the acceleration due to gravity. As gravitational acceleration is constant, Equation (11.1) informs us that the vertical displacement of the CM, and therefore the jump height, will increase with the square of the vertical component of the CM velocity at takeoff. Notice that the total vertical displacement of the CM from the position of upright posture to the peak displacement achieved during the flight phase is further influenced by **takeoff height**—that is, the displacement of the CM above that associated with the upright standing posture at the point of takeoff. This effect is caused by the athlete rising onto the toes, raising the arms (if an arm swing is used during the jump), or raising the non-takeoff leg (if performing a unilateral jump) prior to takeoff (Figure 11.1). During vertical jumps performed from two feet and in the absence of an arm swing, this displacement does not contribute significantly to overall jump height (Moir, 2008). Moreover, if jump height is determined by the peak displacement of a specific body part, such as the hands during a jump and reach task, as opposed to the displacement of the CM alone, then the distance between the body part and the CM will affect the height attained (see Jumping Concept 11.1).

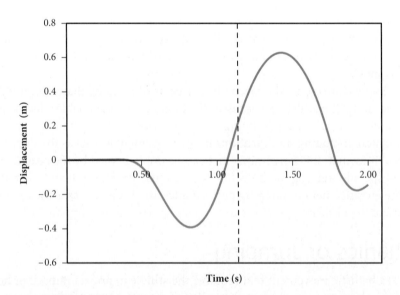

Figure 11.1 The vertical displacement of the center of mass of an athlete during the countermovement vertical jump. The dashed vertical line represents the point of takeoff. Notice that the center of mass has been raised above the starting position, resulting in a takeoff height of 0.11 m.

Jumping Concept 11.1

Differences when reaching with one versus two hands during a vertical jump

When jumping to intercept a ball, the height of the ball above the ground determines the maximal height to which the body part used to intercept the ball must be projected. In most situations, an athlete would select the hand to intercept the ball. Therefore, whether the ball is successfully intercepted will be determined by the height of the hand above the ground, which is further determined by the takeoff height of the CM, the displacement of the CM during the flight phase, and the distance between the CM and the outstretched hand. Given that the position of the CM within the athlete's body will be affected by the location of the body segments about the CM, the athlete can influence the distance between the CM and the outstretched hand by manipulating the number of body segments that are arranged above the CM during the flight phase of the jump. Specifically, if the athlete reaches for the target with both hands, the distance between the CM and the hands will be reduced in comparison to the situation where the athlete reaches for the target with a single hand. This difference reflects the greater number of body segments, and therefore mass, located above the CM during the flight phase when reaching with two hands. Therefore, if the athlete attempts to intercept the target by reaching with one hand during the flight phase of the jump, the vertical position of the hand will be higher above the ground than if the athlete attempted to reach with both hands simultaneously. This has implications for interceptive tasks such as tip-offs and rebounds in basketball and blocks in volleyball.

The horizontal displacement of the CM during the flight phase is somewhat more complicated than that during vertical jumps, involving both vertical and horizontal components of takeoff velocity. Horizontal displacement during flight can be determined from the following equation:

$$s = v\cos\theta \times t$$

Eq. (11.2)

where s is the horizontal displacement, v is the resultant velocity of the CM at takeoff, θ is the takeoff angle, and t is the time of flight. The time of flight, t, can be derived from the following expression:

$$t = \frac{2v\sin\theta}{g}$$

Eq. (11.3)

where t is the time of flight, v is the resultant velocity of the CM at takeoff, θ is the takeoff angle, and g is the acceleration due to gravity. In turn, Equation (11.2) can be rewritten as follows:

$$s = \frac{v^2 2\sin\theta\cos\theta}{g}$$

Eq. (11.4)

where s is the horizontal displacement, v is the resultant velocity of the CM at the point of takeoff, θ is the takeoff angle, and g is the acceleration due to gravity.

Equation (11.4) returns the horizontal displacement when the height of the CM is the same at takeoff as it is upon landing. Typically when athletes perform horizontal jumps, their CM will be higher at takeoff than upon landing. Under such circumstances, the difference in the height of the CM at takeoff and landing, known as the **relative projection height**, needs to be included in the calculations of horizontal displacement. Therefore, Equation (11.4) is rewritten as follows:

$$s = \frac{v^2 \sin\theta\cos\theta + v\cos\theta\sqrt{v^2 \sin^2\theta + 2gh}}{g} \qquad \text{Eq. (11.5)}$$

where s is the horizontal displacement, v is the resultant velocity of the CM at takeoff, θ is the takeoff angle, g is the acceleration due to gravity, and h is the relative projection height. Thus the horizontal displacement undergone during flight depends on the velocity of the CM at takeoff, the takeoff angle, the relative projection height, and gravitational acceleration.

Given a constant gravitational acceleration, Equation (11.5) informs us that the magnitude of the resultant velocity of the CM will have the greatest influence on the horizontal displacement traveled by the CM during flight (the resultant velocity is squared in the equation). Increasing h, the relative projection height, will also increase the horizontal displacement achieved, although this effect will not be as dramatic as that associated with an increase in the magnitude of the velocity. The takeoff angle that optimizes the horizontal displacement is largely dependent upon the relative projection height. Specifically, if the CM is at the same height at takeoff and landing, then the takeoff angle that maximizes horizontal displacement will be 45°. However, if the height of the CM at takeoff is above that upon landing—as is the case in most situations when athletes jump for horizontal distance—then a takeoff angle less than 45° is required; how much less than 45° depends on the relative projection height, with small relative projection heights requiring angles closer to 45° than large relative projection heights. Notice that the takeoff angle is dependent upon the magnitude of the horizontal and vertical velocity components at takeoff (see Jumping Concept 11.2).

Jumping Concept 11.2

Elite long jumpers do not produce optimal takeoff angles

The jumping distance covered during the execution of a horizontal jump is determined from the sum of the takeoff distance (the horizontal distance from the takeoff board to the CM at the point of takeoff), the flight distance (the horizontal distance traveled by the CM during the flight phase of the jump), and the landing distance (the horizontal distance between the CM and the feet upon landing). Of these distances, flight distance contributes approximately 90% to the overall distance of the jump (Hay, 1993). It is this distance, which depends on the kinematic characteristics of CM speed at takeoff, the takeoff angle, and the relative projection height, that is considered here.

Table 11.1

Jump Distances and Kinematic Characteristics of the Center of Mass at Takeoff Recorded from Six Elite Long Jump Athletes and the Optimal Takeoff Angle Calculated for Each

Jump Distance (m)	Takeoff Speed (m/s)	Vertical Velocity (m/s)	Horizontal Velocity (m/s)	Takeoff Angle (degrees)	Optimal Takeoff Angle (degrees)
8.95	9.8	3.9	9.0	23.2	43.3
8.90	9.6	3.9	8.8	24.0	43.3
8.79	10.0	3.2	9.5	18.7	43.4
7.14	8.9	3.0	8.4	19.6	43.0
7.13	9.4	2.5	9.1	15.6	43.2
7.12	8.5	3.2	7.9	22.1	42.8

Note: Optimal takeoff angles are calculated using the takeoff speeds and assuming a relative projection height of 0.60 m. Air resistance is neglected in the calculations.

Data from Hay, J. G. (1993). *The biomechanics of sports techniques.* Englewood Cliffs, NJ: Prentice Hall.

Table 11.1 shows the kinematic variables of distance jumped, takeoff speed, vertical and horizontal velocity of the CM at takeoff, and takeoff angle for elite long jump athletes. Also shown in the table is the optimal takeoff angle for each athlete, calculated mathematically from the takeoff speed and assuming a relative projection height of 0.60 m (i.e., the position of the CM at takeoff is 0.60 m above that upon landing).

A striking feature of the data presented in Table 11.1 is that none of the athletes approaches the optimal takeoff angle. As the takeoff angle is determined by the magnitude of the horizontal and vertical components of CM velocity at takeoff, this situation could be remedied by the athlete reducing the horizontal component of velocity at takeoff. However, this strategy would reduce the magnitude of the resultant velocity, compromising the horizontal displacement of the CM during the flight phase. The other option then becomes increasing the vertical velocity component at takeoff; indeed, a cursory inspection of Table 11.1 demonstrates that none of the athletes is able to generate sufficient vertical velocity while maintaining high horizontal velocity at takeoff. Indeed, the high horizontal velocities of even elite long jumpers appear to be produced at the expense of high vertical velocities of the CM at takeoff, resulting in a suboptimal takeoff angle.

The total distance covered by an athlete during a horizontal jump includes both takeoff and landing distances in addition to the flight distance (Figure 11.2). The **takeoff distance** is defined as the horizontal distance between the takeoff foot and the CM at the point of takeoff (during an event such as the long jump, takeoff distance is defined as the horizontal distance between the takeoff board and the CM at the point of takeoff); the **landing distance** is defined as the horizontal distance between the CM and the feet upon landing (Hay, 1993). Research has shown that the takeoff and landing distances each contribute 5% of the total jumping distance, leaving the horizontal

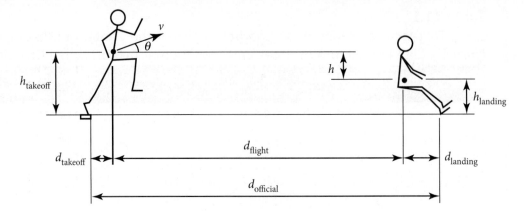

Figure 11.2 Diagram showing the takeoff distance, flight distance, and landing distance that contribute to the official distance jumped by the athlete during a long jump event.

jump distance largely dependent on the displacement undergone by the CM during the flight phase of the jump (Hay, 1993).

From the preceding discussion, it can be determined that performance in both vertical and horizontal jumps is largely determined by the development of CM velocity at takeoff that has the appropriate magnitude and direction relative to the specific demands of the jumping task. Recall that the velocity possessed by the CM is encapsulated in the variables of linear momentum and translational kinetic energy—variables that are changed by the application of an impulse and the performance of work, respectively. Therefore, to develop the appropriate takeoff velocity, the athlete is required to generate an appropriate impulse or to perform work during the **propulsive phase** of the jump, defined as the phase between the first positive vertical motion of the CM when the athlete is in contact with the ground and the takeoff. Given the impulse–momentum relationship and making the assumption that the vertical momentum of the CM at the beginning of the propulsive phase of the jump is zero, we can rewrite Equation (11.1) to determine the influence of the generation of impulse on the vertical velocity of the CM and, therefore, on jump height:

$$s = \frac{(\int F dt \,/\, m)^2}{2g}$$

Eq. (11.6)

where s is the vertical displacement of the CM during the flight phase, $\int F dt$ is the net vertical impulse acting on the CM during propulsion, m is body mass, and g is the acceleration due to gravity. Equation (11.1) can further be rewritten to express the influence of the work done on the CM during propulsion on the total vertical displacement of the CM from the beginning of the propulsion phase to the peak vertical displacement achieved during the flight phase of a vertical jump:

$$s = \frac{(2\,/\,m)\int F ds}{2g}$$

Eq. (11.7)

where s is the total vertical displacement from the beginning of the propulsive phase to the peak vertical displacement achieved during the flight phase, m is body mass, $\int Fds$ is the work done on the CM during the propulsive phase, and g is the acceleration due to gravity. Similar rearrangements can be applied to Equation (11.5) to highlight the importance of the impulse of the force or the work done by the force on the CM in determining the distance covered by the athlete during horizontal jumping tasks. Ultimately, the performance of both vertical and horizontal jumps requires the athlete to develop an appropriate impulse or to perform an appropriate amount of work during the propulsive phase of the jump to satisfy the specific demands of the task—namely, the appropriate vertical or horizontal displacement undergone by the CM during the jump.

Biomechanics of Jumping

A mechanical analysis of jumping informs us that the athlete should generate a takeoff velocity that is commensurate with the demands of the specific task. This section outlines the biomechanical aspects that constrain the jumping performance of athletes. It first considers standing jumps, then running jumps.

Standing Jumps

Standing jumps are initiated from a starting position in which the athlete does not possess any horizontal motion. As with all jumping tasks, the athlete is required to generate a ground reaction impulse with vertical and horizontal components that produce a velocity of the CM at takeoff that is commensurate with the goal of the task (i.e., the appropriate vertical and/or horizontal projection of the CM). Recall that the moments generated at the various joints are transformed into the ground reaction force (GRF) when the athlete is in contact with the ground that acts to accelerate the athlete's CM during a given movement task. During a **standing vertical jump** (SVJ), the magnitude of the moment at the hip joint and the work done by this moment increase as the jump height increases from submaximal to maximal values, with a concomitant increase in the magnitude of the impulse of the GRF (Lees, Vanrenterghem, & De Clercq, 2004a). Little change occurs in the mechanical output at the ankle joint as jump height increases. In contrast, the moment at the knee joint actually decreases with increasing jump height, although the work done by the moment changes little.

The importance of the mechanical output of the hip joint has also been demonstrated in the execution of a **standing long jump** (SLJ), where there is a greater relative contribution by the work done at the hip joint to the overall work generated during the propulsive phase of the jump than the output at either the knee or ankle joints (Horita, Kitamura, & Kohno, 1991). Indeed, the peak moment at the knee joint actually decreases as the athlete changes from executing a SVJ to a SLJ, while the magnitude of the moments at the hip and ankle joint remains unchanged (Jones & Caldwell, 2003). Thus the mechanical output of the hip joint makes a relatively greater contribution to the generation of the impulse of the GRF during both SVJ and SLJ than the knee and ankle joints.

The relative magnitude of the moments at the hip, knee, and ankle joints and the direction of the moments (e.g., extensor or flexor) during a given movement task will determine the location of the center of pressure of the GRF and the direction in which the GRF acts on the athlete during the movement. Specifically, extensor moments exerted at the hip, knee, and ankle joints when the athlete adopts a posture such that the CM is located above the GRF center of pressure will result in the generation of a GRF that acts normal to the supporting surface. However, an increase in the magnitude of the extensor moment at the hip joint with a simultaneous flexor moment at the knee joint when the athlete is in the same posture will result in the generation of a positive horizontal component of the external force, producing a resultant GRF that is directed both forward and upward (Wells & Evans, 1987). Furthermore, this directional control of the GRF conferred by the alteration of the moments at the hip, knee, and ankle joints is largely due to the activation patterns of the biarticular muscles crossing those joints. Specifically, an increase in the activity of the hamstrings and a concomitant decrease in the activity of the rectus femoris have been reported when athletes execute a SLJ compared to a SVJ (Jones & Caldwell, 2003). This alteration in the activation of the biarticular muscles likely reflects the requirement to produce a more forward-directed GRF commensurate with the horizontal projection of the CM associated with the SLJ task.

The biarticular muscles (e.g., hamstrings, rectus femoris, gastrocnemius) serve a further purpose during jumping tasks by transporting the work done by the monoarticular muscles to the distal joints (Umberger, 1998). For example, the positive work performed by the monoarticular gluteus maximus in extending the hip joint can be transported to the knee by the biarticular rectus femoris during the propulsive phase of a jumping task. The rectus femoris, which acts to flex the hip joint and extend the knee joint, will operate under near-isometric conditions during propulsion, given that the hip and the knee are extended almost simultaneously. As such, this muscle will be able to generate a relatively large force due to the force–velocity relationship of skeletal muscle. When the rectus femoris generates a large isometric force, it acts much like a stiff cable, effectively connecting the hip joint with the knee joint; this effect is known as the **tendon function** of a biarticular muscle (Zatsiorsky & Prilusky, 2012). The tendon function of the rectus femoris will result in knee extension when the hip joint is simultaneously extended. In turn, some of the work performed by the monoarticular gluteus maximus in extending the hip joint appears at the knee to extend this joint, transported there by the biarticular rectus femoris. A similar transportation of work occurs between the knee and ankle joints as a result of the biarticular gastrocnemius.

This proximal-to-distal transportation of work between the lower-body joints by the biarticular muscles allows the monoarticular muscles to maximize the amount of work they are able to generate before takeoff during jumping tasks (Bobbert & van Soest, 2000). Indeed, the activation of the monoarticular muscles (e.g., gluteus maximus, vastii group, soleus) follows a proximal-to-distal sequence during the propulsive phase of both standing vertical and long jumps (Jones & Caldwell, 2003). This specific activation sequence of the monoarticular muscles allows the athlete's feet to remain in contact with the ground for a longer duration, thereby delaying takeoff and allowing the monoarticular muscles to generate more work. This work is then transported distally by the tendon function of the biarticular muscles, generating a greater impulse of the GRF than if the monoarticular muscles were activated simultaneously.

Although the activation of the muscles crossing the hip, knee, and ankle joints is generally similar during the execution of both SVJ and SLJ, some differences are seen between the two different jumping tasks. Specifically, the tibialis anterior and rectus femoris muscles are activated earlier during the execution of the SLJ to reduce ankle plantar flexion and increase hip flexion, respectively (Jones & Caldwell, 2003). These actions at the ankle and hip joints, along with the reduced knee extensor moment observed during a SLJ, result in the forward translation of the CM early during ground contact with this type of jump. As a consequence, the CM possesses greater forward momentum at the beginning of the propulsive phase during the SLJ task in comparison to the SVJ task. The forward translation of the CM also increases the horizontal displacement between the CM and the center of pressure of the GRF during propulsion, with the CM being projected in front of the center of pressure. This produces a moment about the CM caused by the ground reaction force that rotates the athlete forward during the propulsive phase, despite the forward-directed GRF (Ashby & Heegaard, 2002). The angular momentum possessed by the athlete as a result of the moment generated by the GRF during the execution of the SLJ must either be reduced prior to takeoff or be controlled by the swinging of the arms during the flight phase (Ashby & Heegaard, 2002), although the extended posture adopted by the athlete at takeoff limits the forward angular velocity by increasing the athlete's mass moment of inertia. However, the angular momentum is advantageous in that the athlete will be rotated forward upon landing, preventing him or her from falling backward and increasing the distance jumped.

The positioning of the CM ahead of the center of pressure of the GRF during the execution of a SLJ can be achieved early when the athlete initiates the task by performing a **countermovement**. A countermovement occurs when there is an initial downward movement of the CM prior to the propulsive phase of the jump. The completion of a countermovement ensures there is little difference in the muscle activation patterns and joint mechanics during the propulsive phase of a SVJ and a SLJ (Jones & Caldwell, 2003). However, if the jumps are executed in the absence of an initial countermovement, then differences in the mechanical output at the hip, knee, and ankle joints will be seen between the SLJ and SVJ tasks. Specifically, the magnitude of the extensor moments at the hip and ankle joints will be reduced, with a concomitant increase observed in the magnitude of the extensor moment at the knee joint in the SLJ compared to the SVJ to initiate the forward motion of the CM (Ridderikhoff, Batelaan, & Bobbert, 1999). In summary, the biomechanical aspects of any jumping task are dependent upon the specific constraints associated with the requirements of the jump (e.g., vertical or horizontal projection of the CM, the performance of an initial countermovement).

Enhancement of Standing Jumps

The enhancement of any standing jump task when the goal is to maximize the displacement of the CM during flight can be reduced to the ability to maximize the impulse of the GRF during the propulsive phase. An athlete can adopt various strategies to achieve this increase in impulse, including performing a countermovement prior to the propulsive phase and swinging the arms during the propulsive phase. Furthermore, the coach can manipulate the constraints associated with the jumping task and the information provided to the athlete to enhance the jumping performance.

Incorporation of a Countermovement

A countermovement is an initial downward movement of the CM prior to the initiation of the propulsive phase of a jumping task. The performance of an initial countermovement results in a greater vertical jump height compared to those jumps performed without a preparatory countermovement (Bobbert, Gerritsen, Litjens, & Van Soest, 1996; Hudson, 1986; Komi & Bosco, 1978; Kubo, Kawakami, & Fukunaga, 1999;

Sanders, McClymont, Howick, & Kavalieris, 1993). For example, the jump height achieved during a **countermovement vertical jump** is approximately 6% greater than that achieved during a **static vertical jump** where the initial countermovement of the CM is absent (Hudson, 1986).

The initial downward motion of the CM associated with the countermovement is believed to eccentrically load the musculotendinous units of the lower-body joints, thereby allowing greater work to be performed during the subsequent propulsive phase of the jump when the contractile elements are operating concentrically and the CM is ascending toward takeoff. This specific pattern of an eccentric muscle action preceding a concentric muscle action is known as the **stretch–shortening cycle** (SSC). The enhancement of jumping performance through the inclusion of the SSC is influenced by the magnitude and rate of eccentric loading. For example, such loading occurs when performing a **drop jump**, as the athlete drops from a height prior to landing and then jumps for maximal height. The jump height achieved during a drop jump is greater than that achieved during a countermovement jump, which is in turn greater than that achieved during a static jump, when such jumps are performed by well-trained athletes (Moran & Wallace, 2007). Moreover, the jump height achieved during the execution of drop jumps tends to increase with the drop height due to the increased eccentric loading (Walsh, Arampatzis, Schade, & Brüggemann, 2004), although the eccentric loading must be within the capabilities of the athlete if these advantages are to be realized (Turner & Jefferys, 2010). The difference in the height achieved during these different jumps provides information about the athlete's ability to utilize the SSC, as reflected in the **eccentric utilization ratio** (McGuigan et al., 2006). The ability to utilize the SSC has been shown to be improved following a period of resistance training (Cormie, McCaulley, & McBride, 2007; McBride, Triplett-McBride, Davie, & Newton, 2002).

The involvement of the SSC during jumps allows a greater amount of work to be performed by the musculotendinous units during the propulsion phase, producing a greater velocity of the CM at takeoff in comparison to those jumps where the SSC is absent. Recall that the following mechanisms serve to produce a greater amount of work during the SSC:

- Increased active state. The greater tension developed during an eccentric action reflects a greater proportion of attached crossbridges, which determine the active state of the muscle. A greater active state at the commencement of the propulsive phase of a jump allows the muscles to perform more work early during the propulsive phase, increasing the takeoff velocity of the CM (Bobbert & Casius, 2005).
- Activation of the stretch reflex. During the initial eccentric action of the SSC, the muscles are stretched, activating the intrafusal fibers. The excitatory connections with the α-motoneurons result in the generation of a greater force, and therefore greater work, during the subsequent concentric action (Komi, 2003).
- Storage and return of strain potential energy. The initial eccentric action of the SSC stretches the series elastic components of the musculotendinous units, particularly the aponeurosis and tendon, allowing them to store strain potential energy. This stored energy can then be returned during the subsequent concentric phase of the SSC, allowing the musculotendinous unit to perform work even when the contractile elements are limited in their ability to perform work by the force–velocity relationship (Komi, 2003).

Table 11.2

Duration of the Countermovement and Propulsive Phases During the Standing Vertical Jump and the Standing Long Jump

Jump Type	Countermovement Phase	Propulsion Phase
Standing vertical jump	601 ms	298 ms
Standing long jump	708 ms	293 ms

Data from Jones, S. L., & Caldwell, G. E. (2003). Mono- and bi-articular muscle activity during jumping in different directions. *Journal of Applied Biomechanics, 19*, 205–222.

■ Interaction of contractile and elastic elements. The lengthening and shortening of the contractile elements during the SCC is limited as a result of the stretch and recoil of the tendinous structures. This limited length change allows the fascicles to operate under near-isometric conditions while the musculotendinous unit as a whole lengthens and shortens, resulting in a greater force being generated during the concentric phase than if the contractile elements were required to shorten (Fukashiro, Hay, & Nagano, 2006). Therefore, more work will be performed during the propulsive phase of a jump when the SSC is involved than if propulsion is initiated without a prior countermovement.

In the discussion of the biomechanics of the SLJ, it was noted that the countermovement provides an opportunity to translate the CM in front of the center of pressure of the GRF. This action increases the horizontal momentum of the CM and the forward angular momentum of the body about the CM at takeoff, which are collectively required to project the CM horizontally (Ashby & Heegaard, 2002; Jones & Caldwell, 2003). Accomplishing this motion of the body during the countermovement allows the athlete to employ a similar pattern of joint dynamics during the propulsive phase of a SLJ as would be used during a SVJ to achieve the goal of the task (Jones & Caldwell, 2003). It also explains the increased duration of the countermovement seen in a SLJ compared to a SVJ (Table 11.2). Thus a preparatory countermovement enhances performance during standing jumping tasks.

Incorporation of an Arm Swing

Swinging the arms during the propulsive phase has been shown to increase vertical jump height, with the enhancement being approximately 10% (Feltner, Fraschetti, & Crisp, 1999; Lees, Vanrenterghem, & De Clercq, 2004b). The arm swing results in greater energy possessed by the CM at takeoff, with both a greater takeoff velocity and a greater takeoff height being observed, although the enhancement of the takeoff velocity greatly exceeds that of the takeoff height (Lees et al., 2004b). The greater takeoff velocity is due to the extra work performed at the shoulder and elbow joints, combined with an enhancement of the work performed at the hip joint (Lees et al., 2004b). Specifically, the arm swing results in greater inclination of the trunk during the initial countermovement of a SVJ, increasing the work done at the hip joint. The work at the hip joint is transferred to the arms, where it increases their energy as the arms move forward and downward during the countermovement. Once the arms begin to swing upward during the propulsive phase, the energy of the arm segments due to the work done at the shoulder and elbow joints as well as that performed at the hip joint is then transferred back to the lower body joints (hip, knee, and ankle) to allow them to perform more work late in the propulsive phase.

An arm swing has also been shown to increase jump height during jumps performed without a preparatory countermovement (Walsh, Waters, Böhm, & Potteiger, 2007). The arms generate a force on the trunk segment acting at the shoulder joint during the upward motion of the arm swing; this force "pulls" the trunk vertically. In this way, it decreases the energy of the arms at takeoff while concomitantly increasing the energy of the CM (Lees et al., 2004b). The pulling effect associated with the arm swing results from the difference in momentum between the arm and trunk segments during propulsion, with the arms possessing greater momentum than the trunk as they are swung forward and upward (Lees & Barton, 1996). Indeed, the greater the difference in momentum between the segments, the greater the pulling effect will be—implying that the greater the velocity of the arms during the swinging motion or the greater the mass of the arms, the greater the enhancement of jump height associated with an arm swing.

Research has shown that male athletes produce a greater enhancement of jump height during a SVJ when incorporating an arm swing compared to female athletes, although the difference appears to be unrelated to the strength of the upper-body musculature (Walsh et al., 2007). However, strengthening the upper-body joints has been shown to increase jump height during a SVJ (Young, MacDonald, & Flowers, 2001). Other researchers have reported that more skilled jumpers produce greater increases in jump height when incorporating an arm swing (Laffaye, Bardy, & Traiar, 2006). Therefore, enhancing jumping performance with an arm swing may require strengthening exercises for the upper-body musculature and practice to ensure the coordination of the arm motion with that of the other segments during the execution of a jump.

An arm swing can also enhance performance during a SLJ. Specifically, the forward rotation of the body about the CM during flight that is associated with horizontal jumps can be reduced by swinging the arms backward during the flight phase (Ashby & Heegaard, 2002). Indeed, restricting the arm swing during horizontal jumps requires that the excessive forward rotation of the body about the CM be eliminated during the ground contact prior to takeoff. This results in a premature decline in the vertical GRF and an increase in the backward-rotating moment of the GRF about the CM at takeoff, limiting jumping distance (Ashby & Heegaard, 2002).

Manipulating Constraints

The performance of any movement is affected by the specific constraints surrounding the athlete's motor system. The coach can manipulate many of these constraints to influence the performance of the specific movement. For example, manipulating the **task constraints** during a jumping task through the use of an overhead goal that the athlete has to aim for has been shown to increase jump height (Ford et al., 2005). The **instructions** provided to the athlete prior to a movement task as well as the feedback provided upon completion of the task represent **informational constraints** that can also be manipulated by the coach to enhance performance. Research has shown that the provision of instructions to the athlete that result in an external focus of attention lead to enhanced performance (jump height/distance) compared to instructions that result in an internal focus of attention (Porter, Ostrowski, Nolan, & Wu, 2010; Wu,

Porter, & Brown, 2010; Wulf & Dukek, 2009). Such an external focus is achieved by having the athlete focus on an external target during the execution of the jump and results in a greater impulse of the GRF (Wulf & Dufek, 2009). Finally, the provision of feedback has been shown to affect the performance during a jumping task. Specifically, feedback in the form of **knowledge of results**, achieved by providing the peak power output attained after each vertical jump performed in a series, has been shown to increase jumping performance compared to when the peak power output information was withheld from the athlete (Staub et al., 2013). The coach can readily manipulate these constraints when athletes are performing jumping tasks to enhance jumping performance.

Running Jumps

In running jumps, the athlete possesses horizontal motion at the beginning of the ground contact phase preceding takeoff. Performance in running jumps exceeds performance in jumps executed from a standing position, with much greater takeoff velocities being achieved. Indeed, the takeoff velocity during a running long jump (RLJ) can be almost three times greater than that during a SLJ due to the approach speed of the athlete; this speed is positively correlated with jump distance during the RLJ (Hay, 1993). In contrast, an inverse relationship is reported between the approach speed and the takeoff angle during a RLJ (Campos et al., 2013), and the vertical takeoff velocity during RLJ is often less than an athlete could achieve during a SVJ. The approach speeds used in the execution of a running vertical jump (RVJ) are typically less than those associated with a RLJ, yet the takeoff velocities during a RVJ exceed those achieved during a SVJ (Ae et al., 2008).

The completion of a run-up prior to takeoff has been shown to increase the eccentric loading and decrease the ground contact time even when compared to a drop jump (Aura & Viitasalo, 1989). Other differences between running and standing jumps exist as well. For example, running jumps are typically performed with an arm swing, which transforms the horizontal velocity of the CM into vertical velocity at takeoff (Dapena & Chung, 1988; Yu & Andrews, 1998). In addition, running jumps are typically performed unilaterally (due to the rules associated with the track and field event of high jump), and the takeoff leg is placed ahead of the CM at the beginning of the ground contact phase preceding takeoff. This results in greater eccentric loading during the ground contact phase than would be achieved during standing jumps, despite the absence of a discernable countermovement during running jumps (Dapena & Chung, 1988; Graham-Smith & Lees, 2005). Specifically, the CM rises throughout the ground contact phase preceding takeoff during running jumps primarily due to the CM pivoting over the takeoff leg in a RLJ (Graham-Smith & Lees, 2005) and the combination of the pivot mechanism and the centripetal force generated by the curved approach adopted during a RVJ (Dapena & Chung, 1988; Tan & Yeadon, 2005). The unilateral ground contact phase also allows the free leg to swing forward and upward during the propulsive phase of the jump, which aids the vertical velocity of the CM at takeoff (Yu & Andrews, 1998).

Jump height following a run-up is greater during bilateral jumps compared to unilateral jumps due to the greater impulse of the GRF (Vint & Hinrichs, 1996). However, this difference is not as great as might be predicted—only 42% higher as opposed to 50% higher. This reduced difference in jump height is likely due to the **bilateral deficit**. The contribution of the motion of the free leg during the propulsive phase of running jumps to the vertical takeoff velocity of the CM is not as great as the contribution of the takeoff leg (Yu & Andrews, 1998). However, the motion of the free leg as it swings up increases the height of the CM at takeoff in both horizontal and vertical jumps (Dapena & Chung, 1988; Vint & Hinrichs, 1996).

Running Long Jumps

When maximizing the horizontal distance during a jump following a run-up, the athlete is required to minimize the loss of horizontal velocity of the CM during the final ground contact phase prior to takeoff while concomitantly attempting to maximize the vertical velocity of the CM. Moreover, the generation of vertical velocity appears to be more important than the minimization of the loss of horizontal velocity during takeoff (Campos et al., 2013; Graham-Smith & Lees, 2005). In an effort to create this effect, the athlete places the takeoff foot in front of the CM at touchdown such that the athlete is actually leaning back, inducing a **braking phase** where the horizontal component of the GRF acts in opposition to the motion of the CM. The backward lean results in the CM being relatively low at touchdown, and the vertical displacement of the CM increases during the ground contact phase until takeoff despite the knee joint initially flexing during the braking phase (Table 11.3).

The rise of the CM during the ground contact phase is caused by the **pivot mechanism**, whereby the CM is rotated about the takeoff leg, allowing the transformation of large horizontal velocity of the CM at touchdown into vertical velocity of the CM takeoff, and increasing the takeoff angle and horizontal distance of the jump (Graham-Smith & Lees, 2005). The pivot mechanism requires high eccentric loading during the braking phase to allow strain potential energy stored in the active musculotendinous

Table 11.3
Kinematic Variables During the Ground Contact Phase Prior to Takeoff for Elite Long Jump Athletes

Mechanical Variable	Events During Unilateral Stance		
	Touchdown	Maximum Knee Flexion	Takeoff
CM horizontal velocity (m/s)	9.93	8.64	8.55
CM vertical velocity (m/s)	−0.18	2.29	3.37
Angle of CM velocity (degrees)	−1	15	22
CM height (m)	0.98	1.04	1.27
Distance from CM to takeoff foot (m)	0.55	0.03	−0.44
Hip angle (degrees)	146	157	201
Knee angle (degrees)	167	140	169

Notes: CM = center of mass. The angle of CM velocity is expressed relative to the right horizontal, with positive values reflecting a counterclockwise direction. Distance from CM to takeoff foot represents the horizontal displacement between the two, with positive values reflecting the CM being behind the takeoff foot.

Reproduced from Campos, J., Gámez, J., Encarnación, A., Guitiérrez-Dávila, M., Rojas, J., & Wallace, E. S. (2013). Three-dimensional kinematics during the take-off phase in competitive long jumping. *International Journal of Sports Science and Coaching, 8,* 395–406.

units to be returned during the subsequent propulsive phase. The braking phase lasts approximately 47 ms in well-trained long jumpers (Campos et al., 2013), and there is a large peak generated in the GRF associated with the impact of the takeoff leg during this phase. High **leg stiffness** is required to prevent the collapse of the takeoff leg, which explains the influence of leg stiffness on the generation of sufficient vertical velocity of the CM at takeoff, and therefore jumping distance, during a RLJ (Seyfarth, Friedrichs, Wank, & Blickhan, 1999). However, the stiffness of the leg must be modulated appropriately to account for changes in the horizontal velocity and the distance that the foot is placed ahead of the CM at touchdown if jump performance is to be maximized (Seyfarth et al., 1999). Each athlete likely has his or her own optimal leg stiffness commensurate with the specific technique adopted during the execution of a RLJ.

The motion of the free limbs during a unilateral RLJ (e.g., arms, contralateral leg) also causes the CM to rise during the ground contact phase. This effect is responsible for transforming the horizontal velocity at touchdown into the vertical velocity at takeoff, although its contribution to this transformation is not as great as the pivot mechanism provided by the takeoff leg (Yu & Andrews, 1998).

The posture adopted by the athlete at takeoff during a RLJ produces a GRF that acts behind the CM in the sagittal plane. This factor, combined with the linear and angular velocities possessed by the segments, results in negative angular momentum of the body about the mediolateral axis at takeoff, which then tends to rotate the athlete forward during the flight phase (Bouchouras, Moscha, Papaiakovou, Nikodelis, & Kollias, 2009). To prevent this rotation, the athlete could increase the mass moment of inertia about the mediolateral axis—an effect achieved through the "hang" technique adopted by some jumpers. Alternatively, the athlete could transfer some of the angular momentum into the arm and leg segments by rotating these segments during flight—an effect achieved through the "hitch-kick" technique (Figure 11.3). The "hitch-kick" technique produces greater negative angular momentum of the body at takeoff compared to the "hang" technique, which in turn prevents the athlete from falling backward upon landing, maximizing the overall jumping distance (Bouchouras et al., 2009).

Running Vertical Jumps

When performing a jump for maximal vertical height following a run-up, there are a number of differences compared to a RLJ. First, the approach speeds are less during a RVJ compared to a RLJ. Second, the athlete typically follows a curved path during a RVJ, such as that observed during the high jump event in track and field. The athlete leans in toward the center of the curve, and the radius of the curve diminishes as the athlete approaches the takeoff point. The increase in centripetal force acting on the athlete due to the reduced radius of this curved path results in an increase in vertical velocity of the CM at takeoff by rotating the athlete about the anterio-posterior axis of the CM (Dapena & Chung, 1988; Tan & Yeadon, 2005). Third, the athlete tends to lean back during the final stance phase prior to takeoff, with the takeoff foot being positioned well ahead of the CM. This increases the eccentric loading of the musculotendinous units as well as the vertical displacement of the CM during the propulsive phase (Dapena & Chung, 1988). The motion of the free limbs (e.g., arms, contralateral leg) acts during ground contact just as it does during the SLJ. Collectively, these actions result in vertical velocities at takeoff in excess of 4.50 m/s in well-trained high jump athletes (Ae et al., 2008).

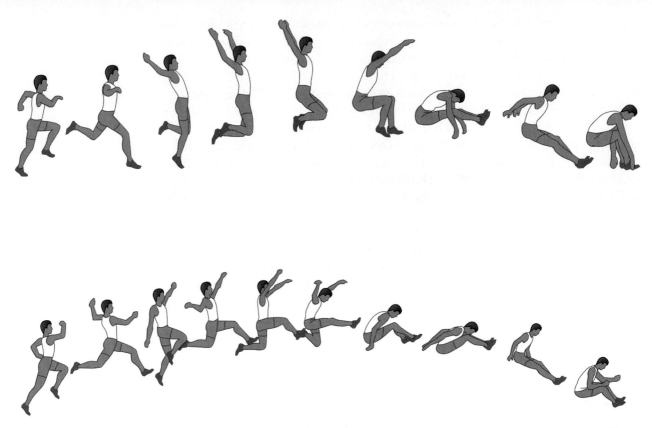

Figure 11.3 The "hang" and the "hitch-kick" techniques used to reduce the rate of rotation of the athlete during the flight phase of a running long jump. The "hang" technique increases the mass moment of inertia of the body, while the "hitch-kick" technique allows the angular momentum of the trunk segment to be transferred into the arms and legs as they rotate during flight.

Predictive Analysis of Jumping

A **predictive approach** to jumping requires the development of computer-generated mathematical models of the human motor system. These simulation models allow researchers to manipulate a wealth of biomechanical variables—including muscular strength, timing of muscle activation, and tendon characteristics—to determine the most important factors influencing jumping performance. Once these "limiting" factors are identified, methods to improve them can be developed.

Most of the simulation models have been developed for a SVJ. When using one such model, Pandy (1990) reported that jump height is most sensitive to increases in the muscular strength-to-body weight ratio. This finding would appear to confirm the dependence of jumping performance on the generation of the impulse of the GRF and the dependence on the GRF on joint moments of force, which themselves depend on the forces generated by the active muscles. However, Bobbert and van Soest (1994) reported that simply increasing muscular strength is not enough to increase jump height and could, in fact, lead to a decrease in jump height. These authors identified that a change in the timing of the activation of the muscles is required to transform the increase in muscular strength into increased jump height. Their findings were confirmed by Nagano and Gerritsen (2001), who reported that simultaneous increases in maximal isometric force, maximal muscle shortening velocity, and maximal activation amplitude of the muscles result in an increase in jump height only when the timing of muscle activation is appropriately altered. These authors also noted that the greatest improvements in jump height are attributable to the strengthening of the knee extensors. Others, however, have reported that the increase in jump height is more sensitive to increasing the strength of the knee and ankle extensors (Cheng, 2008). Strengthening the musculature around the shoulder joint results in the smallest increase in vertical jump height (Cheng, 2008). Collectively, the results of these simulation studies suggest that a training program for improving vertical jump performance should include exercises to increase muscular strength, particularly of the knee and ankle musculature, but also jump-related exercises that allow the athlete to modify his or her technique appropriately to take advantage of the increased muscular strength.

Fewer simulation studies have sought to investigate the biomechanical factors influencing performance during horizontal jumps. Seyfarth, Blickhan, and Van Leeuwen (2000) developed a model of the final ground contact of a RLJ. In this model, jumping performance was insensitive to muscle shortening velocity and tendon compliance. However, the maximal isometric strength of the knee extensor muscles as well as the eccentric strength of these muscles conferred considerable influence on the distance jumped, with increases in these muscular properties resulting in increased jump performance.

Qualitative Analysis of Jumping Performance

In this section, we use the four-stage model of qualitative analysis developed by Knudson and Morrison (2002) to address jumping performance. This model includes four stages: preparation, observation, evaluation/diagnosis, and intervention.

Preparation Stage

In the initial preparation stage of a qualitative analysis, the coach should identify the critical features of the jumping task from biomechanical principles and develop a deterministic model of the skill to aid the analysis of the movement. Table 11.4 identifies some basic biomechanical principles and indicates their application to technique analysis during jumping tasks.

Figure 11.4 provides an example of a deterministic model for performance in a running long jump. Following the identification of the critical features of the jumping task, the coach should identify the movement phases for the observation of the technique. Table 11.5 shows the movement phases for the analysis of running jumps.

Observation Stage

Coaches should place themselves so that they view the performance of the jump from the side, as the major motions of the body segments involved in the execution of a jumping task occur in the sagittal plane. Exceptions to this are running long jumps, where pelvic motion in the frontal plane (lateral pelvic tilt) may occur during the ground contact phase, and certain executions of running vertical jumps, where a curved approach and rotations about the longitudinal axis through the CM can complicate the positioning of the coach during observation. If a video camera is used to supplement the observations of the coach, then ascertaining the fast movements

Table 11.4
Biomechanical Principles That Can Be Applied in the Qualitative Analysis of Jumping Technique

Principle	Application to Jumping Tasks
Use of the stretch–shortening cycle	Assess whether the athlete incorporates a preparatory countermovement (standing jumps) or a braking phase (running jumps) during the ground contact phase prior to takeoff.
Number of body segments	Assess the number of segments accelerated by the athlete during the execution of the jump. For example, determine if an arm swing is incorporated (standing jumps) and assess the action of the free limbs (running jumps) during the ground contact phase prior to takeoff.
Coordination of body segments	Assess the order of rotation of the body segments during the propulsive phase of the ground contact phase prior to takeoff so as to determine the proximal-to-distal sequence at the hip, knee, and ankle joints. Assess the position of the free limbs at the beginning of the propulsive phase; for example, are the arms and the free leg beginning their upward movement?
Maximizing the acceleration path	Determine the change in height of the CM by assessing the position of the pelvis from touchdown to takeoff of the ground contact phase.
Path of projection	Assess the path of the CM during the flight phase by observing the position of the pelvis to establish the height, angle, and speed at takeoff.

Note: CM = center of mass.

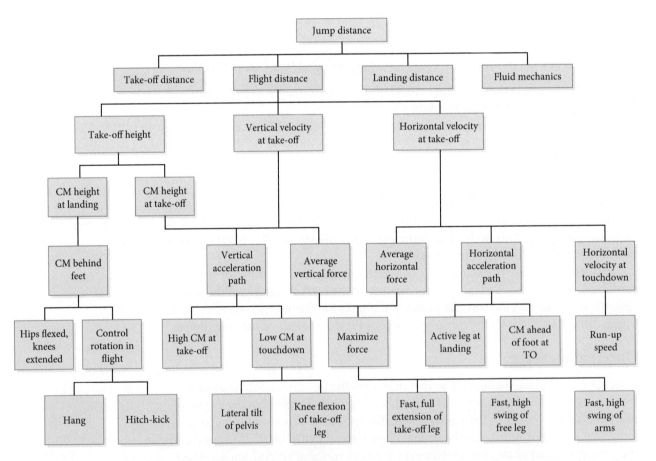

Figure 11.4 A deterministic model highlighting the critical biomechanical features involved in the performance of a running long jump for maximal horizontal distance.

Data from Bartlett, R. (2007). *Introduction to sports biomechanics: Analysing human movement patterns*. London, UK: Routledge.

Table 11.5

Movement Phases for the Analysis of Technique During Running Jumps

Movement Phase	Details
Approach	Ends at touchdown of takeoff leg at the beginning of ground contact.
Ground contact	Begins at touchdown of the takeoff leg.
	Ends with takeoff.
	Contains the phases of braking (touchdown until the point of maximum flexion of the knee joint) and propulsion (end of braking until takeoff).
Flight	Begins at takeoff and ends with landing.
Landing	Begins at contact after flight.

associated with jumping tasks requires a relatively high shutter speed, with a speed of 1/100 s being suggested (Bartlett, 2007).

Evaluation/Diagnosis Stage

The athlete's performance during the execution of a jump can be evaluated by assessing the biomechanical features during each of the movement phases pertinent to the specific jumping task. Table 11.6 outlines a method to evaluate the biomechanical

Table 11.6

Evaluation of the Biomechanical Principles During the Different Movement Phases Associated with the Technique During Running Jumps

Movement Phase	Biomechanical Principle	Evaluation
Ground contact	Use of SSC	Was the takeoff leg placed ahead of the CM at touchdown?
	Number of body segments	Was an arm swing incorporated?
		Was the free leg motion appropriate?
	Coordination of body segments	In horizontal jumps, was the CM projected ahead of the takeoff leg at takeoff?
		Was there proximal-to-distal sequencing of rotations of the trunk, thigh, and leg segments during the propulsive phase?
		Did the arms and the free leg begin their upward motion at the beginning of the propulsive phase?
	Acceleration path	What was the vertical position of the CM at touchdown?
		How much did the CM rise during the braking phase?
		How much did the CM rise during the propulsive phase?
Flight	Path of projection	Did the CM possess appropriate horizontal and/or vertical speed commensurate with the goal of the jump?

Note: SSC = stretch–shortening cycle; CM = center of mass.

principles during the different movement phases associated with the technique during running jumps.

The correction of identified weaknesses in jumping performance can be prioritized as follows:

- Look at the sequence of features for each phase of movement.
- Prioritize critical features that maximize performance improvements.
- Prioritize critical features based on which will be easiest to improve.

Intervention Stage

After identifying the athlete's areas of weakness during the evaluation/diagnosis stage of the qualitative analysis, the strength and conditioning coach needs to develop an intervention to improve jumping performance. Most observations of motor skills are undertaken in situations where the athlete is removed from the typical task and environmental constraints that he or she must operate within during the actual sporting situation. The strength and conditioning practitioner is likely to observe the athlete jumping in a well-controlled environment to ease the analysis of the movement. Consequently, this observed skill may not be representative of how the athlete executes a jumping movement in the actual sport, which may lead to the selection of inappropriate interventions to improve performance.

Interventions to Improve Jumping Performance

A variety of training methods to improve jumping performance can be incorporated into an athlete's wider training program. Given the importance of generating an appropriate ground reaction impulse during any jumping task, methods to improve muscular strength are clearly important. Furthermore, given that the execution of jumping tasks needs to be coupled with environmental information during all sports, training methods that enhance the attunement of the athlete's jumping ability to the relevant environmental information are required as well. This section first addresses jumping-specific methods to improve muscular strength, then discusses representative learning for jumping tasks where task constraints are manipulated to improve jumping performance.

Resistance Training Methods

Table 11.7 displays each of the indices of muscular strength, and identifies the relationship between them and jumping performance. Resistance training has been shown to be an effective method to improve the indices of muscular strength; likewise, resistance training methods, including heavy resistance exercises and plyometric exercise, have been shown to improve jumping performance (Markovic, 2007; Perez-Gomes & Calbet, 2013).

Gains in muscular strength are specific to the resistance training exercises used. Given this fact, the coach should be mindful of the following mechanical variables associated with the resistance training exercises and the jumping task:

- Movement patterns
- Force magnitude

Table 11.7
Indices of Muscular Strength and Their Application to Jumping Performance

Strength Index	Description
Voluntary maximal dynamic strength	Maximal dynamic strength strongly correlated with SVJ performance (Wisløff, Castagna, Helgerud, Jones, & Hoff, 2004).
	Strong positive correlations between 1-RM back squat and PPO in loaded CMJ even under low load conditions (Stone et al., 2003).
Voluntary maximal isometric strength	Peak isometric force during a pulling movement (hip angle 170–175°; knee angle 120–135°) strongly correlated with CMJ and SJ height (Kraska et al., 2009).
	Peak force during a pulling movement (hip angle 124°; knee angle 141°) significantly correlated with CMJ and SJ height (Kawamori et al., 2006).
Speed-strength	Speed-strength strongly correlated with RVJ and SVJ height (Young, Wilson, & Byrne, 1999).
Explosive strength	PRFD recorded during an isometric pulling movement strongly related to both SJ and CMJ height (Kraska et al., 2009).
	Late RFD (more than 250 ms) more strongly correlated than early RFD (Kraska et al., 2009).
	PRFD during single-joint isometric testing significantly correlated with CMJ (Jarić, Ristanovic, & Corcos, 1989).
Reactive strength	Reactive strength correlated with both vertical and horizontal standing jump performance (Ball & Zanetti, 2012).
	Reactive strength, as assessed by DJ performance, more strongly correlated with RVJ than SVJ (Young et al., 1999).

Note: CMJ = countermovement vertical jump; DJ = drop jump; PPO = peak power output; PRFD = peak rate of force development; RFD = rate of force development; RVJ = running vertical jump; SJ = static vertical jump; SVJ = standing vertical jump.

- Rate of force development
- Acceleration and velocity parameters
- Ballistic versus non-ballistic movements

Jumping is a multijoint, closed-kinetic chain movement whereby a force is applied to the ground via the legs during the ground contact phase. Moreover, jumping is ballistic such that the CM possesses momentum at takeoff.

Resistance Training Methods to Increase Maximal Muscular Strength

Increases in maximal muscular strength require the use of heavy external loads (80% or more 1-repetition maximum [RM]) during resistance training exercises, with the completion of multiple sets (Ratamess, 2012). The high intensities involved in maximal strength workouts require relatively long inter-set rest periods.

The resistance training exercises selected should consist of multijoint exercises that are also closed-kinetic chain, requiring large forces to be exerted by the extensor muscles of the hip, knee, and ankle joints. In particular, the back squat and the deadlift exercises are recommended. However, neither of these exercises is ballistic, so their mechanical specificity is limited. For example, back squats have been shown to require a different muscle activation pattern compared to jumping tasks (Robertson, Wilson, & St. Pierre, 2008), presumably due to the different requirements associated with the non-ballistic back squat compared to the ballistic jump. Recall that increases in maximal muscular strength may underpin improvements in other indices of muscular strength. Therefore, both back squats and deadlifts are promoted as a general resistance exercise in the development of muscular strength to enhance jumping performance. Table 11.8 outlines a resistance training workout to increase maximal dynamic muscular strength using the back squat and deadlift.

Eccentric resistance training has been suggested to elicit greater gains in maximal muscular strength than conventional exercises utilizing the SSC (Aagaard, 2010). Furthermore, increased eccentric strength of the knee extensors may potentially improve running long jump performance (Seyfarth et al., 2000). Unfortunately, there is a paucity of research on the appropriate acute program variables for an eccentric resistance

Table 11.8
A Resistance Training Workout to Increase Maximal Dynamic Muscular Strength and Improve Jumping Performance

Acute Program Variable	Description
Exercise selection	Multijoint, closed-kinetic chain exercises including the back squat and the deadlift.
	As these exercises are not ballistic, they can be considered general exercises for jumping performance.
Volume and intensity	80–100% 1-RM for 8–1 repetitions, for multiple sets (≥ 3).
Rest periods	2–3 min between sets.
Repetition velocity	Moderate velocity during barbell descent with attempted high velocity during barbell ascent.
Instructions to athlete	Have the athlete focus on the motion of the barbell throughout the lift.
	Instruct the athlete to exert the force "as fast and as hard as possible" during barbell ascent.
Modifications	Use of chains to increase the force during barbell ascent (chains provide 15–20% of the barbell load at the end of the ascent).
	Use of elastic bands to increase the force during barbell ascent (bands provide 15–30% of barbell load at the end of ascent).
	Perform unilateral exercises.

Note: 1-RM = one-repetition maximum.

training workout for the lower-body musculature; making specific recommendations is, in turn, difficult.

Increases in maximal isometric strength, particularly of the knee extensors and ankle plantar flexors, have been proposed to increase SVJ and RLJ performance (Seyfarth et al., 2000). Isometric resistance training of the ankle plantar flexors has been shown to increase SVJ height (Burgess, Connick, Graham-Smith, & Pearson, 2007). Increases in maximal isometric exercises during multijoint tasks involving the hip, knee, and ankle musculature, such as during isometric back squats or pulling movements, may be effective at improving jumping performance given the near-isometric operation of the biarticular muscles during jumping tasks (Umberger, 1998).

Resistance Training Methods to Increase Speed-Strength

Low-load speed-strength assessed in a jump-specific movement (squat jumps with loads less than 30% back squat 1-RM) has been shown to improve with training involving unloaded vertical jumps (Cormie et al., 2007). In the research study, this training program did not elicit any improvements in high-load speed-strength (squat jumps with loads more than 30% back squat 1-RM), as the principle of mechanical specificity would dictate. Nevertheless, a combination of unloaded jumps and heavy back squats (90% 1-RM) used in the same workout increased both low-load and high-load speed-strength in a jump-specific movement as well as maximal dynamic muscular strength (Cormie et al., 2007).

Table 11.9 outlines a resistance training workout combining low-load squat jump and heavy back squat exercises to elicit improvements in both low-load and high-load speed-strength in jump-specific movements.

Resistance Training Methods to Increase Explosive Strength

Explosive muscular strength is determined by the rate of force development (RFD); RFD, in turn, is divided into early (less than 50 ms) and late (150 ms or longer) periods (Andersen & Aagaard, 2006). This division into early and late RFD relates to the propulsive phases associated with running jumps (approximately 80 ms) and standing jumps (approximately 300 ms), respectively (Campos et al., 2013; Jones & Caldwell, 2003). Late RFD depends more heavily on maximal muscular strength than early RFD; the latter is more influenced by neural factors and myosin heavy chain composition (Andersen & Aagaard, 2006). Indeed, late RFD responds favorably to high-intensity resistance training that elicits an improvement in maximal isometric muscular strength (Andersen, Andersen, Zebis, & Aagaard, 2010). Andersen et al. (2005) reported that a period of detraining following RT resulted in an increased proportion of type IIX fibers, which was paralleled by an increase in RFD. However, a concomitant decrease in muscle mass occurred during the detraining period, which may negate any enhancement in performance due to the fiber type changes. Eccentric resistance training has been proposed as a method to improve RFD (Aagaard, 2010), although specific recommendations for the development of eccentric resistance training workouts are currently lacking in the literature.

Plyometric training exercises, defined as those involving the SSC, have been shown to improve both RFD and vertical jump performance (Burgess et al., 2007). In a review of the extant literature, plyometric training was suggested to elicit greater improvements in SVJ involving a countermovement compared to drop jump

Table 11.9

A Resistance Training Workout Combining Low-Load Squat Jumps and Heavy Back Squats to Increase Both Low-Load and High-Load Speed-Strength and Improve Jumping Performance

Acute Program Variable	Description
Exercise selection	Multijoint, closed-kinetic chain exercises including the squat jumps and back squats. The squat jumps are ballistic; the back squats are non-ballistic.
Volume and intensity	6 repetitions of unloaded squat jumps for 7 sets. 3 repetitions of back squats with 90% 1-RM for 3 sets.
Rest periods	2–3 min between sets.
Exercise order	Squat jumps completed prior to heavy back squats.
Repetition velocity	Squat jumps performed for maximum jump height. Moderate velocity during barbell descent, with attempted high velocity during barbell ascent in the back squat.
Instructions to athlete	Instruct the athlete to jump for maximal height during the squat jumps. Have the athlete focus on the motion of the barbell throughout the lift. Instruct the athlete to exert the force "as fast and as hard as possible" during barbell ascent.
Modifications	Use of an external goal during the jumps to increase jump height. Provision of knowledge of results after each jump via either a contact mat or linear position transducer. Use of chains to increase the force during barbell ascent (chains provide 15–20% of the barbell load at the end of the ascent) of the back squat. Use of elastic bands to increase the force during barbell ascent (bands provide 15–30% of barbell load at the end of ascent) of the back squat. Perform unilateral exercises. Perform the heavy back squats prior to the squat jumps to elicit post-activity potentiation.

Note: 1-RM = one-repetition maximum.

performance, presumably due to the differences in SSC times during each of the movements (Markovic, 2007). A combination of heavy resistance training exercises (56–85% 1-RM), loaded squat jumps (load equivalent to approximately 30% back squat 1-RM), and unloaded vertical jumps has been shown to elicit greater gains in RFD than either of the training modes performed in isolation (de Villareal, Izquierdo, & Gonzalez-Badillo, 2011).

Resistance Training Methods to Increase Reactive Strength

Plyometric training appears to be effective in increasing jump-specific measures of reactive strength (drop jump performance) (Ramirez-Campillo, Andrade, & Izquierdo, 2013), and drop jumps appear to be more effective than other plyometric exercises in increasing reactive strength, as the concept of mechanical specificity would dictate. Table 11.10 describes a plyometric workout using drop jumps to improve reactive strength (Byrne, Moran, Rankin, & Kinsella, 2010). Reactive strength is related to leg

Table 11.10
A Plyometric Training Workout Using Drop Jumps to Improve Reactive Strength

Acute Program Variable	Description
Exercise selection	Drop jumps.
Volume and intensity	3 sets of 10 repetitions from a height that maximizes drop jump height.
Rest periods	2 min between sets; 15 s between jumps.
Repetition velocity	Jumps are performed for maximal height.
Instructions to athlete	Instruct the athlete to "jump for maximal height."
Modifications	Use of an external goal during the jumps to increase jump height.
	Provision of knowledge of results after each jump via either a contact mat or linear position transducer.
	Perform unilateral jumps.
	Perform heavy back squats prior to the jumps to elicit post-activity potentiation.

stiffness, so resistance training methods to improve measures of stiffness are likely to increase jumping performance. A combination of heavy resistance exercises and plyometric exercises can increase knee joint stiffness, while producing a concomitant increase in vertical jump performance (Toumi, Best, Martin, & Poumarat, 2004).

Other Resistance Training Methods to Improve Jumping Performance

Other resistance training methods have also been proposed to improve jumping performance, including assisted jump training and the use of whole-body vibration protocols.

Assisted jump training involves a reduction in body weight via the use of elastic bands attached to the athlete during the execution of the jumps (Tran, Brown, Coburn, Lynn, & Dabbs, 2012). The elastic bands should reduce body weight by 10–40% to elicit improvements in takeoff velocity and jump height that result in improved jumping performance following a period of training with this method.

The application of **whole-body vibration** (WBV) prior to the execution of jumps can improve jumping performance as well (Dabbs, Tran, Garner, & Brown, 2012). Table 11.11 shows a recommended protocol using WBV during a plyometric workout. Note, however, that evidence of the effectiveness of WBV in conjunction with jump training is currently lacking (Perez-Gomes & Calbet, 2013).

Consideration should be given to strengthening the upper-body musculature when developing a resistance training program to enhance jumping performance (Young et al., 2001). Indeed, more skilled jumpers appear to be better able to coordinate the arm swing during jumping tasks so as to take advantage of the enhancement proffered by the arm swing (Laffaye et al., 2006). Therefore, the coach should ensure practice is provided to allow athlete to effectively coordinate arm swing into the movement.

Table 11.11
A Whole-Body Vibration Protocol to Be Used During a Plyometric
Workout to Increase Jumping Performance

Variable	Description
Frequency and amplitude of vibration	30 Hz at an amplitude of 2–4 mm.
	50 Hz at an amplitude of 4–6 mm.
Exercise performed during vibration	30–60 s of quarter-squats at a 5-s cadence.
Rest period prior to jumps	0–4 min.
	The coach should have the athlete complete the protocol with different rest periods to find the optimal periods.

Data from Dabbs, N. C., Tran, T. T., Garner, J. C., & Brown, L. E. (2012). A brief review: Using whole-body vibration to increase acute power output and vertical jump performance. *Strength and Conditioning Journal, 34,* 78–84.

Finally, muscular strength represents an organismic constraint influencing the movements exhibited by the athlete during jumping tasks. In recognition of this factor, the strength and conditioning practitioner should allow athletes to explore their movement capabilities and attune their movements to the sources of environment information relevant to their specific sports.

In many sports, the execution of a jump does not occur in isolation, but rather occurs as part of a sequence of movements. The strength and conditioning practitioner should recognize that these movement sequences will emerge from the confluence of constraints acting upon the athlete during the sport. This understanding requires the practitioner to consider representative learning practices to promote effective perception–action couplings.

Representative Learning Practices for Jumping

The jumps performed by athletes within their sports require that the execution of the movement be coupled with the environmental information available to them. The environmental information to which athletes are required to attune their jumping movements may be derived from the location of a ball to be intercepted or an opponent to avoid, in games such as basketball, volleyball, or soccer. It is unlikely that these jumps will be maximal; instead, the required height of the jump is determined by the location of the projectile or the location of the opponent. Furthermore, the athlete may be required to change direction upon landing from the jump depending on the demands of the task. It is also unlikely that every jump will be performed under optimal mechanical conditions due to the posture of the athlete at the beginning of each jump.

Given these variations, athletes need practices that allow them to recalibrate their action-scaled affordances following improvements in organismic constraints such as muscular strength. As such, representative learning practices where athletes are required to couple their jumping movements to the environmental information experienced in their sports may help improve their performance.

In volleyball, a player has to jump to intercept the ball, either offensively (e.g., spiking) or defensively (e.g., blocking). The player must therefore be able to attune his or her vertical jumps to sources of environmental information including the position of the other players and the motion of the ball. Table 11.12 and Table 11.13 present examples of representative learning practices to enhance perception–action coupling while still having the athlete complete a jumping workout.

Table 11.12

A Representative Learning Practice to Promote Perception–Action Coupling for Volleyball Players Using Spike Jumps

Description of tasks	▪ The coach is positioned at the net and tosses the ball to an individual player, who is required to spike the ball. This requires the athlete to couple the jumps with the motion of the ball. ▪ The balls are tossed at different heights. If the ball is not at a height that permits a jump and spike, then the player is required to set the ball (bump) and spike it. This permits the execution of running jumps or standing jumps depending on the requirement to spike or set, then spike. ▪ The balls are tossed to different positions along the net. This requires the player to modulate the approach speed to successfully intercept the ball. ▪ The individual player begins from a different position on the court such that he or she is required to perform running jumps from different approach speeds.
Volume and intensity	▪ The number of running jumps and standing jumps should be determined by the coach before the workout. ▪ 3 sets of 10 repetitions. ▪ The total volume should vary between 60 and 250 foot contacts for beginners and between 120 and 450 foot contacts for advanced athletes, depending on the time of the season. ▪ Running jumps are considered to be more intense than standing jumps.
Rest periods	▪ 2 min between sets; 15 s between jumps. ▪ During inter-set rest periods, the coach engages the player by asking the following questions to enhance the calibration of action-based affordances: ▪ "What height does the ball need to be to allow you to spike the ball?" ▪ "What is the approach speed that allows you to maximize your jump height?"
Manipulation of task constraints	▪ High ball toss: The player determines that the ball is jumpable and spikes the ball by executing a running vertical jump. ▪ Low ball toss: The player determines that the ball is not jumpable, resets the ball by bumping it, and then spikes the ball by executing a standing vertical jump. ▪ Ball tossed close to the net: The player alters the approach speed accordingly. ▪ Ball tossed over the player: The player alters the takeoff position accordingly. ▪ Starting position of player on court: The player alters the approach speed accordingly.
Coaching analysis	▪ Assess the height achieved (relative to net) during each jump. ▪ Assess the player position (vertical and horizontal) relative to the ball at ball contact. ▪ Assess the depth and speed of the countermovement/braking phase. ▪ Assess the coordination of the arm swing during the countermovement/braking and propulsive phases. ▪ Assess the approach speed. ▪ Assess the location of the ball in the opposing court after it has been spiked.

Table 11.13
A Representative Learning Practice to Promote Perception–Action Coupling for Volleyball Players Using Small-Sided Games

Description of tasks	■ Two players line up on opposite sides of the net. ■ Each court is reduced in size. ■ A rule is instigated that a minimum of two touches are required before the ball crosses the net. ■ A point is awarded only when a jump spike scores.
Volume and rest periods	■ Each game lasts 2 min. ■ 3 games are played, separated by 2 min. ■ During inter-game rest periods, the coach engages the player by asking the following questions: 　■ "What height does the ball need to be to allow you to spike the ball?" 　■ "What is the approach speed that allows you to maximize your jump height?"
Manipulation of task constraints	■ Court dimensions: Increasing the dimensions will result in more running jumps. Decreasing the court dimensions will result in more standing jumps. ■ Number of players: Increasing the number of players requires more accurate spiking, reduces the number of jumps performed by each player, and reduces the number of running jumps.
Coaching analysis	■ Assess the height achieved (relative to net) during each jump. ■ Assess the player position (vertical and horizontal) relative to the ball at ball contact. ■ Assess the depth and speed of the countermovement/braking phase. ■ Assess the coordination of the arm swing during the countermovement/braking and propulsive phases. ■ Assess the approach speed. ■ Assess the location of the ball in the opposing court after it has been spiked.

The general progression of the resistance training methods and representative learning practices that can be used by the strength and conditioning practitioner to develop jumping ability in athletes is shown in Table 11.14.

Chapter Summary

Performance in vertical and horizontal jumps is determined largely by the velocity of the center of mass at takeoff. As a consequence, jump performance is largely determined by the impulse of the ground reaction force or the work done during

Table 11.14

A Continuum of Workouts Incorporating Resistance Training and Representative Practices to Improve Jumping Performance

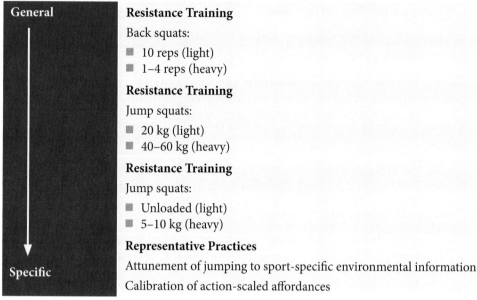

General	**Resistance Training**
	Back squats:
	▪ 10 reps (light)
	▪ 1–4 reps (heavy)
	Resistance Training
	Jump squats:
	▪ 20 kg (light)
	▪ 40–60 kg (heavy)
	Resistance Training
	Jump squats:
	▪ Unloaded (light)
	▪ 5–10 kg (heavy)
	Representative Practices
	Attunement of jumping to sport-specific environmental information
Specific	Calibration of action-scaled affordances

Data from Baker, D. (1996). Improving vertical jump performance through general, special, and specific strength training: A brief review. *Strength and Conditioning Journal, 10*, 131–136.

propulsion. The moments at the lower-body joints are transformed into the resultant GRF, and the monoarticular muscles crossing the lower-body joints perform work and generate energy during the propulsive phase of jumps; meanwhile, the biarticular muscles transport the energy distally while also controlling the direction of the GRF.

Jumping performance can be enhanced by incorporating a countermovement prior to takeoff. Executing a countermovement prior to the propulsive phase of a vertical jump increases the velocity of the CM at takeoff. During a horizontal jump, the countermovement allows the CM to be placed ahead of the GRF prior to takeoff.

Incorporating an arm swing also enhances jumping performance by increasing the velocity of the CM at takeoff during vertical jumps and limiting the reduction in the GRF prior to takeoff in horizontal jumps. An external focus of attention enhances vertical jump performance, as does the provision of feedback about the height achieved during the jump.

Performance during running vertical and horizontal jumps is greater than that achieved during standing jumps due to the increased eccentric loading experienced by the takeoff leg and the motion of the free limbs (arms, contralateral leg). A curved run-up is typically incorporated when executing a running vertical jump that increases the vertical velocity of the CM at takeoff due to the centripetal force acting on the athlete.

Given the influence of the GRF on jumping performance, resistance training methods improve jumping performance. The strength and conditioning practitioner should also incorporate representative learning practices to support enhanced perception–action coupling.

Review Questions and Projects

1. Which mechanical variables influence vertical displacement undergone by the CM during a standing vertical jump?

2. What are the mechanical determinants of horizontal displacement of the CM during a standing long jump?

3. Explain the differences in performing jumps from a run-up versus from a standing position with respect to the jumps' mechanical determinants.

4. Explain the role of the arm swing in enhancing performance during standing jumps.

5. Explain the difference between jumping and reaching with one versus two hands on the height achieved during a vertical jump to intercept a projectile.

6. Describe the roles of takeoff distance, flight distance, and landing distance during horizontal jumps.

7. Explain how a countermovement can affect a standing vertical jump.

8. Explain how a countermovement can affect a standing horizontal jump.

9. Explain the biomechanical differences between bilateral and unilateral jumps.

10. Why does the CM continue to rise throughout the final ground contact phases prior to takeoff associated with running vertical and running long jumps?

11. What is the importance of the free leg during unilateral jumping tasks?

12. Explain how the run-up can be modified when performing a running vertical jump and what the mechanical effects of the modification are.

13. What is the importance of the tendon function of biarticular muscles during jumping tasks?

14. Why is the braking phase prior to propulsion important during the execution of running jumps?

15. Explain why the angular momentum possessed by the athlete during the flight phase of a horizontal jump is beneficial upon landing.

16. Which "limiting factors" have been identified in the predictive analyses of vertical jumping?

17. Explain how a strength and conditioning practitioner can use contact mats and/or linear position transducers to enhance jumping performance.

18. Develop a resistance training workout to improve the jumping performance of a basketball player.

19. Explain the potential problems of performing jumps in isolation during practice for a basketball player.

20. Develop a representative learning practice specific to basketball to enhance the attunement of jumping performance with sources of environmental information.

References

Aagaard, P. (2010). The use of eccentric strength training to enhance maximal muscle strength, explosive force (RFD) and muscular power: Consequences for athletic performance. *Open Sports Sciences Journal, 3*, 52–55.

Abdelkrim, N. B., El Fazaa, S., & El Ati, J. (2007). Time–motion analysis and physiological data for elite under-19-year-old basketball players during competition. *British Journal Sports Medicine, 41*, 69–75. 2007.

Ae, M., Nagahara, R., Ohshima, Y., Koyama, H., Takamoto, M., & Shibayama, K. (2008). Biomechanical analysis of the top three male high jumpers at the 2007 World Championships in athletics. *New Studies in Athletics, 23*, 45–52.

Andersen, L. L., & Aagaard, P. (2006). Influence of maximal muscle strength and intrinsic muscle contractile properties on contractile rate of force development. *European Journal of Applied Physiology, 96*, 46–52.

Andersen, L. L., Andersen, J. L., Magnusson, S. P., Suetta, C., Madsen, J. L., Christensen, L. R., & Aagaard, P. (2005). Changes in the human muscle force–velocity relationship in response to resistance training and subsequent detraining. *Journal of Applied Physiology, 99*, 87–94.

Andersen, L. L., Andersen, J. L., Zebis, M. K., & Aagaard, P. (2010). Early and late rate of force development: Differential adaptive responses to resistance training. *Scandinavian Journal of Medicine and Science in Sports, 20*, 162–169.

Ashby, B. M., & Heegaard, J. H. (2002). Role of arm motion in the standing long jump. *Journal of Biomechanics, 35*, 1631–1637.

Aura, O., & Viitasalo, J. T. (1989). Biomechanical characteristics of jumping. *International Journal of Sports Biomechanics, 5*, 89–98.

Ball, N. B., & Zanetti, S. (2012). Relationship between reactive strength variables in horizontal and vertical drop jumps. *Journal of Strength and Conditioning Research, 26*, 1407–1412.

Bangsbo, J., Mohr, M., & Krustrup, P. (2006). Physical and metabolic demands of training and match-play in elite football players. *Journal of Sports Sciences, 24*, 665–674.

Bartlett, R. (2007). *Introduction to sports biomechanics: Analysing human movement patterns*. London, UK: Routledge.

Bobbert, M. F., & Casius, L. J. (2005). Is the effect of a countermovement on jump height due to active state development? *Medicine and Science in Sports and Exercise, 37*, 440–446.

Bobbert, M. F., Gerritsen, K. G. M., Litjens, M. C. A., & Van Soest, A. J. (1996). Why is countermovement jump height greater than squat jump height? *Medicine and Exercise in Sports and Exercise, 28*, 1402–1412.

Bobbert, M. F., & van Soest, A. J. (1994). Effects of muscle strengthening on vertical jump height: A simulation study. *Medicine and Science in Sports and Exercise, 26*, 1012–1020.

Bobbert, M. F., & van Soest, A. J. (2000). Two-joint muscle offer the solution, but what was the problem? *Motor Control, 4*, 48–52.

Bouchouras, G., Moscha, D., Papaiakovou, G., Nikodelis, T., & Kollias, I. (2009). Angular momentum and landing efficiency in the long jump. *European Journal of Sport Sciences, 9*, 53–59.

Burgess, K. E., Connick, M. J., Graham-Smith, P., & Pearson, S. J. (2007). Plyometric vs. isometric training influences on tendon properties and muscle output. *Journal of Strength and Conditioning Research, 21*, 986–989.

Byrne, P. J., Moran, K., Rankin, P., & Kinsella, S. (2010). A comparison of methods used to identify "optimal" drop height for early phase adaptations in depth jump training. *Journal of Strength and Conditioning Research, 24*, 2050–2055.

Campos, J., Gámez, J., Encarnación, A., Guitiérrez-Dávila, M., Rojas, J., & Wallace, E. S. (2013). Three-dimensional kinematics during the take-off phase in competitive long jumping. *International Journal of Sports Science and Coaching, 8*, 395–406.

Cheng, K. B. (2008). The relationship between joint strength and standing vertical jump performance. *Journal of Applied Biomechanics, 24*, 224–233.

Cormie, P., McCaulley, G. O., & McBride, J. M. (2007). Power versus strength–power jump squat training: Influence on the load–power relationship. *Medicine and Science in Sports and Medicine, 39*, 996–1003.

Dabbs, N. C., Tran, T. T., Garner, J. C., & Brown, L. E. (2012). A brief review: Using whole-body vibration to increase acute power output and vertical jump performance. *Strength and Conditioning Journal, 34*, 78–84.

Dapena, J., & Chung, C. S. (1988). Vertical and radial motions of the body during the take-off phase of high jumping. *Medicine and Science in Sports and Exercise, 20*, 290–302.

de Villareal, E. S., Izquierdo, M., & Gonzalez-Badillo, J. J. (2011). Enhancing jump performance after combined vs. maximal power, heavy-resistance, and plyometric training alone. *Journal of Strength and Conditioning Research, 25*, 3274–3281.

Feltner, M. E., Fraschetti, D. J., & Crisp, R. J. (1999). Upper extremity augmentation of lower extremity kinetics during countermovement vertical jumps. *Journal of Sports Sciences, 17*, 449–466.

Ford, K. R., Myer, G. D., Smith, R. L., Byrnes, R. N., Dopirak, S. E., & Hewett, T. E. (2005). Use of an overhead goal alters vertical jump performance and biomechanics. *Journal of Strength and Conditioning Research, 19*, 394–399

Fukashiro, S., Hay, D. C., & Nagano, A. (2006). Biomechanical behavior of muscle–tendon complex during dynamic human movements. *Journal of Applied Biomechanics, 22*, 131–147.

Graham-Smith, P., & Lees, A. (2005). A three-dimensional kinematic analysis of the long jump take-off. *Journal of Sports Sciences, 23*, 891–903.

Haugen, T. A., Tønnessen, E., & Seiler, S. (2013). Anaerobic performance testing of professional soccer players 1995–2010. *International Journal of Sports Physiology and Performance, 8*, 148–156.

Hay, J. G. (1993). *The biomechanics of sports techniques.* Englewood Cliffs, NJ: Prentice Hall.

Horita, T., Kitamura, K., & Kohno, N. (1991). Body configuration and joint moment analysis during standing long jump in 6-yr-old children and adult males. *Medicine and Science in Sports and Exercise, 23*, 1068–1077.

Hudson, J. L. (1986). Coordination of segments in the vertical jump. *Medicine and Science in Sports and Exercise, 18*, 242–251.

Jarić, S., Ristanovic, D., & Corcos, D. M. (1989). The relationship between muscle kinetic parameters and kinematic variables in a complex movement. *European Journal of Applied Physiology, 59*, 370–376.

Jones, S. L., & Caldwell, G. E. (2003). Mono- and bi-articular muscle activity during jumping in different directions. *Journal of Applied Biomechanics, 19*, 205–222.

Kawamori, N., Rossi, S. J., Justice, B. D., Haff, E. E., Pstilli, E. E., O'Bryantt, H. S., . . . Haff, G. G. (2006). Peak force and rate of force development during isometric and dynamic mid-thigh clean pulls performed at various intensities. *Journal of Strength and Conditioning Research, 20*, 483–491.

Knudson, D. V., & Morrison, C. S. (2002). *Qualitative analysis of human movement.* Champaign, IL: Human Kinetics.

Komi, P. V. (2003). Stretch-shortening cycle. In P. V. Komi (Ed.), *Strength and power in sport* (pp. 184–202). Oxford, UK: Blackwell Science.

Komi, P. V., & Bosco, C. (1978). Utilization of stored elastic energy in leg extensor muscles by men and women. *Medicine and Science in Sports, 10*, 261–265.

Kraska, J. M., Ramsey, M. W., Haff, G. G., Fethke, N., Sands, W. A., Stone, M. E., & Stone, M. H. (2009). Relationship between strength characteristics and unweighted and weighted vertical jump height. *International Journal of Sports Physiology and Performance, 4*, 461–473.

Kubo, K., Kawakami, Y., & Fukunaga, T. (1999). Influence of elastic properties of tendon structures on jump performance in humans. *Journal of Applied Physiology, 87*, 2090–2096.

Laffaye, G., Bardy, B., & Traiar, R. (2006). Upper-limb motion and drop jump: Effect of expertise. *Journal of Sports Medicine and Physical Fitness, 46*, 238–247.

Lees, A., & Barton, G. (1996). The interpretation of relative momentum data to assess the contribution of the free limbs to the generation of vertical velocity in sports activities. *Journal of Sports Sciences, 14*, 503–511.

Lees, A., Vanrenterghem, J., & De Clercq, D. (2004a). The maximal and submaximal vertical jump: Implications for strength and conditioning. *Journal of Strength and Conditioning, 18*, 787–791.

Lees, A., Vanrenterghem, J., & De Clercq, D. (2004b). Understanding how an arm swing enhances performance in the vertical jump. *Journal of Biomechanics, 37*, 1929–1940.

Markovic, G. (2007). Does plyometric training improve vertical jump height? A meta-analytical review. *British Journal of Sports Medicine, 41*, 349–355.

Markovic, G., & Jaric, S. (2007). Is vertical jump height a body size–independent measure of muscle power? *Journal of Sports Sciences, 25,* 1355–1363.

McBride, J. M., Triplett-McBride, T., Davie, A., & Newton, R. U. (2002). The effects of heavy- vs. light-load jump squats on the development of strength, power, and speed. *Journal of Strength and Conditioning Research, 16,* 75–82.

McGuigan, M. R., Doyle, T. L. A., Newton, M., Edwards, D. J., Nimphius, S., & Newton, R. U. (2006). Eccentric utilization ratio: Effect of sport and phase of training. *Journal of Strength and Conditioning Research, 20,* 992–995.

Moir, G. L. (2008). Three different methods of calculating vertical jump height from force platform data in men and women. *Measurement in Physical Education & Exercise Science, 12,* 207–218.

Moran, K. A., & Wallace, E. S. (2007). Eccentric loading and range of knee joint motion effects on performance enhancement in vertical jumping. *Human Movement Science, 26,* 824–840.

Nagano, A., & Gerritsen, K. G. M. (2001). Effects of neuromuscular strength training on vertical jumping performance: A computer simulation study. *Journal of Applied Biomechanics, 17,* 113–128.

Pandy, M. G. (1990). An analytical framework for quantifying muscular action during human movements. In J. M. Winters & S. L-Y. Woo (Eds.), *Multiple muscle systems: Biomechanical and movement organization* (pp. 653–662). New York, NY: Springer-Verlag.

Perez-Gomes, J., & Calbet, J. A. L. (2013). Training methods to improve vertical jump performance. *Journal of Sports Medicine and Physical Fitness, 53,* 339–357.

Porter, J. M., Ostrowski, E. J., Nolan, R. P., & Wu, W. F. (2010). Standing long-jump performance is enhanced when using an external focus of attention. *Journal of Strength and Conditioning Research, 24,* 1746–1750.

Radcliffe, J. C., & Farentinos, R. C. (1999). *High-powered plyometrics.* Champaign, IL: Human Kinetics.

Ramirez-Campillo, R., Andrade, D. C., & Izquierdo, M. (2013). Effects of plyometric training volume and training surface on explosive strength. *Journal of Strength and Conditioning Research, 27,* 2714–2722.

Ratamess, N. (2012). *ACSM's foundations of strength training and conditioning.* Philadelphia, PA: Lippincott Williams & Wilkins.

Ridderikhoff, A., Batelaan, J. H., & Bobbert, M. F. (1999). Jumping for distance: Control of the external force in squat jumps. *Medicine and Science in Sports and Exercise, 31,* 1196–1204.

Robertson, D. G. E., Wilson, J-M. J., & St. Pierre, T. A. (2008). Lower extremity muscle functions during full squats. *Journal of Applied Biomechanics, 24,* 333–339.

Sanders, R. H., McClymont, D., Howick, I., & Kavalieris, L. (1993). Comparison of static and counter movement jumps across a range of movement amplitudes. *Australian Journal of Science and Medicine in Sport, 25,* 3–6.

Seyfarth, A., Blickhan, R., & Van Leeuwen, J. L. (2000). Optimal take-off technique and muscle design for long jump. *Journal of Experimental Biology, 203,* 741–750.

Seyfarth, A., Friedrichs, A., Wank, V., & Blickhan, R. (1999). Dynamics of the long jump. *Journal of Biomechanics, 32,* 1259–1267.

Sheppard, J. M., Gabbett, T., Taylor, K-L., Dorman, J., Lebedew, A. J., & Borgeaud, R. (2007). Development of a repeated-effort test for elite men's volleyball. *International Journal of Sports Physiology and Performance, 2,* 292–304.

Staub, J. N., Kraemer, W. J., Pandit, A. L., Haug, W. B., Comstock, B. A., Dunn-Lewis, C., . . . Häkkinen, K. (2013). Positive effects of augmented verbal feedback on power production in NCAA Division I collegiate athletes. *Journal of Strength and Conditioning Research, 27,* 2067–2072.

Stone, M. H., Sanborn, K., O'Bryant, H. S., Hartman, M., Stone, M. E., Proulx, C., . . . Hruby, J. (2003). Maximum strength–power–performance relationships in collegiate throwers. *Journal of Strength and Conditioning Research, 17,* 739–745.

Tan, J. C. C., & Yeadon, M. R. (2005). Why do high jumpers use a curved approach? *Journal of Sports Sciences, 23,* 775–780.

Toumi, H., Best, T. M., Martin, A., & Poumarat, G. (2004). Muscle plasticity after weight and combined (weight + jump) training. *Medicine and Science in Sports and Exercise, 36,* 1580–1588.

Tran, T. T., Brown, L. E., Coburn, J. W., Lynn, S. K., & Dabbs, N. C. (2012). Effects of assisted jumping on vertical jump parameters. *Current Sports Medicine Reports, 11,* 155–159.

Turner, A. N., & Jefferys, I. (2010). The stretch-shortening cycle: Proposed mechanisms and methods for enhancement. *Strength and Conditioning Journal, 32*, 87–99.

Umberger, B. R. (1998). Mechanics of the vertical jump and two-joint muscles: Implications for training. *Strength and Conditioning Journal, 22*, 70–74.

Vint, P. F., & Hinrichs, R. N. (1996). Differences between one-foot vertical jump performances. *Journal of Applied Biomechanics, 12*, 338–358.

Walsh, M., Arampatzis, A., Schade, F., & Brüggemann, G-P. (2004). The effect of drop jump starting height and contact time on power, work performed, and moment of force. *Journal of Strength and Conditioning Research, 18*, 561–566.

Walsh, M. S., Waters, J. A., Böhm, H., & Potteiger, J. A. (2007). Gender bias in jumping kinetics in National Collegiate Athletic Association Division I basketball players. *Journal of Strength and Conditioning Research, 21*, 958–962.

Wells, R., & Evans, N. (1987). Functions and recruitment patterns of one- and two-joint muscles under isometric and walking conditions. *Human Movement Sciences, 6*, 349–372.

Wisløff, U., Castagna, C., Helgerud, J., Jones, R., & Hoff, J. (2004). Strong correlation of maximal squat strength with sprint performance and vertical jump height in elite soccer players. *British Journal of Sports Medicine, 38*, 285–288.

Wu, W. F., Porter, J. M., & Brown, L. E. (2010). Effects of attentional focus strategies on peak force and performance in the standing long jump. *Journal of Strength and Conditioning Research, 26*, 1226–1231.

Wulf, G., & Dukek, J. S. (2009). Increased jump height with an external focus due to enhanced lower extremity joint kinetics. *Journal of Motor Behavior, 41*, 401–409.

Young, W. B., MacDonald, C., & Flowers, M. A. (2001). Validity of double- and single-leg vertical jumps as tests of extensor muscle function. *Journal of Strength and Conditioning Research, 15*, 6–11.

Young, W., Wilson, G., & Byrne, C. (1999). Relationship between strength qualities and performance in standing and run-up vertical jumps. *Journal of Sports Medicine and Physical Fitness, 39*, 285–293.

Yu, B., & Andrews, J. G. (1998). The relationship between free limb motions and performance in the triple jump. *Journal of Applied Biomechanics, 14*, 223–237.

Zatsiorsky, V. M., & Prilutsky, B. I. (2012). *Biomechanics of skeletal muscle*. Champaign, IL: Human Kinetics.

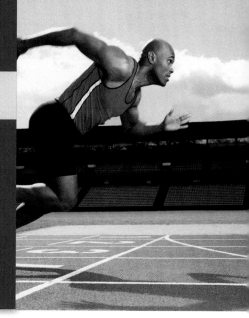

CHAPTER 12

Biomechanics of Fundamental Movements: Landing

Chapter Objectives

At the end of this chapter, you will be able to:

- Describe and explain the mechanical aspects of landing tasks
- Explain the biomechanical aspects of landing tasks
- Explain modifications to technique that can reduce the risk of injury during landing tasks
- Explain modifications to task and informational constraints that a coach can implement to enhance landing performance
- Develop a qualitative analysis of landing tasks to reduce the risk of injury
- Develop specific workouts targeting muscular strength, balance, and technique to reduce the risk of injury
- Develop specific workouts based on representative learning that enhance the attunement of the athletes' landing movements to environmental information

Key Terms

Absorption phase

Effective mass

Explicit learning

Flight phase

Frictional forces

Gravitational potential
energy

Impact phase

Implicit learning

Impulse–momentum
relationship

Informational constraints

Instructions

Knowledge of performance

Leg stiffness

Planned tasks

Preparatory landing tasks

Prevent Injury and Enhance
Performance

Sportsmetrics
Neuromuscular Training
Programs

Stabilization phase

Stationary landing tasks

Translational kinetic energy

Unplanned tasks

Work–energy theorem

Chapter Overview

The execution of jumps is an integral component of many sports, and multiple jumps are typically performed in sports including basketball, soccer, and volleyball. Due to the presence of gravitational acceleration, every jump will necessarily be followed by a landing. During a landing task, the athlete is required to change the motion of the center of mass (CM). For example, the athlete may be required to arrest the motion completely, such as when he or she lands at the completion of a long jump event in track and field. Conversely, the athlete may be required to change the direction of the CM during the landing task to execute another jump so as to avoid an opponent during soccer play or to intercept the ball during a volleyball rally, or the athlete may be required to complete a cutting maneuver upon landing. Success in these scenarios relies on the ability of the athlete to couple his or her movements to the relevant information present in the environment, constraining those movements during the specific landing task. Furthermore, changing the motion of the CM during any landing task presents a considerable risk for injury to the musculoskeletal structures of the lower body, particularly those of the knee joint. Notably, female athletes appear to be at increased risk for incurring injury to the anterior cruciate ligament (ACL) compared to male athletes. The requirement to couple the mechanics of the landing task with the specific stimuli contained within the information-rich environments associated with sport places a considerable constraint on the athletes' technique that can predispose them to injury. It is clear, then, that improving performance in landing tasks will be beneficial for athletes involved in numerous sports.

This chapter introduces the mechanical and biomechanical aspects of landing tasks typically experienced in sport (e.g., landing from a jump, change of direction). Particular attention is given to the factors associated with the risk of incurring a musculoskeletal injury during landing tasks. Technique modifications and training methods that can reduce the risk of incurring an injury during a landing task are highlighted. A qualitative analysis of landing technique is developed. Finally, the role of specific training methods to improve landing performance is discussed, as is the requirement for representative learning practices to enhance performance of sport-specific landing tasks.

Mechanics of Landing

The mechanics of landing can be described using the simple example of landing following the execution of a vertical jump. In such a jump, we can assume that the CM possesses only vertical motion that should be arrested by the ground reaction force (GRF) when the athlete makes contact with the ground upon landing. Here, then, the mechanics of the landing task are straightforward—they are the opposite of the mechanics associated with the execution of the jump. Specifically, jumping performance, defined by the height achieved by the CM during the flight phase, depends on the momentum possessed by the CM at takeoff, and the athlete is required to generate the appropriate impulse during the propulsive phase of the jump to achieve the desired momentum. During the subsequent landing, the momentum of the CM gained at takeoff must be reduced, requiring an impulse acting on the CM that is equal in magnitude to the momentum and that acts in the opposite direction:

$$\int F dt = m v_{\mathrm{f}} - m v_{\mathrm{i}}$$

Eq. (12.1)

where $\int F dt$ is the impulse of the GRF acting on the athlete during the landing, mv_f is the momentum of the CM at the end of landing, and mv_i is the momentum of the CM at the beginning of landing.

Note that the momentum of the CM at the beginning of landing would have a negative sense, as the CM is falling. Furthermore, the height that the CM has fallen from during the flight phase of the jump determines the magnitude of mv_i in Equation (12.1) and, therefore, depends on the impulse generated during the propulsive phase of the jump prior to takeoff. Thus, we can determine that the impulse of the GRF acting on the athlete during landing must be equal to that generated by the athlete during the propulsive phase of the jump if the motion of the CM is to be arrested upon landing from a vertical jump:

$$J_{\text{prop}} = J_{\text{land}} \qquad\qquad \textbf{Eq. (12.2)}$$

where J_{prop} is the impulse of the GRF acting on the athlete during the propulsive phase of the vertical jump and J_{land} is the impulse of the GRF acting on the athlete during the landing. Note that both impulses would have the same positive sense.

Equation (12.2) is predicated on the CM rising and falling the same distance during the flight phase of the jump and, therefore, the height of the CM being the same at takeoff as upon landing. This situation is unlikely given the changes in posture adopted by the athlete at takeoff and landing; that is, the athlete is likely to have a more extended posture at takeoff and greater flexion of the lower-body joints upon landing. If the displacement undergone by the CM as it falls from its highest position during flight until the beginning of landing is known, then the momentum possessed by the CM can be calculated from an equation of motion:

$$mv_i = m(2as)^{0.5} \qquad\qquad \textbf{Eq. (12.3)}$$

where mv_i is the momentum of the CM at the beginning of landing, m is the mass of the athlete, a is the gravitational acceleration, and s is the displacement undergone by the CM from the apex of flight until the beginning of landing.

We can then use the **impulse–momentum relationship** to determine the magnitude of the ground reaction impulse required to arrest the motion of the CM during landing; it will simply be an impulse equal in magnitude but opposite in direction to mv_i in Equation (12.3). Therefore, the impulse acting on the athlete during a landing task varies in proportion to the height from which the athlete has fallen, given that the mass of the athlete and the gravitational acceleration will remain constant during our analysis.

Given that the CM must fall prior to ground contact, it is informative to describe the mechanics of landing using the **work–energy theorem**. When the CM is at the apex of its trajectory during the flight of a jump, it will possess **gravitational potential energy** (E_{GP}). The E_{GP} possessed by the CM will be transformed by the gravitational force into **translational kinetic energy** (E_{TK}) as the athlete falls; it is this energy that must be dissipated by a force acting on the athlete upon landing. The force acting on the athlete during landing does work equivalent to the magnitude of the E_{TK} possessed by the CM at the beginning of landing. Therefore, a landing task that begins when the athlete first contacts the ground involves an initial **absorption phase** whereby the E_{TK} of the CM is dissipated by the work done on the athlete. This absorption phase ends when the E_{TK} becomes zero and the athlete's motion has been arrested. The work done during the absorption phase of landing can be expressed mathematically as follows:

$$\int Fds = \left(\frac{mv_f^2}{2}\right) - \left(\frac{mv_i^2}{2}\right) \qquad \text{Eq. (12.4)}$$

where $\int Fds$ is the work done by the force acting on the athlete during the absorption phase of landing, $\frac{mv_f^2}{2}$ is the E_{TK} of the CM at the end of the absorption phase (0 J), and $\frac{mv_i^2}{2}$ is the E_{TK} of the CM at the beginning of the absorption phase. Note that $\frac{mv_i^2}{2}$ depends on the height from which the athlete has fallen. Thus, the work done during a landing task varies in proportion to the height from which the athlete has fallen, given that the mass of the athlete and the gravitational acceleration will remain constant during our analysis. The practitioner can use this knowledge to select exercises to minimize the load experienced during landing tasks (see Landing Concept 12.1).

The GRF does no work on the CM in the vertical direction during the absorption phase of landing, given that work is the integral of force with respect to the displacement undergone by the point of application of the force (the point of application of the GRF does not undergo any substantial displacement during landing when the

Landing Concept 12.1

Jumping to a box reduces the impulse of the ground reaction force and the required work done during landing when performing plyometric exercises

The impulse–momentum relationship states that the impulse of the ground reaction force to arrest the momentum of the center of mass during landing depends on the CM momentum upon ground contact. The magnitude of the CM momentum depends on the mass of the athlete and the height from which the athlete has fallen (given constant gravitational acceleration). The work–energy theorem informs us that the work done on the athlete during landing to dissipate the translational kinetic energy of the CM again depends on the height from which the athlete has fallen. Therefore, the load experienced by the musculoskeletal structures during landing from a vertical jump, which has implications for injuries, is related to the height jumped.

During lower-body plyometric exercises, the coach may require the athlete to maximize the impulse of the ground reaction force and the work done by the athlete during the propulsive phase of the jump so as to stimulate the appropriate training adaptations, resulting in large jump heights being achieved. However, by having the athlete execute these jumps to a box, the coach reduces the height from which the athlete falls during flight, thereby reducing the magnitude of the ground reaction impulse and the work done during landing. This represents a simple method by which the strength and conditioning coach can maximize the mechanics associated with propulsion while minimizing the loads experienced by the athlete upon landing, reducing the potential for musculoskeletal injuries.

athlete falls vertically unless the surface can be displaced, such as when landing on a crash mat or when landing in sand). However, the human body is a linked segmental system. In turn, intersegmental forces are exerted as the segments are displaced relative to one another during a landing task. It is the sum of these intersegmental forces—mainly those associated with the musculotendinous units crossing the lower-body joints—applied through the displacement associated with the range of motion of each joint that represents the work done to dissipate the energy during the absorption phase of a landing task (Chapman, 2008).

To this point, we have discussed the mechanics associated with a landing task when the athlete possesses only vertical motion, such as during a landing from a vertical jump. However, following the execution of a jump for horizontal distance, the CM will possess horizontal motion upon landing. An effective landing under such circumstances requires sufficient **frictional forces** upon landing to generate an appropriate horizontal impulse of the GRF that will reduce the horizontal momentum. If this frictional force is lacking due to a low coefficient of friction, then the athlete will slip during the landing. Recall that during the execution of horizontal jumps, the athlete also generates angular momentum during propulsion. This angular momentum possessed by the athlete needs to be effectively reduced if the athlete is to remain balanced upon landing (i.e., maintain the gravity line within the base of support). This will require the GRF to produce an appropriate angular impulse upon landing to reduce the angular momentum. The body must be positioned such that the resultant GRF (the vector sum of the horizontal and vertical components) acts at a distance from the CM to generate a moment during the absorption phase or such that the bodyweight force acts to generate the appropriate angular impulse.

If the athlete is required to perform another movement following the landing, such as executing another jump, then the impulse of the GRF generated during landing must exceed the negative momentum possessed by the CM. For example, during the landing associated with a drop–jump, the impulse of the GRF must be sufficient to reduce the negative vertical momentum the athlete possesses upon landing to zero, then increase the positive vertical momentum to an appropriate value at takeoff (commensurate with the height required during the subsequent jump).

From the preceding mechanical analysis, we can differentiate between two types of landing tasks based on different goals. During **stationary landing tasks**, the goal is to arrest the motion of the CM. An example of such a task would be a drop–landing, whereby the athlete falls from a raised box, absorbing the energy during landing before returning to an upright posture. In contrast, the goal of **preparatory landing tasks** is to execute another movement following the absorption phase, such as a drop–jump landing, in which the athlete is required to land and then execute a jump immediately following the absorption phase or during a change of direction task where the athlete executes a cutting movement. Preparatory landing tasks can be further categorized as **planned**, where the athlete has prior knowledge about the movements required following landing (i.e., the direction of the cut), or **unplanned**, where the athlete is unaware of the subsequent movement at the beginning of the task (see Landing Concept 12.2).

We can conclude that during landing tasks, the athlete must contend with two basic mechanical constraints:

- Dissipating the translational kinetic energy of the CM
- Controlling linear and/or angular momentum commensurate with the goal of the landing task (i.e., maintaining balance once the motion has been arrested or executing a jumping or cutting movement)

Landing Concept 12.2

Planned and unplanned tasks

In planned tasks, the performer has prior knowledge of the movements that are required to achieve the goal of the task before initiating the movement. For example, during a preparatory landing task, a performer may be provided with the instructions to "step from the box, land on your dominant leg, and cut to the right." Conversely, during an unplanned task, the performer is unaware of the specific movement that will be required to successfully achieve the goal of the task, requiring the performer to make a decision as to the most appropriate movement and execute it in response to the presentation of a stimulus. For example, during a preparatory landing task, a performer may be provided with the instructions to "step from the box, land on your dominant leg, and cut in the direction of the live opponent positioned across from you." To use the traditional motor learning taxonomy, planned tasks are closed skills, whereas unplanned tasks are open skills (Magill, 2011). In most sports, but especially field and court sports, movements are typically not planned in advance of their execution; thus planned movements are not representative of many sports.

Consideration should be given to the form of the stimulus that the athlete has to respond to during unplanned tasks. For example, some authors have proposed creating unplanned drills where the athlete is required to attend and respond to the coach calling a particular color or pointing in a given direction as the athlete approaches (Dawes, 2012). This type of stimulus is non-sport specific and, therefore, represents generic information. Alternatively, the motion of an opponent may be placed in front of the athlete; it represents sport-specific information.

This distinction is important when we consider that the definition of motor learning is the attunement of the athlete's movements to sport-specific environmental information (Araújo & Davids, 2011). The use of unplanned tasks involving the presentation of sport-specific information is, therefore, more appropriate than tasks where generic information is used when testing or developing movements of athletes. Moreover, some evidence indicates that the dynamics of the movements executed by athletes differ when they are required to respond to a video stimulus compared to the same stimulus presented "live" (Dicks, Button, & Davids, 2010), suggesting that the use of video tasks should be limited if possible.

The role of affordances in movements executed in unplanned tasks must also be taken into consideration. For example, the unplanned preparatory landing task in which the athlete is provided with the instruction to "step from the box, land on your dominant leg, and cut in the direction of the live opponent positioned across from you" incorporates sport-specific information, yet the required movement (a cut) is still specified by the coach in advance of the task. In an actual sporting situation, the movements executed by an athlete to satisfy the task goal will be determined by the athlete's perception of the affordances

(continues)

(continued)

provided by the situation relative to the individual's own capabilities; action-scaled affordances become a very strong determinant of the observed movements executed by the athlete. Therefore, one athlete may choose to execute a cutting movement to achieve the goal of the task given his or her action-scaled affordances and the specific information presented by the scenario, whereas another athlete may choose to execute a straight-line sprint and still achieve a successful outcome. The specification of the required movement to be executed in many unplanned tasks in research studies reflects an element of experimental control on behalf of the investigators to allow them to study the mechanics of the movements executed in the tasks. However, such tasks are not representative of most sporting situations.

The first constraint mainly applies to stationary landing tasks, while the second applies to both stationary and preparatory landing tasks. During preparatory landing tasks, the energy possessed by the CM can be utilized during the subsequent propulsive phase of the task to perform another movement rather than being dissipated.

Biomechanics of Landing

As the preceding analysis of the mechanics of landing tasks indicates, the impulse of the GRF during ground contact is determined by the momentum of the CM upon landing and the goals of the landing task (e.g., a stationary or preparatory landing task). Although the impulse of the GRF acts to change the momentum of the CM during the absorption phase of a landing task, the dynamics of the actual GRF in terms of its peak value and loading rate can be manipulated by the athlete. This is important because the dynamics of the GRF may potentially be injurious to the athlete (see Landing Concept 12.3).

Dynamics of Ground Reaction Force During Landing

A bimodal vertical GRF occurs during bilateral landing tasks (Dufek & Bates, 1990; Zhang, Derrick, Evans, & Yu, 2008). This bimodal pattern arises from the impacts associated with the forefoot and then the heel. The first peak (forefoot impact) is lower than the second peak (heel impact), and both increase with increasing falling height

Landing Concept 12.3

Peak ground reaction force and loading rate are associated with musculoskeletal injuries during landing tasks

Conceptually, an injury occurs when the stress applied to a biological tissue exceeds that tissue's ability to withstand the stress either acutely or chronically (McBain et al., 2012). Stress is a vector that expresses the magnitude of a force applied to the tissue relative to the cross-sectional area of the tissue. In turn, both the magnitude of the applied force and the size of the tissue should be considered when determining injury to biologic tissue. The ground reaction force (GRF), which provides an indication of the forces experienced by the musculoskeletal structures of the athlete during any movement task, represents an important variable in the etiology of many musculoskeletal injuries.

Stress fractures to bone are common in sport, accounting for approximately 20% of all musculoskeletal injuries incurred by athletes (Zadpoor & Nikooyan, 2011). Stress fractures are mainly limited to the lower-body skeleton, with the tibia and the metatarsal representing the most frequently injured sites. Such injuries may occur in response to repetitive submaximal loading applied to the bone with insufficient time for bone remodeling between loading cycles (Zadpoor & Nikooyan, 2011). In a review of the studies investigating the influence of the dynamics of the GRF on stress fractures, the authors concluded that the loading rate of the GRF—rather than the peak GRF—during repetitive landing tasks associated with running was greater in athletes who incurred a stress fracture (Zadpoor & Nikyoon, 2011). This effect is likely due to the fatigue strength of the bone, defined as the number of loading cycles required to induce failure, being lower when the loading rate is increased.

The GRF is an external force applied to an athlete, and the loads transferred to the bones can be attenuated through the action of muscles, tendons, and ligaments. One might expect the dynamics of the GRF to be implicated in injuries to these biological tissues. Landing tasks may involve rapid deceleration of the body and dissipation of energy, both of which are likely to increase the magnitude of the GRF as well as the loading rate associated with the GRF. Muscles dissipate energy when they actively lengthen (Roberts & Konow, 2013), so eccentric actions are experienced as the lower-body joints are accelerated into flexion during the absorption phase of a landing task. Greater forces are generated during eccentric muscle actions compared to concentric actions (Harry, Ward, Heglund, Morgan, & McMahon, 1990). These greater forces experienced during the eccentric actions associated with landing tasks are likely to induce damage to the tissue, ranging from delayed-onset muscle soreness to more severe muscle strains (LaStayo et al., 2003). This relationship highlights the importance of eccentric muscular strength in minimizing injury potential during landing tasks.

Tendons can absorb energy during the lengthening of the musculotendinous units by deforming, although they can only dissipate a very small proportion of energy that they absorb. Fascicles, on the other hand, are able to dissipate large amounts of energy as they lengthen. However, tendons are able to store the energy temporarily and then return it to perform work on the muscle fascicles, lengthening them at a lower rate and with a lower force than if the tendons did not provide this functional energy buffer (Roberts & Konow, 2013). This action of tendons can reduce the potential for damage to the fascicles during landing tasks.

Leg stiffness during a landing task, calculated as the ratio between the peak GRF and the deformation of the leg, can inform us of the potential for injury to the musculotendinous units. Low leg stiffness during landing caused by increased joint displacements increases the reliance on the energy absorbed by the musculotendinous units crossing the hip, knee, and ankle joints, likely increasing the risk of overuse injuries to these tissues (Butler, Crowell, &

(continues)

(continued)

McClay-Davis, 2003). Conversely, high leg stiffness is associated with minimal joint displacements and, therefore, is likely to increase the injury risk for bony and articular cartilaginous structures of the joints given the increased loads applied (Butler et al., 2003). Leg stiffness also appears to increase in proportion to the peak GRF and loading rate during landing task. Finally, peak vertical and posterior components of the GRF during landing tasks have been implicated in injuries to the structures around the knee joint, particularly the anterior cruciate ligament (Hewett et al., 2005; Sell et al., 2007).

The dynamics of the GRF during landing tasks clearly represent an important factor predisposing the athlete to various musculoskeletal injuries. Nevertheless, biological tissues appear to be capable of adapting to the stresses applied to them so long as those stresses do not exceed their mechanical capabilities and sufficient time is provided between loading cycles to allow tissue remodeling.

(Zhang et al., 2008; **Figure 12.1**). (During unilateral landing tasks, only a single peak is observed in the vertical GRF trace [Ali, Robertson, & Rouhi, 2014; Schmitz, Kulas, Perrin, Riemann, & Shultz, 2007].) Notice that both peaks in the vertical GRF occur within 100 ms from the initial ground contact; the CM will still be descending following the occurrence of the second peak, such that the absorption phase of the landing

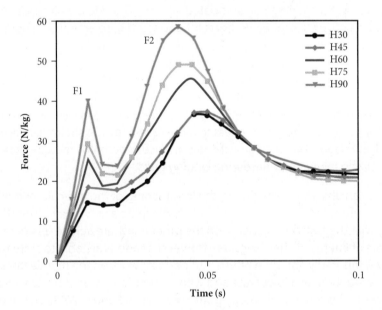

Figure 12.1 The normalized vertical ground reaction force during a stationary landing task performed from different fall heights showing the bimodal pattern. F1 represents toe contact; F2 represents heel contact; H30 is a fall height of 0.30 m; H45 is a fall height of 0.45 m; H60 is a fall height of 0.60 m; H75 is a fall height of 0.75 m; H90 is a fall height of 0.90 m.

Reproduced from Zhang, S., Derrick, T. R., Evans, W., & Yu, Y-J. (2008). Shock and impact reduction in moderate and strenuous landing activities. *Sports Biomechanics, 7*, 296–309. Reprinted by permission of the publisher (Taylor & Francis Ltd, http://www.tandfonline.com).

is not complete. The dynamics associated with the vertical GRF allow the absorption phase to be reduced to two further subphases: the **impact phase** (defined as the first 100 ms from initial ground contact) and the **stabilization phase** (defined as the event from 100 ms after initial ground contact to the lowest vertical position of the CM). These distinct phases have important implications for joint kinetics during landing tasks (Kulas, Schmitz, Shultz, Watson, & Perrin, 2006).

The magnitude of the peak vertical GRF increases with increasing drop height when athletes are performing drop–landings (Ali et al., 2014; Zhang, Bates, & Dufek, 2000). The peak horizontal component of the GRF also increases during stationary landings as athletes land from greater distances associated with horizontal jumps (Ali et al., 2014). These findings have important implications for musculoskeletal injury.

Yet the peak GRF during landing is not always positively correlated with the height of the fall. For example, some athletes can accommodate landing from greater heights by lessening the peak GRF (James, Bates, & Dufek, 2003). The peak GRF can be attenuated by increasing the range of motion undergone at the hip and knee joints during a stationary landing task (Zhang et al., 2000; Zhang et al., 2008). Indeed, greater range of motion at the hip, knee, and ankle joints is typically observed during falls from greater heights (Zhang et al., 2000). Because of the ability to displace segments relative to one another, athletes are able to reduce their **effective mass** during a landing task, modifying the dynamics of the GRF (Derrick, 2004). (See Figure 12.2.) For example, flexion angles at the ankle, hip, and trunk are negatively correlated with the peak vertical and horizontal GRF during stationary landings from various drop

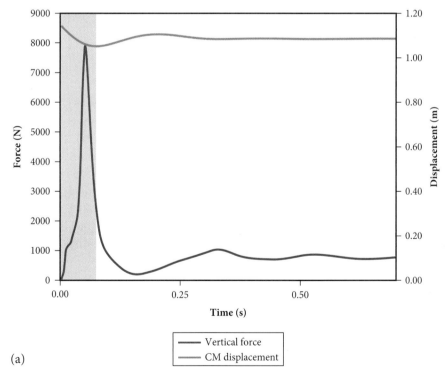

(a)

Figure 12.2 (a) The vertical ground reaction force and the displacement of the center of mass of an athlete who lands and keeps the joints stiff after having stepped from a 0.30-m box. *(continues)*

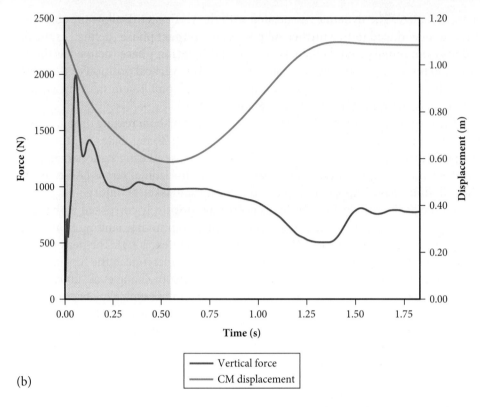

(b)

Figure 12.2 *(continued)* (b) The same athlete landing after having stepped from the same box but flexing the joints of the lower body. The shaded area represents the absorption phase of landing. Note the difference in the peak vertical ground reaction force between the two landing techniques.

heights and horizontal jump distances (Ali, Rouhi, & Robertson, 2013). Even increasing the forward lean of the trunk during a landing task has been shown to reduce the peak vertical GRF (Shimokochi, Ambeganokar, Meyer, Lee, & Shultz, 2013), whereas landing on the forefoot is associated with lower peak GRF and loading rate compared to a heel-to-toe landing due to an increased range of motion at the lower-body joints (Kovacs, Tihanyi, DeVita, Racz, Barrier, & Hortobagyi, 1999). Fatigue induced by previous exercise has been shown to result in greater peak vertical GRF and loading rates (James, Dufek, & Bates, 2006); these changes in dynamics of the GRF are accompanied by less knee flexion at ground contact but a greater angular displacement at the knee during landing.

Dissipating Kinetic Energy During Landing

As noted in the discussion of the mechanics of landing, one of the mechanical constraints associated with landing tasks is dissipation of the E_{TK} of the CM, which occurs during the absorption phase of landing (defined as the event between ground contact and the time of zero vertical motion possessed by the CM). The dissipation of E_{TK} requires work to be done by intersegmental forces acting at the joints as they are displaced during the landing task. These intersegmental forces are largely due to the forces exerted by the musculotendinous units that produce moments across the joints.

The largest moments at the lower-body joints (hip, knee, and ankle) during landing tasks are observed in the sagittal plane, reflecting flexion–extension about a mediolateral axis. As the CM descends during landing, the hip, knee, and ankle joints will flex. Figure 12.3 shows the joint moments in the sagittal plane during a stationary landing task. Notice that the moments are mainly extensor at each of the joints, despite the joints being accelerated into flexion. The integral of the moment at each joint and the angular displacement represents the work done at each joint; the integral returned at the joints during landing has a negative sense, constituting negative work being done

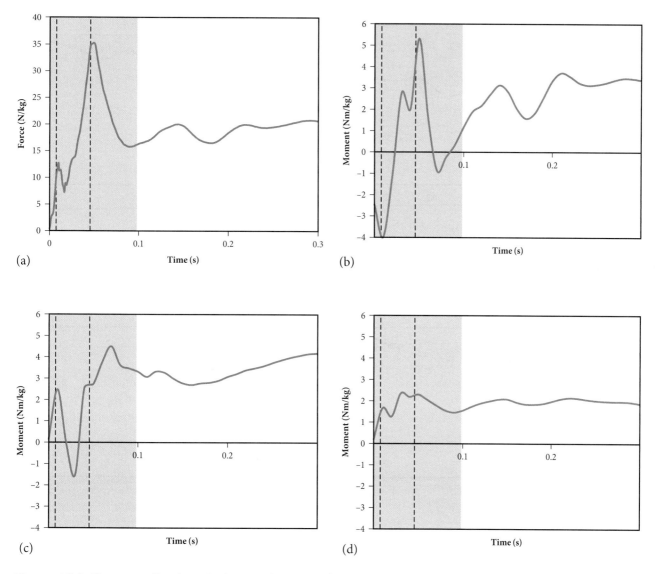

Figure 12.3 The normalized vertical ground reaction force (a) and joint moments in the sagittal plane at the (b) hip joint, (c) knee joint, (d) ankle joint during the absorption phase of a stationary landing task. Positive values for the joint moments reflect extensor moments while negative values represent flexor moments. The colored area on the figures denotes the impact phase of absorption; the first dashed vertical line denotes the time of the first peak of the ground reaction force, reflecting toe contact; the second dashed vertical line denotes the time of the second peak of the ground reaction force, reflecting heel contact.

during absorption. (Figure 12.4 shows the power at each of the joints, calculated as the product of the moment and the angular velocity, which represents the rate at which the joint moment does work during the landing task.) This negative work done at the joints indicates the dissipation of energy during the absorption phase of a landing task by the active lengthening of the musculotendinous units (McNitt-Gray, 1993).

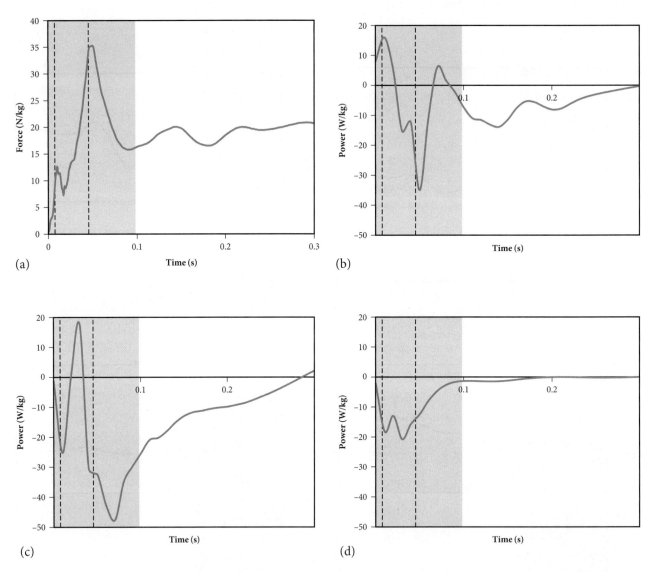

Figure 12.4 The normalized vertical ground reaction force (a) and the power output of the joint moments in the sagittal plane at the (b) hip joint, (c) knee joint, (d) ankle joint during the absorption phase of a stationary landing task. The area under each of the power output curves represents the work done by the joint moment with positive values reflecting the joint moment generating energy (positive work) and negative values reflecting the joint moment absorbing energy (negative work). The colored area on the figures denotes the impact phase of absorption; the first dashed vertical line denotes the time of the first peak of the ground reaction force, reflecting toe contact; the second dashed vertical line denotes the time of the second peak of the ground reaction force, reflecting heel contact.

Therefore, the negative work done by the joint moments during the absorption phase of landing can be used to represent eccentric muscle actions. In fact, this negative work can be utilized during the propulsive phase to enhance jumping performance via the stretch–shortening cycle, although the eccentric loading must be within the capabilities of the athlete if such advantages are to be realized (Turner & Jefferys, 2010). This relationship highlights the importance of sufficient eccentric muscular strength during preparatory landing tasks. The use of the negative work performed during the absorption phase of landing has been shown to reduce the energetic cost of performing repeated jumps (McBride & Snyder, 2012), which has implications for sports in which multiple jump–landing cycles are required (e.g., basketball, soccer, volleyball).

Notice in Figure 12.3 that the extensor moments at the knee and ankle joints reach their first peak shortly after impact, at the time corresponding to toe contact. A large magnitude of negative work is done by the moments at these joints at this time (Figure 12.4). However, the moment at the hip joint is actually a flexor moment after impact, generating some positive work. This difference in the moments at the hip and knee joints likely arises from the action of the biarticular rectus femoris during the impact phase of landing (McNitt-Gray, 2000). At the time associated with the second peak in the vertical GRF, all of the moments at the lower body in the sagittal plane are extensor, with the hip and ankle moments achieving their peak (Figure 12.3). The moments at all joints absorb energy at this time (Figure 12.4).

The magnitude of the moments during landing tasks increases with increased fall height, with the greatest moments typically being generated at the hip joint (Shultz, Schmitz, Nguyen, & Levine, 2010; Zhang et al., 2000). However, the amount of negative work performed by the joint moments during absorption differs between stationary landing tasks and preparatory landing tasks. Overall negative joint work is greater during a preparatory landing task (drop–jump) when compared to that performed during a stationary landing task (drop–landing), mainly due to a greater amount of energy being absorbed at the hip joint (Shultz et al., 2012). Similar amounts of negative work are performed at the knee and hip joints during stationary landing tasks, with the work at these joints exceeding that at the ankle (Zhang et al., 2000). Other sources have reported greater negative work at the knee joint during stationary landing tasks compared to that at the hip and ankle joints (Yeow, Lee, & Goh, 2010; Zhang et al., 2008). During a preparatory landing task (drop–jump), a similar amount of negative work is performed at the hip and ankle joints, but both amounts are greater than the amount of negative work performed at the knee joint (Schultz et al., 2010). This demonstrates the influence of task constraints on the subsequent joint mechanics during landing tasks. Dividing the absorption phase into the subphases of impact and stabilization reveals further differences in the energy absorbed by the lower-body joints during landing. Specifically, during the impact phase of a stationary landing task, the knee and ankle joints make the greatest contributions to energy absorption, while the hip and knee joints provide the greatest contribution to the energy absorbed during the stabilization phase (Kulas et al., 2006; see Figure 12.4).

During the propulsive phase of a vertical jump, energy is transferred from the hip to the knee and from the knee to the ankle joints by the biarticular rectus femoris and gastrocnemius, respectively. The same energy transfer occurs in reverse during landing tasks, thereby allowing the mechanical energy to be distributed across the joints during landing (Prilutsky & Zatsiorsky, 1994). This distal-to-proximal transfer of energy by the biarticular muscles aids the smaller distal monoarticular muscles in dissipating the energy associated with landing by transferring some of it to the larger proximal monoarticular muscles. The magnitude of the energy transferred between the joints is greater during the propulsive phase of a vertical jump compared to a stationary landing task (drop–landing) (Prilutsky & Zatsiorsky, 1994).

Although the work at each joint mainly occurs in the sagittal plane, some work is done in the frontal and transverse planes at the hip, knee, and ankle joints, reflecting abduction–adduction and internal–external rotation moments, respectively. Greater increases in the negative work performed at the hip joint compared to the knee and ankle joints in the frontal plane have been reported as fall height increases during a stationary landing task (Yeow, Lee, & Goh, 2009).

Fatigue Affects Energy Absorption

Fatigue produced by the performance of prior landing tasks results in increased knee extension and ankle plantarflexion at ground contact during stationary landing tasks (Weinhandl, Smith, & Dugan, 2011). This effect is associated with greater energy absorption at the ankle joint and a concomitant decrease in energy absorbed at the knee joint. However, during preparatory landing tasks, such as repeated single-leg hops, fatigue induced via repeated knee extension exercise increases the reliance on energy absorption at the knee joint, with reductions occurring at both the hip and ankle joints (Augustsson et al., 2006). In one study, fatigue induced via aerobic exercise (a VO_{2peak} test followed by 30 min of interval running) resulted in mechanical alterations during a preparatory landing task (stop–jump) that were similar to those following a fatiguing protocol consisting of 5 min of sport-specific agility work in female soccer players (Quammen et al., 2012). Specifically, the players landed with less flexion at the hip and knee joints following the fatiguing protocols. The fatigue that affects the athlete's ability to control the motion of the lower-body joints is central in origin when the athlete is required to make a decision regarding his or her subsequent movements prior to landing (McLean & Samorezov, 2009). See Applied Research 12.1.

Landing Posture Affects Energy Absorption

During the **flight phase** of a jumping task, the athlete is able to position the limbs and activate the muscles as the CM falls. These prelanding alterations in posture can have significant implications for the biomechanical variables during landing. For example, a more extended (upright) posture at landing is associated with greater peak GRF, while adopting a forward lean reduces the peak GRF (Shimokochi et al., 2013). Landing on the forefoot is associated with large knee and ankle moments and negative power at these joints, whereas heel-to-toe landing is associated with large hip and knee moments and negative power (Kovacs et al., 1999).

Whether the participant has prior knowledge about the required movement following landing affects the landing posture and, therefore, the joint mechanics during absorption. During unplanned preparatory landing tasks in which the athlete is required to change direction during landing in response to external visual stimuli, the mechanics during landing are altered. For example, increased abduction and internal rotation moments at the knee caused by the GRF have been reported during an unplanned cutting task where the athletes' direction was signaled by lights, compared to when the athlete had prior knowledge of the required direction change (Bessier, Lloyd, Ackland, & Cochrane, 2001). However, the mechanics during the

Applied Research 12.1
Central fatigue causes changes in the mechanics of lower-body joints during an unplanned preparatory landing task

Twenty female NCAA Division I athletes who participated in volleyball, soccer, and basketball had the kinematic and kinetic variables of the lower-body joints assessed when performing a series of single-leg preparatory landing tasks. The single-leg trials required the athletes to jump forward from a position 2 m behind a force plate, land on either the right or left leg, and then cut to the contralateral side. These tasks were performed under planned and unplanned conditions, whereby the athlete either had knowledge of the cutting direction prior to jumping forward (planned) or was made aware of the required cutting direction only during the propulsive phase of the forward jump (unplanned). Following the completion of unfatigued trials, the athletes were exposed to a fatiguing protocol involving a set of three single-leg squats, after which they performed another single-leg landing task. This protocol was continued until the athlete could no longer complete the squats without assistance. The order of the landing legs and the fatigued legs as well as the planned and unplanned conditions were randomized across the athletes, allowing the effects of unilateral fatigue on the mechanics of the nonfatigued contralateral leg during a preparatory landing task to be investigated.

The investigators reported that fatigue resulted in altered landing mechanics, including an increase in the knee abduction displacement and increased external abduction and internal rotation moments acting at the knee joint. These alterations caused by fatigue were even demonstrated in the nonfatigued contralateral leg during unplanned trials. The findings provide evidence that the mechanical alterations caused by fatigue are centrally mediated during unplanned landing tasks.

McLean, S. G., & Samorezov, J. E. (2009). Fatigue-induced ACL injury risk stems from a degradation in central control. *Medicine and Science in Sports and Exercise, 41,* 1661–1672.

landing associated with unplanned movements are affected by the specificity of the visual information presented to the athlete (Lee, Lloyd, Lay, Bourke, & Alderson, 2013). (See Applied Research 12.2.) Even the presence of a stationary opponent during a preparatory landing task (change of direction) increases flexion and abduction at the hip and knee joints (McLean, Lipfert, & van den Bogert, 2004). These data demonstrate that alterations in task and environmental constraints can influence the mechanics of the movement during landing tasks and have significant implications for the assessment of landing performance as well as the training exercises used to improve landing performance.

Muscle activation occurs during flight so as to dissipate the energy during the absorption phase associated with the landing. Interestingly, earlier activation of the muscles occurs when the athlete is performing a landing from a jump compared to when the athlete is performing a landing following a step from a box (drop–landing task) despite an equivalent fall distance of the CM (Afifi & Hinrichs, 2012). This difference likely reflects a greater flight time associated with the vertical jump (time of CM ascent and descent) compared to the stepping task (time of CM descent only). Moreover, a lower vertical loading rate is associated with both a lower peak GRF and a greater time to peak GRF; greater hip, knee, and ankle flexion angles at the time of peak GRF; and greater muscle activation during the landing from a maximal vertical

Applied Research 12.2
Mechanics during unplanned landing tasks differ when sport-specific visual information is presented to the athlete

In a study conducted by Lee et al. (2013), male soccer players from different competitive levels performed a change of direction task from a running start under four different visual conditions: (1) a planned condition in which the required direction change was displayed by means of a large arrow presented on a screen in front of the athletes from the time that they began their approach; (2) an unplanned condition in which a large arrow identifying the required direction change was presented only during the last stride prior to the cutting movement; (3) an unplanned condition in which athletes were required to change direction in response to a life-size video image of a single defender changing direction; and (4) an unplanned condition in which athletes were required to change direction in response to one of two life-size video images of defenders changing direction. The videos of the opposing players were of a duration that allowed the video defender to change direction at the same time as the athlete was about to execute their cutting movement, and the kinematic and kinetic data from the lower body during the movement were recorded. This experimental design allowed the mechanical effects of planned and unplanned tasks to be investigated as well as the differences caused by the presentation of generic and sport-specific visual information.

The authors reported that the smallest peak external abduction moments at the knee joint occurred during the planned condition. By comparison, the largest peak external abduction moments occurred during the unplanned condition involving the presentation of an arrow (generic information) with the magnitude of the moments during the unplanned task using sport-specific visual information (opposing defender) falling between the two arrow conditions. These findings demonstrate that the mechanics of planned landing tasks differ from those of unplanned tasks where the athlete is required to make a decision in response to visual information. Moreover, the specificity of the visual information in terms of its relationship to the information to which athletes attune their movements in their chosen sport can confer a considerable constraint on athletes' movements. Collectively, these findings suggest that strength and conditioning practitioners should use sport-specific visual stimuli when using unplanned landing tasks in training.

Lee, M. J. C., Lloyd, D. G., Lay, B. S., Bourke, P. D., & Alderson, J. A. (2013). Effects of different visual stimuli on postures and knee moments during sidestepping. *Medicine and Science in Sports and Exercise, 45*, 1740–1748.

jump compared to the drop–landing task. Other sources have reported greater asymmetry in the bilateral peak GRF during the two landing phases associated with a drop–jump task (an initial preparatory landing followed by a stationary landing); specifically, greater asymmetry occurs during the second stationary landing (stationary landing) compared to the first preparatory landing (Bates, Ford, Myer, & Hewett, 2013). There was also less vertical displacement of the CM during the absorption phase of the second landing.

These findings are important because landing tasks experienced by athletes during most sports will occur following the performance of a jump rather than after stepping from a raised obstacle. They highlight the role of task constraints on the mechanics of landing tasks and have implications for both the assessment and training tasks that strength and conditioning practitioners utilize with their athletes.

Controlling Momentum During Landing

Another mechanical constraint associated with landing tasks is the need to control linear and angular momentum of the body commensurate with the goal of the task. During stationary landing tasks, the control of momentum refers to arresting the momenta during the absorption phase. The situation becomes more complicated during preparatory landing tasks, in which the athlete may be required to change the vertical momentum and maintain the horizontal momentum, such as during the landing associated with the running long jump takeoff; to transfer horizontal momentum to vertical momentum while generating angular momentum, such as during the landing associated with the running vertical jump takeoff; or to change the vertical, horizontal, and angular momenta of the body, such as during the landing associated with change of direction tasks.

During stationary landing tasks, the athlete is required to arrest whole-body vertical, horizontal, and angular momentum. A mechanical solution requires that the GRF generate sufficient linear and angular impulse during landing to reduce the linear and angular momenta, respectively. However, if the athlete is to maintain balance during landing, the arrest of momenta needs to be achieved with the CM above the base of support. If the CM falls outside the boundary of the base of support, the body-weight force will produce a moment that acts to increase the angular momentum of the body and rotate it, resulting in an unbalanced posture and a possible fall.

Maintaining balance during stationary landings is important in many sports activities. For example, landing in a balanced posture following a spike in volleyball allows the player to ready himself or herself for the next phase of play; in a sport such as gymnastics, the athlete is actually scored on the balance achieved during the landing. In contrast, in other sports, the loss of balance during a stationary landing may actually enhance performance. For example, during the landing at the completion of the long jump event in track and field, the angular momentum possessed by the athlete generated at takeoff rotates the athlete forward upon landing (Bouchouras, Moscha, Papaiakovou, Nikodelis, & Kollias, 2009). This forward rotation prevents the athlete from falling backward, which would reduce the measured jump distance.

Maintaining balance during landings is dependent upon the whole-body momenta (both linear and angular) upon landing and the linear and angular impulses of the GRF during landing. Horizontal and angular momenta are determined at takeoff, whereas the vertical momentum is determined by the height that the CM has fallen. The posture that the athlete adopts upon landing—specifically, the location of the CM relative to the feet—will greatly affect the linear and angular impulses of the GRF. Furthermore, the orientation of the limbs, the velocity of the joints, and the activation of muscles prior to ground contact will all influence the mechanics during the subsequent landings. Clearly, then, the flight phase preceding landing is important in determining the success of the landing task.

For example, an athlete will possess forward angular momentum (negative rotation) during the flight phase of a running long jump. This angular momentum will remain constant during flight, although the angular velocity of the athlete can be modified by altering the posture and, therefore, the moment of inertia during flight (the "hang" technique) or by rotating the arm and leg segments during flight to take up the angular momentum (the "hitch-kick" technique). Arresting the forward angular momentum requires an angular impulse acting on the athlete that opposes the angular momentum. This could be achieved by the athlete landing with the feet placed ahead of the CM such that the body-weight force acts behind the boundary of the base of support, resulting in the body-weight force producing a moment to oppose the forward angular momentum. The horizontal momentum of the CM upon landing will then translate the CM within the boundary of the base of support, removing the moment caused by the body-weight force. The horizontal and vertical components of the GRF will produce linear impulses to arrest the horizontal and vertical momenta possessed by the CM. If the arrest of the momenta occurs with the CM within the boundaries of the base of support, the athlete will remain balanced.

If the athlete lands with the CM within the boundaries of the base of support while possessing both linear and angular momenta, the athlete can alter the direction of the resultant GRF by manipulating the net joint moments acting about the hip, knee, and ankle joints. Recall that the combination of extensor moments at the hip and ankle joints with a flexor moment at the knee joint produces a resultant GRF that acts in a forward and upward direction. Therefore, landing with this configuration of joint moments will result in the GRF acting anteriorly to the CM, producing an angular impulse to reduce the forward angular momentum of the body. Changing the net moment at each of the joints to an extensor moment will move the resultant GRF back toward the CM. When the GRF acts through the CM, it eliminates the angular impulse that would otherwise reduce the angular momentum of the body; however, the GRF continues to act to reduce the horizontal and vertical components of linear momentum of the CM (Figure 12.5). Again, as long as the momenta are reduced to zero when the CM is within the boundaries of the base of support, the athlete will retain a balanced posture. Evidence shows that the angular momentum is arrested early during landing, mainly during the impact phase, while the retardation of the linear momentum of the CM continues during the stabilization phase as the resultant GRF acts through the CM (Mathiyakom & McNitt-Gray, 2008). The interaction between the lower-body joint moments can be changed accordingly to allow the linear and angular momenta to be altered during a preparatory landing task where the athlete must possess momentum to project him or her into a subsequent flight phase commensurate with the task (e.g., a jump or cutting movement).

Gender Differences in the Biomechanics of Landing

The evidence shows that females tend to incur greater peak normalized GRF during landings compared to males (Chappell, Creighton, Giuliani, Yu, & Garrett, 2007; Kernozek, Torry, Van Hoof, Cowley, & Tanner, 2005; LaPorta et al., 2013; Pappas, Hagins, Sheikhzadeh, Nordin, & Rose, 2007; Schmitz et al., 2007). These gender differences in the dynamics of the GRF are likely due to the differences in the posture adopted at landing, as females tend to land in a more extended posture with greater extension at the hip and knee joints (Decker, Torry, Wyland, Sterett, & Steadman, 2003; Schmitz et al., 2007). This would increase the effective mass of females during landing tasks compared to males. Gender differences have also been reported in the negative work performed at the hip, knee, and ankle joints during landing tasks. For example, although both male and female athletes absorb a greater amount of energy at the hip and ankle joints compared to the knee joint, female athletes absorb a greater amount of energy at the knee joint compared to male athletes (Schmitz & Shultz, 2010; Shultz et al., 2010). Indeed, in one study females absorbed the greatest energy at the knee joint, then the ankle joint, with the least amount of energy absorbed at the hip joint (Decker et al., 2003).

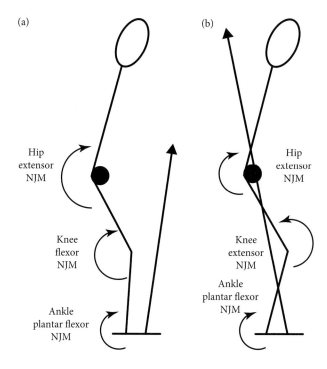

Note: NJM is net joint moment.

Figure 12.5 The effect of net joint moments at the hip, knee, and ankle joint on the direction of the resultant ground reaction force during a stationary landing task where the body possesses positive horizontal and negative vertical linear momentum and negative (forward-rotating) angular momentum. (a) At initial ground contact, a net extensor moment at the hip and ankle joints combined with a net flexor moment at the knee generates an upward and forward-directed resultant ground reaction force. This ground reaction force acts away from the center of mass at this instant, generating an angular impulse to arrest the negative angular momentum of the body. (b) Changing the net joint moments to extensor moments results in the resultant ground reaction force changing direction, such that it now acts through the center of mass. The ground reaction force no longer generates an angular impulse but continues to generate vertical and horizontal impulses to arrest the linear momentum of the center of mass.

It is apparent that female athletes tend to rely on the negative work done by the knee extensors more than their male counterparts. Gender differences are also noted in abduction–adduction moments at the knee joint, with females being reported to produce a lower adduction moment at the knee joint during a stationary landing task (Kernozek et al., 2005). As a result, female athletes demonstrate greater knee abduction angles during a variety of landing tasks (Ford, Myer, & Hewett, 2003; Kernozek et al., 2005; McLean, Walker, & van den Bogert, 2005).

Interestingly, female athletes with limited sagittal plane motion at the lower-body joints tend to demonstrate increased motion in the frontal plane (Pollard, Sigward, & Powers, 2010). Females have also been shown to exhibit decreased hip external rotation but increased knee internal rotation during preparatory landing tasks (Chappell et al., 2007; Nagano, Hirofumi, Akai, & Fukubayashi, 2007).

Finally, gender differences have been identified in the activation of the musculature controlling the moment at the knee joint about the mediolateral axis identified during landing tasks. Specifically, females demonstrate greater activation of the quadriceps and hamstring muscles during a preparatory landing task compared to males (Shultz, Nguyen, Leonard, & Schmitz, 2009). Other researchers have reported that female athletes tend to demonstrate earlier quadriceps activation relative to the hamstrings compared to male athletes prior to landing (Nagano et al., 2007) or reduced hamstrings activation during the absorption phase of landing (Chappell et al., 2007). Furthermore, female athletes appear to respond to increased fall heights with greater quadriceps activation but without similar increases in the activation of the hamstrings (Ford, Myer, Schmitt, Uhl, & Hewett, 2011)—a factor that would explain the greater knee extensor moments demonstrated by females during landing tasks.

These gender differences in the biomechanical variables associated with landing tasks have implications for injuries to the structures that provide support to the knee joint, particularly the ACL (see Landing Concept 12.4).

Landing Concept 12.4

Injury during landing tasks: Noncontact anterior cruciate ligament injuries

The anterior cruciate ligament is a dense band of connective tissue that runs from the medial side of the lateral femoral condyle to insert on the medial tibial eminence (Zantop, Petersen, & Fu, 2005). The anterior-medial course that the ligament follows as it runs through the intercondylar fossa permits it to primarily resist anterior tibial translation, providing 85% of total restraint to the translation of the tibia, with abduction and internal rotation of the tibia relative to the femur also restrained by the ACL (Kweon, Lederman, & Chhabra, 2013; Zantop et al., 2005). Functionally, the ACL is differentiated into anteromedial (AM) and posterolateral (PL) bundles. The AM becomes more taut as the knee is accelerated into flexion and the PL loosens during this motion; the opposite effects occur when the knee is accelerated into extension (Zantop et al., 2005). In addition to the contributions to the stability of the knee joint proffered by the ACL, the mechanoreceptors located within the ligament confer an important proprioceptive function to the ACL (Zantop et al., 2005).

An estimated 250,000 ACL injuries occur annually in the United States (Boden, Griffin, & Garrett, 2000), and injury to the ACL is especially common among athletes. For example, approximately 2000 injuries per year were reported in National Collegiate Athletics Association sports during the period 1988–1989 through 2003–2004 (Renstrom et al., 2008). The majority of these injuries were incurred in noncontact situations (i.e., situations where there is an absence of a direct application of a force from an opposing player) when the player was either landing from a jump or performing a cutting movement (Griffin et al., 2000). An ACL injury requires a potentially lengthy rehabilitation period, and osteoarthritis of the knee joint has been shown to develop in 40% to 50% of individuals within 14 years following an ACL injury regardless of the method of treatment (von Porat, Roos, & Roos, 2004).

The biomechanics of the ACL (restraining anterior tibial translation, abduction, internal rotation) allow the mechanisms for the injury to the ligament during these noncontact situations to be determined. For example, knee flexion greater than 10° in combination with an externally applied abduction moment and anterior tibial translation has been shown to increase the loading on the ACL (Markoff et al., 1995). Indeed, a multiplanar mechanism of injury to the ACL during noncontact situations appears more likely than a single-planar mechanism (Quatman, Quatman-Yates, & Hewett, 2010). Peak strain of the ACL has been predicted to occur during a rapid deceleration of the body, such as that experienced during the impact phase (100 ms or less after ground contact) of landing tasks (Cerulli, Benoit, Lamontagne, Caraffa, & Liti, 2003; Koga et al., 2010; Withrow, Huston, Wojtys, & Ashton-Miller, 2006). This is typically the time of greatest energy absorption at the knee joint (Zhang et al., 2000).

What is noteworthy about the epidemiology of noncontact ACL injuries is that female athletes have been shown to have a 2- to 10-fold greater rate of ACL injury compared to male athletes (Hewett & Myer, 2011). This finding has prompted the investigation of differences between female and male athletes that may be responsible for the gender disparity in noncontact ACL injuries. These differences can be broadly divided into risk factors that are external to the athlete and those that are internal (Table 12.1).

There is likely an interaction between the risk factors presented in Table 12.1 that predisposes a female athlete to a greater chance of incurring an ACL injury, rather than any one risk factor alone being the cause of the gender disparity (McLean & Beaulieu, 2010). For the strength and conditioning practitioner, the important point is to recognize that some of these risk factors are modifiable. Notably, the variables related to differences in the lower-body joint mechanics between female and male athletes during landing tasks should be taken into account. These mechanical differences, described in Table 12.2, can be categorized as landing strategies that are ligament, quadriceps, leg, or trunk dominant in the female athlete (Myer, Brent, Ford, & Hewett, 2011).

Evidence shows that the poor landing mechanics demonstrated by female athletes (and highlighted in Tables 12.1 and 12.2) are already established in prepubertal females (Sigward, Pollard, & Powers, 2012), although some researchers have reported that anatomic and physiological changes during puberty result in the appearance of the biomechanical risk factors (Ford, Shapiro, Myer, Van Den Bogert, & Hewett, 2010; Haas et al., 2003). This implies that any prevention program aimed at improving the poor landing mechanics in female athletes should be instigated at an early age.

(continues)

(continued)

Table 12.1
External and Internal Risk Factors for Noncontact Anterior Cruciate Ligament Injury

Category	Variable	Description
External	Competition in games versus practice	■ Greater risk during competition compared to practice
	Footwear and playing surface	■ Greater risk when performing on surfaces with high coefficient of friction
	Meteorological conditions	■ Greater risk during periods of low rainfall and high evaporation
Internal	Anatomical	*Notch size and ACL geometry* ■ Greater risk with small intercondylar notch ■ Female ACL smaller than male ACL *Posterior tibial slope* ■ Greater risk with greater slope of lateral tibial plateau and lower slope of medial tibial plateau
	Hormonal	*Structure and mechanical properties of ACL* ■ Female ACL has lower tensile stiffness ■ Females have greater knee joint laxity *Menstrual cycle* ■ Greater risk during preovulatory phase of cycle
	Lower-body joint mechanics	*Trunk motion* ■ Females have greater lateral motion of the trunk during landing tasks *Hip joint* ■ Females have less hip flexion at ground contact during landing tasks ■ Females have less hip flexion during absorption phase of landing tasks *Knee joint* ■ Females have less knee flexion at ground contact during landing tasks ■ Females have less knee flexion during absorption phase of landing tasks ■ Females have greater quadriceps electromyography during absorption phase of landing tasks ■ Females have greater anterior tibial shear force during landing tasks ■ Females have greater knee abduction at ground contact during landing tasks ■ Females have greater knee abduction during absorption phase of landing tasks

Data from Hewett, T. E., & Myer, G. D. (2011). The mechanistic connection between the trunk, hip, knee, and anterior cruciate ligament injury. *Exercise and Sport Sciences Reviews, 39*, 161–166; Renstrom, P., Ljungqvist, A., Arendt, E., Beynnon, B., Fukubayashi, T., Garrett, W., . . . Engebretsen, L. (2008). Non-contact ACL injuries in female athletes: An International Olympic Committee current concepts statement. *British Journal of Sports Medicine, 42*, 394–412.

Table 12.2

Mechanical Risk Factors That Predispose Female Athletes to a Higher Risk of Anterior Cruciate Ligament Injury During Landings

Risk Factor Category	Description
Ligament dominance	Imbalance between neuromuscular and ligamentous control of dynamic knee joint stability
Quadriceps dominance	Imbalance between the strength, recruitment, and coordination of the knee flexors and extensors
Leg dominance	Bilateral strength, coordination, and control differences
Trunk dominance	Inability to resist the inertial demands of the trunk
Technique perfection	Ability to maintain the jump–landing sequence across multiple jumps

Data from Myer, G. D., Brent, J. L., Ford, K. R., & Hewett, T. E. (2011). Real-time assessment and neuromuscular training feedback techniques to prevent ACL injury in female athletes. *Strength and Conditioning Journal, 33,* 21–35.

The mechanics of the knee during preparatory landing tasks appear to be more injurious when the task is unplanned and the athlete has to respond to an external stimulus prior to ground contact, compared to when tasks are planned and the athlete has prior knowledge of the specific movements required during the task (McLean, Borotikar, & Lucey, 2010). For example, dancers and cheerleaders do not typically incur noncontact ACL injuries with the same frequency as soccer and basketball players (Didier & Wall, 2011). A plausible explanation for difference is that the movements of dancers and cheerleaders, being choreographed, are preplanned. Moreover, the presentation of generic stimuli during an unplanned cutting task has been shown to induce more injurious knee mechanics than unplanned cutting tasks that require the athlete to attend to sport-specific information (Lee et al., 2013). An analysis of actual ACL injuries incurred in noncontact situations revealed that an opponent was close to the athlete at the time of injury (Krosshaug et al., 2007). This suggests that the close proximity of an opponent may provide sufficient distraction for the athlete to perturb the motor system into producing injurious mechanics.

Collectively, these findings suggest that the assessment of gender differences in noncontact ACL injuries and prevention programs requires the athlete to complete movements that comprise task and environmental constraints specific to the sports, including "distracting elements" such as other players in close proximity (i.e., representative tasks). A closed-skill task such as stepping from a box may not represent a valid assessment tool for a coach to determine potentially injurious mechanics of the athlete or provide an appropriate stimulus to which the athlete must adapt.

Enhancement of Landing

In our discussion of the enhancement of landing, we will focus on the biomechanical aspects of landing tasks that have implications for reducing the risk of injury. Although the range of injuries that an athlete could incur due to landing tasks are numerous, with many associated etiological factors, we will limit our discussion here to biomechanical aspects that attenuate the peak GRF and the loading rate of the GRF (see Landing Concept 12.3), and those that can reduce the risk of incurring an ACL injury (see Landing Concept 12.4). The variables covered in this section relate to the technique used by the athlete, the muscular strength of the athlete (an organismic constraint), the landing surface and footwear during the landing task (environmental constraints), and the instructions provided to the athlete by the coach (task or informational constraints).

Increasing Lower-Body Joint Flexion During Absorption

Increasing the flexion undergone at the hip, knee, and ankle joints during the absorption phase of a landing task would reduce the effective mass of the athlete, thereby decreasing the peak GRF and loading rate during the impact phase. This would decrease the loads applied to the joint structures during a landing task, reducing the risk of injury. For example, peak vertical and horizontal GRF during landing has been associated with greater anterior tibial shear forces (Yu, Lin, & Garrett, 2006), whereas greater combined hip and knee flexion during landing is associated with lower knee abduction and internal rotation (Pollard et al., 2010), likely reducing the load applied to the ACL. However, an increased flexion at the lower-body joints during absorption could potentially increase the risk of overuse injuries by increasing the energy absorption of the musculotendinous units that are in a lengthened position (Butler et al., 2003; Kulas et al., 2006). Moreover, the increased time of absorption that would accompany increased joint flexion during landing, while likely reducing the likelihood of injury, may not be conducive to the rapid movements required in many sports.

Use of Arms During Flight and Absorption

Raising the arms during the flight phase of a jump will raise the CM within the body, but will not raise the CM above the ground in the absence of an external reaction force. This will have the effect of moving the athlete's feet closer to the ground during flight, effectively reducing the height that the CM falls between the apex of flight and the beginning of the landing phase. Raising the arms will, therefore, reduce the E_{TK} of the CM upon landing, thereby decreasing the magnitude of work required during the absorption phase of landing. Moreover, the overall work done to dissipate the E_{TK} of the CM is the sum of the work done at each joint during the landing task. In turn, the more joints that the athlete involves during the landing task, the lower the work required from any individual joint. The inclusion of a downward arm swing during the absorption phase of landing, for example, will reduce the work required at the other joints. Therefore, the motion of the arms both during the preceding flight phase and the landing phase can reduce the risk of injury to the lower-body joints.

Bilateral Compared to Unilateral Landings

Greater peak GRF has been reported during both stationary and preparatory landing tasks performed unilaterally compared with similar tasks performed bilaterally

(Wang, 2011; Weinhandl, Joshi, & O'Conor, 2010). The greater peak forces during the unilateral task are caused by lower flexion angles at the hip and the knee joints (greater effective mass). Greater peak extension and abduction moments as well as greater anterior shear forces at the knee are also evident during unilateral compared to bilateral landing tasks (Wang, 2011), thereby increasing the potential for ACL injuries during the unilateral tasks. The relative contribution of energy absorption at the lower-body joints also differs between bilateral and unilateral landing tasks. Specifically, hip and knee joints are the main energy dissipaters in the sagittal plane (e.g., negative work done by an extensor moment at the joints) during stationary landing tasks performed bilaterally, while the hip and the ankle joint fulfill this role during unilateral performance (Yeow, Lee, & Goh, 2011a). Moreover, the hip is the main energy dissipater in the frontal plane (e.g., negative work done during abduction–adduction) during bilateral landing tasks, whereas the knee becomes the main energy dissipater in the frontal plane during unilateral landing, performing a greater amount of negative work than even during bilateral tasks (Yeow et al., 2011a). This is again likely to increase the risk of incurring an injury to the ACL.

Even when performing bilateral landing tasks, differences are noted in the mechanics associated with the dominant and nondominant legs. Specifically, during a preparatory landing task (stop–jump), there is a greater knee extensor moment in the dominant leg; by comparison, there is a lower peak vertical GRF during a stationary landing task in the dominant leg (Edwards, Steele, Cook, Purdam, & McGhee, 2012). This has implications for injury risk in both legs. In recognition of this fact, the strength and conditioning coach may wish to identify the dominant and nondominant legs of the athlete and minimize any differences in muscular strength.

Muscular Strength

Despite the different indices of muscular strength, investigations into the role of strength in the mechanics of landing have focused on measures of maximal muscular strength. In women, greater maximal isometric strength of the knee extensors predicts greater energy absorption at the knee joint during a preparatory landing task (Schmitz & Shultz, 2010), suggesting that those female athletes with greater muscular strength adopt a landing strategy whereby the knee controls the motion of the CM during the absorption phase. Maximal knee extensor strength has also been shown to be a predictor of greater quadriceps activation during a preparatory landing task (drop–jump) in females but not males (Shultz et al., 2009). However, knee extensor strength did not predict knee motion during the landing task.

Females have been shown to have less muscle mass than males (Wells, 2007), with these differences in muscular strength between male and female athletes then being proposed as an explanation as to why females tend to land with reduced hip and knee flexion angles (Lephart, Ferris, Riemann, Myers, & Fu, 2002). In men, muscular strength (peak isokinetic knee extension and flexor torque normalized to body mass) has been shown to be positively correlated with knee flexion angle at ground contact and knee flexion excursion during the absorption phase of landing during the execution of a single-leg stop–jump task (Nagai, Sell, House, Abt, & Lephart, 2013), yet isokinetic strength does not correlate with knee valgus angles during single-leg drop–landings in male rugby union players (Akins et al., 2013). However, eccentric muscular strength has been shown to correlate positively with the energy absorbed at the hip, knee, and ankle joints in female athletes but not in males (Montgomery, Shultz, Schmitz, Wideman, & Henson, 2012). Furthermore, eccentric strength appears to be an intermediary factor in the relationship between lean mass and energy absorption in the female athletes. Therefore, the strength and conditioning coach may wish to assess both lean mass and eccentric strength of athletes, particularly females.

Finally, stronger athletes are better able to utilize the negative work done during the absorption phase of a repeated drop–jump task, resulting in a higher mechanical efficiency than their weaker counterparts (McBride & Snyder, 2012). This reduction in the energetic cost of performing repeated drop–jumps has implications for athletes involved in sports such as basketball, soccer, and volleyball, in which the athlete is required to execute multiple jumps and landing sequences throughout the game.

Landing Surface and Footwear

Just as the deformation of the lower-body joints influences the dynamics of the GRF acting on the athlete, so, too, does the deformation of the surface onto which the athlete lands. Computer simulations have shown that peak GRF is greater when an athlete lands on a stiff surface with low deformation as compared to an elastic surface that experiences greater deformation (Peikenkamp, Fritz, & Nicol, 2002). When athletes actually perform preparatory landing tasks on surfaces of differing stiffness values, time to peak vertical GRF is shorter when landing on high-stiffness surfaces (e.g., concrete, bitumen) as compared to low-stiffness surfaces (e.g., turf, rubber) despite no differences in the magnitude of the peak force (Steele & Milburn, 1988). This is something that the strength and conditioning practitioner has direct control over when implementing jump–landing exercises, although the surfaces used in competition are often beyond their control.

The expectation that the athlete has of the stiffness of the surface also alters the athlete's mechanics during landing tasks. For example, when athletes were informed of the relative stiffness of the mat upon which they were about to land, researchers observed an increase in knee flexion during a stationary landing task performed onto a stiffer mat, with a concomitant decrease in the time to peak vertical GRF (McNitt-Gray, Yokoi, & Millward, 1993, 1994). During a preparatory landing task (single-leg hopping) onto a surface that was known to be stiff, individuals anticipated ground contact with increased knee flexion and greater ranges of flexion at the hip and ankle joints when compared to the landings performed onto a surface that was known to be less stiff (Moritz & Farley, 2004). Despite these alterations, leg stiffness was increased on the stiffer surface, allowing the individuals to maintain the same magnitude of vertical stiffness (ratio of GRF to displacement of CM) and time to peak force during the landing task. However, when the surface was unexpectedly changed from a low-stiffness surface to a high-stiffness surface, the individuals were able to increase knee flexion during landing and the time to peak force was decreased. These findings demonstrate that the surface upon which the athlete lands has significant effects on the mechanics of the landing task.

The choice of footwear worn by the athlete has been shown to make little difference to the dynamics of the GRF during landing tasks. For example, little difference was observed in the impact force during a stationary landing task when athletes wore tennis shoes, wore minimalist shoes, or performed the task barefoot (LaPorta et al., 2013; Yeow, Lee, & Goh, 2011b). However, joint mechanics can be altered by footwear selection. For example, a greater energy absorption at the knee joint occurs when the athlete wears shoes as compared to going barefoot (Yeow et al., 2011b), while ankle stiffness is greater in barefoot athletes compared to shod athletes during drop–jump landings (Shultz, Schmitz, Tritsch, & Montgomery, 2012). These differences likely result from a conscious alteration in landing posture due to the athlete's anticipation of the landing. Nevertheless, footwear choice has less influence on landing mechanics in terms of energy dissipation than the action of the joint moments during the absorption phase (Zhang, Clowers, Kohstall, & Yu, 2005).

Manipulating Informational Constraints

The instructions provided to the athlete prior to a movement task as well as the feedback provided upon completion of the task represent **informational constraints** that can be manipulated by the coach to enhance performance. Specifically, the provision of specific verbal **instructions** to the athlete prior to a landing task can result in an immediate change in the mechanics of the movement. For example, when females were instructed to "land softly," researchers observed a reduction in peak vertical GRF and an increase in knee flexion when landing from a vertical jump; the instruction to "land with the knees over the toes" also produced greater knee flexion during landing (Milner, Fairbrother, Srivatsan, & Zhang, 2012). The instruction to "land with equal weight distribution" reduced the asymmetry in peak vertical GRF during the same landing task. Other researchers have reported that instructing the athlete to lean forward during landing resulted in an immediate reduction in the peak vertical GRF and knee extensor moment, while concomitantly increasing the hip and ankle extensor moments in both men and women during a single-leg stationary landing task (Shimokochi et al., 2013). Some evidence indicates that the instruction to land softly reduces the peak GRF by causing the athlete to exert lower peak extensor moments at the knee and ankle joints (Zhang et al., 2000).

The provision of feedback has also been shown to affect athletes' performance during landing tasks. Specifically, feedback in the form of **knowledge of performance**, in which athletes review video footage of their own movements during landing, combined with an expert providing verbal corrections and visual demonstrations, has been shown to reduce the peak vertical GRF during landing tasks (Ericksen, Gribble, Pfile, & Pietrosimone, 2013). The provision of feedback appears to be effective at altering the mechanics of landing tasks even when it is delayed by one week after the practice session (Ericksen et al., 2013). Interestingly, providing real-time visual feedback on knee abduction moments does not improve frontal-plane knee mechanics during jumping landings beyond simply performing the task (Beaulieu & Palmieri-Smith, 2013). Furthermore, improved knee mechanics (greater flexion at ground contact, greater flexion during absorption phase) have been reported following an intervention comprising video feedback of both an expert landing correctly (observational learning) and video feedback of the athlete's own performance during the landing associated with a drop jump task; these improvements were maintained for a one-month period, as demonstrated by performance on a retention test (Etnoyer, Cortes, Ringleb, Van Lunen, & Onate, 2013). However, a transfer task was not performed.

Qualitative Analysis of Landing Performance

This qualitative analysis of landing focuses on the biomechanics of stationary landing tasks that influence the dynamics of the GRF (peak and rates of force development of both the vertical and horizontal components) during landing tasks, as these appear to be important risk factors for a number of injuries, including stress fractures, muscle strains, and ACL injuries. To explore this topic, we will use the four-stage model of qualitative analysis of technique during a given motor skill developed by Knudson and Morrison (2002). This model includes the stages of preparation, observation, evaluation/diagnosis, and intervention. Here we discuss each of these four stages as they apply to the analysis of stationary landing tasks.

Preparation Stage

In the initial preparation stage of a qualitative analysis, the coach should identify the critical features of the landing task from biomechanical principles as well as the task and environmental constraints associated with sports performance. This will allow the coach to develop a deterministic model of the skill to aid in the analysis of the movement. Table 12.3 identifies some basic biomechanical principles and their application to the analysis of stationary landing tasks.

Table 12.3
Biomechanical Principles That Can Be Applied in the Qualitative Analysis of Stationary Landing Tasks

Principle	Application to Landing Tasks
Number of body segments	The coach should assess the number of segments accelerated by the athlete during the landing task. For example, determine if a downward arm swing is incorporated during the absorption phase of the landing and the rotation of the trunk, thigh, and leg segments about the hip, knee, and ankle joints.
Coordination of body segments	The coach should assess the motion of the arms, trunk, and lower-body segments prior to landing.
	The coach should assess the order of rotation of the body segments during the absorption phase to analyze the distal-to-proximal sequence at the ankle, knee, and hip joints.
	The coach should assess the orientation of the body segments at ground contact in the sagittal plane (i.e., forward lean of the trunk, flexion at the knee and ankle joints) and the frontal plane (i.e., lateral trunk lean, feet width, knee motion).
	The coach should assess whether the athlete lands with a toe-to-heel sequence and whether the feet make contact simultaneously during bilateral tasks.
Maximizing the deceleration path	The coach should determine the change in height of the CM during the absorption phase by assessing the position of the pelvis from ground contact to its lowest position during landing.
	The deceleration path will be affected by flexion at the hip, knee, and ankle joints during the absorption phase.
Stability	The coach should determine if the CM remains within the base of support during absorption by assessing the position of the pelvis with respect to the feet.
	The coach should assess the motion of the trunk and arms after absorption, along with any forward or backward steps taken by the athlete.

Note: CM = center of mass.

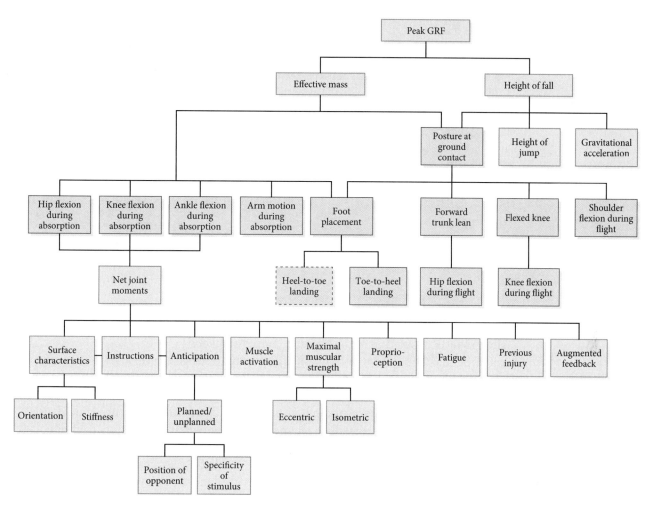

Figure 12.6 A deterministic model of the peak vertical ground reaction force during landing from a vertical jump. The shaded variables are those that the coach can observe during the execution of the task; the variable in the dashed box is associated with the large peak vertical ground reaction force.

Figure 12.6 shows a simple deterministic model developed from investigations of the biomechanical factors affecting the dynamics of the GRF during stationary landing tasks. The coach can observe the variables in the shaded boxes during landings executed by the athlete. The variables relating to the flexion of the joints should be increased to minimize the peak GRF and loading rate, while the athlete should adopt a toe-to-heel landing strategy. The dashed box in Figure 12.6 represents a variable that has been associated with greater peak GRF and loading rates and should be avoided by the athlete. Note that the kinematic variables identified in this model occur in the sagittal plane. When assessing the landing technique to determine the biomechanical risk factors associated with ACL injuries, the mechanics in the frontal plane also need to be assessed (see Worked Examples 12.1 and 12.2 later in this section).

Following the identification of the critical features of the landing task, the coach should identify the movement phases for the observation of the skill. Table 12.4 identifies the movement phases for the analysis of a stationary landing task. Note that

Table 12.4
Movement Phases for the Analysis of Stationary Landing Tasks

Movement Phase	Details
Flight	The airborne phase that precedes the initial contact with the ground.
Absorption	Begins with the initial contact after flight.
	Ends with the CM at its lowest vertical position (or at the time of maximal knee flexion).
	Contains the phases of impact (initial 100 ms of absorption) and stabilization (from 100 ms to the lowest vertical position of the CM).

Note: CM = center of mass.

a preparatory landing task would also include a propulsion phase beginning at the lowest vertical position of the CM and ending at takeoff.

The selection of the specific task is important during the preparation stage of a qualitative assessment of landing technique. Recall that landing from a fall from a box is mechanically different from landing from a jump, and that stationary landings are different from preparatory landings (Afifi & Hinrichs, 2012). The coach should also consider whether the task will be planned or unplanned. If an unplanned landing task will be used, then the coach should consider the specificity of the stimulus presented to the athlete relative to the chosen sport (see Applied Research 12.2).

The coach should also determine whether the landing task will be unilateral or bilateral. If it is bilateral, the coach needs to decide from which side he or she will assess the athlete's technique. When assessing one leg during a bilateral task, the most common approach is to assess the dominant leg, identified through simple question-ing of the athlete (e.g., "Which leg do you kick a ball with?").

Finally, the coach should consider the instructions that are provided to the athlete prior to his or her performance. Recall that instructions represent informational constraints that can alter the mechanics of the athlete (e.g., "land softly," "land with the knees over the toes," "land with equal weight distribution"). In most cases, the coach does not provide any instructions on the specific mechanical aspects of the landing technique of the athlete so as to avoid any alterations that doing so may cause. However, during preparatory landing tasks, an instruction relating to the subsequent movement following landing is required (e.g., "jump for maximal height," "cut as fast as you can").

Observation Stage

Coaches should place themselves so that they can view the performance of the athlete from the side, as the major motions of the body segments involved in the execution of a landing task occur in the sagittal plane. However, a frontal view of the athlete is also required if the coach is concerned with the risk of ACL injury. If a video camera is used to supplement the observations of the coach, then the fast movements associated with landing tasks require relatively high shutter speeds, with a speed of 1/100 s being suggested (Bartlett, 2007).

Evaluation/Diagnosis Stage

The performance during the landing task can be evaluated by determining the accomplishment of the biomechanical features during each of the movement phases pertinent to the specific goal of the task. Table 12.5 outlines a method to evaluate the biomechanical principles during the absorption phase of a stationary landing task.

Examples of qualitative analyses of landing that have been developed for preparatory landing tasks and are specific to identifying the mechanical risk factors for ACL injuries are highlighted in Worked Examples 12.1 and 12.2.

Table 12.5
Evaluation of the Biomechanical Principles During the Absorption Phase Associated with a Stationary Landing Task

Movement Phase	Biomechanical Principle	Evaluation
Flight	Coordination of body segments	Did the athlete raise the arms during flight?
		Did the athlete have forward lean of the trunk and flexion at the hip, knee, and ankle joints prior to landing?
Absorption	Number of body segments	Did the athlete produce flexion at the hip, knee, and ankle joints during landing?
		Did the athlete swing the arms down during landing?
	Coordination of body segments	Was there distal-to-proximal sequencing of rotations of the trunk, thigh, and leg segments during the landing?
		Was the trunk leaning forward at the start of landing?
		Were the hip, knee, and ankle joints flexed at the start of landing?
		Did the athlete land on the toes?
		Did the feet contact simultaneously?
		Did the landing sound soft?
	Deceleration path	How far did the pelvis descend to its lowest position?
	Stability	Was the athlete's pelvis above the feet at the end of the absorption phase?
		Did the athlete use the trunk and arm segments after the absorption phase to maintain balance?
		Did the athlete have to take a step forward or backward to establish balance after absorption?

Intervention Stage

The final stage of a qualitative analysis of landing requires the development of an intervention to improve performance of the landing task. It is important to recognize that most observations of motor skills are undertaken in situations where the

Worked Example 12.1
Using the repeated tuck jump test to perform a qualitative analysis during a preparatory landing task

Myer, Ford, and Hewett (2008) developed the repeated tuck jump test, in which tuck jumps are performed continuously for a period of 10 s, as an assessment tool to identify potentially injurious landing mechanics in athletes. The athlete is instructed to "jump repeatedly for 10 s with high effort, bringing the knees up as high as possible so that both thighs are parallel to the ground, landing softly in the same foot print with each jump, and then immediately begin the next jump." The foot placement is marked on the floor for each athlete, and no feedback is provided regarding the technique. The technique is also videoed from in the sagittal and frontal planes to improve the accuracy of the assessment.

Technique flaws during the tuck jump protocol can be categorized as relating to knee and thigh motion, foot position during landing, and plyometric technique (Table 12.6). Each of the risk factors presented in Table 12.6 can be assigned a score of 1 (present) or 0 (not present) following the viewing of the video footage. An overall score for the athlete can then be provided by summing the individual risk factor scores.

The athlete's performance during the repeated tuck jump test can be used to establish mechanical risk factors associated with ACL injury (Table 12.7). While Myer et al. (2008) reported that the repeated tuck jump protocol has high intra-rater reliability, Dudley

Table 12.6
Technique Flaws Identified During the Repeated Tuck Jump Protocol

Category	Observation
Knee and thigh motion	Knee abduction at landing
	Thighs do not reach parallel (peak of jump)
	Thighs not equal side-to-side (during jump)
Foot position during landing	Foot placement not shoulder-width apart
	Foot placement not parallel (front-to-back)
	Foot contact timing not equal
	Excessive landing contact noise
Plyometric technique	Pause between jumps
	Technique declines prior to 10 s
	Does not land in same footprint (excessive in-flight motion)

Data from Myer, G. D., Ford, K. R., & Hewett, T. E. (2008). Tuck jump assessment for reducing anterior cruciate ligament injury risk. *Athletic Therapy Today, 13*, 39–44.

Table 12.7

Observations Made During the Repeated Tuck Jump Test and the Risk Factors Associated with Noncontact Anterior Cruciate Ligament Injuries

Risk Factor	Description	Observations During Landing Task
Ligament dominance	An imbalance between the neuromuscular and ligamentous control of dynamic knee joint stability	Foot placement greater than shoulder width at ground contact Knee abduction during absorption
Quadriceps dominance	An imbalance between the strength, recruitment, and coordination of the knee flexors and extensors	Fully extended knee at ground contact Minimal knee flexion during absorption Excessively loud contact
Leg dominance	Bilateral strength, coordination, and control differences	Unequal displacement of thighs during flight of each tuck jump Asymmetry in foot contact Nonparallel foot placement
Trunk dominance	Inability to resist the inertial demands of the trunk	Unequal displacement of thighs during each tuck jump Pause between jumps Landing in different foot print
Technique perfection	An ability to maintain jump–landing sequence across multiple jumps	Technique deterioration across 10-s period

Data from Myer, G. D., Brent, J. L., Ford, K. R., & Hewett, T. E. (2011). Real-time assessment and neuromuscular training feedback techniques to prevent ACL injury in female athletes. *Strength and Conditioning Journal, 33*, 21–35.

et al. (2013) identified only poor to moderate intra-rater reliability for this protocol. Furthermore, inter-rater reliability in the scoring of landing technique was improved following a second administration of the protocol, suggesting learning effects with the assessment protocol on behalf of the observer.

athletes are removed from the typical task and environmental constraints that they must operate within in their actual sporting situation; the strength and conditioning practitioner is likely to observe an athlete landing in a well-controlled environment to facilitate analysis of the movement. As a consequence, the observed skill may not be representative of how the athlete executes a landing in the actual sport, which may lead to the selection of interventions to improve performance that may actually be inappropriate. Specific interventions that can be utilized to improve landing performance are the focus of the next section.

Worked Example 12.2
Using the landing error scoring system to perform a qualitative analysis during a preparatory landing task

The Landing Error Scoring System (LESS) requires the athlete to jump forward from a 0.30-m box and land a distance equal to half of the athlete's standing height in front of the box, before then performing a vertical jump for maximal height (Padua et al., 2009). The athlete is instructed to jump as high as possible when landing from the box. No feedback regarding technique is provided. The movement is video-taped in the sagittal and frontal planes.

Table 12.8 shows the scoring system associated with the LESS. Each variable identified is associated with increased risk of ACL injury (Beutler, de la Motte, Marshall, Padua, &

Table 12.8
The Landing Error Scoring System Used in the Qualitative Assessment of Landing Technique for Anterior Cruciate Ligament Injury Risk Factors

Sagittal (Side) View of Landing	Frontal View of Landing
Hip flexion angle at ground contact: hips are flexed	Lateral (side) trunk flexion at contact: trunk is flexed
Yes = 0, No = 1	*Yes = 0, No = 1*
Trunk flexion angle at contact: trunk in front of hips	Knee abduction angle at contact: knees over midfoot
Yes = 0, No = 1	*Yes = 0, No = 1*
Knee flexion angle at contact: greater than 30°	Knee abduction displacement: knees inside of large toe
Yes = 0, No = 1	*Yes = 0, No = 1*
Ankle plantarflexion at contact: toe-to-heel	Foot position at contact: toes pointing out less than 30°
Yes = 0, No = 1	*Yes = 0, No = 1*
Hip flexion at maximum knee flexion angle: greater than at contact	Stance width at contact: less than shoulder width
Yes = 0, No = 1	*Yes = 0, No = 1*
Trunk flexion at maximum knee flexion angle: trunk in front of hips	Stance width at contact: greater than shoulder width
Yes = 0, No = 1	*Yes = 0, No = 1*
Knee flexion displacement: greater than 30°	Initial foot contact: symmetric
Yes = 0, No = 1	*Yes = 0, No = 1*
Sagittal plane joint displacement	
Large motion (soft) = 0	
Average = 1	
Small motion (loud/stiff) = 2	

Table 12.8   (continued)

Overall Impression of Landing
Excellent = 0
Average = 1
Poor = 2

Final Scoring
Excellent (0–3)
Good (4–5)
Moderate (6)
Poor (≥7)

Data from Padua, D. A., Marshall, S. W., Boling, M. C., Thigpen, C. A., Garrett, W. E., & Beutler, A. I. (2009). The Landing Error Scoring System (LESS) is a valid and reliable clinical assessment tool of jump-landing biomechanics: The JUMP-ACL study. *American Journal of Sports Medicine, 37,* 1996–2002.

Boden, 2009; Padua et al., 2009). The LESS has been shown to be both valid and reliable in determining inappropriate landing mechanics (Padua et al., 2009). However, it was unable to predict ACL injuries sustained in a cohort of high school and collegiate athletes (Smith et al., 2012).

Interventions to Reduce the Risk of Injury During Landing Tasks

A variety of effective training methods to reduce the risk of injury during landing tasks can be incorporated into an athlete's wider training program. As a mechanical analysis of landing reveals, the athlete must contend with two basic mechanical constraints during landing tasks: (1) the need to dissipate the E_{TK} of the CM and (2) the need to control the linear and/or angular momentum commensurate with the goal of the landing task (i.e., maintain balance upon arresting the motion or execute a jumping or cutting movement). Dissipating energy is achieved by musculotendinous units performing eccentric actions as the lower-body joints flex during the absorption phase of landing to prevent the forces being transmitted to other musculoskeletal structures. The technique that the athlete uses during a landing task influences the ability of these musculotendinous units to absorb energy. Controlling momentum during landing ensures that the athlete can maintain his or her balance or complete a task following landing. Of course, reducing injury risk during landing tasks is another goal.

Given these requirements of landing, training methods to improve muscular strength, balance, and technique are integral in any intervention developed to reduce the risk of injury during landing. These interventions manipulate organismic and task constraints to achieve the desired improvements.

Resistance Training

An intervention comprising only resistance training has not been found to improve landing performance (Herman et al., 2008). Indeed, six weeks of progressive resistance training combining multijoint and single-joint exercises performed twice per week, which resulted in increased maximal (1-RM deadlift) and explosive (broad jump) muscular strength, actually increased the abduction moments at the knee during an unplanned preparatory landing task (cutting) in men with no history of knee injuries (Jamison et al., 2012). Notably, this resistance training program also worsened trunk control in response to unplanned perturbations. Furthermore, the inclusion of trunk stability exercises in the resistance training program did not change the landing mechanics and was ineffective at improving trunk control.

Another study reported that resistance training combining a single-joint exercise (leg curl) and a multijoint exercise (squat) for the lower body induced an increase in potentially injurious mechanics (increased internal rotation moment, decreased knee flexion) during a preparatory landing task (cutting) in recreationally active men (Cochrane et al., 2010). It would appear that a period of resistance training involving general exercises for the lower body performed with moderate intensities (loads equivalent to approximately 60% of maximal strength) in isolation can increase poor landing mechanics in men. However, it should be noted that the general exercises do not necessarily emphasize the muscular strength indices associated with poor landing mechanics (e.g., eccentric strength, plyometric ability).

Balance Training

An intervention consisting of only balance training incorporating exercises performed on a variety of unstable surfaces (e.g., wobble boards, dura discs, Swiss balls) has been shown to reduce poor mechanics (reduction in knee abduction and internal rotation loads) during a preparatory landing task in recreationally active men (Cocharane et al., 2010). However, it is unclear how this mode of training, which is performed in isolation, affects measures of muscular strength (e.g., maximal strength, explosive strength) and athletic performance (e.g., sprinting) given the low intensities associated with exercises performed on unstable surfaces. It is likely that performing isolated balance training may result in detraining and, in turn, a loss of athletic performance, despite the improvements in landing mechanics associated with this training modality.

Integrated Training Programs

Integrated training programs that combine resistance training exercises, plyometric exercises, balance exercises, and sprint/agility training appear to be more effective at improving landing mechanics than programs in which these exercises are performed in isolation. For example, eight weeks of progressive resistance training exercises for the upper and lower body was not as effective as an intervention combining progressive resistance, trunk stability, power, and agility exercises in terms of improving a qualitative assessment of landing performance (Distefano, Distefano, Frank, Clark, & Padua, 2013).

The addition of balance exercises to a training program including progressive resistance training and sprint training with plyometric training produced improved landing mechanics during a unilateral stationary landing task (reduced peak vertical ground reaction force), whereas the addition of plyometric training to the resistance and sprint training modes actually increased the landing force (Myer, Ford, Brent, & Hewett, 2006). These authors concluded that the inclusion of the balance training, which involved dynamic stabilization exercises (land-hold exercises), is important in attenuating forces during landing tasks. The inclusion of plyometric exercises that involve dynamic stabilization requirements within an integrated training program has also been reported to reduce landing forces (Hewett, Stroupe, Nance, & Noyes, 1996).

In a review of the integrated training programs for improving landing mechanics, Hewett, Ford, and Myer (2006) noted that the most effective programs incorporate the following elements:

- Strength training
- Plyometric training
- Balance training
- Augmented feedback on landing technique
- A minimum duration of six weeks with sessions performed more than one time per week
- High compliance

Sportsmetrics Neuromuscular Training Programs have been developed following these guidelines (Hewett, Lindenfeld, Riccobene, & Noyes, 1999; Hewett et al., 1996). These programs comprise specific warm-up, jump training, flexibility training, and agility, acceleration, speed, and endurance drills specific to the sports of soccer, basketball, and tennis (Table 12.9). As such, each workout requires between 90 and 120 min to complete. The jump training is divided into three phases: technique phase (first two weeks), fundamentals phase (two weeks), and performance phase (two weeks). Athletes are instructed during each session to maintain a neutral alignment from their head to heels during jumps and landings, to exaggerate hip and knee flexion, and to maintain heels under hips with toes and knees pointed forward during all ground phases. Athletes are also encouraged to land on their toes and then transfer the load to their heels. These instructions are emphasized through the use of verbal and visual (video) feedback.

Previous researchers have used these types of interventions, performed three times per week for six weeks, with adolescent female basketball players and reported improved aerobic capacity and jump height as well as improved landing mechanics (Noyes, Barber-Westin, Smith, Campbell, & Garrison, 2012). Specifically, the athletes adopted a more neutral landing posture in the frontal plane during a preparatory landing task (drop–jump) as a result of the intervention (i.e., reduced hip adduction and knee abduction). Other researchers have reported that these improved landing mechanics were retained in the majority of the female athletes (69%) after one year (Barber-Westin, Smith, Campbell, & Noyes, 2010).

In collegiate female volleyball players, a post-season break has been shown to cause alterations in lower-body biomechanics during a preparatory landing task (stop–jump) that could be considered potentially injurious with decreased knee flexion at ground contact (Dai, Sorensen, Derrick, & Gillette, 2012). It was proposed that the more extended knee upon landing was due to a decrease in muscular strength caused by the athletes detraining during the one-month break. However, improvements in landing mechanics (decreased peak GRF) can be accrued following a two-week training intervention emphasizing a reduction in peak GRF during landings,

Table 12.9

Comprehensive Neuromuscular Training Program Developed for Female High School Basketball Players with the Goal of Landing Mechanics

Week and Session	Jump Training	Agility Training	Acceleration, Speed, Aerobic Training	Ladders, Reaction Training, Dot Jump Training
Week 1 Sessions 1–3	Wall jumps (20 s) Tuck jumps (20 s) Squat jumps (10 s) Barrier jumps (20 s each): ■ Side-to-side ■ Forward–backward Broad jumps (5 s) Bounding in place (20 s)	Shuttle drill Maze drill	Mountain climbers Sprint-back pedal Suicides	Ladder: High knees High knee ball toss over barrier Dot drill: Double leg jumps
Week 2 Sessions 4–6	Increase duration of jumps in sessions 1–3 by 5 s Add 5 repetitions to broad jumps	Tip drill Figure 4 drill	Mountain climbers Sprint-back pedal Suicides: ■ Forward ■ Backward	Ladder: Up–up, back–back Double high knee with ball toss Add split leg jumps to dot drills
Week 3 Sessions 7–9	Wall jumps (25 s) Tuck jumps (25 s) Triple broad jump into vertical jump (5 repetitions) Squat jumps (15 s) Barrier hops (25 s each): ■ Side-to-side ■ Forward–backward Single-leg hops (5 repetitions) Scissors jumps (25 s) Bounding for distance (1 run)	Square drill 4-dot drills Quarter eagle	Mountain climbers Quarter eagle sprints Suicides: Defensive slides	Bleacher jumps Add 180° split leg jumps to dot drills
Week 4 Sessions 10–12	Increase duration of jumps in sessions 7–9 by 5 s Add 3 repetitions to triple broad into vertical jump	Defensive slides Shoot and sprint	Mountain climbers Sprint with ground touches Full court relay	Ladder: In–in, out–out Add single-leg hops to dot drills

Table 12.9 (continued)

Week and Session	Jump Training	Agility Training	Acceleration, Speed, Aerobic Training	Ladders, Reaction Training, Dot Jump Training
Week 5 Sessions 13–15	Wall jumps (20 s) Step, jump up, down, vertical (30 s) Squat jumps (25 s) Mattress jumps: ■ Side-to-side ■ Forward–backward Triple single-leg hop, stick (5 repetitions each leg) Jump into bounding (3 runs)	Tip drill Irish "D"	Mountain climbers Sprint 180° Sprint, quick feet	Ladder: ■ Scissors ■ Instructor pointing with quick feet up/down Dot drills: All jumps
Week 6 Sessions 16–18	Same as sessions 13–15 Add 5 repetitions to step, jump up, down, vertical Add 1 run to jump into bounding	T-drills: 5-10-5 Kill the grass	Mountain climbers Sprint 360 Power rebounds relay	Ladder: Icky shuffle Single-leg squat jumps and 180° scissors jumps Dot drills: All jumps

Reproduced from Noyes, F. R., Barber-Westin, S. D., Smith, S. T., Campbell, T., & Garrison, T. T. (2012). A training program to improve neuromuscular and performance indices in female high school basketball players. *Journal of Strength and Conditioning Research, 26,* 709–719.

with physical practice augmented by feedback about the magnitude of the landing force during each landing (Iida, Kanehisa, Inaba, & Nakazawa, 2013). A notable finding from this study was that jump height during the drop–jump task improved as a result of the landing training despite no change in squat jump performance. It would appear that improving the ability to attenuate landing forces actually enhances the ability to take advantage of the negative work performed during the landing task and to utilize it during a subsequent task. Furthermore, the inclusion of balance training in landing interventions and the potential for detraining may require different off-season and in-season interventions.

Warm-up-Based Interventions

In contrast to the comprehensive workouts associated with integrative training programs, some researchers have developed a combination of specific warm-up, stretching, and plyometric and agility exercises that replace a traditional 20-min warm-up completed by athletes prior to practice. The exercises associated with one such warm-up–based intervention, known as the **Prevent Injury and Enhance Performance** (PEP) program, are shown in Table 12.10. The PEP program is designed to be administered

Table 12.10
Exercises Used in the Prevent Injury and Enhance Performance
Warm-up Program for Basketball Players

Category	Exercises	Volume
Jog	Jogging	2 laps around court
Dynamic motion	Traveling exercises	2 lengths of court
	■ Jogging	
	■ Skipping	
	■ Carioca/grapevine	
	■ Side shuffle with arm swing	
	■ Sprint at 75% maximum	
	■ High-knee skipping	
	■ High-knee carioca	
	■ Sprint at 100% maximum	
	■ Backward jog	
	■ Bear crawl	
	■ Butt kickers	
	■ Backward jog half-length, turn sprint	
	■ Diagonal skipping	
	Arm swings: forward and backward	20 repetitions each arm
	Trunk rotations	10 in each direction
	Leg swings	
	■ Front-to-back	10 repetitions each leg
	■ Side-to-side	10 repetitions each leg
Strengthening exercises	Heel raises	
	Squats	
	Plank and side plank	
	Push-ups	
	Lunges	
	■ Forward	
	■ Lateral	
	■ Diagonal	
	Walking lunges	
	■ Forward	
	■ Lateral	
	Prone lifts	
	■ Lift arms and legs together	
	■ Lift opposite arm, leg	
	■ Knees flexed 90°, heels together, hips externally rotated, lift arms/legs	

Table 12.10 (*continued*)

Category	Exercises	Volume
Plyometric exercises	Ankle bounces	10 s (week 1); 20 s (week 2); 30 s (week 3)
	Tuck jumps	
	Jumps in place, rotating 180°	
	Squat jumps	
	Broad jumps: hold landing	5 repetitions
	Jump over 3-inch cone	10 s (week 1); 20 s (week 2); 30 s (week 3)
	■ Front-to-back	
	■ Side-to-side	
	Bounding in place	
	Scissors jump	
	Side-to-side bounding	
	Single-leg hop, hop, stick landing	5 repetitions each leg
	Jump, jump, jump, vertical jump	5 repetitions
	Single-leg jump for distance	5 repetitions each leg
	Jump into bounding	4 court lengths
	Diagonal bounding	2 court lengths
Agility runs	Shuttle run	10 repetitions
	■ Between 2 rows of 5 cones, 50 ft apart	
	■ Sprint to cone, backward jog to next cone	
	Diagonal run	10 repetitions
	■ Between 2 rows of 5 cones, 50 ft apart	
	■ Sprint to cone, turn, sprint to next cone	
	Lateral shuffle	10 repetitions
	■ Between 2 rows of 5 cones, 15 ft apart	
	■ Side shuffle from cone to cone	

Data from LaBella, C. R., Huxford, M. R., Grissom, J., Kim, K-Y., Peng, J., & Christoffel, K. K. (2011). Effect of neuromuscular warm-up on injuries in female soccer and basketball athletes in urban public high schools: Cluster randomized controlled trial. *Archives of Pediatric and Adolescent Medicine, 165*, 1033–1040.

by a strength and conditioning coach following a review of the instructions that accompany the program, which include the correct lower-body alignment during the performance of the exercises in both written instruction and video demonstrations showing "correct" and "incorrect" techniques (observational learning). It does not require the use of any additional equipment. Notice the increase in the volume of some of the exercises between weeks in this program.

After following the PEP program over the course of a season, female soccer players were shown to reduce internal hip rotation and increase hip abduction during a preparatory landing task (drop–jump), although no differences in knee joint kinematics were reported (Pollard, Sigward, Ota, Langford, & Powers, 2006). The PEP program, when performed in the warm-up of NCAA Division I female soccer players three times per week, has been shown to reduce the incidence of ACL injuries during both practices and games (Gilchrist et al., 2008). Similar findings have been reported when these neuromuscular warm-ups are instigated with adolescent female soccer and basketball players (Kiani, Hellquist, Ahlqvist, Gedeborg, & Michaëlson, 2010; LaBella et al., 2011; Mandelbaum et al., 2005; Myklebust et al., 2003; Waldén, Atroshi, Magnusson, Wagner, & Hägglund, 2012).

The warm-up–based interventions have the benefits of ease of administration over the comprehensive interventions highlighted earlier, possibly improving compliance. This outcome is important, given that the efficacy of such interventions is strongly related to the compliance of the players with the program (Soligard et al., 2010; Steffen, Myklebust, Olsen, Holme, & Bahr, 2008). Aerts et al. (2013) implemented a warm-up–based injury-prevention program comprising neuromuscular and proprioceptive training with trained male and female basketball players over a three-month period. In this program, the exercises progressed from those focusing on basic techniques where correct lower-body alignment was emphasized (including the athletic position, lunges, and side-to-side jumps), to fundamental exercises (including tuck jumps, squat jumps, single-leg jumps, and jumps on an unstable surface), and finally to more complex sport-specific movements in the performance phase (including maximal jumps, lay-ups, and running and cutting movements). The intervention lasted three months and the exercises were performed twice a week during the players' warm-up, with each session lasting approximately 10 min (Table 12.11). The authors reported that the intervention resulted in a reduction in lower-extremity injuries incurred by the players. Moreover, the coaches who were tasked with implementing the intervention generally reported that the exercises were highly compatible with their training sessions and believed that the program was a useful addition to their training regimens. Adherence to the program was reported to be 86%. Notice that the actual landing technique of the participants was not recorded during the studies using warm-up–based interventions; rather, the researchers typically used injury rates as a surrogate measure of improved performance.

Representative Learning Practices for Landing

A criticism of the training interventions developed to improve the landing mechanics of athletes is the reliance on **explicit learning** strategies through the instructions and feedback provided to the athlete relating to the specific landing postures required (Benjaminse & Otten, 2011). Explicit learning strategies tend to result in conscious control of movement that can be easily perturbed by factors including anxiety, emotions, and changes in environmental constraints. Therefore, an **implicit learning** strategy may be more effective at producing appropriate landing mechanics when the athlete is in the actual sporting environment.

Furthermore, there is an apparent lack of consideration for the role of informational constraints associated with game situations in contributing to poor landing mechanics. Enhancing the attunement of the athlete's movements to the environmental information may reduce the injurious mechanics associated with landing tasks during game situations. Recall that unplanned landing tasks are more likely to induce poor landing

Table 12.11

Injury-Prevention Warm-up for Basketball Players

Phase	Week	Exercise	Repetitions/ Hold Time (s)	Modifications/Description
Technique	1	Co-contraction	10	Co-contraction of quadriceps and hamstrings
		Wall squat	10	Ensure correct lower-body alignment
		Lateral jump and hold	8	Hold the landing posture
		Front lunge	10	
		Step–hold	8	
	2	Co-contraction	10	Co-contraction of quadriceps and hamstrings
		Squat	10	Ensure correct lower-body alignment
		Step–hold	8	
		Walking lunge	10	
		Lateral hop and hold	8	
	3	Squat	10	
		Lateral jump and hold	8	
		Single tuck jump, soft landing	10	
		Lunge jump	10 s	
		Lateral jump	10	
	4	Squat jump	10	
		Lateral jumps	10 s	
		Double tuck jump	8	
		Broad jump	10	
		Scissors jump	8	
Fundamentals	5	Trunk stability	15	
		Pelvic bridge	10	
		Repeated tuck jumps	10 s	
		Squat jumps	10	
		Jump, single-leg hold	8	
	6	Pelvic bridge, single leg	10	Performed on mat for unstable surface
		Prone bridge (elbow–knee), hip extension, shoulder flexion	10	
		Side-to-side tuck jump	10 s	
		Single-leg lateral hop hold	8	Hold the landing posture
		Hop hold	8	

(continues)

Table 12.11   *(continued)*
Injury-Prevention Warm-up for Basketball Players

Phase	Week	Exercise	Repetitions/ Hold Time (s)	Modifications/Description
	7	Single-leg pelvic bridge	10	Performed on mat for unstable surface
		Prone bridge hip extension	10	
		Side-to-side tuck jumps	10	
		Lateral hop	10 s	
		Two-leg 90°	8	
	8	Single-leg pelvic bridge, ball	10	
		Prone bridge, hip extension, contralateral shoulder flexion	10	Performed on mat for unstable surface
		Lateral hop with ball	10 s	
		Single-leg lateral hop, hold	5	Hold landing posture
		Single-leg 90°	8	
Performance	9	X-hop	6	
		Hop–hop–hold	8	Hold the landing posture
		Mat jump	30 s	The inclusion of the mat provides an unstable surface
		Single-leg squats 90°	8	Performed on mat for unstable surface
		Maximum squat jump hold		Hold the landing posture
	10	Cross-over hop, hop, hold	8	Hold the landing posture
		Single-leg four-way hop, hold	3	Hold the landing posture
				Performed on mat for unstable surface
		Single-leg 90° ball	8	
		Step, jump up, down, vertical jump	5	
		Maximum squat jump, hold	10	Hold the landing posture
	11	Single-leg four-way hop–hold ball	4	
		Single-leg 180°	10	
		Jump, jump, jump, vertical jump	15	
		Mat jumps	40 s	Performed on mat for unstable surface
		Running, jump down single leg, jump	8	
	12	Single-leg 180°	10	
		Jump, jump, jump, vertical jump	15	
		Running, jump down single leg, jump	10	
		Lay-up	10	
		Height jump	10	

Note: One-minute rest between exercises; warm-up performed two times per week.

Reproduced from Aerts, I., Cumps, E., Verhagen, E., Mathieu, N., Van Schuerbeeck, S., & Meeusen, R. (2013). A 3-month jump-landing training program: A feasibility study using the RE-AIM framework. *Journal of Athletic Training, 48,* 296–305.

mechanics (McLean et al., 2010), while the presence of opposing players also appears to perturb the athlete sufficiently to induce poor landing mechanics (Krosshaug et al., 2007). Consequently, landing tasks in game situations are not performed with the same mechanics as used in the closed environments associated with the traditional interventions. Furthermore, the information presented to the athlete during any training exercises should match what the athlete would encounter in the information-rich environment associated with his or her sport (Lee et al., 2013). Enhancing the attunement to appropriate environmental information and incorporating distractions will likely help the transfer of landing mechanics from training to sport.

Table 12.12
A Representative Learning Practice to Promote Correct Mechanics During a Landing Task for Basketball Players Using a Drop–Jump

Description of task	■ The player stands atop a box 2 m from the 3-point line. ■ A ball is placed on the 3-point line. ■ The athlete steps from the box and performs an immediate drop–jump, landing behind the ball. ■ Upon landing, the athlete picks up the ball. This ensures full flexion of the lower-body joints as well as downward motion of the arms during the landing. ■ The arms pass between the knees to retrieve the ball so that the feet are shoulder width apart and the knees do not abduct. ■ The athlete rises with the ball and immediately performs a jump shot, landing appropriately. ■ The coach provides the instructions of "soft landings" and "land with equal weight distribution."
Volume and intensity	■ The number of running jumps and standing jumps should be determined by the coach before the workout. ■ Intensity is determined by the height of the box and the distance from the 3-point line. ■ Perform 3 sets of 10 repetitions. ■ The total volume should vary between 60 and 250 foot contacts for beginners and between 120 and 450 foot contacts for advanced athletes, depending on the time of the season.
Rest periods	■ 2 min between sets; 15 s between repetitions. ■ During inter-set rest periods, the coach engages the player by asking, "How do you land softly?"
Manipulation of task constraints	■ Position a stationary opponent in front of the ball placed on the 3-point line. ■ Have the opponent move to block the jump shot to increase the unplanned nature of the drill and momentum control during landing. ■ Change the height of the box and the location from the 3-point line. ■ Have the player catch the ball during the flight phase of the drop–jump. Catching the ball high above them emphasizes raising the arms during the flight phase of jump. The player should touch the ball on the ground prior to the jump shot to emphasize lower-body joint flexion and downward arm motion. ■ Alter the location of the ball thrown to the player during the drop–jump to emphasize the control of momentum during the initial landing task. ■ Perform the exercise unilaterally.
Coaching analysis	■ Assess the symmetry of the landing during bilateral drills. ■ Assess the width of the feet during bilateral landings. ■ Assess the toe-to-heel and loudness of the landings. ■ Assess the lower-body joint flexion. ■ Assess the trunk motion in the frontal plane. ■ Assess the knee motion in the frontal plane. ■ Video-tape the exercise in the frontal and sagittal planes to provide augmented feedback.

Here we introduce landing exercises that can be included in representative learning practices specific to basketball that enhance perception–action coupling while still having the athlete complete a landing workout emphasizing appropriate mechanics. These exercises emphasize the flexion of the lower-body joints and the downward motion of the arms during landing, which can reduce the magnitude of the GRF, while also preventing abduction at the knee. Explicit instructions relating to these mechanical aspects of landing are avoided in favor of an implicit learning strategy. The specific tasks are outlined in Tables 12.12 and 12.13.

Table 12.13
A Representative Learning Practice to Promote Correct Mechanics During a Landing Task for Basketball Players Using a Stop–Jump

Description of task	▪ A ball is placed on the 3-point line next to the coach. ▪ The player runs up to the 3-point line and another ball is bounced to the player by the coach. ▪ Once the ball is in the player's possession, he or she performs a jump shot by performing a stop–jump at the 3-point line in front of the coach. The coach provides a distracting stimulus during landing. ▪ Upon landing from the jump shot, the player flexes and throws down the arms to pick up the ball placed on the 3-point line and perform an immediate jump shot. ▪ The arms pass between the knees to retrieve the ball so that the feet are shoulder width apart and the knees do not abduct. ▪ The coach provides the instructions of "soft landings" and "land with equal weight distribution."
Volume and rest periods	▪ The number of running jumps and standing jumps should be determined by the coach before the workout. ▪ Perform 3 sets of 10 repetitions. ▪ The total volume should vary between 60 and 250 foot contacts for beginners and between 120 and 450 foot contacts for advanced athletes, depending on the time of the season. ▪ 2 min between sets; 15 s between repetitions. ▪ During inter-set rest periods, the coach engages the player by asking, "How do you land softly?"
Manipulation of task constraints	▪ Have the player alter the run-up speed to change the intensity of the first landing. ▪ Have the player begin the run-up from different positions to alter the initial conditions of the task. ▪ Have the coach move as though blocking the jump shot. ▪ Have opponents run alongside the player in close proximity to increase distraction. ▪ Have the player cut to retrieve another ball upon landing from jump shot 2. ▪ Perform the exercise unilaterally.
Coaching analysis	▪ Assess the symmetry of the landing during bilateral drills. ▪ Assess the width of the feet during bilateral landings. ▪ Assess the toe-to-heel and loudness of the landings. ▪ Assess the lower-body joint flexion. ▪ Assess the trunk motion in the frontal plane. ▪ Assess the knee motion in the frontal plane. ▪ Video the exercise in the frontal and sagittal planes to provide augmented feedback.

Chapter Summary

Landing tasks require the athlete to change the motion of the CM, either arresting it during stationary landing tasks or changing it to perform a subsequent movement during preparatory landing tasks. Preparatory landing tasks can be planned or unplanned, which imposes a substantial constraint on the biomechanical aspects of the task. The dynamics of the vertical GRF acting on the athlete during a landing task (rate of GRF loading, peak GRF) have been implicated in lower-body musculoskeletal injuries, whereas the biomechanics of the lower-body joints during landing tasks can have significant implications for injuries to the structures around the knee joint, particularly the ACL. The greater incidence of noncontact ACL injuries in female athletes compared to male athletes has been suggested to be due to the differences in biomechanics during landing tasks. Interventions to reduce the risk of injury rely on changes in the landing technique through the use of the manipulation of organismic, task, and environmental constraints.

Review Questions and Projects

1. Explain the relationship between the kinetics (i.e., momentum, mechanical energy) of the CM at takeoff and the kinetics upon landing during a vertical jump. Assume that the jump is followed by a stationary landing.

2. How does the analyst use the translational kinetic energy of the CM to determine the absorption phase of a landing task?

3. An athlete with a mass of 70 kg performs a drop–jump from a 0.30-m box. The vertical velocity at takeoff is 2.15 m/s. Calculate the vertical impulse during both landing tasks (the preparatory landing prior to takeoff and the stationary landing following the flight phase of the jump).

4. What are the differences in the dynamics of the GRF during the impact and stabilization subphases of a stationary landing task?

5. How do the joint kinetics differ between the impact and stabilization subphases of a stationary landing task?

6. Which dynamic characteristics of the GRF during landing tasks are implicated in musculoskeletal injuries?

7. Explain how an athlete can attenuate the peak GRF during a stationary landing task.

8. How might female athletes produce greater peak normalized GRF during stationary landing tasks?

9. Describe the five categories of risk factors that are proposed to predispose female athletes to a higher risk of anterior cruciate ligament injury during landing tasks.

10. Explain why the distal-to-proximal transfer of energy via the biarticular muscles crossing the lower-body joints is important during landing tasks.

11. Explain the mechanical differences between landing from a jump and landing during a drop task, and outline their implications for injury.

12. Explain how the arms can be used during the flight and landing phases of a vertical jump to reduce the potential for injury.

13. Explain the influence of the surface on the mechanics of landing.

14. How does the expectation of the landing surface change the mechanics of the lower-body joints during landing tasks?

15. How does the presentation of generic visual information during unplanned preparatory landing tasks influence the joint mechanics during preparatory landing tasks compared to the presentation of sport-specific information?

16. Provide examples of instructions that a strength and conditioning practitioner can use to reduce the magnitude of the athlete's GRF during landing tasks.

17. Which technologies could a strength and conditioning practitioner use to present immediate feedback to an athlete about the forces during landing?

18. Which six elements should be included as part of a comprehensive neuromuscular training program to improve landing mechanics?

19. Present the pros and cons of a warm-up intervention and a comprehensive neuromuscular training program to improve landing mechanics.

20. Outline the steps taken when performing a qualitative analysis of an athlete's landing technique.

References

Aerts, I., Cumps, E., Verhagen, E., Mathieu, N., Van Schuerbeeck, S., & Meeusen, R. (2013). A 3-month jump–landing training program: A feasibility study using the RE-AIM framework. *Journal of Athletic Training, 48*, 296–305.

Afifi, M., & Hinrichs, R. N. (2012). A mechanics comparison between landing from a countermovement jump and landing from stepping off a box. *Journal of Applied Biomechanics, 28*, 1–9.

Akins, J. S., Longo, P. F., Bertoni, M., Clark, N. C., Sell, T. C., Galanti, G., & Lephart, S. M. (2013). Postural stability and isokinetic strength do not predict knee valgus angle during single-leg drop–landing or single-leg squat in elite male rugby union players. *Isokinetics & Exercise Science, 21*, 37–46.

Ali, N., Robertson, D. G., & Rouhi, G. (2014). Sagittal plane body kinematics and kinetics during single-leg landing from increasing vertical heights and horizontal distances: Implications for non-contact ACL injury. *Knee, 21*, 38–46.

Ali, N., Rouhi, G., & Robertson, D. G. (2013). Gender, vertical height and horizontal distance effects on single-leg landing kinematics: Implications for risk of non-contact ACL injury. *Journal of Human Kinetics, 37*, 27–38.

Araújo, D., & Davids, K. (2011). What exactly is acquired during skill acquisition? *Journal of Consciousness Studies, 18*, 7–23.

Augustsson, J., Thomeé, R., Lindén, R., Folkesson, M., Transberg, R., & Karlsson, J. (2006). Single-leg hop testing following fatiguing exercise: Reliability and biomechanical analysis. *Scandinavian Journal of Medicine and Science in Sports, 16*, 111–120.

Barber-Westin, S. D., Smith, S. T., Campbell, T., & Noyes, F. R. (2010). The drop–jump video screening test: Retention of improvement in neuromuscular control in female volleyball players. *Journal of Strength and Conditioning Research, 24*, 3055–3062.

Bartlett, R. (2007). *Introduction to Sports Biomechanics. Analysing Human Movement Patterns*. Oxon, UK: Routledge.

Bates, N. A., Ford, K. R., Myer, G. D., & Hewett, T. E. (2013). Impact differences in ground reaction force and center of mass between the first and second landing phases of a drop vertical jump and their implications for injury risk assessment. *Journal of Biomechanics, 46,* 1237–1241.

Beaulieu, M. L., & Palmieri-Smith, R. M. (2013, January 24). Real-time feedback on knee abduction moment does not improve frontal-plane knee mechanics during jump landings. *Scandinavian Journal of Medicine and Science in Sports.* doi: 10.1111/sms.12051

Benjaminse, A., & Otten, E. (2011). ACL injury prevention, more effective with a different way of motor learning? *Knee Surgery, Sports Traumatology, Arthroscopy, 19,* 622–627.

Bessier, T. F., Lloyd, D. G., Ackland, T. R., & Cochrane, J. L. (2001). Anticipatory effects on knee joint loading during running and cutting maneuvers. *Medicine and Science in Sports and Exercise, 33,* 1176–1181.

Beutler, A. I., de la Motte, S. J., Marshall, S. W., Padua, D. A., & Boden, B. P. (2009). Muscle strength and qualitative jump–landing differences in male and female military cadets: The JUMP-ACL study. *Journal of Sports Science and Medicine, 8,* 663–671.

Boden, B., Griffin, L., & Garrett, W. (2000). Etiology and prevention of noncontact ACL injury. *Physician and Sports Medicine, 28,* 53–60.

Bouchouras, G., Moscha, D., Papaiakovou, G., Nikodelis, T., & Kollias, I. (2009). Angular momentum and landing efficiency in the long jump. *European Journal of Sport Science, 9,* 53–59.

Butler, R. J., Crowell, H. P., & McClay-Davis, I. (2003). Lower extremity stiffness: Implications for performance and injury. *Clinical Biomechanics, 18,* 511–517.

Cerulli, G., Benoit, D. L., Lamontagne, M., Caraffa, A., & Liti, A. (2003). In vivo anterior cruciate ligament strain behavior during a rapid deceleration movement: Case report. *Knee Surgery, Sports Traumatology, Arthroscopy, 11,* 307–311.

Chapman, A. (2008). *Biomechanical analysis of fundamental human movements.* Champaign, IL: Human Kinetics.

Chappell, J. D., Creighton, R. A., Giuliani, C., Yu, B., & Garrett, W. E. (2007). Kinematics and electromyography of landing preparation in vertical stop–jump: Risks for noncontact anterior cruciate ligament injury. *American Journal of Sports Medicine, 35,* 235–241.

Cochrane, J. L., Lloyd, D. G., Besier, T. F., Elliott, B. C., Doyle, T. L. A., & Ackland, T. R. (2010). Training affects knee kinematics and kinetics in cutting maneuvers in sport. *Medicine and Science in Sports and Exercise, 42,* 1535–1544.

Dai, B., Sorensen, C. J., Derrick, T. R., & Gillette, J. C. (2012). The effects of postseason break on knee biomechanics and lower extremity EMG in a stop–jump task: Implications for ACL injury. *Journal of Applied Biomechanics, 28,* 708–717.

Dawes, J. (2012). Quickness drills. In J. Dawes & M. Roozen (Eds.), *Developing agility and quickness* (pp. 93–114). Champaign, IL: Human Kinetics.

Decker, M. J., Torry, M. R., Wyland, D. J., Sterett, W. I., & Steadman, J. R. (2003). Gender differences in lower extremity kinematics, kinetics and energy absorption during landing. *Clinical Biomechanics, 18,* 662–669.

Derrick, T. R. (2004). The effects of knee contact angle on impact forces and accelerations. *Medicine and Science in Sports and Exercise, 36,* 832–837.

Dicks, M., Button, C., & Davids, K. (2010). Examination of gaze behaviours under *in situ* and video simulation task constraints reveals differences in information pick up for perception and action. *Attention, Perception and Psychophysics, 72,* 706–720.

Didier, J. J., & Wall, V. A. (2011). Vertical jumping and landing mechanics: Female athletes and nonathletes. *International Journal of Athletic Therapy and Training, 16,* 17–20.

Distefano, L. J., Distefano, M. J., Frank, B. S., Clark, M. A., & Padua, D. A. (2013). Comparison of integrated and isolated training on performance measures and neuromuscular control. *Journal of Strength and Conditioning Research, 27,* 1083–1090.

Dudley, L. A., Smith, C. A., Olson, B. K., Chimera, N. J., Schmitz, B., & Warren, M. (2013). Interrater and intrarater reliability of the tuck jump assessment by health professionals of varied educational backgrounds. *Journal of Sports Medicine.* ID 483503.

Dufek, J. S., & Bates, B. T. (1990). The evaluation and prediction of impact forces during landings. *Medicine and Science in Sports and Exercise, 22,* 370–377.

Edwards, S., Steele, J. R., Cook, J. L., Purdam, C. R., & McGhee, D. E. (2012). Lower limb movement symmetry cannot be assumed when investigating the stop–jump landing. *Medicine and Science in Sports and Exercise, 44*, 1123–1130.

Ericksen, H. M., Gribble, P. A., Pfile, K. R., & Pietrosimone, B. G. (2013). Different modes of feedback and peak vertical ground reaction force during jump landing: A systematic review. *Journal of Athletic Training, 48*, 685–695.

Etnoyer, J., Cortes, N., Ringleb, S. I., Van Lunen, B. L., & Onate, J. A. (2013). Instruction and jump-landing kinematics in college-aged female athletes over time. *Journal of Athletic Training, 48*, 161–171.

Ford, K. R., Myer, G. D., & Hewett, T. E. (2003). Valgus knee motion during landing in high school female and male basketball players. *Medicine and Science in Sports and Exercise, 35*, 1745–1750.

Ford, K. R., Myer, G. D., Schmitt, L. C., Uhl, T. L., & Hewett, T. E. (2011). Preferential quadriceps activation in female athletes with incremental increases in landing intensity. *Journal of Applied Biomechanics, 27*, 215–222.

Ford, K. R., Shapiro, R., Myer, G. D., Van Den Bogert, A. J., & Hewett, T. E. (2010). Longitudinal sex differences during landing in knee abduction in young athletes. *Medicine and Science in Sports and Exercise, 42*, 1923–1933.

Gilchrist, J., Mandelbaum, B. R., Melancon, H., Ryan, G. W., Silvers, H. J., Griffin, L. Y., . . . Dvorak, J. (2008). A randomized controlled trial to prevent noncontact anterior cruciate ligament injury in female collegiate soccer players. *American Journal of Sports Medicine, 36*, 1476–1483.

Griffin, L. Y., Agel, J., Albolm, M. J., Arendt, E. A., Dick, R. W., Garrett, W. E., . . . Wojtys, E.M. (2000). Noncontact anterior cruciate ligament injuries: Risk factors and prevention strategies. *Journal of the American Academy of Orthopaedic Surgeons, 8*, 141–150.

Haas, C. J., Schick, E. A., Chow, J. W., Tillman, M. D., Brunt, D., & Cauraugh, J. H. (2003). Lower extremity biomechanics differ in prepubescent and postpubescent female athletes during stride jump landings. *Journal of Applied Biomechanics, 19*, 139–152.

Harry, J. D., Ward, A. W., Heglund, N. C., Morgan, D. L., & McMahon, T. A. (1990). Cross-bridge cycling theories cannot explain high-speed lengthening behavior in frog muscle. *Biophysical Journal, 57*, 201–208.

Herman, D. C., Weinhold, P. S., Guskiewicz, K. M., Garrett, W. E., Yu, B., & Padua, D. A. (2008). The effects of strength training on the lower extremity biomechanics of female recreational athletes during a stop–jump task. *American Journal of Sports Medicine, 36*, 733–740.

Hewett, T. E., Ford, K. R., & Myer, G. D. (2006). Anterior cruciate ligament injuries in female athletes. Part 2: A meta-analysis of neuromuscular interventions aimed at injury prevention. *American Journal of Sports Medicine, 34*, 1–9.

Hewett, T. E., Lindenfeld, T. N., Riccobene, J. V., & Noyes, F. R. (1999). The effect of neuromuscular training on the incidence of knee injury in female athletes. *American Journal of Sports Medicine, 27*, 699–706.

Hewett, T. E., & Myer, G. D. (2011). The mechanistic connection between the trunk, hip, knee, and anterior cruciate ligament injury. *Exercise and Sport Sciences Reviews, 39*, 161–166.

Hewett, T. E., Myer, G. D., Ford, K. R., Heidt, R. S., Colosimo, A. J., McLean, S. G., . . . Succop, P. (2005). Biomechanical measures of neuromuscular control and valgus loading of the knee predicts anterior cruciate ligament injury risk in female athletes: A prospective study. *American Journal of Sports Medicine, 33*, 492–501.

Hewett, T. E., Stroupe, A. L., Nance, T. A., & Noyes, F. R. (1996). Plyometric training in female athletes: Decreased impact forces and increased hamstring torques. *American Journal of Sports Medicine, 24*, 765–773.

Iida, Y., Kanehisa, H., Inaba, Y., & Nakazawa, K. (2013). Short-term landing training attenuates landing impact and improves jump height in landing-to-jump movement. *Journal of Strength and Conditioning Research, 27*, 1560–1567.

James, C. R., Bates, B. T., & Dufek, J. S. (2003). Classification and comparison of biomechanical response strategies for accommodating landing impact. *Journal of Applied Biomechanics, 19*, 106–118.

James, C. R., Dufek, J. S., & Bates, B. T. (2006). Effects of stretch shortening cycle exercise fatigue on stress fracture injury risk during landing. *Research Quarterly for Exercise and Sport, 77*, 1–13

Jamison, S. T., McNeilan, R. J., Young, G. S., Givens, D. L., Best, T. M., & Chaudhari, A. M. W. (2012). Randomized controlled trial of the effects of a trunk stabilization program on trunk control and knee loading. *Medicine and Science in Sports and Exercise, 44,* 1924–1934.

Kernozek, T. W., Torry, M. R., Van Hoof, H., Cowley, H., & Tanner, S. (2005). Gender differences in frontal and sagittal plane biomechanics during drop landings. *Medicine and Science in Sports and Exercise, 37,* 1003–1012.

Kiani, A., Hellquist, E., Ahlqvist, K., Gedeborg, R., & Michaëlson, K. (2010). Prevention of soccer-related knee injuries in teenaged girls. *Archives of Internal Medicine, 170,* 43–49.

Knudson, D. V., & Morrison, C. S. (2002). *Qualitative analysis of human movement.* Champaign, IL: Human Kinetics.

Koga, H., Nakamae, A., Shima, Y., Iwasa, J., Myklebust, G., Engebretsen, L., . . . Krosshaug, T. (2010). Mechanisms for noncontact anterior cruciate ligament injuries: Knee joint kinematics in 10 injury situations from female team handball and basketball. *American Journal of Sports Medicine, 38,* 2218–2225.

Kovacs, I., Tihanyi, J., DeVita, P., Racz, L., Barrier, J., & Hortobagyi, T. (1999). Foot placement modifies kinematics and kinetics during drop jumping. *Medicine and Science in Sports and Exercise, 31,* 708–716.

Krosshaug, T., Nakamae, A., Boden, B. P., Engebretsen, L., Smith, G., Slauterbeck, J. R., . . . Bahr, R. (2007). Mechanisms of anterior cruciate ligament injury in basketball: Video analysis of 39 cases. *American Journal of Sports Medicine, 35,* 359–367.

Kulas, A. S., Schmitz, R. J., Shultz, S. J., Watson, M. A., & Perrin, D. H. (2006). Energy absorption as a predictor of leg impedance in highly trained females. *Journal of Applied Biomechanics, 22,* 177–185.

Kweon, C., Lederman, E. S., & Chhabra, A. (2013). Anatomy and biomechanics of the cruciate ligaments and their surgical implications. In G. C. Fanelli (Ed.), *The multiple ligament injured knee: A practical guide to management* (pp. 17–27). New York, NY: Springer Science+Business Media.

LaBella, C. R., Huxford, M. R., Grissom, J., Kim, K-Y., Peng, J., & Christoffel, K. K. (2011). Effect of neuromuscular warm-up on injuries in female soccer and basketball athletes in urban public high schools: Cluster randomized controlled trial. *Archives of Pediatric and Adolescent Medicine, 165,* 1033–1040.

LaPorta, J. W., Brown, L. E., Coburn, J. W., Galpin, A. J., Tufano, J. J., Cazas, V. L., & Tan, J. G. (2013). Effects of different footwear on vertical jump and landing parameters. *Journal of Strength and Conditioning Research, 27,* 733–737.

LaStayo, P. C., Woolf, J. M., Lewek, M. D., Snyder-Mackler, L., Reich, T., & Lindstedt, S. L. (2003). Eccentric muscle contraction: Their contribution to injury, prevention, rehabilitation, and sport. *Journal of Orthopaedic and Sports Physical Therapy, 33,* 557–571.

Lee, M. J. C., Lloyd, D. G., Lay, B. S., Bourke, P. D., & Alderson, J. A. (2013). Effects of different visual stimuli on postures and knee moments during sidestepping. *Medicine and Science in Sports and Exercise, 45,* 1740–1748.

Lephart, S. M., Ferris, C. M., Riemann, B. L., Myers, J. B., & Fu, F. H. (2002). Gender differences in strength and lower extremity kinematics during landing. *Clinical and Orthopedic Related Research, 401,* 162–169.

Magill, R. A. (2011). *Motor learning and Control: Concepts and applications.* New York, NY: McGraw-Hill.

Mandelbaum, B. R., Silvers, H. J., Watanabe, D. S., Knarr, J. F., Thomas, S. D., Griffin, L. Y., . . . Garrett, W. (2005). Effectiveness of a neuromuscular and proprioceptive training program in preventing the incidence of anterior cruciate ligament injuries in female athletes. *American Journal of Sports Medicine, 33,* 1–8.

Markoff, K. L., Burchfield, D. M., Shapiro, M. M., Shepard, M. F., Finerman, G. A., & Slaughterbeck, J. L. (1995). Combined knee loading states that generate high anterior cruciate ligament forces. *Journal of Orthopedic Research, 13,* 930–935.

Mathiyakom, W., & McNitt-Gray, J. L. (2008). Regulation of angular impulse during fall recovery. *Journal of Rehabilitation Research and Development, 45,* 1237–1247.

McBain, K., Shrier, I., Shultz, R., Meeuwisse, W. H., Klügl, M., Garza, D., & Matheson, G. O. (2012). Prevention of sports injury I: A systematic review of applied biomechanics and physiology outcomes research. *British Journal of Sports Medicine, 46,* 169–173.

McBride, J. M., & Snyder, J. G. (2012). Mechanical efficiency and force–time curve variation during repetitive jumping in trained and untrained jumpers. *European Journal of Applied Physiology, 112*, 3469–3477.

McLean, S. G., & Beaulieu, M. L. (2010). Complex integrative morphological and mechanical contributions to ACL injury risk. *Exercise and Sport Sciences Reviews, 38*, 192–200.

McLean, S. G., Borotikar, B., & Lucey, S. M. (2010). Lower limb muscle pre-motor time measures during a choice reaction task associate with knee abduction loads during dynamic single leg landings. *Clinical Biomechanics, 25*, 563–569.

McLean, S. G., Lipfert, S. W., & van den Bogert, A. J. (2004). Effects of gender and defensive opponent on the biomechanics of sidestep cutting. *Medicine and Science in Sports and Exercise, 36*, 1008–1016.

McLean, S. G., & Samorezov, J. E. (2009). Fatigue-induced ACL injury risk stems from a degradation in central control. *Medicine and Science in Sports and Exercise, 41*, 1661–1672.

McLean, S. G., Walker, K. B., & van den Bogert, A. J. (2005). Effect of gender on lower extremity kinematics during rapid direction change: An integrated analysis or three sports movements. *Journal of Science and Medicine in Sport, 8*, 411–422.

McNitt-Gray, J. L. (1993). Kinetics of the lower extremities during drop landings from three heights. *Journal of Biomechanics, 26*, 1037–1046.

McNitt-Gray, J. L. (2000). Subject specific coordination of two- and one-joint muscles during landings suggests multiple control criteria. *Motor Control, 4*, 84–88.

McNitt-Gray, J. L., Yokoi, T., & Millward, C. (1993). Landing strategy adjustments made by female gymnasts in response to drop height and mat composition. *Journal of Applied Biomechanics, 9*, 173–190.

McNitt-Gray, J. L., Yokoi, T., & Millward, C. (1994). Landing strategies used by gymnasts on different surfaces. *Journal of Applied Biomechanics, 10*, 237–252.

Milner, C. E., Fairbrother, J. T., Srivatsan, A., & Zhang, S. (2012). Simple verbal instruction improves knee biomechanics during landing in female athletes. *Knee, 19*, 399–403.

Montgomery, M. M., Shultz, S. J., Schmitz, R. J., Wideman, L., & Henson, R. A. (2012). Influence of lean body mass and strength on landing energetics. *Medicine and Science in Sports and Exercise, 44*, 2376–2383.

Moritz, C. T., & Farley, C. T. (2004). Passive dynamics change leg mechanics for an unexpected surface during human hopping. *Journal of Applied Physiology, 97*, 1313–1322.

Myer, G. D., Brent, J. L., Ford, K. R., & Hewett, T. E. (2011). Real-time assessment and neuromuscular training feedback techniques to prevent ACL injury in female athletes. *Strength and Conditioning Journal, 33*, 21–35.

Myer, G. D., Ford, K. R., Brent, J. L., & Hewett, T. E. (2006). Stabilization and balance training on power, balance, and landing force in female athletes. *Journal of Strength and Conditioning Research, 20*, 345–353.

Myer, G. D., Ford, K. R., & Hewett, T. E. (2008). Tuck jump assessment for reducing anterior cruciate ligament injury risk. *Athletic Therapy Today, 13*, 39–44.

Myklebust, G., Engebretsen, L., Brækken, I. H., Skjølberg, A., Olsen, O-E., & Bahr, R. (2003). Prevention of anterior cruciate ligament injuries in female team handball players: A prospective intervention study over three seasons. *Clinical Journal of Sports Medicine, 13*, 71–78.

Nagai, T., Sell, T. C., House, A. J., Abt, J. P., & Lephart, S. M. (2013). Knee proprioception and strength and landing kinematics during a single-leg stop–jump task. *Journal of Athletic Training, 48*, 31–38.

Nagano, Y., Hirofumi, I., Akai, M., & Fukubayashi, T. (2007). Gender differences in knee kinematics and muscle activity during single limb drop landings. *Knee, 14*, 218–223.

Noyes, F. R., Barber-Westin, S. D., Smith, S. T., Campbell, T., & Garrison, T. T. (2012). A training program to improve neuromuscular and performance indices in female high school basketball players. *Journal of Strength and Conditioning Research, 26*, 709–719.

Padua, D. A., Marshall, S. W., Boling, M. C., Thigpen, C. A., Garrett, W. E., & Beutler, A. I. (2009). The Landing Error Scoring System (LESS) is a valid and reliable clinical assessment tool of jump–landing biomechanics: The JUMP-ACL study. *American Journal of Sports Medicine, 37*, 1996–2002.

Pappas, E., Hagins, M., Sheikhzadeh, A., Nordin, M., & Rose, D. (2007). Biomechanical differences between unilateral and bilateral landings from a jump: Gender differences. *Clinical Journal of Sports Medicine, 17*, 263–268.

Peikenkamp, K., Fritz, M., & Nicol, K., (2002). Simulation of the vertical ground reaction force on sport surfaces during landing. *Journal of Applied Biomechanics, 18*, 122–134.

Pollard, C. D., Sigward, S. M., Ota, S., Langford, K., & Powers, C. M. (2006). The influence of in-season injury prevention training on lower-extremity kinematics during landing in female soccer players. *Clinical Journal of Sports Medicine, 16*, 223–227.

Pollard, C. D., Sigward, S. M., & Powers, C. M. (2010). Limited hip and knee flexion during landing is associated with increased frontal plane knee motion and moments. *Clinical Biomechanics, 25*, 142–146.

Prilutsky, B. I., & Zatsiorsky, V. M. (1994). Tendon function of two-joint muscles: Transfer of mechanical energy between joints during jumping, landing, and running. *Journal of Biomechanics, 27*, 25–34.

Quammen, D., Cortes, N., Van Lunen, B. L., Lucci, S., Ringleb, S. I., & Onate, J. (2012). Two different fatigue protocols and lower extremity motion patterns during a stop–jump task. *Journal of Athletic Training, 47*, 32–41.

Quatman, C. E., Quatman-Yates, C. C., & Hewett, T. E. (2010). A "plane" explanation of anterior cruciate ligament injury mechanisms: A systematic review. *Sports Medicine, 40*, 729–746.

Renstrom, P., Ljungqvist, A., Arendt, E., Beynnon, B., Fukubayashi, T., Garrett, W., . . . Engebretsen, L. (2008). Non-contact ACL injuries in female athletes: An International Olympic Committee current concepts statement. *British Journal of Sports Medicine, 42*, 394–412.

Roberts, T. J., & Konow, N. (2013). How tendons buffer energy dissipation by muscle. *Exercise and Sport Sciences Reviews, 41*, 186–193.

Schmitz, R. J., Kulas, A. S., Perrin, D. H., Riemann, B. L., & Shultz, S. J. (2007). Sex differences in lower extremity biomechanics during single leg landings. *Clinical Biomechanics, 22*, 681–688.

Schmitz, R. J., & Shultz, S. J. (2010). Contribution of knee flexor and extensor strength on sex-specific energy absorption and torsional joint stiffness during drop jumping. *Journal of Athletic Training, 45*, 445–452.

Sell, T. C., Ferris, C. M., Abt, J. P., Tsai, Y-S., Myers, J. B., Fu, F. H., & Lephart, S. M. (2007). Predictors of proximal tibia anterior shear force during a vertical stop–jump. *Journal of Orthopaedic Research, 25*, 1589–1597.

Shimokochi, Y., Ambeganokar, J., Meyer, E., Lee, S., & Shultz, S. (2013). Changing sagittal plane body position during single-leg landings influences the risk of non-contact anterior cruciate ligament injuries. *Knee Surgery, Sports Traumatology, and Arthroscopy, 21*, 888–897.

Shultz, S. J., Nguyen, A-D., Leonard, M. D., & Schmitz, R. J. (2009). Thigh strength and activation as predictors of knee biomechanics during a drop jump task. *Medicine and Science in Sports and Exercise, 41*, 857–866.

Shultz, S. J., Schmitz, R. J., Nguyen, A-D., & Levine, B. J. (2010). Joint laxity is related to lower extremity energetics during a drop jump landing. *Medicine and Science in Sports and Exercise, 42*, 771–780.

Shultz, S. J., Schmitz, R. J., Tritsch, A. J., & Montgomery, M. M. (2012). Methodological considerations of task and shoe wear on joint energetics during landing. *Journal of Electromyography and Kinesiology, 22*, 124–130.

Sigward, S. M., Pollard, C. D., & Powers, C. M. (2012). The influence of sex and maturation on landing biomechanics: Implications for anterior cruciate ligament injury. *Scandinavian Journal of Medicine and Science in Sports, 22*, 502–509.

Smith, H. C., Johnson, R. J., Shults, S. J., Tourville, T., Holterman, L. A., Slauterbeck, J., . . . Beynnon, B. D. (2012). A prospective evaluation of the Landing Error Scoring System (LESS) as a screening tool for anterior cruciate ligament injury. *American Journal of Sports Medicine, 40*, 521–526.

Soligard, T., Nilstad, A., Steffen, K., Myklebust, G., Holme, I., Dvorak, J., . . . Andersen, T. E. (2010). Compliance with a comprehensive warm-up programme to prevent injuries in youth football. *British Journal of Sports Medicine, 44*, 787–793.

Steele, J. R., & Milburn, P. D. (1988). Effect of different synthetic sport surfaces on the ground reaction forces at landing in netball. *International Journal of Sport Biomechanics, 4*, 130–145.

Steffen, K., Myklebust, G., Olsen, O. E., Holme, I., & Bahr, R. (2008). Preventing injuries in female youth football: A cluster-randomized controlled trial. *Scandinavian Journal of Medicine and Science in Sports, 18*, 605–614.

Turner, A. N., & Jefferys, I. (2010). The stretch-shortening cycle: Proposed mechanisms and methods for enhancement. *Strength and Conditioning Journal, 32*, 87–99.

von Porat, A., Roos, E. M., & Roos, H. (2004). High prevalence of osteoarthritis 14 years after an anterior cruciate ligament tear in male soccer players: A study of radiographic and patient relevant outcomes. *Annals of Rheumatic Diseases, 63*, 269–273.

Waldén, M., Atroshi, I., Magnusson, H., Wagner, P., & Hägglund, M. (2012). Prevention of acute knee injuries in adolescent female football players: Cluster randomized controlled trial. *British Medical Journal, 344*, e3042.

Wang, L-I. (2011). The lower extremity biomechanics of single- and double-leg stop–jump tasks. *Journal of Sports Science and Medicine, 10*, 151–156.

Weinhandl, J. T., Joshi, M., & O'Conor, K. M. (2010). Gender comparisons between unilateral and bilateral landings. *Journal of Applied Biomechanics, 26*, 444–453.

Weinhandl, J. T., Smith, J. D., & Dugan, E. L. (2011). The effects of repetitive drop jumps on impact phase joint kinematics and kinetics. *Journal of Applied Biomechanics, 27*, 108–115.

Wells, J. C. (2007). Sexual dimorphism of body composition. *Best Practice and Research: Clinical Endocrinology and Metabolism, 21*, 415–430.

Withrow, T. J., Huston, L. J., Wojtys, E. M., & Ashton-Miller, J. A. (2006). The effect of an impulsive knee valgus moment on *in vitro* relative ACL strain during a simulated jump landing. *Clinical Biomechanics, 21*, 977–983.

Yeow, C. H., Lee, P. V., & Goh, J. C. (2009). Effects of landing height on frontal plane kinematics, kinetics and energy dissipation at lower extremity joints. *Journal of Biomechanics, 42*, 1967–1973.

Yeow, C. H., Lee, P. V., & Goh, J. C. (2010). Sagittal knee joint kinematics and energetics in response to different landing heights and techniques. *Knee, 17*, 127–131.

Yeow, C. H., Lee, P. V. S., & Goh, J. C. H. (2011a). An investigation of lower extremity energy dissipation strategies during single-leg and double-leg landing based on sagittal and frontal plane biomechanics. *Human Movement Science, 30*, 624–635.

Yeow, C. H., Lee, P. V., & Goh, J. C. (2011b). Shod landing provides enhanced energy dissipation at the knee joint relative to barefoot landing from different heights. *Knee, 18*, 407–411.

Yu, B., Lin, C. F., & Garrett, W. E. (2006). Lower extremity biomechanics during the landing of a stop–jump task. *Clinical Biomechanics, 21*, 297–305.

Zadpoor, A. A., & Nikooyan, A. A. (2011). The relationship between lower-extremity stress fractures and the ground reaction force: A systematic review. *Clinical Biomechanics, 26*, 23–28.

Zantop, T., Petersen, W., & Fu, F. H. (2005). Anatomy of the anterior cruciate ligament. *Operative Techniques in Orthopaedics, 15*, 20–28.

Zhang, S., Bates, B. T., & Dufek, J. S. (2000). Contributions of lower extremity joints to energy dissipation during landings. *Medicine and Science in Sports and Exercise, 32*, 812–819.

Zhang, S., Clowers, K., Kohstall, C., & Yu, Y-J. (2005). Effects of various midsole densities of basketball shoes on impact attenuation during landing activities. *Journal of Applied Biomechanics, 21*, 3–17.

Zhang, S., Derrick, T. R., Evans, W., & Yu, Y-J. (2008). Shock and impact reduction in moderate and strenuous landing activities. *Sports Biomechanics, 7*, 296–309.

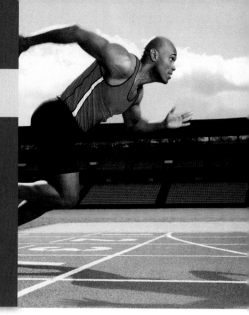

CHAPTER 13

Biomechanics of Fundamental Movements: Sprint Running

Chapter Objectives

At the end of this chapter, you will be able to:

- Explain the multidimensional nature of sprint running and its implications for training and testing
- Describe the mechanical aspects of sprint running
- Describe the biomechanical aspects of sprint running
- Explain the etiology of some of the common musculoskeletal injuries associated with sprint running
- Develop a qualitative analysis of sprint running
- Develop specific workouts targeting muscular strength commensurate with the biomechanical aspects of sprint running
- Explain agility performance and its importance in sport
- Develop specific workouts based on representative learning that enhance the attunement of the athlete's sprinting and agility movements to environmental information

Key Terms

Acceleration

Active leg motion

Attainment of maximal speed

Downhill sprinting

Explosive strength

High-load speed-strength

Leg stiffness

Low-load speed-strength

Maximal dynamic muscular strength

Maximal isometric muscular strength

Multidimensional skill

Reactive strength

Reciprocal ponderal index

Repeated-sprint activities

Rotation–extension strategy

Small-sided games

Stance distance

Stance time

Stride frequency

Stride length

Takeoff distance

Torque treadmills

Touchdown distance

Uphill sprinting

Chapter Overview

Sprint running is an integral movement required in most sports. Like jumping, sprint running can be an event in itself, such as the sprint events in track and field (100 m, 200 m, and 400 m). In these events, the athlete who is able to achieve the greatest average running speed over the duration of the event will win; thus the sprinting ability of the athlete is key to his or her success. However, sprint running is also required to satisfy the strategic/tactical elements in sports such as rugby and soccer, where the athlete may execute a sprint to intercept a ball or avoid an opponent. For example, rugby players have been shown to execute approximately 30 sprints during a game (Duthie, Pyne, & Hooper, 2003), while elite soccer players have been shown to complete as many as 35 sprints during a game, depending on the player's position (DiSalvo et al., 2010). These sprints are performed over a variety of distances and at a variety of speeds, ranging from submaximal to maximal, and are repeated throughout the game (Table 13.1). Each sprint is typically of a short duration (less than 10 s) separated by short recovery periods (less than 60 s), giving rise to **repeated-sprint activities** associated with sports such as basketball, rugby, soccer, and tennis (Bishop & Girard, 2011).

During these repeated-sprint activities, performance is determined by the ability to maintain the highest possible speed during each of the repeated sprints and is largely dependent upon the ability to resynthesize phosphocreatine (PCr) stores during the recovery periods (Glaister, 2005). This places large demands on energy provision for each successive sprint.

The better players in repeated-sprint sports, including soccer and rugby, are able to sprint faster than their lower-level counterparts (Duthie et al., 2003; Haugen, Tønnessen, & Seiler, 2013). This highlights the need for such athletes to develop their sprinting abilities. These sports also require the athlete to change the direction of sprinting in response to environmental information. Moreover, sprints in these sports are likely to be executed with the athlete holding or in contact with a ball, which may influence the speed achieved. Specific training incorporating these environmental and task constraints is required to attune the athlete's sprinting movements to these sport-specific situations.

In this chapter, we introduce sprint running as a multidimensional skill, comprising distinct phases with specific mechanical requirements. We focus on the acceleration and maximal-speed phases of sprint running and discuss the implications for the assessment and training of athletes. We then introduce the biomechanical aspects associated with the acceleration and maximal-speed phases. The importance of muscular strength is discussed before the development of a qualitative analysis of sprint

Table 13.1
Duration, Distance Covered, and Recovery Times Between Runs of More Than 5.50 m/s by Professional Soccer Players During Competitive Games

Duration (s)	Distance (m)	Recovery Time (s)
2.7 ± 0.7	16.5 ± 4.9	13.6 ± 4.4

Values are means ± standard deviations.

Data from Carling, C., Le Gall, F., & Dupont, G. (2012). Analysis of repeated high-intensity running performance in professional soccer. *Journal of Sports Sciences, 30*, 325–336.

running performance. Finally, we will discuss effective training methods that can be used to develop sprint running performance, including representative learning practices that will allow athletes to attune their sprinting movements to relevant environmental information.

Sprint Running as a Multidimensional Skill

Figure 13.1 shows the speed–time curve for an elite athlete performing a 100-m sprint. The biexponential curves reflect distinct phases that an athlete traverses when sprinting from a stationary start:

- Acceleration phase—denoted by the positive slope of the curve over the initial 60 m
- Attainment of maximal-speed phase—denoted by the peak of the curve
- Maintenance of maximal-speed phase—denoted by the negative slope of the curve over the final 40 m

The identification of these distinct phases of sprint running is acknowledged by researchers and coaches alike, although there is some debate on the number of phases that should be included (Delecluse et al., 1995; Jones, Bezodis, & Thompson, 2009; Volkov & Lapin, 1979).

The three sprint phases can be applied to athletes of differing abilities, with the duration of each phase adjusted accordingly. For example, untrained sprinters have been shown to achieve maximal sprinting speed between 10 m and 35 m from the beginning of a 100-m sprint (Delecluse et al., 1995), while elite sprinters achieve their

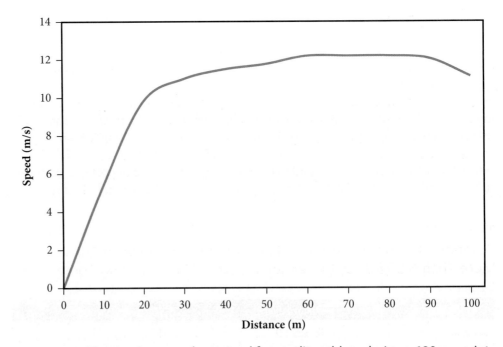

Figure 13.1 The running speeds attained for an elite athlete during a 100-m sprint.

Data from Krzysztof, M., & Mero, A. (2013) A kinematic analysis of three best 100 m performances ever. *Journal of Human Kinetics, 36*, 149–161.

maximal speed between 60 m and 80 m in the same event (Ae, Ito, & Suzuki, 1992; Majumdar & Robergs, 2011).

The distinct phases also have implications for different positional players within a given sport. For example, attackers and wide-midfielders in soccer execute significantly more sprints of distances greater than 20 m than central defenders (DiSalvo et al., 2010). Because central defenders are unlikely to achieve maximal running speeds during their sprints executed during competitive games, development of the accelerative capabilities of these players should be the focus in training. Rugby union backs may perform as many as six sprints per game where they are able to cover a distance that allows them to attain maximal running speed (Duthie, Pyne, Marsh, & Hooper, 2006), necessitating the inclusion of training to develop maximal speed as well as acceleration capabilities. It should be noted that elite sprinters are able to achieve a high percentage of their maximal running speed over short distances (Table 13.2).

The distinct sprint phases have other important implications for the strength and conditioning coach: Because the mechanical requirements of each phase differ, different training strategies will be required to enhance performance during each phase. For example, the performance in each of the phases are not perfectly correlated (Baker & Nance, 1999; Mero, 1988), implying that different factors may contribute to performance in the distinct phases. Indeed, performance in each of the distinct phases of sprint running is limited by specific biomechanical constraints, highlighting the fact that sprint running is a **multidimensional skill** (Delecluse, 1997). The multidimensional nature of sprint running means that specific exercises and modes of training are required to improve performances in the distinct sprint phases, but complications may arise. For example, it has been shown that improvements gained in one phase of sprinting may interfere with performance in other phases (Delecluse et al., 1995).

The different phases of sprint running can be elucidated only if instantaneous speeds are assessed via Global Positioning System (GPS) devices or if split times are recorded during sprint assessments via timing gates. Recording the time taken for an

Table 13.2
Percentage of Maximal Speed Achieved by an Elite Sprinter During 10-m Intervals of a 100-m Race

Interval (m)	Time (s)	Speed (m/s)	Percentage of Maximal Speed
0–10	1.89	5.26	43
10–20	0.99	10.20	83
20–30	0.90	10.87	88
30–40	0.86	12.05	98
40–50	0.83	11.90	96
50–60	0.82	12.19	99
60–70	0.81	12.19	99
70–80	0.82	12.34	100
80–90	0.83	12.05	98
90–100	0.83	12.05	98

Data from Krzysztof, M., & Mero, A. (2013). A kinematic analysis of three best 100 m performances ever. *Journal of Human Kinetics, 36*, 149–161.

athlete to complete a set distance of 100 m, for example, does not provide the strength and conditioning practitioner with sufficient information to develop an effective training program to develop the sprinting ability of the athlete. Furthermore, little information can be gleaned about sprint performance in field-sport athletes beyond a 20-m distance (Brechue, 2011). Here we will focus on the sprint phases of **acceleration** and the **attainment of maximal speed**.

Mechanics of Sprint Running

During the acceleration phase of sprint running, the horizontal velocity of the center of mass (CM) increases per unit time. This requires a net positive horizontal impulse acting on the athlete, as per the impulse–momentum relationship:

$$\int F_{prop} dt + \int F_{ret} dt > 0 \qquad\qquad \textbf{Eq. (13.1)}$$

where F_{prop} is the horizontal propulsive force generated by the athlete, t is the time of force application, and F_{ret} is the sum of the horizontal forces acting to reduce the velocity of the CM (e.g., braking force, drag force). At constant running speeds, such as when the athlete achieves maximal running speed, the horizontal impulses acting on the CM must sum to zero:

$$\int F_{prop} dt + \int F_{ret} dt = 0 \qquad\qquad \textbf{Eq. (13.2)}$$

During both the acceleration and the attainment of maximal speed phases of sprint running, the athlete is required to support his or her body weight such that the vertical impulse generated by the athlete must equal that produced by gravity:

$$\int F_{vert} dt = \int mg dt \qquad\qquad \textbf{Eq. (13.3)}$$

where F_{vert} is the vertical force generated by the athlete, t is the time of force application, m is the mass of the athlete, and g is gravitational acceleration.

The mechanics of sprint running, then, appear to be straightforward. During acceleration, the athlete is required to generate a propulsive impulse that exceeds the impulse associated with the retarding forces acting on the athlete; when the athlete is unable to achieve this, he or she has attained the maximal running speed. The athlete is also required to exert a vertical force to support body weight. However, how the athlete achieves the mechanics associated with the aforementioned equations is important for a strength and conditioning coach to understand.

Biomechanics of Sprint Running

Now that we have introduced the basic mechanics that determine sprint running performance during the acceleration and maximal-speed phases of sprint running, we turn our attention to how an athlete is able to satisfy the specific mechanical demands by investigating the biomechanics of sprint running. The biomechanical aspects of sprint running have been assessed using both over-ground and treadmill protocols, which has implications for the data collected (see Sprint Running Concept 13.1). An athlete attains a sprint running speed through alternating phases of stance and flight associated with each running stride. A stride is defined as the event between touchdown of the stance leg and the next ipsilateral touchdown (DeVita, 1994). Thus it comprises two stance phases, in which the athlete is in contact with the supporting surface, and two aerial phases, in which the athlete is in flight. The presence of aerial phases makes sprint running a ballistic movement. Mathematically, sprint running speed is a product of **stride length** (SL), defined as the distance between ipsilateral stance phases, and **stride frequency** (SF), defined as the inverse of stride time (the sum of stance and flight time).

Sprint Running Concept 13.1

Comparison of treadmill and over-ground sprint running

The assessment of the biomechanical aspects of sprint running can be simplified if the movement is performed on a treadmill, as multiple consecutive strides can be recorded with this approach. Nevertheless, certain differences between treadmill and over-ground running may alter the biomechanics of the movement. For example, the absence of drag forces during treadmill sprinting may allow for the attainment of greater maximal running speeds compared to over-ground running. However, Lakomy (1987) reported that the maximal sprinting speeds achieved by athletes running on a non-motorized treadmill were actually lower than those achieved over ground. This result may have been due to a greater braking impulse acting on the athlete during each stance phase as a result of the frictional forces exerted onto the treadmill belt. The same effect would also be apparent when using conventionally motor-driven treadmills.

To counter this issue, **torque treadmills** have been developed. These treadmills have servo-motors that act to minimize the loss of belt speed during each stance phase caused by friction. In a comparison of sprinting performance on a conventionally motor-driven treadmill and a torque treadmill, McKenna and Riches (2007) reported longer stance phases, longer braking during stance, a more extended knee at touchdown, and a greater hip extension velocity on the conventional treadmill. Moreover, the mechanics of sprint running performed on the torque treadmill were not substantially different from those achieved in over-ground trials performed at the same speed (7 m/s). Other authors have reported that the maximal sprinting speed achieved on a torque treadmill is slightly lower than that achieved over ground (Chelly & Denis, 2001; Morin & Sève, 2011). Furthermore, the maximal running speeds are achieved with a relatively large net positive horizontal force being exerted by the athlete (Morin & Sève, 2011), likely due to the servo-motor generating a torque to minimize the loss of belt speed during stance. However, the maximal speeds achieved on the torque treadmill were highly correlated with those achieved over ground, leading the authors to conclude that although treadmill running cannot reproduce the exact biomechanics of the over-ground sprint running, it can be used to interpret over-ground sprinting performance (Morin & Sève, 2011).

Another potential limitation of using treadmills to assess sprint running is that these devices typically preclude the natural acceleration observed when

(continues)

(continued)

running over ground from a stationary starting position. Indeed, some protocols to assess maximum running speeds require the performer to lower himself or herself onto the treadmill belt while it is moving (Bundle, Hoyt, & Weyand, 2003; Kivi, Maraj, & Gervais, 2002). This might explain some of the kinematics differences associated with sprint running performed on a treadmill. For example, Kivi et al. (2002) reported kinematic decrements in the running movement when the speed exceeded 90% of the maximum the athlete was able to attain on the treadmill. These authors proposed that the increased variability of the sagittal plane joint data (e.g., joint angles and velocities) indicated a "mechanical breakdown" of running technique and advised that any sprint training undertaken on a treadmill should not be performed at speeds in excess of 90% of maximum.

Botwell, Tan, and Wilson (2009) developed a mechanical feedback system to be used on treadmills whereby the speed of the treadmill belt is automatically altered in response to the position and speed of the performer relative to the front of the treadmill. This treadmill allows the performer to accelerate from walking up to maximum running speeds that are actually 11.5% greater than those achieved in over-ground running trials. Such a system may have implications for training sprint athletes.

Table 13.3 shows the kinematic variables of sprinting speed, SL, SF, and stance and flight times for a well-trained sprinter during the acceleration, attainment of maximal speed, and maintenance of maximal speed phases of a 100-m sprint. These values represent averages calculated during the different sprint phases.

Notice in Table 13.3 that this athlete attains the maximal running speed by increasing SL, with a slight reduction in SF from the acceleration phase. Researchers have long debated the relative importance of SL and SF on running speed in an attempt to determine which of these two variables limits performance. However, there is conflicting evidence. For example, field-sport athletes demonstrating greater acceleration produce higher SF (Murphy, Lockie, & Coutts, 2003), while Hunter, Marshall, and McNair (2004) have reported a strong relationship between SL and sprint time over a 16-m distance

Table 13.3
Average Kinematic Variables During the Strides Associated with Acceleration, Maximum Velocity, and Maintenance Phase of a 100-m Sprint by a Well-Trained Sprinter

Sprint Phase	Speed (m/s)	Stride Length (m)	Stride Frequency (Hz)	Stance Time (s)	Flight Time (s)
Acceleration	9.80	4.16	2.36	0.10	0.12
Maximal speed	10.46	4.48	2.34	0.08	0.13
Maintenance	9.85	4.36	2.26	0.10	0.13

Reproduced from Cunha, L., Alves, F., & Veloso, A. (2002). *The touch-down and takeoff angles in different phases of 100 m sprint running.* Presentation at the International Symposium on Biomechanics in Sport, Cáceres-Extremadura, Spain.

in a group of heterogeneous athletes. For maximal-speed sprinting, some authors have argued that SL imposes a limit (Brechue, 2011; Gajer, Thépaut-Mathieu, & Lehénaff, 1999), whereas others promote SF as the limiting factor (Luhtanen & Komi, 1978; Mann & Herman, 1985). Identifying the limiting variable would enable effective training methods to be developed that increase either SL or SF. However, Salo, Bezodis, Batterham, and Kerwin (2011) recently reported that the reliance upon either SL or SF is highly individual, even in a group of well-trained sprinters. Therefore, a strength and conditioning practitioner should determine the contribution of SL and SF for each individual athlete and tailor the training program accordingly.

Goodwin (2011) has proposed that focusing solely on the interaction of SL and SF, while mathematically appealing, could be misleading when developing interventions to increase maximal running speed. SL, this author notes, is largely a consequence of running speed rather than a cause of it; this is due to SL mainly being affected by the distance that the CM travels during the flight phase, such that it is largely influenced by the factors determining horizontal jumping distance. What is more informative about sprinting speed are the variables of **stance distance** and **stance time** (Goodwin, 2011). Stance distance is the horizontal distance traveled by the CM during each stance phase, while stance time is the duration of the stance phase. The ratio of the two provides a measure of running speed during each stance phase:

$$\text{Speed} = \frac{d_{\text{stance}}}{t_{\text{stance}}} \qquad\qquad \textbf{Eq. (13.4)}$$

where d_{stance} is horizontal distance traveled by the CM during the stance phase and t_{stance} is the duration of the stance phase. Stance distance is the sum of **touchdown distance** (the horizontal distance between the stance foot and the CM at touchdown) and **takeoff distance** (the horizontal distance between the stance foot and the CM at takeoff) (Figure 13.2).

As an athlete accelerates up to maximal running speed, the duration of each stance phase decreases while stance distance slightly increases. For example, an increase in stance distance from 0.85 m during the acceleration phase to 0.90 m at

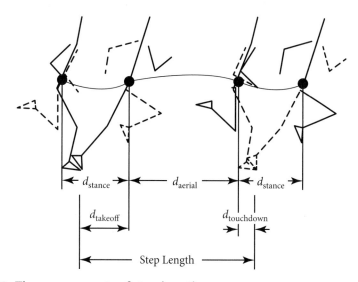

Figure 13.2 The components of step length.

maximal running speed has been reported in well-trained sprinters (Cuhna, Alves, & Veloso, 2002). This effect would explain the increased average running speeds recorded as the athlete accelerates to maximal speed. However, stance distance is no different between athletes who exhibit high versus low magnitudes of acceleration (Hunter et al., 2004), nor does it differ between athletes who achieve high versus low maximal running speeds (Weyand, Sternlight, Bellizzi, & Wright, 2000). The difference between fast and slow sprinters, therefore, appears to be largely due to the shorter stance times exhibited by the faster athletes as opposed to greater stance distances, irrespective of the phase of sprinting (Bushnell & Hunter, 2007; Hunter et al., 2004; Weyand, Sandell, Prime, & Bundle, 2010). Indeed, trained sprinters produce shorter stance durations than distance runners even when running at the same submaximal speeds (Bushnell & Hunter, 2007). This factor is important because the stance phase represents the only time during a running stride when the athlete is able to exert a force to the ground and can change the momentum of the CM through the application of an impulse associated with the ground reaction force (GRF). (During the flight phase of a running stride, the CM will experience the retarding forces of gravity and drag.) The reduced stance time associated with faster sprinting represents a considerable biomechanical constraint associated with sprint running performance.

Biomechanics of Accelerative Sprint Running

Table 13.4 shows the kinematic characteristics of the first 10 steps during the acceleration phase for a trained sprinter. Notice that step length (the horizontal distance traveled between stance and the next ipsilateral stance) and step frequency

Table 13.4
Step Length, Stance Time, and Aerial Time During the First 10 Steps During the Acceleration Phase for a Trained Sprinter

Step	Step Length (m)	Step Frequency (Hz)*	Speed (m/s)	Stance Time (s)	Aerial Time (s)†
1	1.03	4.93	5.08	0.172	0.031
2	0.99	5.41	5.36	0.142	0.043
3	1.33	5.52	7.34	0.141	0.040
4	1.36	5.41	7.36	0.130	0.055
5	1.58	6.49	10.25	0.111	0.043
6	1.55	5.99	9.28	0.117	0.050
7	1.71	5.81	9.94	0.129	0.043
8	1.77	5.78	10.23	0.117	0.056
9	1.86	6.90	12.83	0.099	0.046
10	1.86	5.92	11.01	0.117	0.052

* Step frequencies are calculated from the inverse of step time (stance time + aerial time).

† Aerial times are calculated by halving the flight times provided.

Data from Čoh, M., Tomažin, K., & Štuhec, S. (2006). The biomechanical model of the sprint start and block acceleration. *Physical Education and Sport, 4*, 103–114.

(the inverse of step time) increase with each step taken. Also notice that the stance time decreases with each step.

Recall that stance represents the time when the athlete is able to generate an impulse of the GRF to change his or her horizontal momentum and that a net positive horizontal impulse is required during the acceleration phase of sprinting (Equation 13.1). During the second stance phase after a block start, there is a net positive horizontal impulse of 87 Ns in trained sprinters (Mero, 1988). This horizontal impulse comprises a small braking impulse (–3 Ns) and a much greater propulsive impulse (90 Ns). The small braking impulse occurs despite the CM being ahead of the stance foot at touchdown and is caused by the forward movement of the stance foot with respect to the ground. Indeed, for the first two steps following a sprint start, the CM is ahead of the stance foot at touchdown, but falls behind the stance foot by the third step (Mero, Komi, & Gregor, 1992). The small braking impulses acting on the CM during each stance of accelerative sprinting do not influence running speed over short distances (5 m) (Sleivert & Taingahue, 2004). In contrast, the magnitude of the propulsive impulse of the GRF is strongly correlated to accelerative sprinting speed (Hunter, Marshall, & McNair, 2005; Mero, 1988; Sleivert & Taingahue, 2004).

As the athlete progresses through the acceleration phase, the duration of each stance decreases (Table 13.4), while the relative proportion of the stance comprising braking increases. For example, 11% of the second stance phase from the start consists of braking (Mero, 1988), whereas 32% of stance at mid-acceleration (16 m) is braking (Hunter et al., 2004). The increased braking experienced during stance is caused by the stance foot being placed ahead of the CM at touchdown, with a touchdown distance of 0.28 m being recorded at mid-acceleration (Hunter et al., 2004). At this stage of accelerative sprint running, the magnitude of the braking impulse affects the athlete's speed, with the faster athletes demonstrating smaller braking impulses (Hunter et al., 2004). The propulsive impulse still exceeds the braking impulse at this stage of the sprint, resulting in a net positive horizontal impulse to maintain the acceleration of the CM, yet the magnitude of the net horizontal impulse is less than that recorded during initial acceleration; the acceleration of the athlete decreases as he or she moves away from the start of the sprint and toward the maximal running speed. As stance time decreases and the athlete approaches the maximal running speed, less time is available for the athlete to generate the necessary propulsive impulse. Furthermore, the posture of the athlete changes from a forward lean of the trunk during the early steps associated with accelerative sprinting to a more upright posture, such that the stance foot contacts the ground ahead of the CM; this action increases the retardation of velocity through the increased braking impulse.

The change from a forward lean to an upright posture as the athlete progresses through the acceleration phase to attain maximal running speed is related to the need to provide a vertical force to support body weight and propel the CM during the progressively shorter stance phases (Equation 13.3). Moreover, the vertical force exerted during stance should be sufficient to project the CM into the subsequent aerial phase, requiring the CM to possess vertical velocity at takeoff. However, the vertical velocity of the CM at takeoff during accelerative sprint running, and therefore the net vertical impulse of the GRF during stance, has been reported to limit running speed (Hunter et al., 2004). For this reason, excessive vertical impulse during the stance phases of accelerative sprint running should be avoided.

Given the requirement for a large net horizontal impulse and a vertical impulse to support body weight and project the CM into flight, we can now establish that performance during the acceleration phase of sprint running requires a forward-directed

GRF during stance, as has been identified in the literature (Kawamori, Nosaka, & Newton, 2013; Kugler & Janshen, 2010; Morin et al., 2012; Morin, Edouard, & Samonzino, 2011). Yet the existence of a braking force early during stance demands that the direction of the resultant GRF change throughout the stance. The control exerted over the direction of the resultant force to achieve high horizontal velocity of the CM represents a significant biomechanical constraint to accelerative sprint running and requires a specific activation sequence of the muscles crossing the hip, knee, and ankle joints. Control over the direction of the GRF during movement tasks is achieved by the distribution of net joint moments across the lower-body joints. The specific distribution of net joint moments is, in turn, determined by the activity of the biarticular muscles. At touchdown during the initial acceleration phase of sprinting, there is a large net extensor moment at the hip joint and a small flexor moment at the knee joint, but only a very small moment at the ankle joint (Jacobs & van Ingen Schenau, 1992). These moments at the hip and knee joint tend to pull the stance foot backward, reducing the braking force during early stance (Figure 13.3a). As the stance phase progresses, the moment at the knee changes to a small extensor moment, with a very large extensor moment generated at the ankle joint, while an extensor moment continues to be generated at the hip (Jacobs & van Ingen Schenau, 1992). This distribution of joint moments will produce a forward-directed GRF, commensurate with the mechanical demands of the task. However, early during stance, the resultant GRF actually acts anterior to the CM (Figure 13.3b).

The resultant GRF acting anterior to the CM increases the positive angular momentum of the athlete, tending to accelerate the individual upward and backward, and contravening the requirements of the task. Activation of the hamstrings and gluteus maximus early during the stance phase produces the net extensor moment at the hip joint: The biarticular function of the hamstrings, however, limits the magnitude of the knee extensor moment at this time and prevents the resultant GRF from increasing in magnitude (Jacos & van Ingen Schenau, 1992; Figure 13.3b). At this time during stance, the CM is rotated forward about the stance foot, resulting in positive horizontal velocity of the CM.

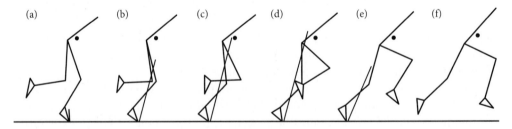

Figure 13.3 The rotation–extension strategy used to control the direction of the ground reaction force relative to the center of mass during the stance phase of accelerative sprint running (a). During early stance, the GRF acts anterior to the center of mass, decreasing the negative angular momentum of the athlete (b). The center of mass is then rotated about the stance foot, and the GRF now acts behind the center of mass, increasing the negative angular momentum (c). The athlete now begins the forceful extension of the stance leg to maximize the horizontal velocity of the center of mass at takeoff (d through f).

As this rotation continues, the activation of the hamstrings is reduced while that of the rectus femoris increases (Jacobs & van Ingen Schenau, 1992). This reciprocal activation of the biarticular hamstrings and rectus femoris increases the magnitude of the extensor moment at the knee, in turn increasing the angular velocity of the joint. Furthermore, the gluteus maximus remains active, so the rectus femoris is able to transport energy from this muscle to the knee joint. The extension of the hip and knee joints contributes to the increase in the magnitude of the resultant GRF, which, while still being directed forward, now acts behind the CM (Jacobs & van Ingen Schenau, 1992; Figures 13.3c and 13.3d). At this time the GRF acts to increase the negative angular momentum of the athlete, increasing the horizontal velocity of the CM while minimizing the vertical velocity of the CM at takeoff. (Notice in Figure 13.3 that the mass moment of inertia of the body about the CM has been increased during stance due to the extension of the stance leg, so the negative angular momentum at takeoff will be relatively small.)

Once the CM has been rotated about the stance foot, the extension of the stance leg makes the greatest contribution to the horizontal velocity of the CM (Jacobs & van Ingen Schenau, 1992). This extension late during stance, once the CM has been rotated about the stance foot, produces a large takeoff distance of 0.65 m during accelerative sprinting (Hunter et al., 2004). The **rotation–extension strategy** during the stance phases associated with accelerative sprint running, whereby the horizontal velocity of the CM is produced first by rotating the CM about the stance foot before the forcible extension of the stance leg, results from the reciprocal activation of the biarticular hamstrings and rectus femoris muscles and satisfies the requirements of maximizing the horizontal velocity and minimizing the vertical velocity of the CM at takeoff (Jacobs & van Ingen Schenau, 1992). The activation of the hamstrings early during stance, followed by later activation of the rectus femoris, also allows the proximal-to-distal transport of energy liberated by the monoarticular muscles, satisfying the geometric and anatomic constraints associated with generating a GRF. Note that the reciprocal activation of the hamstrings and rectus femoris muscles and the amount of energy transported by these muscles during the stance phase of accelerative sprint running differ from the corresponding effects observed during the propulsive phase of a vertical jump (Jacobs, Bobbert, & van Ingen Schenau, 1996). The rotation–extension strategy associated with accelerative sprint running is, therefore, likely to demand specific training exercises to elicit improvements in accelerative sprinting performance.

Joint Kinematics and Kinetics During Accelerative Sprint Running

During the initial acceleration phase of a sprint, the hip joint extends throughout stance, with the angular velocity of the joint increasing rapidly after approximately 40% of stance (Jacobs & van Ingen Schenau, 1992). The increase in extension velocity is caused by a net extensor moment at the hip joint, which persists through approximately 70% of stance, but changes to a flexor moment thereafter (Bezodis, Salo, & Trewartha, 2012; Jacobs & van Ingen Schenau, 1992). This change in the net hip moment arises from the reciprocal activity of the hamstrings and rectus femoris muscles during stance (Jacobs & van Ingen Shencau, 1992). The continued extension of the hip with a net flexor moment during the final 30% of stance means that the hip moment absorbs energy prior to takeoff. However, over the duration of stance, the net moment at the hip generates energy of approximately 110 J (Bezodis, Salo, & Trewartha, 2012).

Similar to the hip joint, the knee joint extends throughout the majority of the stance phase during accelerative sprinting, with flexion occurring prior to takeoff (Jacobs & van Ingen Schenau, 1992). The extension angular velocity at the knee remains relatively low during the first 30% of stance primarily due to the hamstrings activity at this time, which also accounts for the initial net flexor moment at the knee. The net moment then changes to extensor due to the reciprocal activity of the hamstrings and rectus femoris and the increased activity of the vastii group, resulting in increased extension velocity of the joint (Jacobs & van Ingen Schenau, 1992). The net extensor moment is reduced or changed to a net flexor moment at the time of takeoff (Bezodis et al., 2012; Jacobs & van Ingen Schenau, 1992). This effect is caused by a decrease in the activation of the vastii and an increase in the activity of the gastrocnemius (Jacobs & van Ingen Scheau, 1992). Thus the net moment at the knee joint absorbs energy initially, before generating energy until approximately 80% of stance. Over the duration of stance, a net generation of energy occurs at the knee (approximately 70 J). Not all athletes exhibit this behavior, however—some demonstrate a net energy absorption (Bezodis et al., 2012).

The ankle joint is accelerated into dorsiflexion during the initial 30% of stance, with plantarflexion occurring thereafter (Jacobs & van Ingen Schenau, 1992). The net moment at the ankle joint remains plantarflexion throughout stance, reaching a peak value at approximately 50% of stance, corresponding to an increase in the activity of the soleus (Bezodis et al., 2012; Jacobs & van Ingen Schenau, 1992). Over the first 30% of stance, the net joint moment absorbs energy, generating energy throughout the remainder of stance. The overall result is a net energy generation at the ankle joint (approximately 85 J) over the duration of stance during the acceleration phase of sprint running (Bezodis et al., 2012).

The rapid increase in angular velocity at the hip, knee, and ankle joints after approximately 30% of stance corresponds to the extension of the stance leg. This effect contributes to the horizontal velocity of the CM, as per the rotation–extension strategy associated with accelerative sprint running (Jacobs & van Ingen Schenau, 1992).

Biomechanics of Maximal-Speed Sprint Running

In contrast to accelerative sprinting, the attainment of maximal running speed requires that the net horizontal impulse acting on the CM be equal to zero during each stride, such that the propulsive impulse generated by the athlete is equal to that associated with the retarding impulse (e.g., braking forces, drag; see Equation (13.2). This requirement for a net zero horizontal impulse acting on the CM applies across an entire sprinting step or stride. During the aerial phase of each step, the athlete will decelerate due to the retarding effects of drag. Thus, during each stance phase, the athlete will be required to exert a sufficient impulse to offset any losses of speed experienced during the aerial phases as well as those experienced during stance.

The notion that maximal running speed is achieved when the braking and propulsive impulses acting on the CM during stance are equal is merely theoretical. Yet because of the braking forces experienced during stance as the athlete attains maximal running speed, the athlete is still required to exert a propulsive impulse. The athlete experiences greater braking forces during stance as he or she approaches maximal running speed compared to accelerative sprinting, partly due to the greater touchdown distances associated with the increased running speeds (Alcaraz, Palao, Elvira, & Linthorne, 2008; Girard, Miscallef, & Millet, 2011; Ito, Fukuda, & Kijima, 2008).

(See Table 13.5.) Meanwhile, the drag forces acting to retard the athlete during stance are also greater due to the athlete's speed.

In Table 13.5, notice that the net positive horizontal impulse during the acceleration phase of sprint running is much greater than that when the athlete attains the maximal speed (Girard et al., 2011). However, the propulsive impulse required during maximal-speed sprinting is still relatively large due to the greater braking impulse experienced by the athlete during stance. Furthermore, this propulsive impulse has to be generated in a much shorter stance time. This relationship highlights the importance of horizontal force production even during maximal-speed running (Brughelli, Cronin, & Chaouachi, 2011; Morin et al., 2012). An obvious method to reduce the magnitude of the required horizontal impulse during stance is to minimize the braking impulse.

In addition to generating a propulsive impulse to offset the braking impulse experienced early during stance, the athlete is required to generate a vertical impulse during each stance phase to support body weight and prevent the CM from falling (Equation 13.3). During maximal-speed sprinting, the CM descends during the braking phase of stance, but then ascends during the remaining time such that the height of the CM at touchdown is approximately equal to that at takeoff (Girard et al., 2011; Weyand et al., 2010). Notice in Table 13.5 that there is little difference between the vertical impulse generated by the athlete during accelerative sprinting compared to that associated with maximal-speed sprinting. However, the athlete has less time available to generate this impulse due to the shorter stance times associated with maximal-speed sprinting. The requirement to exert sufficient vertical impulse to support body weight and project the CM into the subsequent aerial phase in short stance times has

Table 13.5
Kinematic and Kinetic Variables During Steps in the Acceleration and Maximal-Speed Phases of Sprint Running in Untrained Sprinters

Kinematic and Kinetic Variables	Acceleration Phase	Maximal-Speed Phase
Distance (m)	5–10	30–35
Speed (m/s)	6.54	8.01
Stride length (m)	3.23	4.20
Stride frequency (Hz)	2.03	1.91
Stance time (s)	0.154	0.135
Flight time (s)	0.106	0.127
Braking time (s)	0.036	0.057
Propulsive time (s)	0.118	0.078
Braking impulse (Ns)	–2.1	–13.6
Propulsive impulse (Ns)	26.0	15.1
Vertical impulse (Ns)	169	174

Reproduced from Girard, O., Miscallef, J.-P., & Millet, G. P. (2011). Changes in spring-mass model characteristics during repeated running sprints. *European Journal of Applied Physiology, 111*, 125–134, with kind permission from Springer Science and Business Media.

been identified as a substantial biomechanical constraint that limits the attainment of maximal running speed (Weyand et al., 2010; Weyand et al., 2000).

Beginning with the theoretical assumptions that the propulsive impulse during stance associated with maximal-speed sprinting is equal to the braking impulse, and that the height of the CM is the same at touchdown and takeoff, sprinting speed can be expressed in terms of the net vertical force during each stance phase and the kinematic variables of stance distance, stance time, and the duration of the aerial phase (Weyand et al., 2010):

$$\text{Speed} = \left(\left[\frac{F_{\text{vert}}}{F_{\text{BW}}} \right] \times d_{\text{stance}} \right) \times (t_{\text{stance}} + t_{\text{aerial}})^{-1} \qquad \textbf{Eq. (13.5)}$$

where F_{vert} is the average vertical GRF during the stance phase, F_{BW} is the body-weight force, d_{stance} is stance distance, t_{stance} is the duration of the stance phase, and t_{aerial} is the duration of the aerial phase (the time between contralateral stance phases). Equation (13.5) informs us that maximal running speed is directly proportional to the net vertical force applied by the athlete during the stance phase and stance distance, and inversely proportional to the sum of the duration of the stance and aerial phases (i.e., step frequency).

A stance distance of approximately 0.90 m has been reported during maximal-speed sprinting (Alcaraz et al., 2008; Paradisi & Cooke, 2001) and is largely determined by leg length, whereas the duration of the aerial phase differs little between the fastest sprinters and their slower counterparts (Weyand et al., 2000). As noted elsewhere, the duration of the stance phases is shorter in the fastest sprinters—a factor that appears to be an important mechanical variable determining maximal running speed. However, the ability to generate sufficient vertical force to support body weight and project the CM into the aerial phase where the leg is repositioned for the next stance phase is compromised as stance time decreases. Therefore, a mechanical limitation to maximal running speed is imposed by the vertical forces that can be applied to the ground during short stance phases and thereby provide the minimum aerial time to reposition the leg for the subsequent ipsilateral stance (Weyand et al., 2010; Weyand et al., 2000). (See Applied Research 13.1.) Indeed, reducing the times required to reposition the limbs during flight actually reduces the magnitude of the vertical force required during the stance phase (Weyand et al., 1999). But recall that there is little difference in the aerial times for fast and slow sprinters—the mechanics associated with the stance phase would appear to limit the attainment of maximal running speeds in athletes. This relationship explains why posture changes from a forward lean during acceleration to an upright posture when running at maximal speed. An inability to exert sufficient GRF during stance is responsible for the greater maximal running speeds that are achieved when sprinting along a straight path as opposed to around a curve (see Sprint Running Concept 13.2).

Exerting the required vertical impulse during shorter stance phases results in greater peak vertical forces generated as the athlete approaches maximal running speed compared to those vertical forces generated during accelerative sprinting, while the horizontal forces decrease (Figure 13.4). These demands relate to the distinct biomechanical constraints associated with accelerative and maximal-speed sprint running—namely, the rotation–extension strategy and the application of large vertical support forces, respectively.

Applied Research 13.1

Vertical force production during short stance phases imposes a limit on maximal sprinting speed

Weyand et al. (2010) investigated whether maximal sprinting speeds were limited by the greatest vertical force that the sprinter is able to generate versus the minimum time associated with stance required to generate the force. To do so, they had track athletes (jumpers and sprinters) hop forward and sprint forward and backward at a variety of speeds up to maximal on a high-speed treadmill. The treadmill had a force plate embedded to allow the investigators to record the ground reaction force during the different movements.

Greater maximal speeds were achieved in the forward sprinting task. However, the authors reported that the average and peak vertical GRF was greater during the hopping task than during the forward sprinting task at comparable speeds, although the stance times were longer. The vertical GRF and stance times were equivalent during forward and backward sprinting at comparable speeds.

The authors concluded that maximal sprinting speed is limited by the vertical GRF that the athlete can apply in the short stance times, necessitating a high rate of force development. They suggested that if an athlete were capable of generating the same magnitude of vertical force in the short stance phases associated with maximal-speed sprinting as the athlete could generate during the forward hopping task, then a sprinting speed of approximately 19 m/s would be possible (assuming no changes in stance distance or the aerial time required to reposition the swing leg).

Weyand, P. G., Sandell, R. F., Prime, D. N. L., & Bundle, M. W. (2010). The biological limits to running speed are imposed from the ground up. *Journal of Applied Physiology, 108*, 950–961.

Sprint Running Concept 13.2

Humans achieve greater maximal running speeds along straight paths compared to flat curves

Comparisons of humans sprinting along straight paths compared to around curved paths have demonstrated a loss in maximum speed around flat curves (Chang & Kram, 2007; Usherwood & Wilson, 2006). Indeed, an analysis of the times for 200-m races in track and field performed on straight tracks revealed a 0.4-s improvement when compared to the event performed on a curved track (Jain, 1980). Furthermore, the difference depends on the magnitude of the radius associated with the curved path, with greater radii conferring less of a decrement in race time (Jain, 1980). This finding has significant implications for the lane assignment during track and field races performed around the curves of the track.

The limitations to maximum running speed around a curved path are biomechanical in nature. It has been proposed that the requirement for centripetal force to allow the athlete to negotiate the bend, and the associated lean into the bend adopted by the athlete to achieve this force, reduces the athlete's ability to generate sufficient vertical force during each stance phase to support body weight and project the CM; in turn, the athlete must increase the duration of each stance phase when running along a curved path to allow sufficient

(continues)

(continued)

vertical force to be generated (Usherwood & Wilson, 2006). As the distance traveled during each stance remains unchanged, the increased duration of stance results in reduced running speeds.

Such a hypothesis is predicated on a "constant limb force" being exerted by an athlete when running along either a straight or curved path. However, Chang and Kram (2007) demonstrated that the assumption of a constant limb force is erroneous, with the magnitude of the resultant GRF exerted during each stance phase declining as the radius of curvature followed during the sprint decreased. These authors proposed that the joint moments in the frontal plane during each stance phase actually limit the ability of the athlete to exert sufficiently large GRF, thus limiting the maximal speed that can be achieved. Specifically, the requirement to exert muscular forces to stabilize the lower-limb joints in the frontal plane during each stance phase as the athlete leans into the bend (a requirement to exert the necessary centripetal force) precludes the attainment of large muscular forces in the sagittal plane, limiting vertical force production. This biomechanical constraint is suggested to be particularly limiting for the inside leg as the athlete runs around a curve (Chang & Kram, 2007).

Joint Kinematics and Kinetics During Maximal-Speed Sprint Running

The hip joint extends throughout each stance phase when sprinting at maximal speed, with low angular velocity during the braking phase and an increase in extension velocity during propulsion (Bezodis, Kerwin, & Salo, 2008). The net moment at the hip joint is extensor during the first 80% of stance, reaching a large peak after 20%. This is largely due to the activation of the hamstrings and gluteus maximus that begins prior to touchdown, but then declines during stance (Kuitunen, Komi, & Kyröläinen, 2002). During the final 20% of stance there is a net flexor moment through takeoff, which accelerates the stance leg into the swinging motion required during the flight phase. The generation of energy by the hip moment during the first 80% of stance and the energy absorption during the remaining stance results in a net energy generation at the hip (approximately 30 J) during stance when sprinting at maximal speed (Bezodis et al., 2008).

The knee undergoes flexion during the first half of stance when sprinting at maximal speed, extending during the remainder of the phase (Bezodis et al., 2008). Some investigators have reported that knee extension continues after takeoff (Bezodis et al., 2008), while others have reported flexion at the knee at takeoff (Bushnell & Hunter, 2007). The flexion observed at the knee prior to takeoff may reduce the duration of stance, potentially increasing running speed. It has also been proposed that the abbreviated stance caused by knee flexion does not interfere with force production because little force is generated after midstance when running at maximal speed (Mann & Sprague, 1980). However, during this time the propulsive force is generated to offset the braking forces experienced during early stance. A large net extensor moment has been reported at the knee during stance by some researchers, most likely due to the activation of the vastii muscles (Kuitunen et al., 2002). Others have reported more complicated changes in the net moment at the knee throughout stance, although the amplitudes are very small (Bezodis et al., 2008). Furthermore, there is considerable inter-athlete variability in the energy absorbed and generated at the knee joint during stance (Bezodis et al., 2008).

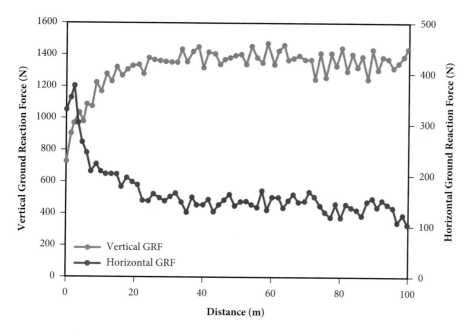

Figure 13.4 The horizontal and vertical components of the ground reaction force as an athlete sprints 100 m on a treadmill. Notice that the magnitude of the horizontal component decreases, while the magnitude of the vertical component increases as the athlete accelerates up to maximum running speed. The horizontal component actually remains positive even once the athlete has achieved the maximum running speed during this protocol due to the use of a torque-treadmill (see Running Concept 13.1).

Reproduced from Morin, J-B., & Sève, P. (2011). Sprint running performance: Comparison between treadmill and field conditions. *European Journal of Applied Physiology, 111,* 1695–1703, with kind permission from Springer Science and Business Media.

Dorsiflexion at the ankle joint has been reported during the first half of stance, with the joint extending during the remainder of stance (Bezodis et al., 2008; Kuitunen et al., 2002). The net moment is plantarflexion for the duration of stance as a result of the activity of the soleus and gastrocnemius (Kuitunen et al., 2002). It absorbs energy initially before generating energy later, resulting in a net energy absorption (approximately 29 J) at the joint (Bezodis et al., 2008).

The leg is rotated forward during the flight phase of maximal-speed sprinting due to the net flexor moments at the hip and knee joints (Kuitunen et al., 2002). The iliopsoas has been shown to be important in generating the flexor moment at the hip joint at takeoff (Dorn, Schache, & Pandy, 2012). Toward the end of the flight phase as touchdown approaches, the activation of the hamstrings and gluteus maximus generates a large net extensor moment at the hip joint (Kuitunen et al., 2002). A net flexor moment is also generated at the knee joint at this time. The combined extensor and flexor moments at the hip and the knee, respectively, act to reduce the forward velocity of the foot and pull it back prior to touchdown. This action, which reduces the braking force during stance, is termed an **active leg motion**. (Note the contrast here with the general technique associated with accelerative sprinting: Athletes "push" themselves during the acceleration phase and "pull" themselves over the stance leg when sprinting at maximal speed.) The biarticular hamstrings have been implicated in the active leg prior to touchdown (Dorn et al., 2012; Wiemann & Tidow, 1995) and may be predisposed to strain injury during maximal-speed sprinting as a result (see Sprint Running Concept 13.3).

Sprint Running Concept 13.3

Hamstring injuries during sprinting

Hamstring strain injuries (HSI) are the most prevalent noncontact musculoskeletal injury in sports including American football, Australian football, rugby union, and soccer (Heiderscheit, Sherry, Silder, Chumanov, & Thelen, 2010; Opar, Williams, & Shield, 2012). In contrast to other common musculoskeletal injuries sustained in these sports, the rate of HSI does not appear to be declining.

The hamstrings muscle is located at the posterior of the thigh and comprises the biceps femoris (long and short heads), semimembranosus, and semitendinosus. The long head of the biceps femoris (BF_{LH}) along with the semimembranosus and semitendinosus cross both the hip and knee joints, meaning that the length of the biarticular hamstrings at any time is a function of the hip and knee joint angles. The moment arm of the hamstrings is greater at the hip joint compared to the knee joint (Thelen et al., 2005). Both the semimembranosus and the semitendinosus display greater activation when they are operating at short muscle lengths, whereas the BF_{LH} shows greater activation at longer lengths (Onishi et al., 2002). The hamstrings are proposed to be injured when the muscle is activated while being lengthened. The largest number of HSI occur during running activities, although the greatest severity of injuries are sustained during kicking activities (Freckleton & Pizzari, 2013). Furthermore, the BF_{LH} is the muscle most often injured among the hamstrings group (Heiderscheit et al., 2010).

The mechanisms of a strain injury to a musculotendinous unit include the fibers being strained during lengthening of an active muscle and the negative energy absorbed by the muscle (Lieber & Friden, 2001). This implicates eccentric muscle actions in such injuries. However, evidence also shows that muscle strain injuries are possible during concentric muscle actions (Uchiyama, Tamaki, & Fukuda, 2001). Whatever the specific mechanism, muscle strain injuries are characterized by disruption to the structure and functioning of the specific muscle. Indeed, the severity of the disruption is used to categorize strain injuries: Grade I strains are characterized by minor microscopic tears and some loss of functioning, whereas grade III strains involve the complete rupture of the muscle and a complete loss of functioning (Blankenbaker & Tuite, 2010).

During sprint running at maximal speed, a HSI is most likely to occur during the late swing phase. Schache et al. (2012) provided evidence from a forward dynamic computer simulation of sprint running that the maximum lengthening of the BF_{LH}, semimembranosus, and semitendinosus occurs at the same time during the late swing phase as the leg is decelerated in preparation for the stance phase. As a consequence, the requirement for an active leg motion to reduce the braking forces when running at maximal speed may provide a mechanism to induce a HSI. Furthermore, Thelen et al. (2005) have presented evidence that the BF_{LH} undergoes a greater strain than the semimembranosus or the semitendinosus during the late swing of maximal-speed sprinting, providing a possible explanation for the greater prevalence of HSI involving this muscle. Others have proposed that HSI are more likely to occur during the early stance phase of maximal-speed sprinting due to the greater forces acting on the muscle at this time (Orchard, 2012). Chumanov, Heiderscheit, and Thelen (2011) reported that the hamstrings are lengthened at touchdown when sprinting at maximal speed, but all three muscles are shortened during stance into early swing. Thereafter, all three muscles experience lengthening. Large forces are generated by the muscles during stance and during late swing, with the forces generated by the BF_{LH} and semimembranosus being greater during the swing phase. Furthermore, the energy absorbed by these muscles during late swing as they are being lengthened exceeds that generated by them during stance as they shorten. The authors proposed that these mechanics of the hamstrings during late swing are consistent with the mechanisms of muscle strain injuries.

An understanding of the mechanisms associated with HSI has led to the search for factors that predispose an athlete to incurring this injury. Age has consistently been shown to be a risk factor for HSI, with an age greater than 23 or 24 years being associated with a greater risk (Dallinga, Benjaminse, & Lemmink, 2012; Freckleton & Pizzari, 2013; Heiderscheit et al., 2010; Liu, Garrett, Moorman, & Yu, 2012; Opar et al., 2012). Possible reasons for this association include increased body weight, reduced muscle mass, reduced flexibility, or nerve impingement with increased age, although the evidence to support any of these factors is limited. A previous HSI has also been shown to be a significant risk factor for a future HSI, possibly because the scar tissue from the original injury alters the muscle lengthening mechanics and eccentric strength of the muscle (Liu et al., 2012; Opar et al., 2012). Some evidence shows that the volume of injured tissue associated with the original injury affects the risk of future injury (Freckleton & Pizzari, 2013). Other risk factors include muscular strength imbalances (e.g., a low hamstrings:quadriceps strength ratio, bilateral hamstring asymmetry), low flexibility, and increased fatigue, although the evidence to support these variables' relationship with HSI is largely inconclusive (Freckleton & Pizzari, 2013; Liu et al., 2012; Opar et al., 2012). Nevertheless, these proposed risk factors can be modified through specific interventions, in comparison with the nonmodifiable risk factors of age and previous injury. Mendiguchia, Alentorn-Geli, and Brughelli (2012) propose that the current understanding of risk factors for HSI is limited because previous researchers have examined the risk factors in isolation; it is more likely that these risk factors are interconnected and interact with one another to predispose an athlete to HSI.

Interventions to prevent HSI typically involve either muscle strengthening or flexibility training. In general, findings regarding the effectiveness of interventions that utilize eccentric strength training are inconclusive at present (Opar et al., 2012). This is likely due to the inclusion of ineffective exercises that do not provide sufficient hip flexion with concurrent knee extension to lengthen the

(continues)

(continued)

muscle as it is being loaded. For example, the inclusion of Nordic hamstrings exercise has been criticized, whereas use of the stiff-legged deadlift has been encouraged (Opar et al., 2012). There is limited evidence that flexibility training can prevent HSI, mainly due to the poor design of the studies performed to date (Opar et al., 2012). Furthermore, flexibility has not been consistently reported as a risk factor for HSI.

McHugh and Cosgrave (2010) provide a rationale for the inclusion of stretching exercises performed as part of a warm-up routine in reducing the risk of HSI. They note that flexibility is an intrinsic factor, while engaging in stretching is an extrinsic factor. These authors propose that static stretches of the hamstrings groups can render the muscles more compliant when the stretches are held for a sufficient duration (60 s or longer). Such a mechanical alteration would result in a shift of the torque–angle relationship, allowing a greater relative force to be generated at longer muscle lengths and possibly conferring a protective effect against HSI. McHugh and Cosgrave (2010) propose a warm-up including the application of four or five stretches to pain tolerance held for 60 s bilaterally to the hamstrings, followed by the completion of dynamic drills to mitigate the potential force loss associated with static stretches.

Verrall, Slavotinek, and Barnes (2005) performed an intervention over the course of a two-year period with elite Australian football players. In this group, training was altered to incorporate a greater proportion of repeated-sprint activities and thereby better reflect the physiological demands of the game. Moreover, the players performed sprint training drills where they were required to accelerate with an accentuated forward lean of the trunk (achieved by chasing a ball rolling along the ground in front of the player), thereby lengthening the hamstrings muscles in a sport-specific manner. Finally, the players were encouraged to perform static stretches of the hamstrings during breaks within their workouts. The authors reported that the number of HSI incurred within competitive games was significantly reduced as a result of this intervention, falling below the average number of HSI reported by other professional teams.

A decrease in the magnitude of the braking force during stance through an active leg motion reduces the requirement for a propulsive force during the short stance phases associated with maximal-speed sprint running. It has also been shown that the contralateral leg swinging forward is the only segment that contributes to offset the retardation of the CM velocity during the braking phase of the stance leg (Mero, Luhtanen, & Komi, 1986). The athlete can minimize the braking force, thereby allowing for a net positive horizontal force during stance, through the rapid rotation of the swinging leg. Indeed, sprinters tend to have a short horizontal distance between the knees of the swing and stance legs at touchdown, suggesting a more rapid forward rotation of the swinging leg (Bushnell & Hunter, 2007). This emphasizes the importance of the hip flexor muscles, especially the iliopsoas, in maximal-speed sprinting (Dorn et al., 2012).

Arm Action During Sprint Running

Given the importance of the GRF during both accelerative and maximal-speed sprint running, the role of the arms requires consideration. Typically, the arms swing in opposition to the legs during a running stride. The role of the swinging arms has been suggested to be necessary to offset the rotation of the trunk caused by the forward motion of the contralateral leg as it is recovered in preparation for stance (Mann, 1981).

Recall that the inclusion of an arm swing during the propulsive phase of a vertical jump increases jump height. The arm swing is believed to store energy that is later returned to the CM at takeoff, increasing takeoff velocity, while the swinging arms also exert a "pulling" action on the CM toward takeoff (Lees, Vanrenterghem, & De Clercq, 2004). It is possible that the arm swing could fulfill a similar mechanical role during sprint running. It has been reported that the arm swing contributes to the vertical momentum of the CM at takeoff during distance running (Hinrichs, 1990). A similar contribution during maximal sprinting speed might enhance performance given the limitation imposed by vertical force production during this phase of sprinting, allowing the stance leg to generate a horizontal propulsive impulse. The forward lean of the trunk associated with accelerative sprint running might then direct the force exerted by the arms on the CM to a more forward direction, enhancing performance during this phase (Young, Benton, Duthie, & Pryor, 2001), although there is no research to support this proposition. The contribution of the arm swing to the horizontal velocity of the CM when sprinting at maximal speed has been shown to be small (Mero et al., 1986), but sprint times have been shown to increase by between 3% and 10% when the arms have been constrained during maximal-speed running (Wiemann & Tidow, 1995).

Other researchers have reported minimal muscular contributions at the shoulder and elbow joints during maximal-speed sprinting (Mann, 1981). In addition, constraining the motion of the legs through addition of mass to the limbs has been shown to impede maximal running speed to a much greater extent than constraining the motion of the arms (Ropret, Kukolj, Ugarkovic, & Matavulj, 1998). Although leg motion appears to be more important, the arms serve an important function of balancing the action of the legs while sprinting, and their integration into the sprinting technique is required to enhance performance.

The Relationships Between Measures of Muscular Strength and Sprint Running

From our discussion of the biomechanical aspects associated with sprint running, it should be apparent that the generation of an appropriate GRF is required. We should therefore expect muscular strength to have a significant influence on sprinting performance. Indeed, faster sprinters demonstrate greater strength than their slower counterparts (Mero, Luhtanen, Viitasalo, & Komi, 1981).

The acceleration and maximal-speed phases have specific constraints associated with them. The rotation–extension strategy during the acceleration phase allows the development of a forward-directed GRF, in contrast to the requirement for generating sufficient vertical force to support body weight and project the CM during the shorter stance times when running at maximal speed. It is therefore informative to investigate the relationships between different indices of muscular strength and performance during the acceleration and maximal-speed phases of sprint running. Many indices of muscular strength exist and most assessments of muscular strength that have been employed when investigating the relationship with sprinting require vertical force application (e.g., squat, vertical jump). As such, the magnitude of the correlations is typically greater when investigating the relationships with performance in the maximal-speed phase compared to the acceleration phase. Moreover, the assessments of muscular strength are typically bilateral, whereas sprint running requires unilateral force generation.

Measures of **maximal dynamic muscular strength** normalized to body mass demonstrate larger correlations to maximal-speed sprinting than to acceleration (Baker & Nance, 1999). Absolute **maximal isometric muscular strength** has been shown to be correlated to both accelerative and maximal-speed sprinting (Mero et al., 1981; Young, McLean, & Ardagna, 1995).

Large correlations have been demonstrated between measures of **low-load speed-strength** (e.g., vertical jumps with a load less than 30% 1-RM) and both accelerative and maximal-speed sprinting performance (Baker & Nance, 1999; Hennessy & Kilty, 2001; Kale, Aşçi, Bayrak, & Açikada, 2009; Mero, Luhtanen, & Komi, 1983; Mero et al., 1981). Interestingly, large correlations have been reported between unloaded horizontal jumps and accelerative sprinting (Mero et al., 1983), but not between these measures of low-load speed-strength and maximal-speed sprinting (Hennessy & Kilty, 2001; Kale et al., 2009; Mero et al., 1981), perhaps reflecting the different mechanical constraints associated with accelerative and maximal-speed sprinting. Measures of **high-load speed-strength** (e.g., power output during vertical jumps with a load more than 30% 1-RM) normalized to body mass have demonstrated large to very large correlations with both accelerative sprinting and maximal-speed sprinting performance (Baker & Nance, 1999; Sleivert & Taingahue, 2004), although López-Segovia, Marques, van den Tillar, and Gonzàlez-Badillo (2011) reported small to moderate correlations between absolute measures of high-load speed-strength and accelerative performance, with very large correlations observed between absolute high-load speed-strength and maximal-speed sprinting.

Large to very large correlations between normalized measures of **explosive strength** (e.g., rate of force development during squats) and both accelerative sprinting and maximal-speed sprinting have been reported (Sleivert & Taingahue, 2004; Young et al., 1995). Very large correlations have been reported between **reactive strength** (e.g., drop–jump performance) and sprinting performance during both the acceleration phase and the maximal-speed phase (Hennessy & Kilty, 2001; Kale et al., 2009; Mero et al., 1983; Mero et al., 1981).

Leg stiffness, which is related to reactive strength, has been shown to have very large correlations to maximal-speed sprinting, whereas the correlation between leg stiffness and accelerative sprinting was quite small (Bret, Rahmani, Dufour, Messonnier, & Lacour, 2002; Chelly & Denis, 2001). This finding likely reflects the greater braking forces and the short stance durations experienced as the athlete attains maximal speed. The importance of leg stiffness is highlighted by the greater knee and ankle joint stiffness demonstrated by sprint-trained athletes compared to distance runners (Hobara et al., 2008).

The use of appropriate training methods to improve the specific indices of muscular strength is likely to improve sprint running performance. Combining the evidence presented here with the known biomechanical constraints associated with the acceleration and maximal-speed phases of sprint running, it can determined that maximal muscular strength and low-load speed-strength are important during both sprinting phases, although the horizontal projection of the CM is more important during the acceleration phase. High-load speed-strength and leg stiffness become greater determinants of sprinting performance as the athlete attains his or her maximal sprinting speed. Samonzino, Rejc, Di Prampero, Belli, and Morin (2012) noted that the optimal force–velocity profile for an athlete requiring the horizontal projection of the CM is characterized by greater velocity capabilities, while the vertical projection of the CM requires greater force capabilities. Basic mechanics would suggest that an increase in the athlete's muscular strength relative to his or her body mass would allow for a greater improvement in sprinting performance than absolute increases in muscular strength, given the relationship between acceleration, the net force applied to a body, and the mass of the body. By comparison, an increase in the average vertical force normalized to body weight applied by the athlete during stance would allow for attainment of higher maximal sprinting speeds (Weyand et al., 2010). However, while there is evidence to suggest that absolute measures of muscular strength have smaller relationships with sprinting performance (Baker & Nance, 1999), this is not always the case (Mero et al., 1983; Young et al., 1995). Furthermore, a positive relationship exists between body mass and sprint performance (see Sprint Running Concept 13.4).

Sprint Running Concept 13.4

Anthropometric characteristics and their influence on running performance

When observing runners who specialize in different running events, it is clear that they have different anthropometric characteristics. For example, the sprint runners tend to be more massive than the distance runners, irrespective of gender. A relationship between increases in the maximum running speeds associated with sprint running world records and increases in the anthropometric dimensions of body mass and height has been noted (Charles & Bejan, 2009). As the average vertical force normalized to body weight exerted during the stance phase of running increases with running speed (Weyand et al., 2010), the faster athletes require greater muscle mass to exert the required forces and larger anatomic structures to transmit these forces (e.g., tendons, bones). Indeed, sprinters have a greater muscle mass than distance runners and have greater muscle cross-sectional area (Lorentzon, Johansson, Sjostrom, Fagerlunds, & Fugl-Meyer, 1988; Maughan, Watson, & Weir, 1983; Spenst, Martin, & Drinkwater, 1993). However, the masses of sprinters tend to be greater than those of distance runners, yet smaller than those of bodybuilders of similar statures (Weyand & Davis, 2005).

The positive relationship between the increased height of the fastest athletes and sprint running records may be due to the theoretical influence of the height of the CM on the generation of high maximal running speeds (Bejan, Jones, & Charles, 2010). This might have implications for the upper-body hypertrophy that is often observed in the fastest sprinters, which would tend

(continues)

(continued)

to raise the height of the CM. Taller athletes are likely to have longer legs, and stance distance has been shown to be largely dependent upon leg length (Hunter et al., 2004). While leg length is essentially an unmodifiable anthropometric characteristic, Weyand and Bundle (2010) have considered the potential improvements in maximal running speeds by leg lengthening through artificial limbs. In addition to the increase in leg length that would be possible with such prosthetics, these authors have proposed that the reduction in mass associated with artificial limbs would lead to reduced minimum swing times required to reposition the legs, thereby reducing the magnitude of the normalized average vertical force to be generated during stance and enhancing sprinting performance.

The interaction of body mass and height of an athlete is encapsulated in the **reciprocal ponderal index** (RPI), calculated as a ratio of height to scaled body mass (height/body mass$^{2/3}$), providing a measure of the "shape" of the athlete (Watts, Coleman, & Nevill, 2012). The greater the RPI, the more linear the athlete's shape. A positive relationship has been demonstrated between the average running speeds associated with world record performance in the 100 m event and the RPI in both female and male athletes in the past 70 years (Watts et al., 2012). In other words, while the fastest sprinters appear to be increasing in body mass, they are also becoming taller. The shape of the athlete can, therefore, exert an influence on the maximal running speeds attained.

Qualitative Analysis of Sprint Running Performance

The four-stage model of qualitative analysis of performance developed by Knudson and Morrison (2002) includes the stages of preparation, observation, evaluation/diagnosis, and intervention. Here we discuss each of these four stages as they apply to the analysis of sprint running.

Preparation Stage

In the initial preparation stage of a qualitative analysis, the coach should differentiate the critical features of the sprinting task from biomechanical principles and develop a deterministic model of the skill to facilitate the analysis of the movement. Table 13.6 identifies some basic biomechanical principles and their application to the analysis of sprinting.

Figures 13.5 and 13.6 display deterministic models for step length and step frequency during sprint running, respectively. Notice that the vertical impulse is an important mechanical variable affecting both step length and step frequency. However, excessive vertical impulse generated during the stance phases of accelerative sprinting is likely to interfere with the optimal interaction of step length and step frequency (Hunter et al., 2004), and the rotation–extension strategy that is required to maximize the propulsive impulse.

Table 13.6
Biomechanical Principles That Can Be Applied in the Qualitative Analysis of Sprint Running

Principle	Application to Sprinting Tasks
Use of the stretch–shortening cycle	Assess the change in vertical position of the pelvis during the first half of stance.
Number of body segments	Assess the athlete's arm swing and the motion of the swinging leg, particularly during stance.
Coordination of body segments	Assess the position of the foot relative to the CM at touchdown and the forward lean of the trunk at takeoff during acceleration.
	Assess the minimum hip and knee angle of the swinging leg as it is recovered during flight.
	Assess the "clawing" action of the leg as it approaches touchdown (active leg) and the horizontal distance between the swing and stance knees at touchdown.
	Assess the knee extension at takeoff.
	Proximal-to-distal sequencing of the hip, knee, and ankle joint rotations will allow monoarticular muscles to maximize their work during stance.
Maximizing the acceleration path	Assess the change in vertical position of the pelvis during the second half of stance.
	Notice that an excessive vertical acceleration path during maximal speed sprinting may be indicative of low leg stiffness.
	Assess the change in the horizontal distance of the pelvis during stance.
Path of projection	Assess the path of the CM during the flight phase by observing the position of the pelvis to establish the height, angle, and speed at takeoff.
	Avoid too much vertical velocity during the accelerative sprinting, but recognize when this velocity is sufficient when sprinting at maximal speed to allow repositioning of the swing leg.

Note: CM = center of mass.

Following the identification of the critical features of sprinting, the coach should identify the movement phases for the observation of the task. Table 13.7 outlines the movement phases for the analysis of sprint running steps.

Observation Stage

The coach should decide if the performance will take place on a track or on a treadmill. If observing the athlete sprinting on a track, the coach should place himself or herself so that the coach can view the performance of the sprint from the side, as the major motion of the body segments involved in the execution of sprint running occur in the sagittal plane. The coach needs to consider where to view the athlete so as to capture steps during the acceleration and maximal-speed phases. If a video camera is used to supplement the observations of the coach, then the fast movements associated with sprinting tasks require a relatively a high shutter speed, with a speed of 1/100 s being suggested (Bartlett, 2007).

Evaluation/Diagnosis Stage

The performance during sprinting can be evaluated by determining the accomplishment of the biomechanical features during each of the movement phases pertinent to

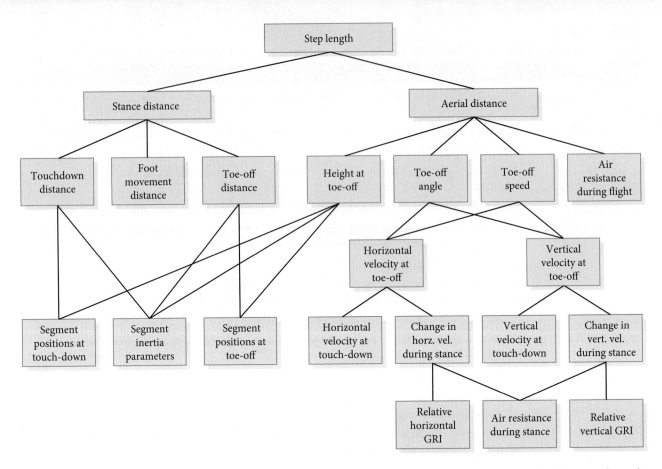

Figure 13.5 A deterministic model highlighting the critical biomechanical features involved in step length during sprint running.

Note: GRI = ground reaction impulse.

Reproduced from Hunter, J. P., Marshall, R. N., & McNair, P. J. (2004). Interaction of step length and step rate during sprint running. *Medicine and Science in Sports and Exercise, 36,* 261–271.

the specific sprinting task. Table 13.8 outlines a method to evaluate the biomechanical principles during the different movement phases of an accelerative sprinting step. Table 13.9 provides a method to evaluate the biomechanical principles during the different movement phases of a maximal sprinting speed step.

The following methods may be used to prioritize the correction of identified weaknesses in sprinting performance:

- Look at the sequence of features as per phases of movement.
- Prioritize critical features that maximize performance improvements.
- Prioritize critical features based on which will be the easiest to improve.

Intervention Stage

After having identified the athlete's areas of weakness from the evaluation/diagnosis stage of the qualitative analysis, the strength and conditioning coach must then develop an intervention to improve sprinting performance. It is important to recognize that most observations of motor skills are undertaken in situations where the

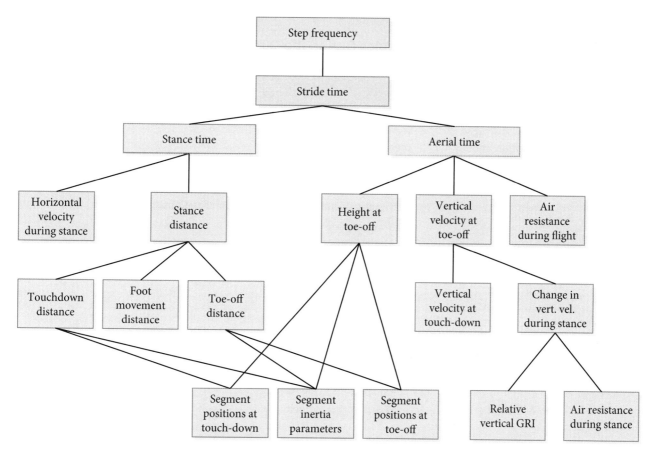

Figure 13.6 A deterministic model highlighting the critical biomechanical features involved in step frequency during sprint running.

Note: GRI = ground reaction impulse.

Reproduced from Hunter, J. P., Marshall, R. N., & McNair, P. J. (2004). Interaction of step length and step rate during sprint running. *Medicine and Science in Sports and Exercise, 36,* 261–271.

athlete is removed from the typical task and environmental constraints within which he or she must operate in the actual sporting situation; specifically, the strength and conditioning practitioner is likely to observe the athlete sprinting alone in a well-controlled environment to ease the analysis of the movement. Because the observed skill may not be representative of how the athlete executes a sprint in the actual sport, it might potentially lead to the selection of interventions to improve performance that are actually inappropriate.

Table 13.7
Movement Phases for the Analysis of a Sprinting Step

Movement Phase	Details
Stance	Begins with touchdown of the foot.
	Ends with takeoff of the foot.
Aerial	Begins at takeoff and ends with ipsilateral touchdown.

Table 13.8
Evaluation of the Biomechanical Principles During the Different Movement Phases Associated with a Step During Accelerative Sprinting

Movement Phase	Biomechanical Principle	Evaluation
Stance	Number of body segments	Arm swing and motion of the swing leg
	Coordination of body segments	Touchdown distance
		Forward lean at takeoff
		Hip and knee extended at takeoff
		Proximal-to-distal sequencing for joint rotations
		Vigorous motion of swing leg
		Takeoff distance
		Time of stance
	Maximizing the acceleration path	Change in vertical position of the pelvis during stance
Aerial	Number of body segments	Arm swing
	Coordination of body segments	Minimum knee angle during recovery (less in sprinters)
		Minimum hip angle during recovery (less in sprinters)
		Active leg motion prior to touchdown
	Path of projection	Too much vertical velocity of CM at takeoff interfering with horizontal velocity

Note: CM = center of mass.

Table 13.9
Evaluation of the Biomechanical Principles During the Different Movement Phases Associated with a Step During Maximal-Speed Sprinting

Movement Phase	Biomechanical Principle	Evaluation
Stance	Number of body segments	Arm swing and motion of swing leg
	Coordination of body segments	Touchdown distance
		Distance between swing and stance knees at touchdown
		Proximal-to-distal sequencing for joint rotations
		Vigorous motion of swing leg
		Knee flexed at takeoff
		Takeoff distance
		Time of stance
Aerial	Number of body segments	Arm swing
	Coordination of body segments	Minimum knee angle during recovery (less in sprinters)
		Minimum hip angle during recovery (less in sprinters)
		Active leg motion prior to touchdown
	Path of projection	Sufficient vertical velocity at takeoff to allow time to reposition swing leg

Interventions to Improve Sprint Running Performance

The interventions that are available to the strength and conditioning practitioner to improve sprinting performance can be divided into those that focus on developing the organismic constraints of the athlete, including resistance training methods, and those that develop the attunement of the sprinting movement to the task and environmental information specific to an athlete's sport, as exemplified by representative learning practices. (Metabolic conditioning is not considered here.) It is the responsibility of the strength and conditioning practitioner to select training methods that will address the specific weaknesses of the athlete when developing an intervention to improve sprinting performance. Most of the data presented on the efficacy of these methods have been drawn from studies where the methods have been used in isolation over relatively short durations; it is very difficult to determine the effects of combining the methods over an entire training program for a given athlete.

Resistance Training Methods

Sprint running performance is dependent upon muscular strength. Given this relationship, resistance training should be an appropriate method to improve sprint running performance. The adaptations to a period of resistance training are specific to the exercises used, and the acceleration and maximal-speed phases of sprinting have specific biomechanical constraints associated with them. Therefore, it might be expected that a period of resistance training will produce differential effects on these two disparate phases.

In one study, an eight-week periodized resistance training program resulted in a reduction in sprint times during the 0- to 10-m interval, while there was no change over the 0- to 20-m interval (Moir, Sanders, Button, & Glaister, 2007). These two intervals may have reflected different phases for the individuals involved—that is, acceleration and maximal speed. The resistance training exercises used involved vertical force production (e.g., squat, power clean), so that they were more specific to the maximal-speed phase of sprinting. Furthermore, the resistance training program had differential effects on the kinematic stride variables during the initial 10-m interval, increasing step length while concomitantly reducing step frequency (see Applied Research 13.2).

The gains in measures of muscular strength are generally greater than any changes in sprinting performance following a period of resistance training. Indeed, Cronin, Ogden, Lawton, and Brughelli (2007) concluded that an increase of approximately 23% in maximal muscular strength was required to elicit an improvement in sprinting performance of more than 2%.

The intensity of the resistance training exercise as determined by the external load has been shown to influence the effectiveness of the program in improving sprinting speed. For example, McBride, Triplett-McBride, Davie, and Newton (2002) reported that an eight-week resistance training program comprising jump squats performed with loads equivalent to 30% of 1-RM back squat resulted in greater accelerative sprint performance, whereas jump squats performed with loads equivalent to 80% 1-RM actually slowed the athletes. These findings were explained in terms of mechanical specificity, with the higher movement velocities associated with the low-load jump squats transferring to the sprinting movement. Other investigators have also reported the effectiveness of high-velocity resistance training for improving sprinting (Delecluse et al., 1995).

Applied Research 13.2
Resistance training may have different effects on the different sprint phases

Moir et al. (2007) investigated the effects of a periodized resistance training program on 20-m sprint performance in a group of men. Resistance training was performed three times per week for eight weeks, with the program including multijoint exercises for both the upper body (e.g., bench press) and the lower body (e.g., back squats, power cleans). A mixed-method program was used where heavy, medium, and light days were completed within each training week, with different exercises performed on the medium training days. The program followed a block periodized model, with the intensity and repetitions in the first four weeks promoting strength endurance, but then switching to a maximal strength/power focus in the final four weeks. No sprint running sessions were completed by the participants during the time of the study.

The resistance training resulted in significant increases in measures of maximal muscular strength as well as increases in both low- and high-load speed-strength. There was no change in 20-m sprint time. However, the sprint times for the initial 10 m were slower following the training, while those for the second 10 m were actually faster. An analysis of the kinematics over the initial 10 m using a two-dimensional motion analysis system revealed an increase in stride length and a greater reduction in stride frequency.

The authors postulated that the resistance training exercises may have interfered with the rotation–extension strategy required to optimize accelerative sprinting performance by promoting vertical force production. The greater vertical force production during each stance phase may have contributed to the decreased sprint times recorded over the second 10-m phase of the sprint, as this is likely to represent the maximal-speed phase of the sprint for these participants.

Moir, G., Sanders, R. H., Button, C., & Glaister, M. (2007). The effect of periodized resistance training on accelerative sprint performance. *Sports Biomechanics, 6,* 285–300.

Given the requirement to develop maximal muscular strength to enhance the gains in explosive and speed-strength, some authors have promoted a mixed-method approach where high-intensity (heavy-load) and lower-intensity (lower-load) resistance training exercises are combined to improve sprinting speed, given the current lack of consensus regarding the most appropriate intensities to use (Cronin et al., 2007). Moreover, an initial assessment of the athlete's strength capability will guide the development of an appropriate resistance training program. Table 13.10 provides an example of a mixed-method resistance training program that was effective at improving accelerative and maximal sprinting speed (McMaster, Gill, McGuigan, & Cronin, 2014). This resistance training program was effective at increasing maximal muscular strength (both absolute and relative values) as well as improving measures of low- and high-load speed strength.

Plyometric exercises are often promoted as being more specific to sprinting than traditional resistance training methods, allowing the strength and power gained from traditional training methods to be transferred into the sprinting movement (Young, 2006). The mechanical characteristics of stepping and hopping plyometric exercises appear to replicate those associated with the stance phase of sprinting (Mero & Komi, 1994). Sprint drills such as high knee exercises (e.g., marching A's, A skips, running A's) should also be viewed as plyometric exercises, rather than as the technical drills that they are often claimed to be (Sheppard, 2013). Table 13.11 provides an example of a four-week plyometric program to improve sprinting performance.

Table 13.10

Five-Week Mixed-Method Resistance Training Program Combining High-Force and High-Velocity Exercises to Improve Sprinting Performance

Training Day			
Monday	Tuesday	Thursday	Friday
Countermovement jumps*	Bench press†	Back squat†	Incline dumbbell press†
Countermovement bench throws*	Concentric-only bench throws*	Quarter-jump squats*	Alternative arm dumbbell bench press*
Power cleans*	Weighted chin-ups†	Bulgarian split squats†	Box squats*
One-arm jammer press†	High pulls*	Speed lunge*	Hip thrusts†
One-arm dumbbell snatch*	One-arm dumbbell rows†		Calf raises†

Progressions					
	Week 1	Week 2	Week 3	Week 4	Week 5
High force† (sets, reps, intensity)	6 × 6, 85% 1-RM	6 × 6, 85% 1-RM	8 × 2–3, 95–98% 1-RM	8 × 2–3, 95–98% 1-RM	4 × 2–3, 97–99% 1-RM
High velocity* (sets, reps, intensity)	6 × 8, 15–30% 1-RM	6 × 5, 30% 1-RM	8 × 7–8, 15% 1-RM	8 × 6–7, 30% 1-RM	5 × 8, 15% 1-RM

Note: 1-RM = one-repetition maximum

Reproduced from McMaster, D., Gill, N., McGuigan, M., & Cronin, J. (2014). Effects of complex strength and ballistic training on maximum strength, sprint ability and force–velocity–power profiles of semi-professional rugby union players. *Journal of Australian Strength and Conditioning, 22*, 17–30. http://www.strengthandconditioning.org/

Table 13.11

Four-Week Plyometric Training Program to Develop Sprinting Speed Performed Three Times per Week

	Sets and Repetitions			
	Week 1	Week 2	Week 3	Week 4
Vertical jumps	15, 10	20, 10	25, 10	25, 10
Bounds	3, 10	4, 10	5, 10	5, 10
Broad jump	5, 8	5, 10	7, 10	8, 10
Drop jump	3, 5	5, 9	6, 15	6, 15
Rest	1–2 min between sets; 15–30 s between repetitions			

Reproduced from Impellizzeri, F. M., Rampinini, E., Castagna, C., Martino, F., Fiorini, S., & Wisløff, U. (2008). Effects of plyometric training on sand versus grass on muscle soreness and jumping and sprinting ability in soccer players. *British Journal of Sports Medicine, 42*, 42–46, with permission from BMJ Publishing Group Ltd.

Resisted and Assisted Sprint Training Methods

Resisted and assisted sprint training methods include exercises that are performed to develop muscular strength using sprint-specific movements. Resisted sprint training methods involve the execution of sprints against a retarding force provided by a sled that is towed, a parachute, or even sprinting up a hill. These methods require the athlete to increase the forward lean of the body and exert greater forces during propulsion to "push" the body—mechanical characteristics that are specific to the acceleration phase of sprinting. Assisted sprint training methods involve the athlete being propelled forward by an external force other than the GRF, such as when the athlete is towed by a mechanical winch or bungee, or when sprinting downhill where some of the gravitational force acts to propel the athlete forward. Given the greater speeds observed during assisted sprint training methods, these methods are used to develop maximal sprinting speed.

Resisted Sprint Training Methods

A common method of providing resistance to an athlete while sprinting is to use a weighted sled that is towed by the athlete. The use of sled loads equivalent to 12.6% and 32.2% body mass have been shown to reduce sprinting speed compared to the speeds achieved without resistance, with the greatest reductions associated with the greater loads (Lockie, Murphy, & Spinks, 2003). The reduced speeds are caused largely by a reduction in step length, although step frequency is also reduced. Furthermore, stance duration and forward trunk lean are increased with the sled towing sprints, while the greatest sled loads result in a greater range of motion at the hip joint (caused by greater hip flexion) and a greater extension at the knee joint at takeoff (Lockie et al., 2003).

The alterations in the kinematics of the body segments with this training technique are likely to lead to improvements in accelerative sprinting. However, a negative transfer may potentially occur when training involves excessive loads that interfere with the sprinting movement—specifically, a 10% reduction in sprint speed should be avoided to rule out negative transfer. Lockie et al. (2003) provide the following equation to allow the determination of the mass of a towed sled to elicit a given reduction in maximal sprinting speed:

$$\text{Sled load} = (-1.96 \times \%_{vel}) + 188.99 \qquad \text{Eq. (13.6)}$$

where sled load is the mass of the sled expressed as a percentage of body mass and $\%_{vel}$ is the required sprinting speed expressed as a percentage of maximal sprinting speed.

In a study reported by Spinks, Murphy, Spinks, and Lockie (2007), eight weeks of resisted sprint training with sled loads that did not reduce sprinting speed by more than 10% of the maximal speed resulted in improved sprinting performance in the acceleration phase. The resisted sprint training led to nonsignificant decreases and increases in step length and step frequency, respectively, but it was no more effective than unresisted sprint training of equivalent volume. Other researchers have reported that resisted sprint training via sled towing does not improve either accelerative or maximal-speed sprinting (Clark, Stearne, Walts, & Miller, 2010).

The combination of horizontal sprinting with resisted sprinting (sled towing) has been shown to improve sprinting performance during both the acceleration and maximal-speed phases (West et al., 2013). Table 13.12 provides an example of a six-week combined horizontal and resisted sprint training program.

Another method of increasing the resistance experienced by the athlete while sprinting is to have the athlete sprint up a slope. The resistance during **uphill sprinting** comes from some of the gravitational force acting to retard the horizontal motion of the CM, with the magnitude of this force being proportional to the inclination of the slope. Uphill sprinting has been reported to result in lower sprinting speeds compared to sprinting on a horizontal surface due to either decreased step length or a combination of decreased step length and step frequency (Paradisis & Cooke, 2001; Slawinski et al., 2008). A greater stance duration, a shorter touchdown distance, a

Table 13.12
Six-Week Combined Horizontal and Resisted Sprint Training Program Performed Two Times per Week

Sprint distance	20 m
Sled load	12.6% body mass
Sets and repetitions	2×3
Sprint order	Resisted sprints set (3×20 m) completed before horizontal sprint set (3×20 m)
Rest intervals	2 min between repetitions; 8 min between sets

Data from West, D. J., Cunningham, D. J., Bracken, R. M., Bevan, H. R., Crewther, B. T., Cook, C. J., & Kilduff, L. P. (2013). Effects of resisted sprint training on acceleration in professional rugby union players. *Journal of Strength and Conditioning Research, 27*, 1014–1018.

greater takeoff distance and a greater forward lean of the trunk at touchdown and takeoff have also been reported. Moreover, sprinting uphill results in a lower activation of the hamstrings compared to horizontal sprinting (Slawinski et al., 2008). Although these acute changes would seem to favor improved sprint performance during the acceleration phase, there are currently no data to support this contention. Six weeks of uphill sprint training was not reported to elicit a significant improvement in maximal sprinting speed (Paradisis & Cooke, 2006).

Assisted Sprint Training Methods

Various methods may be used to tow an athlete while sprinting. For example, a mechanical winch can be attached to the athlete. Such a method has been shown to increase the maximal sprinting speed achieved by athletes by 8.4% compared to sprinting without assistance, with the increased speed being largely due to an increase in step frequency (Mero, Komi, Rusko, & Hirvonen, 1987). Other methods of towing use the energy stored in elastic bungees to perform work on the athlete as he or she sprints, increasing the kinetic energy of the CM. Clark et al. (2009) reported that the greater sprinting speeds achieved when being towed in this manner are due to large increases in step length, with less of an increase in step frequency. However, stance durations are reduced when the athletes are towed despite greater touchdown distances.

The greater touchdown distances resulting from towing methods are likely to result in an increased braking impulse of the GRF (Mero & Komi, 1986). Although the increased braking force associated with towing methods has resulted in researchers questioning the relative merits of such methods (Clark et al., 2009; Corn & Knudson, 2003), the strength and conditioning practitioner should remember the proposed importance of leg stiffness in maximal velocity sprinting (Bret et al., 2002; Chelly & Denis, 2001). Such a stimulus may result in increased leg stiffness that can improve maximal-speed sprinting, although no data have been published to confirm this effect. Four weeks of assisted sprint training has been reported to elicit greater improvements in sprinting performance during the acceleration phase (4.6 m and 13.7 m times) and maximal-speed phase (36.6 m time) compared to the same volume of training performed unassisted in female soccer players (Upton, 2011).

Downhill sprinting represents another assisted sprint training method. Greater sprinting speeds are achieved when sprinting downhill compared to on a horizontal surface due to the gravitational force aiding in the horizontal propulsion of the CM. Ebben

Table 13.13

Eight-Week Sprint Training Program Comprising Uphill and Downhill Sprints Performed Three Times per Week

Week	Workout
1–4	6 × 80 m sprints; 10 min rest
	Each sprint is executed along a specially designed 80-m platform that consists of 20 m horizontal, 20 m up a 3° incline, 10 m horizontal, 20 m down a 3° decline, and 10 m horizontal
5–8	An additional repetition is added to each workout for the remaining three weeks such that 10 repetitions are completed during the final week

Data from Paradisis, G. P., Bissas, A., & Cooke, C. B. (2009). Combining uphill and downhill sprint running training is more efficacious than horizontal. *International Journal of Sports Physiology and Performance, 4,* 229–243.

(2008) reported that the optimal slope for downhill sprinting is 5.8°, with this strategy resulting in sprint times that are 6.5% faster than horizontal sprinting. Paradisis and Cooke (2001) reported that the increased running speeds when sprinting downhill are achieved largely due to an increased step length compared to sprinting on a horizontal surface. Athletes also exhibit an increased touchdown distance and a more extended knee at touchdown, and the trunk is more upright when sprinting downhill.

Although there are currently no data available to determine the effect of downhill sprint training on horizontal sprinting performance, a combination of uphill and downhill sprint training in one study resulted in greater improvements in maximal sprinting speed compared to horizontal sprint training (Paradisis, Bissas, & Cooke, 2009). These improvements were largely due to increased step frequency and decreased stance duration. Table 13.13 provides an example of a sprint training program combining uphill and downhill sprints.

Representative Learning Practices for Sprinting

Representative practices require that task and environmental constraints imposed on the athlete during practice adequately reflect those experienced during the actual performance of the sport (Pinder, Davids, Renshaw, & Araújo, 2011). The equipment used by athletes in specific sports will constrain the sprinting performance of the athlete. For example, football players sprint more slowly when wearing equipment (e.g., helmet, pads) (Brechue, Mayhew, & Piper, 2005), while hockey players sprint more slowly when running with hockey sticks (Wdowski & Gittoes, 2013). Walsh, Young, Hill, Kittredge, and Horn (2007) reported that maximal sprinting speed of both beginner and experienced rugby players is adversely affected when carrying a ball. Therefore, the strength and conditioning coach should ensure that athletes practice sprints with sporting equipment.

The sprints performed by athletes within their sports require that the execution of the movement be coupled with the environmental information available to them. For the strength and conditioning practitioner, it is important to recognize that the information to which the athlete attends to initiate a sprint is sport specific rather than generic. For example, tennis players initiate their movement toward the ball after 127 ms when reacting to a live player hitting the ball (sport-specific information), whereas the movement initiation time increases to 197 ms when reacting to a ball machine (generic information) (Shim, Chow, Carlton, & Woen-Sik, 2005). The difference in the movement initiation time reflects a 1.2-m greater court coverage by the athlete when sport-specific information is presented compared to generic information.

The relative velocity between an attacker and a defender during one-versus-one subphases of a soccer game has been shown to represent sport-specific information that constrains the players' subsequent movements and the outcome of the task (Clemente, Couceiro, Martins, Dias, & Mendes, 2013; Duarte et al., 2010). The movements of the players emerge from these player interactions rather than being prescribed in advance, but the sprinting capabilities of the athletes involved impose a constraint on the observed movements and, therefore, represent an important determinant of the success of the task (scoring a goal for the attacker, preventing a goal for the defender).

Moreover, sprinting speed for the soccer players can be viewed as an action-scaled affordance (Fajen, Riley, & Turvey, 2008); an increase in sprinting speed brought about through specific training methods will require perceptual–motor *recalibration* to allow the athlete to attune his or her altered action capabilities (sprinting speed) to the relevant task information (relative motion of the attacker–defender dyad). The process of recalibration can be achieved through the use of **small-sided games** where the soccer players are exposed to sport-specific information. Furthermore, the strength and conditioning practitioner can use small-sided games as a method to develop sprinting speed. By manipulating the playing area in small-sided games, the strength and conditioning practitioner is able to promote the execution of sprints. For example, increasing the size of the playing area during five-versus-five soccer games has been shown to increase the distance covered by the players at high speed and the number of sprints executed, as well as to produce greater maximal sprinting speeds (Casamichana & Castellano, 2010).

The instructions presented to the players can also influence the sprinting speeds achieved. For example, the presentation of instructions to the attacker that the team is losing and that the game will soon end, necessitating a goal to be scored quickly, results in greater speeds being achieved by the players in a one-versus-one subphase of a game compared to when the attacker is instructed to attack whenever a scoring opportunity is presented (Clemente et al., 2013). This emphasizes the role of instructions as informational constraints to movement.

Small-sided games have been suggested to result in greater improvements in sport-specific skills (e.g., ball control, passing) than typical drills based on repetitious technical instruction due to the inherent variability associated with small-sided games (Gabbett, Jenkins, & Abernethy, 2009). We can use this information to develop a representative learning practice for soccer that promotes sprinting (Table 13.14).

Agility Performance

In many field and court sports, the athlete is required to change direction when sprinting to avoid another player, to intercept another player, to intercept a ball, or to remain within the playing area. The mechanical requirements associated with change of direction tasks include the control of the linear and angular momenta during ground contact. Many of the muscular requirements proposed to underpin change of direction performance (e.g., maximal muscular strength, speed strength, reactive strength) are also strongly correlated with sprinting performance; indeed, sprinting speed is proposed to be a determinant of change of direction ability (Brughelli, Cronin, Levin, & Chaouachi, 2008; Sheppard & Young, 2006). However, a strong relationship between sprinting speed and change of direction ability is not always apparent in the research, implying that each represents a distinct skill likely requiring specific and

Table 13.14
A Representative Learning Practice Using Small-Sided Games to Develop Sprinting in Soccer Players

Description of task	■ The small-sided game format involves two teams of five outfield players and a goalkeeper. ■ The dimensions of the playing area (length/width) are 62 × 44 m, providing a playing area of 2728 m² and an area of 272.8 m² per player. ■ There is no offside rule.
Volume and intensity	■ Three 8-min games are played, with 5 min rest between each game. ■ This format results in the players covering approximately 1000 m during each game and the completion of approximately 6 sprints. ■ Skills including headers, tackles, and passing are also executed.

Manipulation of task constraints	■ Include rules that promote sprinting:
	  ■ "No more than one touch allowed" (encourage players to sprint to find space)
	  ■ "Extra points earned when running past a defender with the ball" (encourage players to sprint with the ball)
	  ■ "A player is not allowed to receive the ball unless he or she has traveled a minimum of 20 m since the player last passed it" (encourage players to sprint for space after having passed)
	  ■ "Team A is behind by 4 goals; goals need to be scored quickly" (encourage players on Team A to sprint when in possession, players on Team B to play conservatively when in possession; switch the instructions)
	■ Decreasing the size of playing area will decrease the number of sprints executed and increase the number of interceptions and dribbles.
	■ Decreasing the number of players will reduce the number of opportunities for the players to pass.

Coaching analysis	■ Use GPS and video analysis to record the players' movements. ■ Observe the times that the athlete chooses to sprint and note the outcome. ■ Provide augmented feedback to attune the player's sprinting movements to relevant information. ■ Consider the action-scaled affordances perceived by the player. ■ Use heart rate monitors to record the physiological load of the workout and change the task constraints accordingly.

Note: GPS = Global Positioning System.

Data from Casamichana, D., & Castellano, J. (2010). Time–motion, heart rate, perceptual and motor behavior demands in small-sides soccer games: Effects of pitch size. *Journal of Sports Sciences, 28*, 1615–1623; Dellal, A., Chamari, K., Owen, A. L., Wong, D. P., Lago-penas, C., & Hill-Haas, S. (2011). Influence of technical instructions on the physiological and physical demands of small-sided games. *European Journal of Sport Science, 11*, 341–346.

distinct methods of training (Sheppard & Young, 2006). Not all researchers agree on this point, however (see Sprint Running Concept 13.5).

When an athlete changes direction during a sport, he or she does so in response to a sport-specific stimulus, which is typically visual. Furthermore, the required movements that will result in a successful outcome in a given situation can be numerous and are not preplanned, requiring the athlete to make an appropriate decision. For a change of direction task to be representative of a given sport, then, it must include the presentation of sport-specific information to which the athlete has to attend to change direction—an understanding that leads to the concept of agility. Extending the definition of Sheppard and Young (2006), we can define agility as a rapid whole-body movement with change of velocity or change of direction in response to a sport-specific stimulus in which the required movement of the athlete to accomplish the task is unplanned. Although agility performance is influenced by change of direction ability and even straight-line sprinting ability, it appears that the decision-making component

Sprint Running Concept 13.5

Are straight-line sprint running and change of direction distinct skills?

Some researchers have reported that straight-line sprinting speed does not correlate strongly with change of direction performance (Young, Hawken, & McDonald, 1996). In one study, six weeks of straight-line sprint training that improved straight-line sprinting performance had no effects on change of direction performance, but the converse was true for change of direction training (Young, McDowell, & Scarlett, 2001). These data imply that straight-line sprinting speed is a distinct skill from change of direction and, therefore, requires different training methods for its improvement. However, some investigators have reported strong relationships between straight-line sprinting speed and change of direction performance (Glaister et al., 2009; Sheppard, Young, Doyle, Sheppard, & Newton, 2006), while still others have reported that resistance training that elicits an improvement in sprint running speed also improves change of direction performance (Markovic, Jukic, Milanovic, & Metikos, 2007). Differences in the individuals included in the various studies, the sprint distances used, and the complexity of the change of direction tasks (e.g., number of changes of direction, angle of the change of direction) complicate the interpretation of the findings; even so, it is not clear that straight-line sprinting and change of direction ability are distinct skills.

Moreover, change of direction tasks do not adequately discriminate between different levels of athletes involved in sports that ostensibly involve many changes of direction (Sheppard et al., 2006). This is likely due to the planned nature of such tests and the presentation of generic information (e.g., a cone denoting the change of direction) rather than sport-specific information (e.g., the relative motion and posture of an opponent).

The issue of the distinction between straight-line sprinting and change of direction ability should really be replaced with the issue of the validity of typical change of direction assessments and exercises. The inclusion of generic stimuli to which the athlete has to attune his or her movements limits the usefulness of these change of direction tasks.

in agility tasks differentiates athletes at different performance levels (Farrow, Young, & Bruce, 2005; Sheppard et al., 2006). See Applied Research 13.3.

The decision-making component largely relies on the ability of the athlete to react appropriately to sport-specific stimuli. It requires the athlete to attend to appropriate stimuli presented in an environment replete with information. Evidence shows that elite performers attend to different visual stimuli and execute different visual search strategies compared to novice performers (Savelsbergh, Williams, Van Der Kamp, & Ward, 2002). Thus a key element in developing agility performance is to have the athlete attend to relevant information during an agility task; the strength and conditioning practitioner should strive to attune the athlete's movements to sport-specific information.

A number of options for agility training are available to the strength and conditioning practitioner. One is the use of practices that incorporate video footage of sport-specific

Applied Research 13.3
Decision-making ability rather than change of direction speed differentiates elite athletes from their lower-level counterparts

Sheppard et al. (2006) investigated the difference between high-level and lower-level Australian football players in terms of their performance in a change of direction task and an agility task. The change of direction task required the players to sprint forward to a point marked 1.5 m ahead, and then change direction and sprint at an approximate right angle to a finish line positioned 5 m to the left or right, depending on the instructions provided prior to initiating the trial. Thus the change of direction task was planned. The agility task required the player to follow the same path, but the change of direction was determined by the movements of a live opponent positioned ahead and facing the player; that is, the player had to respond to the opponent's direction change. The agility trial was therefore unplanned.

Timing gates were placed at the start and the end of the course to allow the determination of change of direction speed. During the agility trials, the opponent was positioned on a contact mat that was synchronized with the timing gates such that the time for the trial began when the opponent stepped from the mat to initiate his or her movement; the time ended when the player crossed the finish line.

The authors reported that there was little difference between the two groups of players in the change of direction task, although the lower-level players were actually slightly faster. By comparison, the high-level players were much faster in the agility task. The authors concluded that the decision-making component of the agility task that required the players to attend to sport-specific information (the movement of an opponent) is an important variable distinguishing between high- and low-level players.

Sheppard, J., Young, W., Doyle, T., Sheppard, T., & Newton, R. (2006). An evaluation of a new test of reactive agility and its relationship to sprint speed and change of direction speed. *Journal of Science and Medicine in Sport, 9,* 342–349.

scenarios to which the athlete has to attend. Research shows that movement initiation times are delayed when athletes are required to respond to a video stimulus compared to the same stimulus presented "live" (Dicks, Button, & Davids, 2010). Furthermore, gaze behavior (where the athlete's gaze is directed) differs between video and live conditions, demonstrating that the information used by the athlete to guide his or her movements is specific to the task constraints (Dicks et al., 2010). Therefore, to better attune the athlete's movements to relevant information, the strength and conditioning practitioner should employ live, sport-specific scenarios—for example, in exercises with live opponents and small-sided games. In such workouts, the athlete is tasked with exploring successful movement solutions to achieve the goals of the task rather than following specific movements prescribed by the coach, such as would occur with the use of typical "agility" drills that rely on cones, ladders, and hurdles (see Sprint Running Concept 13.6). An athlete is able to recalibrate his or her action-scaled affordances to sport-specific information during exercises involving live opponents and small-sided games.

The strength and conditioning practitioner can manipulate the task constraints associated with small-sided games to promote changes of direction. For example, increasing the density of small-sided games by increasing the number of players or reducing the playing area has been shown to increase the number of change of direction movements executed by the players (Davies, Young, Farrow, & Bahnert, 2013). Small-sided games are more effective at developing agility performance in field-sport athletes because they promote decision making based on sport-specific information (Young & Rogers, 2014). Furthermore, the use of small-sided games represents a very efficient training method to improve agility performance (see Applied Research 13.4).

Sprint Running Concept 13.6

Should cone, ladder, and hurdle drills be used to develop agility?

Agility is a rapid whole-body movement with change of velocity or change of direction in response to a sport-specific stimulus in which the required movement of the athlete to accomplish the task is unplanned. The traditional drills that are promoted to develop agility, which typically involve cones, ladders, and hurdles, do not conform to this definition, as they involve generic stimuli and are planned. Such drills are likely to develop change of direction ability, which is itself an important component of agility, so they do have a role in the development of agility. The strength and conditioning practitioner should consider cone, ladder, and hurdle drills as plyometric exercises that can be specific to change of direction performance. Furthermore, their use with novice athletes may promote some important technical adaptations that will underpin improvements in change of direction performance (e.g., effective body positions, foot placement). However, to develop agility performance the drills should include the presentation of sport-specific stimuli in an unplanned manner.

Applied Research 13.4
Small-sided games are an efficient training method to improve agility performance

Young and Rogers (2014) investigated the effects of seven weeks of small-sided games compared to change of direction drills on agility performance in a group of elite junior Australian Rules Football players. One group of players participated in small-sided games training two times per week; these games typically involved four-versus-four scenarios on a 20- × 23-m field or two-versus-two scenarios on a 15- × 15-m field. All games were performed for between 30 and 45 s, with the workouts lasting a total of 15 min. The players in the change of direction group completed drills requiring one to five changes of direction or running speed such that these workouts also lasted 15 min.

Players from both groups were tested in a change of direction task (planned) and an agility task that required them to react to the movements of a video-based opponent. The authors reported that neither group demonstrated improvements in the change of direction task. However, members of the agility training group were significantly faster in the agility task following the training intervention, whereas the change of direction group did not exhibit any change. The improvement in agility performance by the agility group was attributed to substantially shorter decision-making times.

The authors further reported that the mean number of change of direction maneuvers performed by the change of direction group was 43.7 across the entire training period, while the agility group completed only an average of 24.7 change of direction maneuvers during their workouts. It is apparent that small-sided games represent a sport-specific and time-efficient method of developing agility performance in field-sport players.

Young, W., & Rogers, N. (2014). Effects of small-sided game and change-of-direction training on reactive agility and change-of-direction speed. *Journal of Sports Sciences, 32*, 307–314.

Table 13.15 provides an example of a representative learning practice for soccer that promotes agility.

The decision-making capabilities that underpin agility performance can also be developed through the use of evasion exercises (Young & Farrow, 2013). Evasion exercises involve a very small number of players (i.e., one versus one), such that the athlete must attend to fewer stimuli than in small-sided games that incorporate more players (evasion exercises are less complex than small-sided games). This format allows players to better determine the task-relevant information that they should be attending to while they explore their affordances. It may be pertinent for the strength

Table 13.15
A Representative Learning Practice Using Small-Sided Games to Develop Agility in Soccer Players

Description of task	▪ The small-sided game format involves two teams of four outfield players and a goalkeeper. ▪ The dimensions of the playing area (length/width) are 30×20 m, providing a playing area of 600 m² and an area of 75 m² per player. ▪ There is no offside rule.
Volume and intensity	▪ Four 4-min games are played, with 3 min rest between each game. ▪ This format results in the players covering approximately 665 m during each game and the completion of approximately six one-versus-one situations. ▪ Skills including headers, tackles, and passing are also executed.
Manipulation of task constraints	▪ Include rules that promote sprinting: "Extra points earned when dribbling past a defender with the ball" (encourage players to change direction when in control of ball). ▪ Decreasing the number of players will decrease the number of opportunities to execute change of direction movements while also decreasing the number of interceptions and dribbles. ▪ Instigating rules such as "Only one touch allowed" will decrease the number of one-versus-one situations.
Coaching analysis	▪ Use GPS and video analysis to record the players' movements. ▪ Observe the times that the athlete chooses to change direction and note the outcome. ▪ Provide augmented feedback to attune the player's agility movements to relevant information. ▪ Consider the action-scaled affordances perceived by the player. ▪ Use heart rate monitors to record the physiological load of the workout and change the task constraints accordingly.

Note: GPS = Global Positioning System.

Data from Casamichana, D., & Castellano, J. (2010). Time–motion, heart rate, perceptual and motor behavior demands in small-sides soccer games: Effects of pitch size. *Journal of Sports Sciences, 28,* 1615–1623; Dellal, A., Chamari, K., Owen, A. L., Wong, D. P., Lago-penas, C., & Hill-Haas, S. (2011). Influence of technical instructions on the physiological and physical demands of small-sided games. *European Journal of Sport Science, 11,* 341–346.

and conditioning practitioner to develop the athlete's agility performance during evasion exercises before progressing to small-sided games. It is also easier for the coach to control the number of repetitions completed in evasive exercises compared to small-sided games (Young & Farrow, 2013).

The general progression of resistance training methods and representative learning practices that can be used by the strength and conditioning practitioner to develop sprinting and agility abilities in athletes is shown in Table 13.16.

Table 13.16
Continuum of Workouts Incorporating Resistance Training and Representative Practices to Improve Sprinting Performance

General → Specific	
	Resistance Training
	Back squats:
	▪ 10 reps (light)
	▪ 1–4 reps (heavy)
	Resistance Training
	Jump squats:
	▪ 20 kg (light)
	▪ 40–60 kg (heavy)
	Resisted sprints:
	▪ Sled towing (loads conferring more than a 10% reduction in speed)
	▪ Uphill sprints (more than 3° incline)
	Assisted sprints:
	▪ Bungee towing (more than a 10% increase in speed)
	▪ Downhill sprints (6° or greater decline)
	Plyometric exercises:
	▪ Bounding, drop–jumps
	▪ Change of direction exercises for agility
	Resistance Training
	Resisted sprints:
	▪ Sled towing (loads conferring more than a 10% reduction in speed)
	▪ Uphill sprints (3° incline)
	Assisted sprints:
	▪ Bungee towing (less than a 10% increase)
	▪ Downhill sprints (less than 6° decline)
	Plyometric exercises:
	▪ Stepping and hopping
	▪ Sprint drills
	▪ Change of direction exercises for agility
	Representative Practices
	Sprinting and agility with sport-specific equipment
	Evasion exercises and small-sided games:
	▪ Attunement of sprinting and agility to sport-specific environmental information
	▪ Calibration of action-scaled affordances

Chapter Summary

Sprint running is a multidimensional skill consisting of acceleration, attainment of maximal speed, and maintenance of maximal speed phases that are demarcated by the athlete's speed. These phases are characterized by different mechanical demands, such that they impose different biomechanical constraints on the athlete. The acceleration phase requires that the athlete generate a large propulsive GRF during each stance, necessitating a rotation–extension strategy. When the athlete attains the maximal speed, the short stance durations require the generation of large vertical GRF to support body weight and project the CM. These different biomechanical constraints associated with the acceleration phase and the maximal-speed phase result in different running actions: The athlete leans forward and "pushes" from the ground during acceleration, but is more upright and "pulls" himself or herself over the stance leg at maximal speed.

The different biomechanical constraints also necessitate different training methods to improve performance during each of the sprint phases. The strength and conditioning practitioner should recognize that the decision to execute a sprint in sport is based on the attunement of the athlete to specific environmental information, which requires the use of representative practices. Many field and court sports require the athlete to sprint and change direction. Agility is the ability to change velocity or direction in response to a sport-specific stimulus in which the required movement is unplanned. Both change of direction speed and straight-line sprinting speed appear to be important determinants of agility performance. However, decision making is a very important element of agility, and the strength and conditioning practitioner can use evasion exercises and small-sided games to develop agility performance in a sport-specific and time-efficient manner.

Review Questions and Projects

1. Explain the importance of viewing sprint running as a multidimensional skill for the purposes of testing and training.

2. A female athlete approaches a strength and conditioning practitioner to develop a training program to improve her 100-m performance. She has a personal record of 11.26 s. Describe the training methods you would implement to improve this athlete's sprinting performance.

3. Explain the biomechanical differences between treadmill and over-ground sprinting.

4. Explain the biomechanical constraint to accelerative sprinting.

5. What are the implications of the biomechanical constraint associated with accelerative sprinting for training?

6. Explain the biomechanical constraint to maximal-speed sprinting.

7. What are the implications of the biomechanical constraint associated with maximal-speed sprinting for training?

8. Why do sprinters achieve greater running speeds on a straight track compared to when running around a flat curve?

9. A male athlete wants to improve his maximal sprinting speed. Which should he focus on—stride length or stride frequency?

10. Explain the importance of the stance phase of a sprinting step.

11. What is the active leg motion during a sprinting step, and why is it important during both the accelerative and maximal-speed phases?

12. Describe the role of the hamstrings in maximal-speed sprinting, and explain its implications for strain injuries.

13. How might the arms influence the mechanics of sprinting?

14. What is the reciprocal ponderal index, and what are its implications for sprinters?

15. Describe the mechanical differences between sprinting uphill and downhill.

16. Explain the role of resistance training in improving the performance in the different phases of sprint running.

17. Explain the application of resisted sprint training modes to the different phases of sprint running.

18. Explain the application of assisted sprint training modes to the different phases of sprint running.

19. Discuss the role of traditional sprint drills (e.g., A, B drills) in improving sprinting performance.

20. Develop a training drill to attune a tennis player's sprinting movements to environmental information.

References

Ae, M., Ito, A., & Suzuki, M. (1992). The men's 100 meters: Scientific research project at the III World Championship in Athletics, Tokyo 1991. *New Studies in Athletics, 7,* 47–52.

Alcaraz, P. E., Palao, J. M., Elvira, J. L. L., & Linthorne, N. P. (2008). Effects of three types of resisted devices on the kinematics of sprinting at maximum velocity. *Journal of Strength and Conditioning Research, 22,* 890–897.

Baker, D., & Nance, S. (1999). The relation between running speed and measures of strength and power in professional rugby league players. *Journal of Strength and Conditioning Research, 13,* 230–235.

Bartlett, R. (2007). *Introduction to sports biomechanics: Analysing human movement patterns.* London, UK: Routledge.

Bejan, A., Jones, E. C., & Charles, J. D. (2010). The evolution of speed in athletics: Why the fastest runners are black and swimmers white. *International Journal of Design and Nature, 5,* 1–13.

Bezodis, I. N., Kerwin, D. G., & Salo, A. I. T. (2008). Lower-limb mechanics during the support phase of maximum-velocity sprint running. *Medicine and Science in Sports and Exercise, 40,* 707–715.

Bezodis, N. E., Salo, A. I. T., & Trewartha, G. (2012). Modeling the stance leg in two-dimensional analyses of sprinting: Inclusion of the MTP joint affects joint kinetics. *Journal of Applied Biomechanics, 28,* 222–227.

Bishop, D., & Girard, O. (2011). Repeated-sprint ability (RSA). In M. Cardinale, R. Newton, & K. Nosaka (Eds.), *Strength and conditioning: Biological principles and practical applications* (pp. 223–241). West Sussex, UK: Wiley-Blackwell.

Blankenbaker, D. G., & Tuite, M. J. (2010). Temporal changes of muscle injury. *Seminars in Musculoskeletal Radiology, 14*, 176–193.

Botwell, M. V., Tan, H., & Wilson, A. M. (2009). The consistency of maximum running speed measurements in humans using a feedback-controlled treadmill, and a comparison with maximum attainable speed during overground locomotion. *Journal of Biomechanics, 42*, 2569–2574.

Brechue, W. F. (2011). Structure–function relationships that determine sprint performance and running speed in sport. *International Journal of Applied Sports Sciences, 23*, 313–350.

Brechue, W. F., Mayhew, J. L., & Piper, F. C. (2005). Equipment and running surface alter sprint performance of college football players. *Journal of Strength and Conditioning Research, 19*, 821–825.

Bret, C., Rahmani, A., Dufour, A., Messonnier, L., & Lacour, J. (2002). Leg strength and stiffness as ability factors in 100 m sprint running. *Journal of Sports Medicine and Physical Fitness, 42*, 274–281.

Brughelli, M., Cronin, J., & Chaouachi, A. (2011). Effects of running velocity on running kinetics and kinematics. *Journal of Strength and Conditioning Research, 25*, 933–939.

Brughelli, M., Cronin, J., Levin, G., & Chaouachi, A. (2008). Understanding change of direction ability in sport: A review of resistance training studies. *Sports Medicine, 38*, 1045–1063.

Bundle, M. W., Hoyt, R. W., & Weyand, P. G. (2003). High speed running performance: A new approach to assessment and prediction. *Journal of Applied Physiology, 95*, 1955–1962.

Bushnell, T., & Hunter, I. (2007). Differences in technique between sprinters and distance runners at equal and maximal speeds. *Sports Biomechanics, 6*, 261–268.

Casamichana, D., & Castellano, J. (2010). Time–motion, heart rate, perceptual and motor behavior demands in small-sides soccer games: Effects of pitch size. *Journal of Sports Sciences, 28*, 1615–1623.

Chang, Y-H., & Kram, R. (2007). Limitations to maximum running speed on flat curves. *Journal of Experimental Biology, 210*, 971–982.

Charles, J. D., & Bejan, A. (2009). The evolution of speed, size and shape in modern athletics. *Journal of Experimental Biology, 212*, 2419–2425.

Chelly, S. M., & Denis, C. (2001). Leg power and hopping stiffness: Relationship with sprint running performance. *Medicine and Science in Sports and Exercise, 33*, 326–333.

Chumanov, E. S., Heiderscheit, B. C., & Thelen, D. G. (2011). Hamstring musculotendon dynamics during stance and swing phases of high-speed running. *Medicine and Science in Sports and Exercise, 43*, 525–532.

Clark, D. A., Sabick, M. B., Pfeiffer, R. P., Kuhlman, S. M., Knigge, N. A., & Shea, K. G. (2009). Influence of towing force magnitude on the kinematics of supramaximal sprinting. *Journal of Strength and Conditioning Research, 23*, 1162–1168.

Clark, K. P., Stearne, D. J., Walts, C. T., & Miller, A. D. (2010). The longitudinal effects of resisted sprint training using weighted sleds vs. weighted vests. *Journal of Strength and Conditioning Research, 24*, 3287–3295.

Clemente, F. M., Couceiro, M. S., Martins, F. M. L., Dias, G., & Mendes, R. (2013). Interpersonal dynamics: 1v1 sub-phases at sub-18 football players. *Journal of Human Kinetics, 36*, 181–191.

Corn, R. J., & Knudson, D. (2003). Effect of elastic-cord towing on the kinematics of the acceleration phase of sprinting. *Journal of Strength and Conditioning Research, 17*, 72–75.

Cronin, J., Ogden, T., Lawton, T., & Brughelli, M. (2007). Does increasing maximal strength improve sprint running performance? *Strength and Conditioning Journal, 29*, 86–95.

Cuhna, L., Alves, F., & Veloso, A. (2002). *The touch-down and take-off angles in different phases of 100 m sprint run.* Presentation at International Symposium on Biomechanics in Sport, Cáceres-Extremadura, Spain.

Dallinga, J. M., Benjaminse, A., & Lemmink, K. A. P. M. (2012). Which screening tools can predict injury to the lower extremities in team sports? *Sports Medicine, 42*, 791–815.

Davies, M. J., Young, W., Farrow, D., & Bahnert, A. (2013). Comparison of agility demands of small-sided games in elite Australian football. *International Journal of Sports Physiology and Performance, 8*, 139–147.

Delecluse, C. H. (1997). Influence of strength training on sprint running performance: Current findings and implications for training. *Sports Medicine, 24*, 147–156.

Delecluse, C. H., van Coppenolle, H., Willems, E., Diles, R., Goris, M., van Leemputte, M., & Vuylsteke, M. (1995). Analysis of 100 m sprint performance as a multi-dimensional skill. *Journal of Human Movement Studies, 28*, 87–101.

DeVita, P. (1994). The selection of a standard convention for analyzing gait data based on the analysis of relevant biomechanical factors. *Journal of Biomechanics, 27*, 501–508.

Dicks, M., Button, C., & Davids, K. (2010). Examination of gaze behaviours under *in situ* and video simulation task constraints reveals differences in information pick up for perception and action. *Attention, Perception and Psychophysics, 72*, 706–720.

DiSalvo, V., Baron, R., González-Haro, C., Gormasz, C., Pigozzi, F., & Bachl, N. (2010). Sprinting analysis of elite soccer players during European Champions League and UEFA Cup matches. *Journal of Sports Sciences, 28*, 1489–1494.

Dorn, T. W., Schache, A. G., & Pandy, M. G. (2012). Muscular strategy shift in human running: Dependence of running speed on hip and ankle muscle performance. *Journal of Experimental Biology, 215*, 1944–1956.

Duarte, R., Araújo, D., Gazimba, V., Fernandes, O., Folgado, H., Marmeleira, J., & Davids, K. (2010). The ecological dynamics of 1v1 sub-phases in Association Football. *Open Sports Sciences Journal, 3*, 16–18.

Duthie, G., Pyne, D., & Hooper, S. (2003). Applied physiology and game analysis of rugby union. *Sports Medicine, 33*, 973–991.

Duthie, G. M., Pyne, D. B., Marsh, D. J., & Hooper, S. L. (2006). Sprint patterns in rugby union players during competition. *Journal of Strength and Conditioning Research, 20*, 208–214.

Ebben, W. P. (2008). The optimal downhill slope for acute overspeed running. *International Journal of Sports Physiology and Performance, 3*, 88–93.

Fajen, B. R., Riley, M. A., & Turvey, M. T. (2008). Information, affordances, and the control of action in sport. *International Journal of Sport Psychology, 40*, 79–107.

Farrow, D., Young, W., & Bruce, L. (2005). The development of a test of reactive agility for netball: A new methodology. *Journal of Science and Medicine in Sport, 8*, 52–60.

Freckleton, G., & Pizzari, T. (2013). Risk factors for hamstring muscle strain injury in sport: A systematic review and meta-analysis. *British Journal of Sports Medicine, 47*, 351–358.

Gabbett, T., Jenkins, D., & Abernethy, B. (2009). Game-based training for improving skill and physical fitness in team sport athletes. *International Journal of Sports Science and Coaching, 4*, 273–283.

Gajer, B., Thépaut-Mathieu, C., & Lehénaff, D. (1999). Evolution of stride and amplitude during course of the 100 m event in athletics. *New Studies in Athletics, 14*, 43–50.

Girard, O., Miscallef, J.-P., & Millet, G. P. (2011). Changes in spring-mass model characteristics during repeated running sprints. *European Journal of Applied Physiology, 111*, 125–134.

Glaister, M. (2005). Multiple sprint work: Physiological responses, mechanisms of fatigue and the influence of aerobic fitness. *Sports Medicine, 35*, 757–777.

Glaister, M., Hauck, H., Abraham, C. S., Merry, K. L., Beaver, D., Woods, B., & McInnes, G. (2009). Familiarization, reliability, and comparability of a 40-m maximal shuttle run test. *Journal of Sports Science and Medicine, 8*, 77–82.

Goodwin, J. (2011). Maximum velocity is when we can no longer accelerate: Using biomechanics to inform speed development. *UK Strength and Conditioning Association, 21*, 3–9.

Haugen, T. A., Tønnessen, E., & Seiler, S. (2013). Anaerobic performance testing of professional soccer players 1995–2010. *International Journal of Sports Physiology and Performance, 8*, 148–156.

Heiderscheit, B. C., Sherry, M. A., Silder, A., Chumanov, E. S., & Thelen, D. G. (2010). Hamstring strain injuries: Recommendations for diagnosis, rehabilitation, and injury prevention. *Journal of Orthopaedic and Sports Physical Therapy, 40*, 67–81.

Hennessy, L., & Kilty, J. (2001). Relationship of the stretch-shortening cycle to sprint performance in trained female athletes. *Journal of Strength and Conditioning Research, 15*, 326–331.

Hinrichs, R. N. (1990). Whole body movement: Coordination of arms and legs in walking and running. In J. M. Winters & S.L.-Y. Woo (Eds.), *Multiple muscle systems: Biomechanics and movement organization* (pp. 694–705). New York, NY: Springer-Verlag.

Hobara, H., Kimura, K., Omura, K., Gomi, K., Muraoko, T., Iso, S., & Kanosue, K. (2008). Determinants of difference in leg stiffness between endurance- and power-trained athletes. *Journal of Biomechanics, 41*, 506–514.

Hunter, J. P., Marshall, R. N., & McNair, P. J. (2004). Interaction of step length and step rate during sprint running. *Medicine and Science in Sports and Exercise, 36*, 261–271.

Hunter, J. P., Marshall, R. N., & McNair, P. J. (2005). Relationships between ground reaction force impulse and kinematics of sprint-running acceleration. *Journal of Applied Biomechanics, 21*, 31–43.

Ito, A., Fukuda, K., & Kijima, K. (2008). Mid-phase sprinting movements of Tyson Gay and Asafa Powell in the 100-m race during the 2007 IAAF World Championships in Athletics. *New Studies in Athletics, 23*, 39–43.

Jacobs, R., Bobbert, M. F., & van Ingen Schenau, G. J. (1996). Mechanical output from individual muscles during explosive leg extensions: The role of biarticular muscles. *Journal of Biomechanics, 29*, 513–523.

Jacobs, R., & van Ingen Schenau, G. J. (1992). Intermuscular coordination in a sprint push-off. *Journal of Biomechanics, 25*, 953–965.

Jain, P. C. (1980). On a discrepancy in track race. *Research Quarterly in Exercise and Sport, 51*, 432–436.

Jones, R., Bezodis, I., & Thompson, A. (2009). Coaching sprinting: Expert coaches' perception of race phases and technical constructs. *International Journal of Sports Science and Coaching, 4*, 385–396.

Kale, M., Aşçi, A., Bayrak, C., & Açikada, C. (2009). Relationships among jumping performances and sprint parameters during maximum speed phase in sprinters. *Journal of Strength and Conditioning Research, 23*, 2272–2279.

Kawamori, N., Nosaka, K., & Newton, R. U. (2013). Relationships between ground reaction impulse and sprint acceleration performance in team sport athletes. *Journal of Strength and Conditioning Research, 27*, 568–573.

Kivi, D. M. R., Maraj, B. K. V., & Gervais, P. (2002). A kinematic analysis of high-speed treadmill sprinting over a range of velocities. *Medicine and Science in Sports and Exercise, 32*, 662–666.

Knudson, D. V., & Morrison, C. S. (2002). *Qualitative analysis of human movement.* Champaign, IL: Human Kinetics.

Kugler, F., & Janshen, L. (2010). Body position determines propulsive forces in accelerated running. *Journal of Biomechanics, 43*, 343–348.

Kuitunen, S., Komi, P. V., & Kyröläinen, H. (2002). Knee and ankle joint stiffness in sprint running. *Medicine and Science in Sports and Exercise, 34*, 166–173.

Lakomy, H. K. A. (1987). The use of a non-motorised treadmill for analyzing sprint performance. *Ergonomics, 30*, 627–637.

Lees, A., Vanrenterghem, J., & De Clercq, D. (2004). Understanding how an arm swing enhances performance in the vertical jump. *Journal of Biomechanics, 37*, 1929–1940.

Lieber, R. L., & Friden, J. (2001). Mechanisms of muscle injury gleaned from animal models. *American Journal of Physical Medicine and Rehabilitation, 81*, S70–S79.

Liu, H., Garrett, W. E., Moorman, C. T., & Yu, B. (2012). Injury rate, mechanism, and risk factors of hamstring strain injuries in sports: A review of the literature. *Journal of Sport and Health Science, 1*, 92–101.

Lockie, R. G., Murphy, A. J., & Spinks, C. D. (2003). Effects of resisted sled towing on sprint kinematics in field-sport athletes. *Journal of Strength and Conditioning Research, 17*, 760–767.

López-Segovia, M., Marques, M. C., van den Tillar, R., & Gonzàlez-Badillo, J. J. (2011). Relationships between vertical jump and full squat power outputs with sprint times in U21 soccer players. *Journal of Human Kinetics, 30*, 135–144.

Lorentzon, R., Johansson, C., Sjostrom, M., Fagerlunds, M., & Fugl-Meyer, A. R. (1988). Fatigue during muscle contractions in male sprinters and marathon runners: Relationships between performance, electromyographic activity, muscle cross-sectional area and morphology. *Acta Physiologica Scandinavica, 132*, 531–536.

Luhtanen, P., & Komi, P. V. (1978). Mechanical energy states during running. *European Journal of Applied Physiology, 38*, 41–48.

Majumdar, A. S., & Robergs, R. A. (2011). The science of speed: Determinants of performance in the 100 m sprint. *International Journal of Sports Science and Coaching, 6*, 479–493.

Mann, R. V. (1981). A kinetic analysis of sprinting. *Medicine and Science in Sports and Exercise, 13*, 325–328.

Mann, R., & Hermann, J. (1985). Kinematic analysis of Olympic sprint performance: Men's 200 meters. *International Journal of Sport Biomechanics, 1*, 240–252.

Mann, R., & Sprague, P. (1980). Kinetic analysis of the ground leg during sprint running. *Research Quarterly for Exercise and Sport, 51*, 334–348.

Markovic, G., Jukic, I., Milanovic, D., & Metikos, D. (2007). Effects of sprint and plyometric training on muscle function and athletic performance. *Journal of Strength and Conditioning Research, 21*, 543–549.

Maughan, R. J., Watson, J. S., & Weir, J. (1983). Relationships between muscle strength and muscle cross-sectional area in male sprinters and endurance runners. *European Journal of Applied Physiology, 50*, 309–318.

McBride, J. M., Triplett-McBride, T., Davie, A., & Newton, R. U. (2002). The effect of heavy- vs. light-load jump squats on the development of strength, power, and speed. *Journal of Strength and Conditioning Research, 16*, 75–82.

McHugh, M. P., & Cosgrave, C. H. (2010). To stretch or not to stretch: The role of stretching in injury prevention and performance. *Scandinavian Journal of Medicine and Science in Sports, 20*, 169–181.

McKenna, M., & Riches, P. E. (2007). A comparison of sprinting kinematics on two types of treadmill and over-ground. *Scandinavian Journal of Medicine and Science in Sports, 17*, 649–655.

McMaster, D., Gill, N., McGuigan, M., & Cronin, J. (2014). Effects of complex strength and ballistic training on maximum strength, sprint ability and force–velocity–power profiles of semi-professional rugby union players. *Journal of Australian Strength and Conditioning, 22*, 17–30.

Mendiguchia, J., Alentorn-Geli, E., & Brughelli, M. (2012). Hamstring strain injuries: Are we heading in the right direction? *British Journal of Sports Medicine, 46*, 81–85.

Mero, A. (1988). Force–time characteristics and running velocity of male sprinters during the acceleration phase of sprinting. *Research Quarterly for Exercise and Sport, 59*, 94–98.

Mero, A., & Komi, P. V. (1986). Force–, EMG–, and elastic–velocity relationships at submaximal, maximal, and supramaximal running speeds in sprinters. *European Journal of Applied Physiology, 55*, 553–561.

Mero, A., & Komi, P. V. (1994). EMG, force, and power analysis of sprint-specific strength exercise. *Journal of Applied Biomechanics, 10*, 1–13.

Mero, A., Komi, P. V., & Gregor, R. J. (1992). Biomechanics of sprint running: A review. *Sports Medicine, 13*, 376–392.

Mero, A., Komi, P. V., Rusko, H., & Hirvonen, J. (1987). Neuromuscular and anaerobic performance of sprinters at maximal and supramaximal speed. *International Journal of Sports Medicine, 8*, 55–60.

Mero, A., Luhtanen, P., & Komi, P. V. (1983). A biomechanical study of the sprint start. *Scandinavian Journal of Sports Science, 5*, 20–28.

Mero, A., Luhtanen, P., & Komi, P. V. (1986). Segmental contribution to velocity of center of gravity during contact at different speeds in male and female sprinters. *Journal of Human Movement Studies, 12*, 215–235.

Mero, A., Luhtanen, P., Viitasalo, J. T., & Komi, P. V. (1981). Relationships between the maximal running velocity, muscle fiber characteristics, force production and force relaxation of sprinters. *Scandinavian Journal of Sports Science, 3*, 16–22.

Moir, G., Sanders, R. H., Button, C., & Glaister, M. (2007). The effect of periodized resistance training on accelerative sprint performance. *Sports Biomechanics, 6*, 285–300.

Morin, J.-B., Bourdin, M., Edouard, P., Peyrot, N., Samozino, P., & Lacour, J.-R. (2012). Mechanical determinants of 100-m sprint running performance. *European Journal of Applied Physiology, 112*, 3921–3930.

Morin, J.-B., Edouard, P., & Samozino, P. (2011). Technical ability of force application as a determinant factor of sprint performance. *Medicine and Science in Sports and Exercise, 43*, 1680–1688.

Morin, J-B., & Sève, P. (2011). Sprint running performance: Comparison between treadmill and field conditions. *European Journal of Applied Physiology, 111*, 1695–1703.

Murphy, A. J., Lockie, R. G., & Coutts, A. J. (2003). Kinematic determinants of early acceleration in field sport athletes. *Journal of Sports Science and Medicine, 2*, 144–150.

Onishi, H., Yagi, R., Oyama, M., Akasaka, K., Ihashi, K., & Handa, Y. (2002). EMG–angle relationship of the hamstring muscles during maximum knee flexion. *Journal of Electromyography and Kinesiology, 12*, 399–406.

Opar, D. A., Williams, M. D., & Shield, A. J. (2012). Hamstring strain injuries: Factors that lead to injury and re-injury. *Sports Medicine, 42*, 209–226.

Orchard, J. W. (2012). Hamstrings are most susceptible to injury during the early stance phase of sprinting. *British Journal of Sports Medicine, 46*, 88–89.

Paradisis, G. P., Bissas, A., & Cooke, C. B. (2009). Combining uphill and downhill sprint running training is more efficacious than horizontal. *International Journal of Sports Physiology and Performance, 4*, 229–243.

Paradisis, G. P., & Cooke, C. B. (2001). Kinematic and postural characteristics of sprint running on sloping surfaces. *Journal of Sports Sciences, 19*, 149–159.

Paradisis, G. P., & Cooke, C. B. (2006). The effects of sprint running training on sloping surfaces. *Journal of Strength and Conditioning Research, 20*, 767–777.

Pinder, R. A., Davids, K., Renshaw, I., & Araújo, D. (2011). Representative learning design and functionality of research and practice in sport. *Journal of Sport and Exercise Psychology, 33*, 146–155.

Ropret, R., Kukolj, M., Ugarkovic, D., & Matavulj, D. (1998). Effects of arm and leg loading on sprint performance. *European Journal of Applied Physiology, 77*, 547–550.

Salo, A. I. T., Bezodis, I. N., Batterham, A. M., & Kerwin, D. G. (2011). Elite sprinting: Are athletes individually step-frequency of step-length reliant? *Medicine and Science in Sports and Exercise, 43*, 1055–1062.

Samozino, P., Rejc, E., Di Prampero, P. E., Belli, A., & Morin, J.-B. (2012). Optimal force–velocity profile in ballistic movements—*altius: citius* or *fortius? Medicine and Science in Sports and Exercise, 44*, 313–322.

Savelsbergh, G. J. P., Williams, A. M., Van Der Kamp, J., & Ward, P. (2002). Visual search, anticipation and expertise in soccer. *Journal of Sports Sciences, 20*, 279–287.

Schache, A. G., Dorn, T. W., Blanch, P. D., Brown, N. A. T., & Pandy, M. G. (2012). Mechanics of the human hamstring muscles during sprinting. *Medicine and Science in Sports and Exercise, 44*, 647–658.

Sheppard, J. (2013). Technical development of linear speed. In I. Jeffreys (Ed.), *Developing speed* (pp. 31–60). Champaign, IL: Human Kinetics.

Sheppard, J. M., & Young, W. B. (2006). Agility literature review: Classifications, training and testing. *Journal of Sports Sciences, 24*, 919–932.

Sheppard, J., Young, W., Doyle, T., Sheppard, T., & Newton, R. (2006). An evaluation of a new test of reactive agility and its relationship to sprint speed and change of direction speed. *Journal of Science and Medicine in Sport, 9*, 342–349.

Shim, J., Chow, J. W., Carlton, L. G., & Woen-Sik, C. (2005). The use of anticipatory visual cues by highly skilled tennis players. *Journal of Motor Behavior, 37*, 164–175.

Slawinski, J., Dorel, S., Hug, F., Couturier, A., Fournel, V., Morin, J.-B., & Hanon, C. (2008). Elite long sprint running: A comparison between incline and level training sessions. *Medicine and Science in Sports and Exercise, 40*, 1155–1162.

Sleivert, G., & Taingahue, M. (2004). The relationship between maximal jump-squat power and sprint acceleration in athletes. *European Journal of Applied Physiology, 91*, 46–52.

Spenst, L. F., Martin, A. D., & Drinkwater, D. T. (1993). Muscle mass of competitive male athletes. *Journal of Sports Science, 11*, 3–8.

Spinks, C. D., Murphy, A. J., Spinks, W. L., & Lockie, R. G. (2007). The effects of resisted sprint training on acceleration performance and kinematics in soccer, rugby union, and Australian Football players. *Journal of Strength and Conditioning Research, 21*, 77–85.

Thelen, D. G., Chumanov, E. S., Hoerth, D. M., Best, T. M., Swanson, S. C., Li, L., . . . Heiderscheit, B. C. (2005). Hamstring muscle kinematics during treadmill sprinting. *Medicine and Science in Sports and Exercise, 37*, 108–114.

Uchiyama, Y., Tamaki, T., & Fukuda, H. (2001). Relationship between functional deficit and severity of experimental fast-strain injury of rat skeletal muscle. *European Journal of Applied Physiology, 85,* 1–9.

Upton, D. E. (2011). The effects of assisted and resisted sprint training on acceleration and velocity in Division IA female soccer athletes. *Journal of Strength and Conditioning Research, 25,* 2645–2652.

Usherwood, J. R., & Wilson, A. M. (2006). Accounting for elite indoor 200 m sprint results. *Biology Letters, 2,* 47–50.

Verrall, G. M., Slavotinek, J. P., & Barnes, P. G. (2005). The effect of sports specific training on reducing the incidence of hamstring injuries in professional Australian Rules football players. *British Journal of Sports Medicine, 39,* 363–368.

Volkov, N. I., & Lapin, V. I. (1979). Analysis of the velocity curve in sprint running. *Medicine and Science in Sports and Exercise, 11,* 332–337.

Walsh, M., Young, B., Hill, B., Kittredge, K., & Horn, T. (2007). The effect of ball-carrying technique and experience on sprinting in rugby union. *Journal of Sports Sciences, 25,* 185–192.

Watts, A. S., Coleman, I., & Nevill, A. (2012). The changing shape characteristics associated with success in world-class sprinters. *Journal of Sports Sciences, 30,* 1085–1095.

Wdowski, M. M., & Gittoes, M. J. R. (2013). Kinematic adaptations in sprint acceleration performance without and with the constraint of holding a field hockey stick. *Sports Biomechanics, 12,* 143–153.

West, D. J., Cunningham, D. J., Bracken, R. M., Bevan, H. R., Crewther, B. T., Cook, C. J., & Kilduff, L. P. (2013). Effects of resisted sprint training on acceleration in professional rugby union players. *Journal of Strength and Conditioning Research, 27,* 1014–1018.

Weyand, P. G., & Bundle, M. W. (2010). Point:counterpoint: Artificial limbs do/do not make artificially fast running speeds possible. *Journal of Applied Physiology, 108,* 1011–1012.

Weyand, P. G., & Davis, J. A. (2005). Running performance has a structural basis. *Journal of Experimental Biology, 208,* 2625–2631.

Weyand, P. G., Lee, C. S., Marinez-Ruiz, R., Bundle, M. W., Bellizzi, M. J., & Wright, S. (1999). High-speed running performance is largely unaffected by hypoxic reductions in aerobic power. *Journal of Applied Physiology, 86,* 2059–2064.

Weyand, P. G., Sandell, R. F., Prime, D. N. L., & Bundle, M. W. (2010). The biological limits to running speed are imposed from the ground up. *Journal of Applied Physiology, 108,* 950–961.

Weyand, P. G., Sternlight, D. B., Bellizzi, M. J., & Wright, S. (2000). Faster top running speeds are achieved with greater ground forces not more rapid leg movements. *Journal of Applied Physiology, 81,* 1991–1999.

Wiemann, K., & Tidow, G. (1995). Relative activity of hip and knee extensors in sprinting: Implications for training. *New Studies in Athletics, 10,* 29–49.

Young, W. B. (2006). Transfer of strength and power training to sport performance. *International Journal of Sports Physiology and Performance, 1,* 74–83.

Young, W., Benton, D., Duthie, G., & Pryor, J. (2001). Resistance training for short sprints and maximum-speed sprints. *Strength and Conditioning Journal, 23,* 7–13.

Young, W., & Farrow, D. (2013). The importance of a sport-specific stimulus for training agility. *Strength and Conditioning Journal, 35,* 39–43.

Young, W. B., Hawken, M., & McDonald, L. (1996). Relationship between speed, agility, and strength qualities in Australian Rules Football. *Strength and Conditioning Coach, 4,* 3–6.

Young, W. B., McDowell, M. H., & Scarlett, B. J. (2001). Specificity of sprint and agility training methods. *Journal of Strength and Conditioning Research, 15,* 315–319.

Young, W., McLean, B., & Ardagna, J. (1995). Relationships between strength qualities and sprinting performance. *Journal of Sports Medicine and Physical Fitness, 35,* 13–19.

Young, W., & Rogers, N. (2014). Effects of small-sided game and change-of-direction training on reactive agility and change-of-direction speed. *Journal of Sports Sciences, 32,* 307–314.

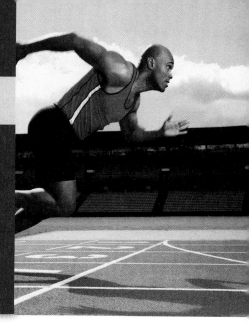

APPENDIX 1

Système Internationale d'Unités

The scientific community uses standardized units associated with the Système Internationale d'Unités (SI) when measuring and recording physical quantities. The SI is an extension of the centimeter/gram/second system proposed in 1873, the meter/kilogram/second system proposed in 1901, and the meter/kilogram/second/ampere system proposed in 1950 (Van Assendelft, 1987).

The SI uses base 10 (decimal) and has the base units of the second, kilogram, and meter for the dimensions of time, mass, and length, respectively, from which other physical quantities are derived (Table A1.1). For example, linear velocity has the dimensions of length and time, while force has the dimensions of mass–length–time^2.

The units associated with the base units of time and length are standardized by naturally occurring phenomena that remain constant. For example, a second is defined as 9,192,631,770 oscillation periods of the hyperfine transitions between the ground state of the cesium-133 atom, while a meter is defined as the distance traveled by light in a vacuum in 1/299,792,458 s (Kibble & Berkshire, 2009). Conversely, the unit of mass, the kilogram, is standardized by the mass of a quantity of platinum and iridium kept at Sèvres in France. Because this measure is not based on a natural constant, its permanence has been recently questioned; the standardized mass has actually fluctuated by 30 billionths of a kilogram (30 nanograms) in the last 100 years (Sobel, 2009). This has led to calls to replace the measure of mass with a natural constant such as the Planck constant.

A supplemental quantity of plane angle is included in the SI measurement scheme. The quantity of plane angle has the SI unit of the radian, defined as the ratio of the length of the radius on a circle to the length of the arc subtended by the radius length. Given that this unit has the dimension of a length divided by a length, it is dimensionless. Being dimensionless, the radian acts as a conversion factor between linear and angular motion; in turn, it is often used in biomechanics. However, plane angles are often measured in biomechanical analyses using the degree, a unit with which coaches (and probably most biomechanists) are more familiar.

The practitioner needs a means to convert between these units. Table A1.2 shows the factors used to convert between the units that are commonly used in biomechanical analyses associated with the SI and U.S. measurement systems.

Table A1.1
Common Physical Quantities Used in Biomechanics, Their Symbols, Dimensions, SI and U.S. Units, and Conversion Factors

Quantity	Symbol	Dimensions	SI units	U.S. Units
Time	t	fundamental	second (s)	second (s)
Mass	m	fundamental	kilogram (kg)	slug (sl)
Length	l	fundamental	meter (m)	foot (ft)
Linear velocity	v	lt^{-1}	meter/second (m/s)	foot/second (ft/s)
Linear acceleration	a	lt^{-2}	meter/second^2 (m/s^2)	foot/second^2 (ft/s^2)
Plane angle	θ	dimensionless	radian (rad)	degree (°)
Force	F	mlt^{-2}	newton (N)	pound-force (lbf)
Linear momentum	p	mls^{-1}	kilogram-meter/second (kg m/s)	slug-foot/second
Impulse of force	J	mls^{-1}	newton-second (Ns)	pound-force second (lbf s)
Work	W	ml^2t^{-2}	joule (J)	pound-force foot (lbf ft)
Energy	E	ml^2t^{-2}	joule (J)	pound-force foot (lbf ft)
Power	P	ml^2t^{-3}	watt (W)	pound-force foot/second (lbf ft/s)
Moment of force	M	ml^2t^{-2}	newton-meter (Nm)	pound-force foot (lbf ft)

The dimensions can give rise to the units of measurement associated with some of the physical quantities, with linear velocity being an example. Other relationships are less intuitive. The scale on which the physical quantity is measured is determined by the dimension, while the units relate more to the resolution and datum associated with the specific scale (Vogel, 2003). The impulse of a force has the same dimensions as linear momentum, but different units. The dimensional equivalence of these variables reflects their relationship to each other, which is

Table A1.2
Factors for Converting Between SI and U.S. Units

Quantity	SI to U.S. Units	U.S. to SI Units
Mass	kilogram × 14.5939	slug ÷ 14.5939
Length	meter ÷ 3.280839895	foot × 3.280839895
Plane angle	radian × (180/π)	degree ÷ (180/π)
Force	newton × 0.224808943	pound-force ÷ 0.224808943
Work	joule × 0.737562149	pound-force foot ÷ 0.737562149
Moment of force	newton-meter × 0.737562149	pound-force foot ÷ 0.737562149

summarized in the impulse–momentum relationship; the impulse of a force is equal to the change in momentum produced. Similarly, work and energy have the same dimensions (translational kinetic energy and gravitational potential energy both have the dimensions of ml^2s^{-2}). However, these variables actually have the same units as well, reflecting their connection as expressed in the work–energy theorem: The work done by a force is equal to the change in mechanical energy produced. Work and moment of force have the same dimensions but different units—joule and newton-meter, respectively. Both the dimensions and the scales appear to be equivalent in this case but they are very different variables; a moment of force that causes a rotation of a body can do work, but does not reflect the work done. Work and the moment of force are actually calculated differently from the same vector variables of force and displacement. Work is calculated as the dot product of the vectors, resulting in a scalar, while the moment of force is calculated from the cross product of the vectors, resulting in a vector variable (see the *Vector Analysis* appendix).

Some variables that are encountered in a mechanical analysis of human movements have no dimensions. The coefficient of friction, the drag and lift coefficients, strain, and mechanical advantage are all numbers that inform our analyses, and all are dimensionless, being ratios of variables derived from the same dimensions.

An issue related to the resolution of the scale associated with the measurement of a physical quantity is the number of significant figures typically reported in biomechanics. Most equipment used in biomechanical analyses proffers measurements to a large number of significant figures, determined by the number of decimal places. When taking a measurement of a physical quantity, however, the result is simply an estimate of the true measure; the accuracy of the recorded measurement relative to the true value depends, in part, on the resolution of the scale being used. Most biomechanical analyses report measurements to three significant figures when possible (Enoka, 2008). For example, the mass of an athlete would be recorded as 78.6 kg, even though the reading from the digital scale was 78.56 kg; the athlete's height would be recorded as 1.86 m even though the stadiometer read 1.856 m. However, some measurements do not lend themselves to three significant figures. A power output of 3126.78 W would be recorded as 3127 W; the decimal places are not required in such a large measure. Furthermore, some measurements have specific prefixes to denote larger or smaller units (Table A1.3).

Table A1.3
Typical Prefixes Denoting Larger and Smaller Units Used in Biomechanical Analyses

Prefix	Symbol	Multiplier
giga-	G	1 billion times ($10^9 \times$)
mega-	M	1 million times ($10^6 \times$)
kilo-	k	1 thousand times ($10^3 \times$)
milli-	m	1 thousandth of ($10^{-3} \times$)
micro-	μ	1 millionth of ($10^{-6} \times$)
nano-	n	1 billionth of ($10^{-9} \times$)

Accordingly, the vertical stiffness of 3246 Nm for an athlete measured during a drop–jump would be recorded as 32.5 kNm. The prefixes are arranged in three orders of magnitude, with a practical consequence being that the millimeter is allowed as a unit of length within the SI scheme, yet the centimeter is not.

The formulae used in this text refer not to units of measurement, but rather to the physical quantities being measured. These quantities are displayed in italicized font throughout the text, whereas the units are non-italicized; for example, J refers to joules (the unit of work and energy), whereas J refers to the impulse of a force.

References

Enoka, R. M. (2008). *Neuromechanics of human movement*. Champaign, IL: Human Kinetics.

Kibble, T. W. B., & Berkshire, F. H. (2009). *Classical mechanics*. London, UK: Imperial College Press.

Sobel, D. (2009, March 8). The kilogram isn't what it used to be: It's lighter. *Discover, 20*. http://discovermagazine.com/2009/mar/08-kilogram-isnt-what-it-used-to-be-its-lighter

Van Assendelft, O. W. (1987). The International System of Units (SI) in historical perspective. *American Journal of Public Health, 77*, 1400–1403.

Vogel, S. (2003). *Comparative biomechanics: Life's physical world*. Princeton, NJ: Princeton University Press.

Scalars and Vectors

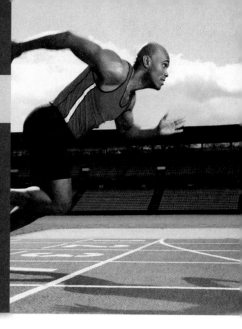

A scalar variable is one that can be fully described by its magnitude, whereas a vector variable requires both a magnitude and a direction to fully describe its mechanical action. In a more formal sense, a scalar variable is one that is unaffected by a transformation of the reference frame in which it operates.

Mass is a scalar. If a body has a mass of 70 kg, it does not matter if we rotate the reference frame in which we are making the recording. Furthermore, it makes little sense to discuss the direction that the mass acts in; if the body is moved in any direction within the reference frame, it will still contain 70 kg of matter.

Conversely, moving 5 m along the y-axis of a reference frame is very different from moving 5 m along the z-axis. Linear displacement is a vector quantity where both the magnitude of the movement and the direction within the reference frame in which the movement occurs are equally important in describing the variable.

Table A2.1 lists scalar and vector variables commonly used in biomechanical analyses.

Some variables noted in Table A2.1 are combinations of scalars and vectors. Indeed, some variables are combinations of the *same* scalars and vectors. For example, the product of the mass of a body (a scalar) and its linear velocity (a vector) results in the vector variable of linear momentum, whose directionality is provided by velocity. However, if we multiply half-mass by the square of the linear velocity of a body, then we have a scalar of kinetic energy. The squaring of the linear velocity in this case eliminates the directionality of the variable.

The mechanical action of scalars can be analyzed using simple algebra and arithmetic, while vectors must be added, subtracted, and multiplied following specific rules (see the *Vector Analysis* appendix). Vectors, however, can be represented graphically as arrows with the length corresponding to the magnitude of the variable and the direction within the specified reference frame determining its line of action.

The lack of dependence upon direction associated with our definition of a scalar does not preclude the occurrence of negative values associated with them. For example, a body can have a temperature of $-5°C$ irrespective of its direction of motion within a reference frame. The sense of the variable simply indicates the location of the physical quantity of temperature on a scale of real numbers. Other scalar quantities, such as mass and volume, are always positive. Therefore, the value of the scalar is determined relative to the datum associated with the particular measurement scale employed.

Table A2.1

Scalar and Vector Variables Commonly Encountered in Biomechanical Analyses of Human Movements, Their Symbols, and SI Units

Physical Quality	Symbol	SI Units
Scalar Variables		
Time	t	seconds, s
Mass	m	kilogram, kg
Translational kinetic energy	E_{TK}	joule, J
Gravitational potential energy	E_{GP}	joule, J
Work	W	joule, J
Power	P	watt, W
Vector Variables		
Linear displacement	s	meter, m
Linear velocity	v	meters per second, m/s
Linear acceleration	a	meters per second per second, m/s^2
Linear momentum	p	kilogram-meter per second, kg m/s
Force	F	newton, N
Impulse	J	newton-second, Ns
Moment of force	M	newton-meter, Nm

Work is a scalar variable. That is, work is defined in terms of the resulting change in energy produced, as per the work–energy theorem, and energy is a scalar; therefore, work must also be a scalar. This explanation is somewhat circular. Another explanation is that work is calculated as the dot product of the force and displacement vectors associated with the body under analysis, and the dot product always returns a scalar (see the *Vector Analysis* appendix). This rationale is mathematically correct, but still rather unsatisfying.

A less formal explanation would be that the change of energy associated with the work done on an object does not depend on the direction that the work is performed. However, Bartlett (2007) notes that some scalars, such as work, can be designated as having a "direction" in which they move during an analysis. For example, when an athlete raises a barbell during a bench press exercise, the individual is performing work on the surroundings and the work done is considered "positive" by convention. Conversely, when the athlete lowers the barbell to the chest, "negative" work is said to be done; that is, the barbell does work on the athlete.

The "direction" in which the work is done has important consequences for the underlying musculotendinous mechanics, and will certainly impact metabolic energy consumption and the adaptive response associated with the muscular contractions during these phases of the movement. Indeed, the "negative work" can be absorbed by the musculotendinous tissue and used subsequently. Technically, work remains a scalar variable throughout the movement. However, the designation of a "direction" associated with the work done does provide some practical meaning for the analyst.

References

Bartlett, R. (2007). *Introduction to sports biomechanics: Analysing human movement patterns.* Oxford, UK: Routledge.

Vector Analysis

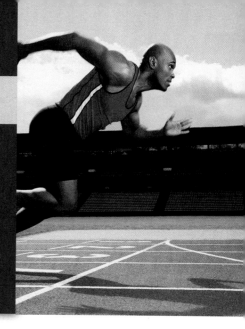

Key Terms

Law of cosines	Resultant vector	Vector composition
Law of sines	Scalar product	Vector product
Parallelogram method	Unit vectors	Vector resolution

Scalar variables used in biomechanical analyses require only magnitude to describe them, being represented by real numbers. In a formal mathematical sense, scalar variables are invariant to transformations of the reference frame. In contrast, vector variables used in biomechanical analyses require reference to both the magnitude and direction to fully describe their mechanical effect. A transformation of the reference frame affects a vector. Vectors are directed line segments within space that can be represented graphically as arrows, with the magnitude of the vector denoted by the length of the arrow and the direction of the vector within space determined by the orientation of the arrow within a specified reference frame.

Addition of Vectors

Vector analysis is important in biomechanical analyses because we may wish to determine the effect of several vectors acting in different directions. Figure A3.1 shows the ground reaction force acting along the horizontal (y) and vertical (z) axes as an athlete runs over a force plate. At each time point during the movement, we could represent the two orthogonal force components as vectors within two-dimensional space (Figure A3.2). The two force components can be added together to reveal a single **resultant vector** in a procedure called **vector composition** (the forces acting along the y- and z-axes are, therefore, known as the components of the

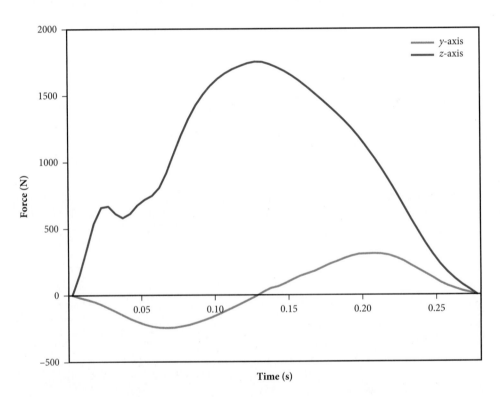

Figure A3.1 The horizontal and vertical components of the ground reaction force measured as an athlete runs over a force plate.

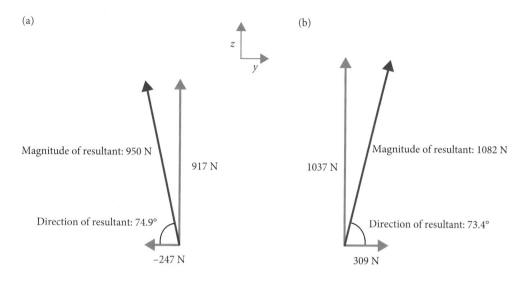

Figure A3.2 The two orthogonal vectors representing the horizontal and vertical components of the ground reaction force at time = 0.065 s (a) and time = 0.205 (b) as an athlete runs over a force plate. The resultant vectors are shown in red. Notice that the resultant force vector changes in both magnitude and direction from time = 0.065 s to time = 0.205 s. When placing the component vectors tail-to-tail, the resultant vector can be represented graphically as the diagonal of the parallelogram that is formed by joining the orthogonal vectors with parallel elements.

resultant force). The magnitude of the resultant vector can be determined using the Pythagorean theorem:

$$F_R = \sqrt{F_y^2 + F_z^2}$$

Eq. (A3.1)

where F_R is the magnitude of the resultant force vector, F_y is the magnitude of the force vector acting along the y (horizontal) axis, and F_z is the magnitude of the force vector acting along the z (vertical) axis. The direction of the resultant vector can be determined using an appropriate trigonometric function:

$$\theta = \tan^{-1} \frac{F_z}{F_y}$$

Eq. (A3.2)

where θ is the angle of the resultant force vector, F_z is the magnitude of the force vector acting along the z (vertical) axis, and F_y is the magnitude of the force vector acting along the y (horizontal) axis. (Note that because the angles are presented with respect to the right horizontal, with counterclockwise being positive, the angle of the resultant force vector in Figure A3.2a is actually $180 - \theta = 105.1°$.) Notice in Figure A3.2 that the orthogonal components have been placed tail-to-tail in each case, such that the resultant vector becomes the diagonal across the parallelogram formed from this arrangement. This represents a graphic method to determine the resultant vector from two component vectors known as the **parallelogram method**.

Vector composition can also be performed on vectors that are not orthogonal. Consider the force vectors representing two muscles shown in Figure A3.3a. By placing the tail of one vector onto the head of the other, we can establish the resultant force vector that acts at the tendon that both muscles innervate. To calculate the magnitude of the resultant force vector, we can use the **law of cosines**:

$$F_R^2 = F_1^2 + F_2^2 - (2 \times F_1 \times F_2 \times \cos \beta)$$ Eq. (A3.3)

where F_R is the magnitude of the resultant force vector acting at the tendon, F_1 is the magnitude of the force vector associated with muscle 1 (500 N), F_2 is the magnitude of the force vector associated with muscle 2 (250 N), and β is the angle between the two vectors (180 − [15 + 10] as per Figure A3.3b). Using the values shown in Figure A3.3, we get

$$F_R = 734.2 \text{ N}$$ Eq. (A3.4)

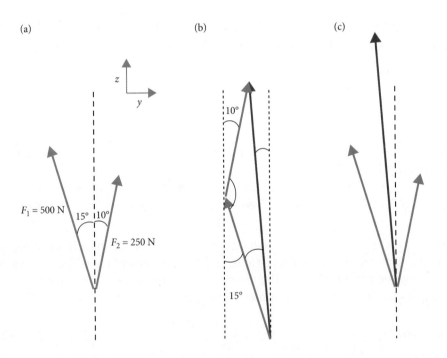

Figure A3.3 (a) Non-orthogonal vectors representing the forces associated with two muscles that innervate a common tendon. The vertical dashed line represents the line of action of the common tendon. (b) The addition of the vectors is represented graphically by placing the tail of F_2 on the head of F_1; the resultant vector is shown in red. The magnitude of the resultant vector can be determined from the law of cosines, while the internal angle γ can be determined from the law of sines. (c) The resultant force vector from the addition of F_1 and F_2.

The **law of sines** can be used to determine the magnitude of the internal angle γ:

$$\frac{\sin \beta}{F_R} = \frac{\sin \gamma}{F_2}$$

Eq. (A3.5)

where β is the angle between the two force vectors associated with muscles 1 and 2, F_R is the magnitude of the resultant force vector acting at the tendon, γ is the internal angle, and F_2 is the magnitude of the force associated with muscle 2. Equation (A3.5) can then be rearranged to solve for the internal angle γ:

$$\gamma = \sin^{-1}\left(F_2 \times \frac{\sin \beta}{F_R}\right)$$

Eq. (A3.6)

$$\gamma = 8.27°$$

Eq. (A3.7)

The internal angle $\gamma = 8.27°$ can then be used to determine angle θ given that F_1 is 15° from the vertical:

$$\theta = 15 - 8.27$$

Eq. (A3.8)

$$\theta = 6.73°$$

Eq. (A3.9)

Therefore, the addition of vectors F_1 and F_2 associated with the two muscles shown in Figure A3.3 produces a resultant force vector acting on the tendon that has a magnitude of 734.2 N and acts at an angle of 96.73°. (Note again that the direction provided by the angle is always expressed relative to the right horizontal in the reference frame with the counterclockwise direction as positive.)

Unit vectors are often used in vector analysis to express the number of units along each of the axes associated with the reference frame that are required to describe the vectors being analyzed. The terms i, j, and k are used to denote unit vectors along the y-, z-, and x-axes, respectively. For example, the vector associated with F_1 in Figure A3.3 can be described by the unit vectors $-129.4i$ and $483.0j$; that is, if we start at the origin (the point in Figure A3.3 where the tail of vector F_1 joins the vertical dashed line associated with the common tendon) and move -129.4 force units along the y-axis (to the left) and 483.0 force units along the z-axis (upward), we will arrive at the head of the vector. (The number of force units along each axis was calculated using trigonometric functions given the hypotenuse of the right triangle of 500 units and the angle of 15°.) The vector associated with F_2 in Figure A3.3 can be described by the unit vectors $43.4i$ and $246.2j$. We can use the unit vectors to determine the resultant force vector produced when we add F_1 and F_2 by first adding the unit vectors along the y-axis (i) and then adding the unit vectors along the z-axis (j). Expressed algebraically, the addition of the two muscle forces using unit vectors becomes

$$F_1 + F_2 = (-129.4 + 43.4)i + (483.0 + 246.2)j$$

Eq. (A3.10)

$$F_1 + F_2 = (-86.0)i + (729.2)j$$

Eq. (A3.11)

Equation (A3.11) informs us that the head of the resultant vector is located – 86.0 force units along the y-axis and 729.2 force units along the z-axis when beginning from the origin (where the two force vectors join the common tendon). We can use trigonometric functions to calculate the horizontal (sine) and vertical (cosine) components associated with the resultant force vector given the hypotenuse of 734.2 N and the angle θ of 6.73° and arrive at the same magnitudes of the components as shown in Equation (A3.11), although the sense of the components will both be positive. The procedure for determining the components of a vector is known as **vector resolution** and is the converse of vector composition.

Multiplication of Vectors

Vectors can be multiplied through one of two different procedures that are named after the character of the resultant vector. The first procedure, known as the **scalar product** (also known as the dot product) of vectors, results in a scalar quantity. The scalar product of two vectors can be expressed as follows:

$$a \cdot b = \|a\|\|b\|\cos\theta$$

Eq. (A3.12)

where $\|a\|$ and $\|b\|$ are the magnitudes of the vectors a and b, respectively, and θ is the angle between the two vectors.

Figure A3.4 shows the average force vector F and displacement vector s associated with a barbell ascending during a bench press exercise in a Smith machine.

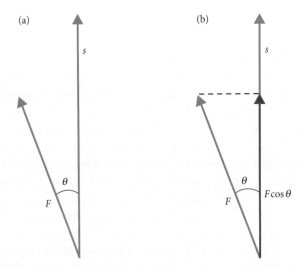

Figure A3.4 (a) The average force (F) and displacement (s) vectors associated with the barbell ascent during a bench press exercise performed in a Smith machine as viewed in the sagittal plane. The athlete exerts a force against the barbell that is directed upward and toward the head; the displacement of the barbell is purely vertical due to the mechanical constraints imposed by the Smith machine such that the angle between the two vectors is θ. (b) The scalar product of the two vectors returns the magnitude of F that acts in the direction of s, denoted by the red vector $F\cos\theta$.

Notice that the athlete actually exerts a force against the barbell that is directed both upward and backward, yet the displacement of the barbell is purely vertical given the mechanical constraints associated with the Smith machine.

If $F = 800$ N, $s = 1.03$ m, and $\theta = 15°$, then we can rewrite Equation (A3.12) as follows:

$$s \cdot F = 1.03 \times 800 \times \cos 15 \qquad\qquad \text{Eq. (A3.13)}$$

$$s \cdot F = 796 \qquad\qquad \text{Eq. (A3.14)}$$

The scalar quantity of 796 represents the work done by the force exerted on the barbell that acts in the direction of the displacement (the units would be joules). Therefore, the work done by a force can be calculated from the scalar product of a displacement and force vector.

The second procedure for multiplying vectors is the **vector product** (also known as the cross product). As its name suggests, the vector product returns a vector quantity. The vector product of two vectors can be expressed as follows:

$$a \times b = \|a\|\|b\|\sin\theta \qquad\qquad \text{Eq. (A3.15)}$$

where $\|a\|$ and $\|b\|$ are the magnitudes of the vectors a and b, respectively, and θ is the angle between the two vectors. The vector resulting from this procedure acts normal (perpendicular) to the plane containing vectors a and b.

Figure A3.5 shows the force (F) applied to a bicycle crank and the position that this vector acts from the crank axis (r). The angle between the two vectors

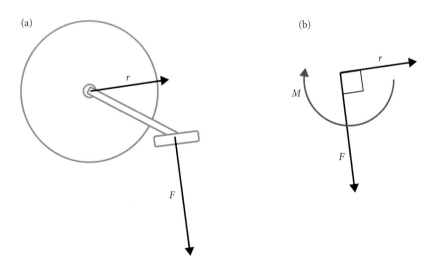

Figure A3.5 (a) The force (F) applied to a bicycle crank and the position that this vector acts from the crank axis (r) at one instant during a revolution of the crank. (b) The vector product of r and F returns the moment of force (M) acting along the axis about which the crank would rotate due to the action of the applied force.

is θ. If $F = 150$ N, $r = 0.30$ m, and $\theta = 90°$, then we can use Equation (A3.16) to determine the vector product:

$$r \times F = 0.30 \times 150 \times \sin 90 \qquad\qquad \text{Eq. (A3.16)}$$

$$r \times F = 45 \qquad\qquad \text{Eq. (A3.17)}$$

The vector quantity of 45 represents the moment of force acting on the crank at this time during the movement and the units would be newton-meters. (In the strict mechanical sense, the vector quantity would represent a torque given that the crank would experience pure rotation as a result of the action of the applied force. However, to maintain consistency with the rest of the text we have referred to the vector quantity as the moment of force here.) This vector acts along the axis about which the crank would rotate due to the action of the applied force and is represented as a curved arrow in Figure A3.5.

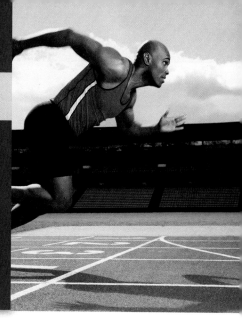

APPENDIX 4

Calculus

© GlobalStock/iStockphoto.com

Key Terms

Chord

Coefficient

Differential calculus

Exponent

First central difference

First derivative

Fundamental theorem of calculus

Integrative calculus

Monomial function

Parabola

Power rule

Second central difference

Second derivative

Tangent

Trapezoid rule

Calculus is concerned with the mathematics of change. Consequently, the mathematical procedures associated with calculus should hold great significance for the biomechanical study of human movements, where the variables of interest (e.g., velocity, force) can change rapidly with respect to time. There are two parts to the mathematics of calculus, **differential calculus** and **integrative calculus**. Both are related by the fundamental theorem of calculus, and both are used in biomechanical analyses of human movements. We begin with a discussion of limits, which are important concepts within calculus.

Limits

Figure A4.1 shows variable y as a function of x. This curve forms part of a **parabola** and is described in the following **monomial function**:

$$f(x) = x^4$$

Eq. (A4.1)

This function provides us with a means of calculating any value of y for a corresponding value of x. For example, using the function in Equation (A4.1), we can determine that $y = 16$ when $x = 2$. A limit provides a method whereby one can focus in on a specific, and small, part of a curve. For example, let us determine the value of y as x approaches 4. Looking at Figure A4.1, we can see that as x increases from a value of 3 toward 4, y increases from approximately 100 to 200, whereas as x decreases from 5 toward 4, y decreases from approximately 600 to 200. As such, at $x = 4$, y is approximately 200. (We can, of course, use the monomial function in Equation (A4.1) to determine the exact value of y when $x = 4$ and find $y = 256$.) What we have determined is the limit of $f(x)$ when x approaches 4. We write this as follows:

$$\lim_{x \to 4} f(x) = 256$$

Eq. (A4.2)

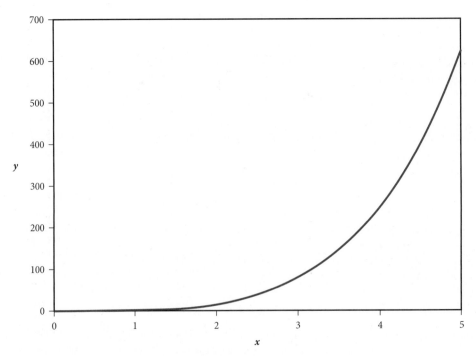

Figure A4.1 The graph of the function $y = x^4$.

Table A4.1

The Linear Displacement Undergone by a Body Falling Under the Influence of Gravity

Time (s)	0	1	2	3	4	5	6
Displacement (m)	0	−4.91	−19.62	−44.15	−78.48	−122.63	−176.58

Limits allow us to define a y value when the change in x is an infinitesimally small value such that x approaches 0 ($x \to 0$). As x refers to time in most biomechanical analyses, limits allow us to determine the value of a dependent variable (y) associated with infinitesimally small changes in time (as the change in time approaches zero). A biomechanist is likely to be interested in determining the slope of a curve or the area under a curve as the change in time approaches zero.

Consider the theoretical case of a body being dropped from a height of 200 m. If we ignore the fluid force of drag, we can calculate the linear displacement undergone in a given time using the following equation of motion:

$$s = \frac{1}{2}at^2$$

Eq. (A4.3)

where s is the linear displacement, a is the acceleration due to gravity (−9.81 m/s²), and t is the time. Table A4.1 shows the linear displacement of the ball after each second of flight. These data are displayed graphically in Figure A4.2.

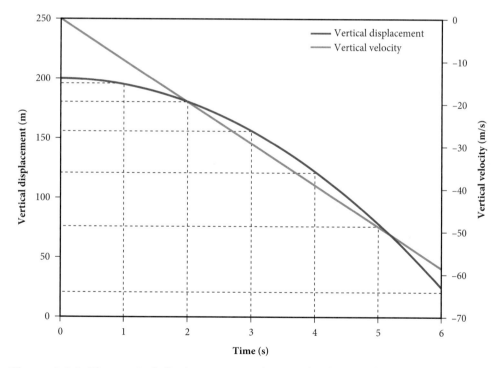

Figure A4.2 The vertical displacement and vertical velocity of a body falling from a height of 200 m. The dashed lines can be used to determine the vertical displacement after each 1-s period of the analysis. Notice that the displacement undergone between consecutive 1-s periods increases with time.

Table A4.2

The Average Velocity of a Falling Body Calculated over Different
Changes in Time

Δt (s)	1	0.5	0.25	0.10	0.05
$\overline{v}$ (m/s)	-14.71	-12.25	-11.02	-10.25	-9.96

Let us attempt to calculate the velocity of the ball at exactly 1 s after the beginning
of the fall. This velocity is the slope of the displacement–time curve at $t = 1$. We could
use the following equation for average velocity:

$$\overline{v} = \frac{\Delta s}{\Delta t}$$

Eq. (A4.4)

where $\overline{v}$ is the average linear velocity of the system during the time of analysis, Δs
is the change in linear displacement over the time of analysis, and Δt is the time
taken to undergo the change in linear displacement. In relation to Figure A4.2,
Equation (A4.4) will determine the slope of the curve associated with the specified change in time. We could then calculate the velocity between the times of
$t = 1$ and $t = 2$, which yields $\overline{v} = -14.71$ m/s. However, we know that the velocity
is increasing as a function of time, and the average velocity calculated over a 1-s
period does not provide a satisfactory answer. By reducing the time interval over
which the velocity value is calculated to 0.5 s (i.e., displacement at 1 s = –4.91 m;
displacement at 1.5 s = –11.04 m), $\overline{v} = -12.25$ m/s. Notice that this is still an average velocity—it has just been calculated over a shorter duration.

Table A4.2 shows the average velocity values calculated over changes in time
from 1 to 0.05 s. Notice that as the change in time approaches 0 s, $\overline{v}$ approaches the
value of –9.81 m/s, which we would expect because the ball is experiencing a constant
acceleration of –9.81 m/s^2 associated with the gravitational force. What we have established is that the instantaneous velocity of a body can be determined as a limiting case
as the change in time approaches zero ($t \to 0$); we have focused in on a specific, and
small, part of the curve shown in Figure A4.2 at 1 s and described the behavior of the
system at that instant. (If we were faced with the problem of determining the instantaneous velocity of a body after 1 s of flight, we could simply use the equation of motion
$v_f = v_i + at$ to arrive at our answer of –9.81 m/s. The preceding example was used
merely to demonstrate the value of limits in calculus.)

Differential Calculus

Differential calculus is used to calculate the rate of change in a variable with respect
to another variable to which it has a functional relationship. The velocity of a body is
defined as the rate of change in displacement; it is calculated as the ratio of the change
in displacement and the change in time. Velocity, therefore, is the **first derivative** of
displacement with respect to time. Graphically, if displacement is plotted on the y-axis
and time is on the x-axis, then velocity is the slope of this curve. As already noted,
instantaneous velocity can be calculated in terms of the limiting case as the change in
time approaches zero ($\Delta t \to 0$), which can be written as follows:

$$v = \lim_{\Delta t \to 0} \frac{\Delta s}{\Delta t}$$

Eq. (A4.5)

In the notation of differential calculus, this expression is written as follows:

$$v = \frac{ds}{dt}$$ Eq. (A4.6)

where v is the instantaneous velocity and ds is an infinitesimally small change in linear displacement caused by an infinitesimally small change dt in time.

A graphic example can be used to highlight what this means. Figure A4.3 shows a curve of the function $y = x^4$ from before. We will attempt to determine the derivative of y at point $x = 4$. This derivative is given by the slope of the **tangent** (a line that touches a curve at only one point) to the curve, as shown in Figure A4.3. Therefore, if y is the displacement of a body and x is the time of analysis, the velocity of the body at any instant is simply the slope of the tangent line at that instant in time.

Consider point $x = 4$ on the curve in Figure A4.3. The instantaneous slope at that point, and therefore the derivative of y, is the slope of the tangent line shown. This slope can be approximated by calculating the slope of the **chord** (a line that touches a curve at two points) joining the points $x = 4$ and $x = 5$, as shown in Figure A4.4.

Notice that in Figure A4.4, the chord $x = 4$, $x = 5$ does not accurately represent the slope of the tangent at $x = 4$. However, if we were to slide point $x = 5$ down the curve toward point $x = 4$, the slope of the chord would get closer to the slope of the tangent. Moving point $x = 5$ closer to point $x = 4$ would require a reduction in the interval between the two points. As the change in interval approaches zero, we will be able to approximate the slope of the tangent from the chord and, therefore, calculate the instantaneous velocity; we will have a time limiting case where $x \to 0$.

Figure A4.5 shows the chord of $x = 3$, $x = 5$. Notice that this chord more closely approximates the slope of the tangent line at point $x = 4$. It crosses two finite intervals

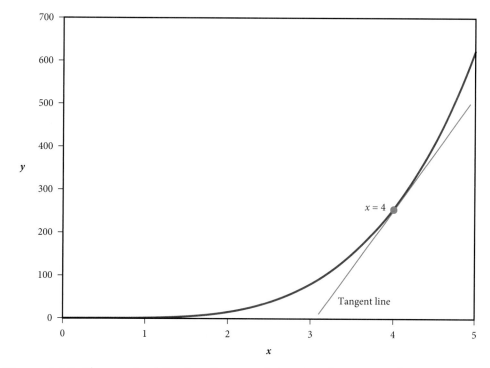

Figure A4.3 The graph of the function $y = x^4$ showing the tangent line at point $x = 4$.

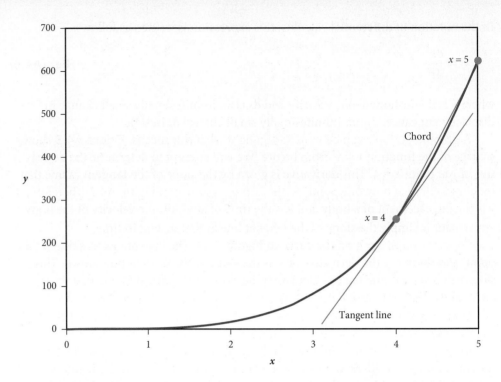

Figure A4.4 The graph of the function $y = x^4$ showing the chord joining points at $x = 4$ and $x = 5$.

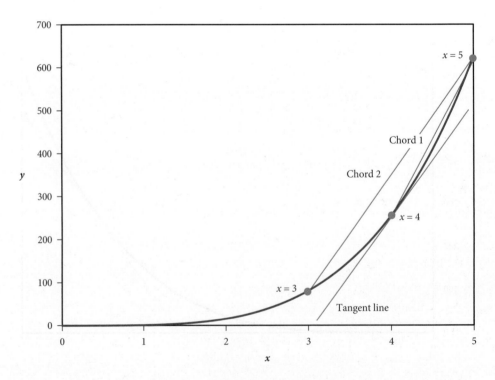

Figure A4.5 The graph of the function $y = x^4$ showing the chord joining points at $x = 4$ and $x = 5$ (Chord 1) and the chord joining points at $x = 3$ and $x = 5$ (Chord 2).

from x_{i-1} to x_{i+1} (where x_i refers to $x = 4$). Knowing the value of y for each value of x, we can determine the slope of the chord x_{i-1}, x_{i+1}, and therefore the derivative of y at $x = 4$, from the following equation:

$$\dot{y}_{x=4} = \frac{y_{i+1} - y_{i-1}}{2\Delta x}$$ Eq. (A4.7)

where $\dot{y}_{x=4}$ is notation for the first derivative of $y_{x=4}$, y_{i+1} is the value of y at $x = 5$, y_{i-1} is the value of y at $x = 3$, and Δx is the change in x between consecutive data points. The term $y_{i+1} - y_{i-1}$ is referred to as the **first central difference**.

Rewriting Equation (A4.7) in terms of velocity and displacement, we have

$$v_i = \frac{s_{i+1} - s_{i-1}}{2\Delta t}$$ Eq. (A4.8)

where v_i is the instantaneous velocity of the data point of interest, s_{i+1} is the displacement data point one time interval after the data point of interest, s_{i-1} is the displacement data point one time interval before the data point of interest, and Δt is the time interval between consecutive data points (Δt can easily be determined as the reciprocal of the sampling frequency used to collect the biomechanical data). Notice that Equation (A4.8) is the same as Equation (A4.7) but that $\dot{y}$ has been replaced with v_i, y has been replaced with s, and x has been replaced with t; instantaneous velocity is the first derivative of displacement with respect to time and is represented as the instantaneous slope of the displacement–time curve.

The **second derivative** of displacement with respect to time is acceleration. In the notation of differential calculus, we write

$$a = \frac{d^2 s}{dt^2}$$ Eq. (A4.9)

where a is the instantaneous acceleration, and ds is an infinitesimally small change in linear displacement caused by an infinitesimally small change dt in time. Referring to the curve in Figure A4.5, the second derivative of $y_{x=4}$ can be estimated using the following equation:

$$\ddot{y}_{x=4} = \frac{y_{i+1} - 2y_i + y_{i-1}}{\Delta t^2}$$ Eq. (A4.10)

where $\ddot{y}_{x=4}$ is notation for the second derivative of $y_{x=4}$, y_{i+1} is the value of y at $x = 5$, y_i is the value of y at $x = 4$, y_{i-1} is the value of y at $x = 3$, and Δx is the change in x. The term $y_{i+1} - 2y_i + y_{i-1}$ is referred to as the **second central difference**. Rewriting Equation (A4.10) in terms of acceleration and displacement, we have

$$a_i = \frac{s_{i+1} - 2s_i + s_{i-1}}{\Delta t^2}$$ Eq. (A4.11)

where a_i is the instantaneous acceleration of the data point of interest, s_{i+i} is the displacement data point one time interval after the point of interest, s_i is the displacement data point of interest, s_{i-1} is the displacement data point one time interval before the point of interest, and Δt is the time interval between consecutive data points.

The equations shown here for calculating instantaneous velocities (Equation A4.8) and accelerations (Equation A4.11) use linear displacement as input. These equations are also appropriate for angular variables, with the linear displacement data simply being replaced by the angular displacement data. Furthermore, differentiation is used for more than calculating velocity and acceleration data in biomechanics. A derivative simply expresses the rate at which one variable changes with respect to another to which it has a functional relationship: Force is the first derivative of momentum with respect to time; power is the first derivative of work with respect to time. As a consequence, the first and second central difference methods used in differentiation have biomechanical applications beyond the calculation of velocities and accelerations.

Another method of calculating the derivative of a known function is to use the **power rule**. In this method, the **exponent** (power) in the term is taken and multiplied by the **coefficient**, and then the power in the term is reduced by 1. For example, consider the following monomial function:

$$f(x) = 2x^4 \qquad \text{Eq. (A4.12)}$$

where the exponent is 4 and the coefficient is 2. Using the power rule, we can determine that the derivative, $f'(x)$, is $8x^3$.

The power rule can be used on polynomial functions (functions that contain multiple terms) as well. For example, consider the following polynomial function:

$$f(x) = 4x^3 + 3x^2 \qquad \text{Eq. (A4.13)}$$

Using the power rule, the derivative is $f'(x) = 12x^2 + 6x$.

The power rule can be useful in calculating the derivatives of variables when the polynomial functions are known. For example, Figure A4.6 shows the vertical

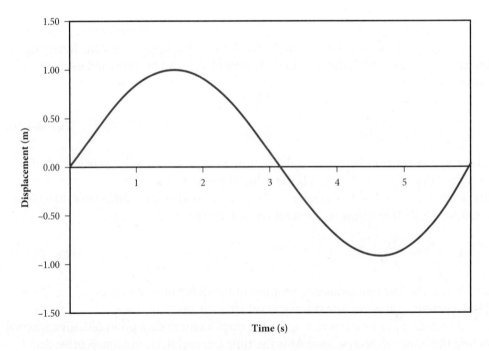

Figure A4.6 The vertical displacement of an oscillating body.

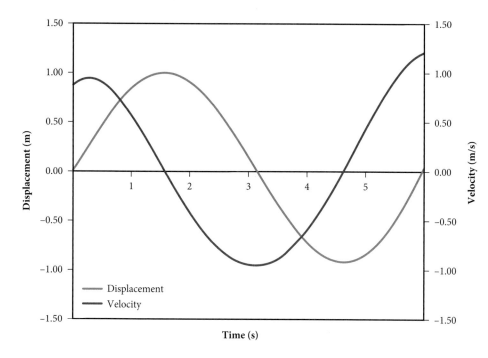

Figure A4.7 The vertical displacement of an oscillating body and the vertical velocity calculated by differentiating the polynomial function in Equation (A4.14) using the power rule.

displacement of an oscillating body. The curve can be approximated from the following polynomial function:

$$s = -0.0056 \times t^5 + 0.0886 \times t^4 - 0.4015 \times t^3$$
$$+ 0.2859 \times t^2 + 0.8617 \times t + 0.0158$$

Eq. (A4.14)

where s is the vertical displacement and t is the time. Using the power rule, the derivative—that is, instantaneous vertical velocity—can then be calculated:

$$v = 5 \times -0.0056 \times t^4 + 4 \times 0.0886 \times t^3 - 3 \times 0.4015 \times t^2$$
$$+ 2 \times 0.2859 \times t + 0.8617 + 0.0158$$

Eq. (A4.15)

The two curves of displacement and velocity are shown in Figure A4.7. The first central finite difference method, as seen in Equation (A4.8), returns almost exactly the same curve as that provided by Equation (A4.15) (see Figure A4.8).

Integrative Calculus

Whereas a derivative is the slope of a curve between specified points, an integral is the area under a curve between specified points. The two concepts of derivatives and integrals are related by the **fundamental theorem of calculus**, which allows one to determine that the change in a dependent variable y in a specified time x is

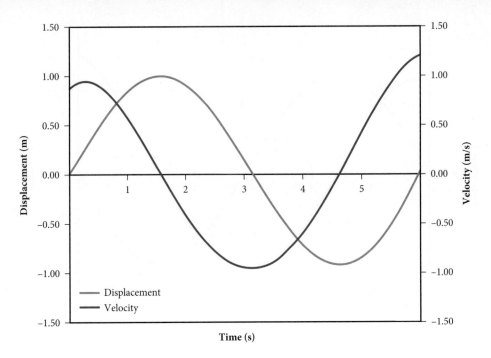

Figure A4.8 The vertical displacement of an oscillating body and the vertical velocity calculated by differentiating the data using the first central difference method.

proportional to the area under the $y = f(x)$ curve during that same specified time. In practical terms, this relationship allows us to determine that if velocity is the first derivative of displacement with respect to time (velocity is the slope of the displacement–time curve), then displacement is the integral of velocity with respect to time (displacement is the area under the velocity–time curve). In one sense, the fundamental theorem of calculus tells us that differentiation and integration are the opposite of each other.

Figure A4.9 shows the instantaneous velocity of a body as it falls under the influence of gravity (the fluid force of drag has been ignored). We can see that the curve has a negative slope throughout. If we were to calculate the gradient of the slope across any time interval, the value would be –9.81. We know that the slope of the velocity–time curve is acceleration (acceleration is the derivative of velocity with respect to time), so we can determine that the acceleration of the body is –9.81 m/s², that associated with the gravitational force. This is determined mathematically using differentiation. By integrating the velocity–time curve, we can determine the displacement undergone by the ball in a given period of time. All we do is calculate the area under the curve during the specified time. For example, the area between $t = 0$ and $t = 1$, denoted by the colored triangle in Figure A4.9, is 4.905; it represents the displacement moved through by the body during this 1-s period. This area is calculated using the **trapezoid rule**:

$$A = 0.5 \times h(a_1 + a_2)$$

Eq. (A4.16)

where A is the area of the trapezoid, h is the height of the trapezoid, and a_1 and a_2 are the sides of the trapezoid. Relating Equation (A4.16) to Figure A4.9, h is

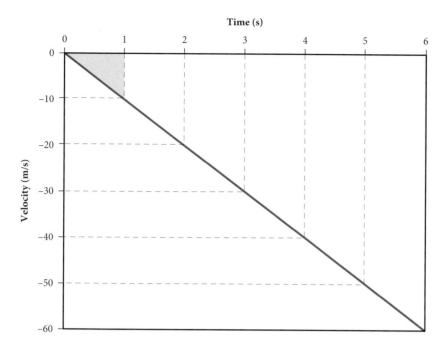

Figure A4.9 The instantaneous vertical velocity of a body falling under the influence of gravity. The dashed lines can be used to determine the vertical velocity after each 1-s period of the analysis. The difference between consecutive horizontal dashed lines corresponds to the acceleration experienced by the body, which remains constant. The area between $t = 0$ and $t = 1$ denoted by the colored triangle represents the displacement undergone by the body in the specified time period.

the change in time, a_1 represents the velocity at time $t = 0$, and a_2 represents the velocity at time $t = 1$. Because the velocities have a negative sense, the area of the trapezoid is actually –4.905, reflecting the negative displacement undergone by the falling body.

From Figure A4.9, we can determine that the velocity at time $t = 1$ is –9.81 m/s. The relationship between displacement and velocity can be established from the following equation of motion:

$$v^2 = 2as \qquad \text{Eq. (A4.17)}$$

where v is velocity, a is the acceleration due to gravity (–9.81 m/s²), and s is the linear displacement. Rearranging Equation (A4.17), we get

$$s = \frac{v^2}{2a} \qquad \text{Eq. (A4.18)}$$

which confirms the displacement of –4.905 m undergone in the period of 1 s. Therefore, integrating the velocity–time curve over the specified time, we get the accumulation of displacement during that time period.

In the notation of integrative calculus, the integral of function $f(x)$ is written as follows:

$$\int_{a}^{b} = f(x)\,dx \qquad\qquad \text{Eq. (A4.19)}$$

where $\int$ is the symbol for the integral, a and b refer to the boundaries of integration, and dx is an infinitesimally small change in x. For the linear displacement calculated in Figure A4.9, we can write the following expression:

$$s = \int_{t_i}^{t_f} v\,dt \qquad\qquad \text{Eq. (A4.20)}$$

where s is the linear displacement of the body, t_i is the time of the start of the integration process, t_f is the time of the end of the integration process, v is the instantaneous linear velocity of the body, and dt is an infinitesimally small change in time. Notice that we can calculate the area under the curve during any time interval specified by t_i and t_f simply by summing consecutive areas. For example, returning to the data shown in Figure A4.9, we can calculate the displacement undergone by the falling body after 5 s:

$$\int_{t=0}^{t=5} v\,dt = -122.63 \qquad\qquad \text{Eq. (A4.21)}$$

The displacement of -122.63 m can be confirmed using Equation (A4.18), given that the instantaneous velocity is -49.05 m/s at time $t = 5$.

Various methods can be used to calculate the area under a curve (e.g., Riemann sums, Simpson's approximation, trapezoid rule). All require the summation of infinitely small areas across the specified period of integration, but all differ in the calculation of the infinitely small areas. However, the trapezoid rule is typically used in biomechanical analyses.

Recall from the discussion of differential calculus that if the function that describes a curve is known, then the power rule can be used to calculate the derivative. Given that integrative calculus is the opposite of differential calculus, we can also calculate the integral of a known function by reversing the power rule. For example, consider the following monomial function:

$$f(x) = 2x^4 \qquad\qquad \text{Eq. (A4.22)}$$

In differential calculus, we could use the power rule to establish that the derivative is $8x^3$ as a result of first multiplying the coefficient in the term by the exponent and then reducing the exponent by a value of 1. When we come to calculate the integral of a function, we simply reverse the order in which we perform the operations associated with the power rule. Specifically, to integrate $8x^3$, we first increase the exponent by 1

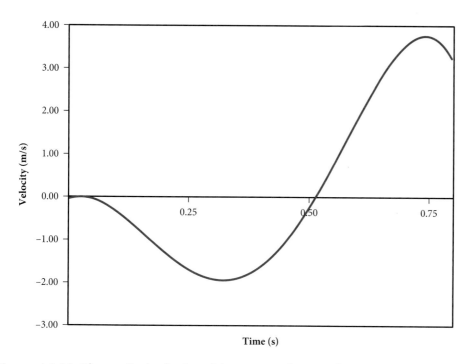

Figure A4.10 The vertical velocity of the center of mass of an athlete performing a countermovement vertical jump.

and then divide the coefficient by the new exponent, such that $8x^3$ becomes $2x^4$. In the notation of integrative calculus, we write

$$\int 8x^3 dx = 2x^4$$

Eq. (A4.23)

The same process can be applied to polynomial functions. For example, Figure A4.10 shows the curve representing the vertical velocity of the center of mass of an athlete performing a countermovement vertical jump. The curve in Figure A4.10 can be approximated by the following polynomial function:

$$v = -71.384 \times t^5 - 83.423 \times t^4 + 229.47 \times t^3 - 93.685$$
$$\times t^2 + 4.016 \times t - 0.0457$$

Eq. (A4.24)

Using the reverse power rule, we can then integrate Equation (A4.24) to obtain the vertical displacement:

$$s = 0.16 \times -71.384 \times t^6 - 0.20 \times 83.423 \times t^5 + 0.25 \times 229.47$$
$$\times t^4 - 0.33 \times 93.685 \times t^3 + 0.50 \times 4.016 \times t^2 - 0.0457$$

Eq. (A4.25)

The coefficients 0.16, 0.20, 0.25, 0.33, and 0.50 that appear in Equation (A4.25) reflect 1/6, 1/5, 1/4, 1/3, and 1/2, respectively, required as part of the reverse power rule.

The curves for both vertical velocity and vertical displacement are shown in Figure A4.11. Notice how similar the vertical displacement curve is to that shown in Figure A4.12, which has been calculated using the trapezoid rule.

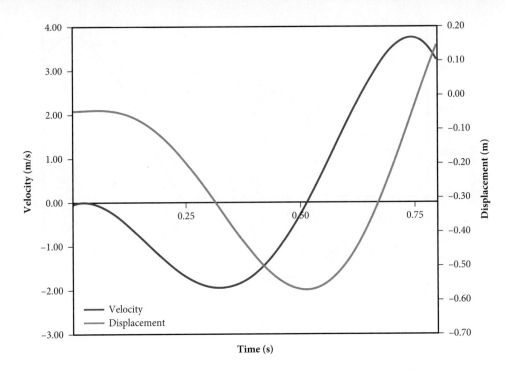

Figure A4.11 The vertical velocity and the vertical displacement of the center of mass of an athlete performing a countermovement vertical jump. The vertical displacement is the integral of vertical velocity calculated from the polynomial function shown in Equation (A4.24) using the reverse power rule.

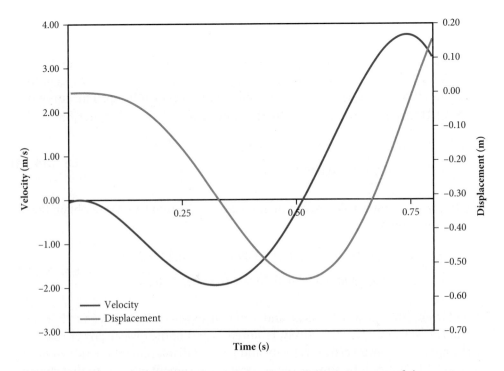

Figure A4.12 The vertical velocity and the vertical displacement of the center of mass of an athlete performing a countermovement vertical jump. The vertical displacement is the integral of vertical velocity calculated using the trapezoid rule.

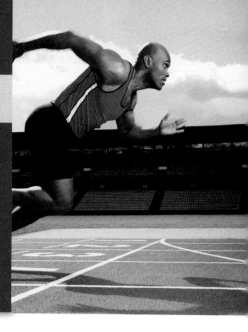

APPENDIX 5

Anatomic Terminology

Key Terms

Anatomic position	Frontal plane	Mediolateral axis	Transverse plane
Anteroposterior axis	Longitudinal axis	Sagittal plane	

The analysis of human movement requires a standardized framework that includes a reference position, planes and axes of rotation, and terminology that is used to describe spatial relations and positions of anatomic structures. The **anatomic position** represents a standardized reference position from which all movements of the human body and the associated body segments are described (Figure A5.1). Three imaginary planes pass through the body in which the body or the body segments move (Figure A5.1): the **frontal plane** (dividing the body into anterior and posterior halves), the **sagittal plane** (dividing the body into left and right halves), and the **transverse plane** (dividing the body into superior and inferior halves). Each anatomic plane has an associated axis of rotation that acts perpendicular to the plane: The **anteroposterior axis** is perpendicular to the frontal plane, the **mediolateral axis** is perpendicular to the sagittal plane, and the **longitudinal axis** is

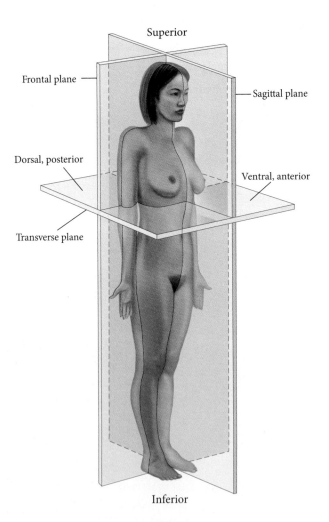

Figure A5.1 The human body in the anatomic position with the anatomic planes of motion shown.

perpendicular to the transverse plane. Rotations in the frontal plane therefore take place about the anteroposterior axis, while rotations in the sagittal plane take place about the mediolateral axis, and rotations in the transverse plane take place about the longitudinal axis.

Table A5.1 presents some commonly used terms that are used to describe the location of anatomic structures and their spatial orientation in relation to the anatomic position. Joint motion terminology used throughout this text is presented in Table A5.2.

Table A5.1
Terminology Used to Describe the Location and Spatial Relations of Anatomic Structures in Relation to the Anatomic Position

Term	Definition
Anterior	The front of the body; ventral
Posterior	The back of the body; dorsal
Superficial	Located close to or on the body surface
Deep	Below the surface
Proximal	Closer to any reference point
Distal	Farther from any reference point
Superior	Toward the head; higher (cephalic)
Inferior	Away from the head; lower (caudal)
Medial	Toward the midline of the body
Lateral	Away from the midline of the body
Ipsilateral	On the same side
Contralateral	On the opposite side
Unilateral	One side
Bilateral	Both sides
Prone	Lying face down
Supine	Lying face up
Valgus	Distal segment of a joint deviates laterally
Varus	Distal segment of a joint deviates medially
Arm	The segment from the shoulder joint to the elbow joint
Forearm	The segment from the elbow joint to the wrist joint
Thigh	The segment from the hip joint to the knee joint
Leg	The segment from the knee joint to the ankle joint

Reproduced from American College of Sports Medicine. *ACSM's Resources for the Personal Trainer,* 4th ed. Baltimore: Lippincott Williams & Wilkins, 2014; 109–176.

Table A5.2
Joint Motion Terminology

Term	Description	Example Exercises
Flexion	Movement resulting in a decrease in joint angle The segment rotates in the sagittal plane	Shoulder joint: upward movement of the barbell during a bench press Elbow joint: upward movement of the dumbbell during a biceps curl Hip joint: the descent during a squat Knee joint: the descent during a squat
Extension	Movement resulting in an increase in joint angle The segment rotates in the sagittal plane	Shoulder joint: downward movement of the barbell during a bench press Elbow joint: downward movement of the dumbbell during a biceps curl Hip joint: the ascent during a squat Knee joint: the ascent during a squat
Abduction	Movement away from the midline of the body The segment rotates in the frontal plane	Shoulder joint: upward movement of the bar during a latissimus pull-down exercise Hip joint: movement of the thigh away from the body during a side-lunge exercise
Adduction	Movement toward the midline of the body The segment rotates in the frontal plane	Shoulder joint: downward movement of the bar during a latissimus pull-down exercise Hip joint: movement of the thigh toward the body during a side-lunge exercise

Table A5.2 (continued)

Term	Description	Example Exercises
Internal rotation	Rotation toward the midline of the body The segment rotates in the transverse plane	Shoulder joint: movement of the hand toward the body during a cable internal row Hip joint: rotation of the hip of the back foot during the backswing of a golf swing
External rotation	Rotation away from the midline of the body The segment rotates in the transverse plane	Shoulder joint: movement of the hand away from the body during a cable internal row Hip joint: rotation of the hip of the back foot during the downswing of a golf swing
Pronation*	Rotation of the radius on the ulna resulting in the hand moving from the palm-up to the palm-down position The forearm rotates in the transverse plane	Radioulnar joint: rotation of the dumbbell from the anatomic position to begin a hammer curl
Supination†	Rotation of the radius on the ulna resulting in the hand moving from the palm-down to the palm-up position The forearm rotates in the transverse plane	Radioulnar joint: opposite to above
Dorsiflexion	Movement of the ankle joint resulting in a decrease in joint angle The foot rotates in the sagittal plane‡	Ankle joint: the descent during a squat
Plantarflexion	Movement of the ankle joint resulting in an increase in joint angle The foot rotates in the sagittal plane ‡	Ankle joint: the ascent during a squat
Horizontal abduction	Movement of the arm in the transverse plane away from the midline of the body	Shoulder joint: downward movement of the barbell during a bench press

(continues)

Table A5.2 *(continued)*
Joint Motion Terminology

Term	Description	Example Exercises
Horizontal adduction	Movement of the arm in the transverse plane toward the midline of the body	Shoulder joint: upward movement of the barbell during a bench press
Elevation	Upward or superior movement of the scapula	Shoulder girdle: upward movement during shoulder-shrug exercises
Depression	Downward or inferior movement of the scapula	Shoulder girdle: downward movement during shoulder-shrug exercises
Upward rotation	Rotating the scapula so that the glenoid fossa moves upward The shoulder girdle rotates in the frontal plane	Shoulder girdle: grasping the bar to begin a latissimus pull-down exercise
Downward rotation	Rotating the scapula so that the glenoid fossa moves downward The shoulder girdle rotates in the frontal plane	Shoulder girdle: pulling the bar down during a latissimus pull-down exercise

*Pronation also occurs at the ankle as a combination of ankle dorsiflexion, subtalar eversion, and forefoot abduction.

†Supination also occurs at the ankle as a combination of ankle plantarflexion, subtalar inversion, and forefoot adduction.

‡ Because the foot is fixed against the floor during movements such as the squat, it appears that the leg rotates in the sagittal plane.

Reproduced from Moir, G., & Bladen, T. L. (2011). Anatomy, kinesiology, and biomechanics for group exercise instructors. In G. DeSimone (Ed.), *ACSM's resources for the group exercise instructor* (pp. 198–225). Philadelphia, PA: Lippincott, Williams & Wilkins.

Resources for Practitioners: Academic Journals

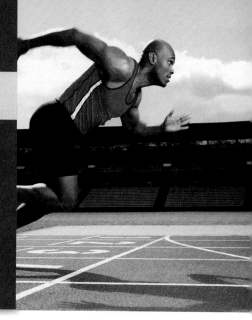

Key Term

Level of evidence

The search for available evidence has been promoted in the application of an evidence-based approach to strength and conditioning, which is defined as a systematic approach to training based on the current best evidence from peer-reviewed research and professional reasoning (English, Amonette, Graham, & Spiering, 2012). There are approximately 130 academic journals in which research relating to sport and exercise science is published annually. The influence and importance of these academic journals are often determined from a metric known as the Impact Factor. However, inherent biases in this measure preclude its use in establishing the quality of a given research article published in a given journal. As a consequence, the practitioner must be able to critique each research article on an individual basis.

The Journal Impact Factor

The Impact Factor (IF) was developed by Thomson Reuters to provide a quantitative means of evaluating and comparing journals. It is calculated by dividing the number of citations from a given journal by the total number of articles that are citable in the journal during a given time period (typically two years). For example, an IF of 2 for a journal indicates that the "average article" within that particular journal was cited twice annually. As such, the IF provides a measure of the relative importance and influence of a journal within a given field (indeed, not all journals qualify for an IF). However, the IF is not without criticism. For example, it has been criticized for its inability to distinguish different shapes of citation distribution curves given the metric relating to the "average article" within a given journal, the inherent bias in the measure caused by the publication of review articles, the influence of the size of the scientific field on the measure, the manipulation of the measure caused by editorial practices such as self-citations, and the lack of clarification as to what determines a "citable" article (Blow, 2014; Misteli, 2013; *PLoS Medicine* editors, 2006; Yang & Zhang, 2013). Use of the IF also leads to the erroneous assumption that the frequency of citations corresponds to the "quality" of the articles published within a given journal. Despite these criticisms, the IF remains an often-used measure to evaluate the importance and influence of a journal within a scientific field.

Table A6.1 lists 22 journals pertinent to the areas of strength and conditioning, biomechanics, and skill acquisition, along with their 2013 IF and the website address for each.

Table A6.1
Impact Factors and Website Addresses for 22 Journals Pertinent to the Areas of Strength and Conditioning, Biomechanics, and Skill Acquisition

Journal	Impact Factor*	Website Address
British Journal of Sports Medicine	3.7	http://bjsm.bmj.com/
European Journal of Applied Physiology	2.7	http://www.springer.com/biomed/human+physiology/journal/421
European Journal of Sport Science	1.2	http://www.tandfonline.com/toc/tejs20/current#
Exercise and Sport Sciences Reviews	5.3	http://journals.lww.com/acsm-essr/
Human Movement Science	2.1	http://www.journals.elsevier.com/human-movement-science/
International Journal of Sports Physiology and Performance	2.3	http://journals.humankinetics.com/ijspp
International Journal of Sports Science and Coaching	< 1.0	http://www.multi-science.co.uk/sports-science&coaching.htm
Journal of Applied Biomechanics	1.3	http://journals.humankinetics.com/jab
Journal of Applied Physiology	3.5	http://jap.physiology.org/front
Journal of Biomechanics	2.7	http://www.jbiomech.com/
Journal of Motor Behavior	1.0	http://www.tandfonline.com/toc/vjmb20/current#
Journal of Physiology	4.4	http://jp.physoc.org/
Journal of Science and Medicine in Sport	2.9	http://www.jsams.org/
Journal of Sports Sciences	2.1	http://www.tandfonline.com/toc/rjsp20/current#
Journal of Strength and Conditioning Research	1.8	http://journals.lww.com/nsca-jscr/
Medicine and Science in Sports and Exercise	4.5	http://journals.lww.com/acsm-msse/
Motor Control	1.4	http://journals.humankinetics.com/mc
Research Quarterly for Exercise and Sport	1.1	http://www.tandfonline.com/toc/urqe20/current#
Scandinavian Journal of Medicine and Science in Sports	3.2	http://onlinelibrary.wiley.com/journal/10.1111/(ISSN)1600-0838
Sports Biomechanics	< 1.0	http://www.tandfonline.com/toc/rspb20/current#
Sports Medicine	5.2	http://link.springer.com/journal/40279
Strength and Conditioning Journal	< 1.0	http://journals.lww.com/nsca-scj/

Critiquing a Research Article

The IF provides a measure of the influence of a journal within a given field, but does not inform the practitioner about the quality of the manuscripts that are published within the journal; thus the quality of a published manuscript must be determined on an individual basis. The academic journals listed in Table A6.1 require that the manuscripts undergo the scholarly peer-review process prior to publication. This regulatory process is performed by experts within the field of study to ensure the quality and credibility of the research prior to publication. However, assessments of the process have revealed that intentional errors placed within articles are often under-reported by expert reviewers (Godlee, Gale, & Martyn, 1998). Another problem noted with the scholarly peer-review process is publication bias, whereby positive findings are more likely to be favorably reviewed and published more quickly than negative or null findings (Hopewell, Loudon, Clarke, Oxman, & Dickersin, 2009). This issue is important because Bayesian probability would suggest that the more novel and surprising the findings presented in a research article are, the more likely they are to be incorrect (Freedman, 2010). It is therefore necessary for practitioners to have a framework that they can use to critique research articles.

An initial step when critiquing a research article is to identify the **level of evidence** associated with the manuscript. The level of evidence can be established by using a hierarchical rating system, as shown in Table A6.2 (Wright, Swiontkowski, & Heckman, 2003). Although no single research study can be accepted as providing definitive evidence in any situation given that the practitioner is required to synthesize the evidence from a range of sources, notice that the design of the study greatly influences the position of the article within the proposed hierarchy. Indeed, the design of a study represents a potent bias leading to the surprising probability that most published research findings are more likely to be false (Ioannidis, 2005). In relation to the levels of evidence

Table A6.2
A Hierarchical Rating System to Establish the Level of Evidence of Published Research

Level of Evidence	Description
Level I	1. Randomized-controlled trial
	2. Systematic review of Level I randomized-controlled trials
Level II	1. Prospective cohort study
	2. Poor-quality randomized controlled trial (less than 80% follow-up)
	3. Systematic review of Level II studies
Level III	1. Case-control study
	2. Retrospective cohort study
	3. Systematic review of Level III studies
Level IV	Case series (no, or historical, control group)
Level V	Expert opinion

Reproduced from Wright, J. G., Swiontkowski, M. F., & Heckman, J. D. (2003). Introducing levels of evidence to the journal. *Journal of Bone and Joint Surgery, 85*, 1–3; with data from OCEBM Levels of Evidence Working Group. The Oxford 2011 Levels of Evidence. Oxford Centre for Evidence-Based Medicine. http://www.cebm.net/index.aspx?o=5

presented in Table A6.2, it should be noted that randomized-controlled trials are rare in the fields of biomechanics, strength and conditioning, and skill acquisition.

Following the establishment of the level of evidence associated with the research article, the practitioner can use the extensive checklist presented in Table A6.3 as a guide to evaluate the article.

Table A6.3
Guidelines for Evaluating Research Articles

Section of Article	Description of Evaluation Criteria
Title	▪ Is the title concise and understandable? ▪ Does the title accurately reflect the purpose, design, results, and conclusions of the study?
Abstract	▪ Is this a succinct, clear, and comprehensive summary of the main text of the article? ▪ Is there enough detail for the reader to understand the purpose of the study, what was measured, and how the measures were obtained? ▪ Is the content (e.g., data, conclusion) consistent with what is presented in the main text? ▪ Are data or other key information presented here but not in the main text (or vice versa)?
Introduction	▪ Does the Introduction succinctly state what is known about the topic? ▪ Are any important findings from previous studies omitted or misrepresented? ▪ Is the functional, biological, and/or clinical significance of the topic established? ▪ Is the specific experimental question, goal, or aim to be addressed stated? ▪ Are previous experimental observations linked together to establish a formally stated and testable working hypothesis? Does the hypothesis clearly indicate the direction of the postulated effect? ▪ If previous reports have addressed the same topic, are their strengths and limitations described such that the need for further study is established? Is it clear how the experimental approach used in the present study is likely to yield more definitive or unique insight than these previous studies? ▪ Is there explanation/justification for the expected outcomes that are based on scientific principles?
Methods	▪ Are the participants adequately described? ▪ Is the participant population appropriate for the question posed? ▪ Is the number of participants sufficiently large to provide the necessary statistical power to show a difference if it is really present (i.e., preventing a Type II error)? ▪ Will the participant population allow extensive or limited generalizability? ▪ Was the assignment of participants to conditions randomized? ▪ Does the experimental design allow the hypothesis to be tested in a rigorous scientific manner? Is there a more appropriate scientific method that could have been employed? ▪ Do the experimental design and the protocols employed control for all potential confounding factors? ▪ Was each methodology described in sufficient detail for others to replicate the study? If not, do the authors provide an appropriate (i.e., peer-reviewed) reference that would provide such details? ▪ Were the correct variables selected to test the anticipated outcomes? ▪ Are the measurement techniques used sufficiently reliable, precise, and valid? ▪ Is the rationale for making each measurement either obvious or explained? ▪ Have the data been analyzed in an appropriate manner? Were the investigators properly "blinded" in the analysis to eliminate possible bias? ▪ Are the details as to how the data were calculated adequately explained so that they can be confirmed by the reviewer and replicated by future investigators? ▪ Is it clear how the data will be interpreted to either support or refute the hypothesis? ▪ Are the statistical techniques used appropriate for the experimental design? ▪ Are any critical assumptions of the statistical techniques (e.g., independence, homogeneity, normality) violated?

Table A6.3 *(continued)*

Section of Article	Description of Evaluation Criteria
Results	▪ Are the data reported in a clear, concise, and well-organized manner?
	▪ Are the data reported so that the reader can observe the values and a corresponding measure of variability (e.g., standard deviation)?
	▪ Where necessary, are the standard deviations reported for each variable? Is there excessive variability in one or more of the measurements for a particular condition compared to the others?
	▪ Are data presented on any measurement that was not described in the Methods section? Are the data on all of the measurements described in the Methods section presented?
	▪ Have the data been presented in the appropriate units (e.g., absolute unit changes versus percentage changes) or properly adjusted statistically (e.g., when differences in the baseline values could confound the interpretation of the data)?
	▪ Have tables, figures, and text been used effectively?
	▪ Are all the figures and tables needed?
	▪ Are the tables and figures appropriately labeled with the correct units?
	▪ Are any data presented more than once in the same form?
	▪ Do the data seem reasonable from a physiological/biomechanical perspective?
	▪ How do the group differences or responses shown compare with the measurement variability?
Discussion	▪ Are the major new findings of the study clearly described and properly emphasized?
	▪ Are the key conclusions adequately supported by the experimental data?
	▪ Is there any other way to interpret and/or explain the data other than that suggested by the authors?
	▪ Is the significance of the present results described? Is it clear how the findings extend previous knowledge in a meaningful way?
	▪ Are important experimental observations from previous reports described in the context of the present results?
	▪ Are the justifications for the anticipated outcomes presented in the Discussion the same as those presented in the Introduction?
	▪ Do the authors support their statements with appropriate references?
	▪ Do the authors discuss their data in a manner that provides insight beyond that presented in previous sections?
	▪ Are the unique aspects and other experimental strengths of the study properly highlighted?
	▪ Are the important experimental limitations of the study described so that the reader will be able to interpret the findings appropriately?
	▪ Do the authors make suggestions as to how the results of their study need to be extended in the future to learn more the issue in question?
	▪ Are recommendations made to extend the results of the study in future research efforts?
	▪ Are the results generalized within the boundaries of the outcomes reported and participants used?
General	▪ Is the paper well written, properly organized, and easy to follow?
	▪ Is the information presented in an open-minded and objective manner?
	▪ Is there significant conflict of financial of scientific interest?

Reproduced from Seals, D. R., & Tanaka, H. (2000). Manuscript peer review: A helpful checklist for students and novice referees. *Advances in Physiology Education, 23*, 52–58; Simpson, K. (2008). Reviewing an original research manuscript for the International Journal of Exercise Science: A guide for students and professionals. *International Journal of Exercise Science, 1*, 43–49.

References

Blow, N. S. (2014). Should we eliminate the Impact Factor? *BioTechniques, 56*, 105.

English, K. L., Amonette, W. E., Graham, M., & Spiering, B. A. (2012). What is "evidence-based" strength and conditioning? *Strength and Conditioning Journal, 34*, 19–24.

Freedman, D. H. (2010). *Wrong*. New York, NY: Little, Brown.

Godlee, F., Gale, C. R., & Martyn, C. N. (1998). Effect on the quality of peer review of blinding reviewers and asking them to sign their reports. *Journal of the American Medical Association, 280*, 237–240.

Hopewell, S., Loudon, K., Clarke, M. J., Oxman, A. D., & Dickersin, K. (2009). Publication bias in clinical trials due to statistical significance or direction of trial results. *Cochrane Data System Reviews, 1*. doi: 10.1002/14651858.MR000006.pub3

Ioannidis, J. P. (2005). Why most published research findings are false. *PLoS Medicine, 2*, e124. doi: 10.1371/journal.pmed.0020124

Misteli, T. (2013). Eliminating the impact of the Impact Factor. *Journal of Cell Biology, 201*, 651–652.

PLoS Medicine editors. (2006). The Impact Factor game. *PLoS Medicine, 3*, e291.

Wright, J. G., Swiontkowski, M. F., & Heckman, J. D. (2003). Introducing levels of evidence to the journal. *Journal of Bone and Joint Surgery, 85*, 1–3.

Yang, Z.-G., & Zhang, C.-T. (2013). A proposal for a novel impact factor as an alternative to the JCR Impact Factor. *Scientific Reports, 3*, 3410. doi: 10.1038/srep03410

Resources for the Practitioner: Useful Websites

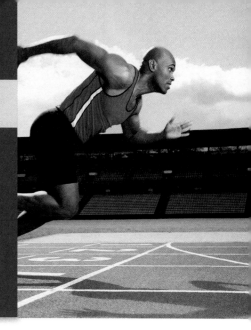

Table A7.1 contains the website addresses for professional organizations and resources for searching and locating research relevant to strength and conditioning, biomechanics, and skill acquisition. The website addresses for companies that manufacture products for the assessment and training of athletes are presented in Table A7.2.

Table A7.1

Website Addresses for Professional Organizations and Resources for Searching and Locating Research Relevant to Strength and Conditioning, Biomechanics, and Skill Acquisition

Organization	Description	Website Address
American College of Sports Medicine (ACSM)	ACSM is the world's largest sports medicine and exercise science organization. The website contains information about ACSM's publications (including *Medicine and Science in Sports and Exercise* and *Exercise and Sport Sciences Reviews*) and educational information on a variety of topics. Membership and certification information is also provided.	http://acsm.org/
American Society of Biomechanics	The American Society of Biomechanics was founded to encourage and foster the exchange of information and ideas among biomechanists working in different disciplines (biological sciences, exercise and sports science, health sciences, ergonomics and human factors, and engineering and applied science) and to facilitate the development of biomechanics as a basic and applied science. The website contains information about conferences and biomechanics degree programs. Membership information is also provided.	http://www.asb-biomech .org/
Australian and New Zealand Society of Biomechanics	The Australian and New Zealand Society of Biomechanics was founded to encourage the exchange of information and ideas among biomechanists working in Australia and New Zealand. The website contains information about conferences and membership information.	http://www.anzsb.asn.au/
Australian Strength and Conditioning Association (ASCA)	ASCA was founded to oversee the professional development of strength and conditioning coaches in Australia. The website contains information about ASCA's publication (*Journal of Australian Strength and Conditioning*) and educational information. Membership and certification information is also provided.	https://www .strengthandconditioning .org/
British Association of Sport and Exercise Sciences (BASES)	BASES was founded to oversee the professional development of sport and exercise scientists in the United Kingdom. The website contains information about BASES's publications (*The Sport and Exercise Scientist*, *Journal of Applied Case Studies in Sport and Exercise Sciences*) and educational information on a variety of topics. Membership and certification information is also provided.	http://www.bases.org.uk/
Canadian Society for Biomechanics	The Canadian Society for Biomechanics was founded to foster research and the interchange of information on the biomechanics of human physical activity. The website contains information about conferences and biomechanics degree programs. Membership information is also provided.	http://www.health .uottawa.ca/biomech/csb/
European College of Sport Science (ECSS)	ECSS was founded to promote science and research, with special attention to the interdisciplinary fields of sport science and sports medicine. The website contains information about ECSS's publication (*European Journal of Sport Science*) and educational information on a variety of topics. Membership information is also provided.	http://sport-science.org/

Table A7.1 (continued)

Organization	Description	Website Address
European Society of Biomechanics	The European Society of Biomechanics was founded to encourage research, disseminate knowledge, and promote progress in biomechanics. The website contains information about conferences and membership information.	http://www.esbiomech.org/
Google Scholar	Google Scholar is a resource for searching and locating research.	http://scholar.google.com/
International Society of Biomechanics	The International Society of Biomechanics was founded to promote the study of all areas of biomechanics at the international level, with special emphasis given to the biomechanics of human movement. The website contains information about conferences and educational programs. Membership information is also provided.	http://isbweb.org/
International Society of Biomechanics in Sport	The International Society of Biomechanics in Sport was founded to provide a forum for the exchange of ideas among sports biomechanics researchers, coaches, and teachers and to bridge the gap between researchers and practitioners. The website contains information about the organization's journal (*Sports Biomechanics*) as well as information regarding conferences and membership.	http://www.isbs.org/
International Society of Motor Control	The International Society of Motor Control was founded to promote basic and applied research in the area of control of movements in biological systems. The website contains information about conferences and membership.	http://i-s-m-c.org/
National Strength and Conditioning Association	The National Strength and Conditioning Association promotes research and education for strength and conditioning professionals. The website contains information about the organization's publications (including *Journal of Strength and Conditioning Research* and *Strength and Conditioning Journal*) and educational information on a variety of topics. Membership and certification information is also provided.	http://www.nsca.com/
Ovid	Ovid is a resource for searching and locating academic journals.	http://www.ovid.com/
PubMed	PubMed is a resource for searching and locating research.	http://www.ncbi.nlm.nih.gov/
Sportscience	Sportscience is a peer-reviewed website for research in sport science. It contains information relating to training, testing and technology, statistics, and nutrition.	http://www.sportsci.org/
Sport Information Resource Centre	The Sport Information Resource Centre is a resource for searching and locating research.	http://www.sirc.ca/
U.K. Strength and Conditioning Association	The U.K. Strength and Conditioning Association was founded to establish and maintain high professional standards for U.K. strength and conditioning practitioners, and to promote and disseminate good practice, knowledge, and research appropriate to strength and conditioning practitioners. The website contains information about the organization's publication (*Professional Strength and Conditioning*) and educational information on a variety of topics. Membership and certification information is also provided.	http://www.uksca.org.uk/uksca/

Table A7.2
Website Addresses for Companies That Manufacture Products for the Assessment and Training of Athletes

Company	Overview of Products	Website Address
Actigraph	Accelerometer technology	http://www.actigraphcorp.com/
AMTI	Force sensor technology for force plates and other applications	http://www.amti.biz/
Bertec	Force sensor technology for force plates and other applications	http://bertec.com/
Brower Timing	Photocell technology for timing gates and vertical jump tests	http://www.browertiming.com/
Catapult Sports	Global Positioning System technology for movement analysis	http://www.catapultsports.com
Dartfish	Motion analysis technology	http://www.dartfish.com
Delsys	Electromyographic sensors and accelerometers	http://www.delsys.com/
GPSports	Global Positioning System technology for movement analysis	http://www.gpsports.com
Innervations	Force plates, force treadmills, linear position transducers, and photocell technologies	http://www.innervations.com/
Kistler	Force sensor technology for force plates and other applications	http://www.kistler.com/
Motion Analysis Corporation	Motion analysis technology	http://www.motionanalysis.com/
Myotest	Accelerometer technology	http://www.myotest.com/
Noldus	Manual video-based time–motion analysis technology	http://www.noldus.com
Noraxon	Electromyographic and force sensors, pressure, and motion analysis technologies	http://www.noraxon.com/
Optojump	Photocell technology for timing gates, vertical jump tests, and stride analyses	http://www.optojump.com/
Prozone	Automated video-based time–motion analysis technology	http://www.prozonesports.com
Qualisys	Motion analysis technology	http://www.qualisys.com/
RS Scan	Pressure sensor technology for gait analysis	http://www.rsscan.co.uk/
Siliconcoach	Motion analysis technology	http://www.siliconcoach.com
Sportstec	Manual video-based time–motion analysis technology	http://www.sportstec.com
Swift Performance Equipment	Photocell technology for timing gates	http://www.spe.com.au/
Tekscan	Pressure sensor technology for gait analysis	http://www.tekscan.com/
Tendo Sports Machines	Linear position transducer technology	http://www.tendosports.com/
Vicon Motion Systems	Motion analysis technology	http://www.vicon.com/

Glossary of Terms

Absolute maximum strength   A measure of maximal muscular strength whereby an electrical stimulus is superimposed upon a maximal voluntary contraction to determine the maximal force of the stimulated muscles. Such protocols provide information about the intrinsic properties of the stimulated muscles.

Absorption phase   A phase during a landing task when the kinetic energy of the center of mass is dissipated. It begins when the athlete first contacts the ground, and it ends when the kinetic energy becomes zero and the athlete's motion is arrested. The absorption phase can be divided into the impact phase (defined as the first 100 ms from initial ground contact) and the stabilization phase (defined as the event from 100 ms after initial ground contact to the lowest vertical position of the center of mass).

Acceleration   The rate of change of velocity; the second derivative of position with respect to time. The SI unit of measurement of linear acceleration is meters per second^2 (m/s^2) and is represented by the symbol a. The SI unit of measurement of angular acceleration is radian per second^2 (rad/s^2) and is represented by the symbol α.

Acceleration phase   In the context of sprint running, the initial phase that is identified by a positive slope of the speed–time curve.

Accelerometer   A device that records the acceleration of a body to which it is attached by converting a mechanical signal (an acceleration) into an electrical signal (a voltage).

Acetyl-coenzyme A (Acetyl-CoA)   A coenzyme that is degraded to carbon dioxide and hydrogen ions in the citric acid cycle as part of oxidative phosphorylation.

Acetylcholine   A neurotransmitter that is released into the synaptic cleft in response to an action potential arriving at the neuromuscular junction during the activation of a skeletal muscle.

Actin   One of three contractile proteins (myofilaments) that are responsible for the tension developed within a sarcomere. The other contractile proteins are myosin and titin.

Action potential   A stimulus used by the central nervous system; it is caused by the movement of ions across an excitable membrane resulting in a change in the electrical potential.

Action-scaled affordances   Affordances that represent the relation between the perception of an athlete's physical capabilities and the possibility for movement.

Active leg motion   The act of reducing the forward velocity of the foot and pulling the leg back prior to touchdown, caused by the activation of the hamstrings and gluteus maximus, when sprinting at maximal speed to reduce the magnitude of the braking force during stance.

Active methods   In the context of warm-up routines, activities that involve volitional movements performed by the athlete.

Adaptation   The process of attaining a new functional capacity in response to the exposure to an exercise stimulus that results in performance enhancements during specific movement tasks. The adaptation process is typically underpinned by cellular and molecular responses, although other factors can contribute to the enhanced performance as a result of adaptation. *See also* Perceptual attunement.

Adenosine-5′-triphosphate (ATP)   The molecule that is hydrolyzed to provide the chemical energy required to sustain the physiological functioning of the skeletal muscles during exercise.

Adenylate kinase reaction   A reversible chemical reaction in which two adenosine diphosphate molecules produce adenosine triphosphate and adenosine monophosphate. The reaction is catalyzed by the adenylate kinase enzyme. The adenylate kinase reaction is one of three reactions that are collectively referred to as the phosphagen system, with the others being the creatine kinase reaction and the AMP deaminase reaction.

Aerial phase   In the context of a running step, the event when the athlete is airborne between takeoff and the next contralateral touchdown.

Afferent   In reference to action potentials, the transmission of the action potential from a receptor or sensory organ (e.g., muscle spindle) toward the central nervous system.

Affordance   An opportunity for movement provided by the environment as perceived by the performer. Affordances are detected by the performer so as to select an appropriate movement solution to achieve the goal of the task. Affordances, which are task specific and learned through the process of perceptual attunement, are central to ecological psychology.

Agility   A rapid whole-body movement with a change of velocity or a change of direction in response to a sport-specific stimulus in which the required movement of the athlete to accomplish the task is unplanned. Although agility performance is influenced by change of direction ability and straight-line sprinting ability, the decision-making component in agility tasks differentiates athletes from different performance levels. Small-sided games are more effective at developing agility performance in field-sport athletes than change of direction drills, as the former promote decision making based on sport-specific information.

Agonist   A muscle whose action produces a specific motion observed at a joint.

Agonist–antagonist pairs   Pairs of resistance training exercises that alternate between the agonist and the antagonist muscles about a given joint (e.g., alternating between sets of bench pulls and bench press). Agonist–antagonist pairs provide a time-efficient method of developing muscular strength and power output.

Agonist–contract technique   A proprioceptive neuromuscular facilitation stretching technique requiring that a joint be moved to a predetermined range of motion before the opposing muscle (the agonist of the joint motion) is activated by the participant while the joint is slowly moved further.

Alactic glycolysis   Glycolysis ending with pyruvate being converted to acetyl-coenzyme A.

Allometric scaling   A method of normalization that is predicated upon geometric similarity—that is, the notion that all human bodies have the same shape, differing only in size. The allometric scaling parameter of body mass$^{2/3}$ has been proposed to normalize measures of muscular strength.

α-motoneuron   A nerve cell originating in the ventral horn of the spinal cord that transmits an action potential to a skeletal muscle during the activation of the muscle.

AMP deaminase reaction   A chemical reaction in which adenosine monophosphate and hydrogen produce inosine monophosphate and ammonium. The reaction is catalyzed by the AMP deaminase enzyme, which maintains the activity of the adenylate kinase reaction in generating ATP. The AMP deaminase reaction is one of three reactions that are collectively referred to as the phosphagen system, with the others being the creatine kinase reaction and the adenylate kinase reaction.

Anatomic cross-sectional area   The area of the section of a muscle that reflects the circumference of the muscle.

Anatomic position   A standardized reference position from which all movements of the human body and the associated body segments are described. In the anatomic position, the body is upright with the feet together, the arms hanging at the sides, and the palms facing forward with the fingers extended and the thumbs facing away from the body. This universally accepted reference position is used in kinesiology to describe spatial relations between body segments and to identify orientations of the body segments during specific movements.

Angle–angle diagram   A plot of two joint angles on the same graph. The topological characteristics of angle–angle diagrams reveal information about the coordination of the degrees of freedom during the execution of a motor skill in the event space.

Angular displacement   The change in angular position of a rotating body within an angular reference frame. The SI unit of measurement of angular position is the radian (rad), which is represented by the symbol θ. There are $180/\pi$ degrees in a radian.

Antagonist   A muscle whose action opposes that of the agonist.

Anteroposterior axis   An axis of rotation that is perpendicular to the frontal plane.

Aponeurosis   The extension of the external tendon that runs within a pennate muscle that the muscle fibers innervate.

Assistance exercises   Single-joint resistance training exercises.

Assisted resistance training exercises   Resistance training exercises that allow the athlete to achieve supra-maximal movement velocities through the use of elastic bands attached to the athlete or the load. In contrast to the use of elastic bands in variable resistance training methods, the bands are placed such that they aid the motion of the external load during assisted resistance training exercises.

Assisted sprint training methods   Training methods whereby the motion of the athlete when sprinting is assisted by means of a mechanical winch, elastic bungee, or running downhill.

Atrophy   A decrease in the cross-sectional area of muscle fibers as a result of protein breakdown exceeding protein synthesis.

Attainment of maximal speed phase   In the context of sprint running, the second phase that is characterized by the attainment of maximal speed as identified by the peak in the speed–time curve.

Attentional focus   The location of the sources of information to which an athlete attends during the execution of a motor skill. *See also* External attentional focus; Internal attentional focus.

Attractor state   Stable coordination patterns observed during the execution of a motor skill due to the intrinsic dynamics of the motor system. Attractor states may compete or cooperate with the to-be-learned coordination pattern to satisfy the goal of a movement task, providing an explanation as to why some individuals may learn at different rates compared to others. The transitions between attractor states occur as a consequence of variations in specific control parameters. Attractor states reside in the perceptual-motor workspace.

Augmented eccentric resistance training exercises   Resistance training exercises that involve the completion of both eccentric and concentric muscle actions during the exercise, but in which the eccentric load is made greater than the subsequent concentric load via the removal of some of the load during the concentric phase.

Autogenic inhibition   The reduced excitability of an active or passively stretched muscle as a result of the activation of Ib-inhibitory interneurons associated with Golgi tendon organs.

Axis   An imaginary line of a reference frame along which the position of the body under analysis can be measured.

Axis of rotation   An imaginary line about which a body rotates.

Ballistic resistance training exercises   Resistance training exercises that require the external load to be projected or released at the end of the concentric phase, removing the constraint of ensuring that the momentum of the load is zero at the end of the movement. This allows for the generation of greater force and power compared to non-ballistic exercises.

Basal lamina   An extracellular matrix that connects the endomysium to the sarcolemma of a muscle fiber. Satellite cells are located in the basal lamina of muscle fibers.

β-alanine   An amino acid that limits the rate of carnosine synthesis in skeletal muscle. Supplementation with β-alanine increases muscle carnosine content, thereby increasing the buffering capacity of the muscle.

Beta-oxidation   The first stage of fatty acid catabolism during which fatty acids are broken down to acetyl-coenzyme A.

Bilateral   Any task in which the mechanical output is generated from both limbs acting concomitantly.

Bilateral deficit   A phenomenon whereby the mechanical output from both limbs acting concurrently (bilateral tasks) is less than the sum of the output of the limbs acting separately (unilateral task). The bilateral deficit is likely due to neural inhibition during symmetrical bilateral muscle activation.

Bioenergetics   The processes involved in the energy transfer associated with the metabolic reactions to sustain the physiological functioning of the human motor system.

Biomechanical principles   A series of biomechanical concepts that can guide the selection of critical features to observe in a qualitative analysis of technique.

Biomechanics   The discipline concerned with the application of mechanics to the study of living organisms, whereby the action of forces is studied relative to the anatomic and functional aspects of biological organisms.

Blocked periodization   A form of periodization of resistance training involving specialized mesocycles ("blocks"), each directed at a minimal number of physical capacities that are sequenced such that the adaptations in one mesocycle potentiate the adaptations in the following mesocycle.

Blocked practice   A practice structure in which a single skill is executed.

Body-scaled affordances   Affordances that represent the relation between a measurable dimension of an athlete's body and a property of the environment that determines whether a movement is possible.

Body weight   The force exerted by a body on to a supporting surface. Body weight is the product of the mass of the body and gravitational acceleration and is a distributed force, with the net effect acting at the body's center of mass.

Braking phase   The initial phase of ground contact (stance) associated with running and jumping in which the foot is placed ahead of the center of mass, resulting in the horizontal component of the ground reaction force acting in opposition to the direction of motion of the center of mass. The magnitude of the braking force can be reduced by an active leg motion.

Ca²⁺ calmodulin-dependent kinase/calcineurin   An intracellular signaling pathway that is involved in muscle fiber hypertrophy.

Center of mass   The virtual point about which the mass of the body is evenly distributed. The human body can be reduced to a point–mass system in many biomechanical analyses, with the center of mass becoming the reference for motion and the action of forces external to the body.

Center of pressure   The virtual point on the supporting surface where the resultant ground reaction force acts. When referring to fluid dynamic forces, the center of pressure represents the virtual point where the drag and lift forces act on the body passing through a fluid.

Central difference method   Formulae taken from finite difference calculus that are used in biomechanics to differentiate variables. *See also* First central difference method and Second central difference method.

Central fatigue   Mechanisms of fatigue that are associated with the processes within the central nervous system.

Centripetal force   A force directed toward the center of a curved path followed by a body that is responsible for changing the direction of the velocity vector of the body, thereby keeping it moving along the curved path.

Challenge-point framework   A concept relating to the design of practices for athletes. The challenge-point framework holds that learning is optimized when the learner is appropriately challenged, with too much difficulty in the practice tasks or too little difficulty hindering the learning process. Manipulation of the practice structure, instructions, and feedback can be used to alter the challenge faced by the learner, thereby influencing the learning process.

Chord   A line that touches a curve at two points.

Citric acid cycle   One part of oxidative phosphorylation involving a series of reactions in which acetyl coenzyme A is degraded to carbon dioxide and hydrogen ions. This cycle takes place in the mitochondria and generates the high-energy reducing equivalents NADH and $FADH_2$, which are transported to the electron transport chain.

CK–PCr shuttle   The creatine kinase–phosphocreatine shuttle. The shuttle refers to the movement of creatine (Cr) and phosphocreatine (PCr) within the cytosol, with creatine moving from the sites of adenosine-5′-triphosphate (ATP) consumption to the sites of ATP resynthesis, and with PCr moving in the opposite direction. The role of PCr as a spatial energy buffer can be determined from the CK–PCr shuttle.

Closed motor skill   A motor skill that is performed in a stable and predictable environment.

Cluster sets   In the context of resistance training workouts, the insertion of short rest intervals (20–130 s) between consecutive repetitions so as to ameliorate the decreases in movement velocity and power output caused by fatigue.

Coactivation   The simultaneous activation of an antagonistic pair of muscles about a joint.

Coefficient   A number that acts as a multiplicative factor in a term of a polynomial.

Coefficient of friction   A dimensionless number that is determined by the characteristics of the surfaces of the two bodies in contact, including the relative roughness, hardness, temperature, lubricating material interposed between the surfaces, and relative velocity of the bodies.

Collision   An event in which two or more bodies in motion make contact and exert forces during the time of contact. During an elastic collision, kinetic energy is conserved such that each body may continue in motion following the collision (although the direction of motion may have changed). During an inelastic collision, total energy remains conserved during the collision even if the two bodies adhere to each other and their kinetic energy is dissipated; the energy is transformed from that due to the motion of the bodies to other forms (heat energy, sound energy), but total energy remains conserved.

Complex pairs   In the context of a resistance training workout, the performance of a high-intensity resistance exercise before performing a mechanically similar but lower-intensity exercise following minutes of recovery. These exercise couplings are proposed to elicit postactivation potentiation.

Complex system   Any system that consists of many independent components operating at different structural and functional levels. The human motor system can be regarded as a complex system whose independent components (e.g., limb segments, joints, muscles, motor units) need to be coordinated and controlled to successfully execute the movements required to accomplish the goal of a motor skill.

Compression   A pushing force.

Computerized myotonometer   A device for estimating muscle stiffness by exerting a small constant mechanical force via an indenter probe that moves at a constant speed until a predetermined force is achieved. From the force and tissue depth measurements recorded, the work done by the device on the tissue can be determined, with the work done correlating inversely with tissue stiffness.

Concentric muscle action   A muscle action in which the muscle exerts tension while shortening.

Conservation laws   Laws that can be applied to certain mechanical variables that remain unchanged over the period of analysis under certain mechanical conditions (mainly, the removal of nonconstant external forces such as friction, air resistance, etc.). *See also* Conservation of mechanical energy and Conservation of momentum.

Conservation of mechanical energy   A principle explaining that the sum of the mechanical energy of a body remains conserved when the only forces acting on the body are constant.

Conservation of momentum   A principle explaining that the sum of the momenta of two bodies remains conserved during a collision.

Constraint   A variable that limits the configuration of the motor system, guiding the movements of the performer as he or she executes a motor skill. The constraints that surround the motor system can be categorized as organismic, environmental, and task constraints.

Constraints-led approach   A theoretical approach to explain the coordination and control of movements during the execution of motor skills, which emphasizes the influence constraints associated with the organism, the environment, and the task. It is from the confluence of the constraints acting on the performer that the coordination and control of the movement emerges. *See also* Dynamical systems theory; Ecological psychology.

Contact mat   A device that uses micro switches to record the time between consecutive activations caused by pressure applied to the mat, allowing running speed or jumping height to be calculated.

Contextual interference   A performance disruption generated by performing multiple skills or variations of a skill within the context of practice. The *contextual interference effect* is the learning benefit resulting from performing multiple skills in a high contextual interference practice structure (random practice) rather than performing skills in a low contextual interference structure (blocked practice).

Continuous motor skill   A motor skill that has an arbitrary beginning and ending.

Continuous relative phase   A method of quantifying the coordination between two joints or body segments calculated as the difference between the phase angle associated with the proximal joint/segment and that associated with the distal joint/segment.

Contract–relax technique   A proprioceptive neuromuscular facilitation stretching technique requiring that a joint be moved to a predetermined range of motion before the participant performs an isometric action of the target muscle (that being stretched), usually maximally, before the joint is slowly moved further.

Control   The ability of an athlete to vary the parameters of a coordination pattern in relation to the specific task constraints during the execution of motor skills.

Control parameter   A variable that moves the motor system through different states of coordination, although it does not contain any specific information regarding the organization of the system. Control parameters can be considered as constraints surrounding the motor system.

Control space   The three-dimensional space in which a body segment is located during a motor skill. *See also* Event space and State space.

Coordination   The patterning of body and limb motions relative to the patterning of environmental objects and events. The topological characteristics of coordination patterns are revealed in angle–angle diagrams and phase portraits.

Coordinative structure   A temporary organization of the available degrees of freedom during the execution of a motor skill that emerges through the process of self-organization under constraint. Coordinative structures are intentional, being influenced by the goal of the specific motor skill; soft-assembled, existing only until the goal of the motor skill is achieved; and autonomous, emerging from the intrinsic dynamics of the performer and the constraints imposed on the motor system.

Core exercises   Multijoint resistance training exercises.

Countermovement An initial downward movement of the center of mass prior to the propulsive phase of a jump. A countermovement allows for the involvement of the stretch–shortening cycle during the execution of a jump.

Countermovement vertical jump A vertical jump that involves a countermovement prior to takeoff. Countermovement jumps are considered slow stretch–shortening cycle tasks.

Creatine kinase reaction A reversible chemical reaction in which phosphocreatine, adenosine diphosphate, and hydrogen produce adenosine triphosphate and creatine. The reaction is catalyzed by the creatine kinase enzyme. The creatine kinase reaction is one of three reactions that are collectively referred to as the phosphagen system, with the others being the adenylate kinase reaction and the AMP deaminase reaction.

Creep Viscoelastic behavior of a material whereby the strain experienced by the material increases over time in response to the application of a constant load.

Critical features In the context of a motor skill, those features that influence performance. Critical features are revealed through predictive, qualitative, and quantitative methods as part of a technique analysis.

Crossbridge The globular head of the myosin protein.

Damped free oscillation A technique for measuring the passive stiffness of a musculotendinous unit in which a perturbing force is manually applied to the limb, resulting in an oscillation that decays over time. A stiffer musculotendinous unit will produce a greater initial acceleration or force in response to the perturbing force and will oscillate at a higher frequency.

Degeneracy The process whereby the coordination of different independent components (degrees of freedom) of the motor system can result in the same movements being produced. Degeneracy is a property of complex systems and confers adaptability and flexibility on the human motor system, allowing the goal of movement tasks to be achieved in the face of changing environmental conditions and/or characteristics of the performer.

Degree of freedom Each independent component of the human motor system (e.g., limb segments, joints, muscles, motor units) that can be organized in many different ways during goal-directed movements. Controlling the large number of degrees of freedom when acquiring motor skills is known as the "degrees of freedom problem."

Degrees of freedom problem A problem faced by the human motor system when learning motor skills related to how the many degrees of freedom are coordinated and controlled during goal-directed movements.

Depolarization The act of the electrical potential associated with an excitable membrane (i.e., muscle fiber membrane, motoneuron membrane) becoming less negative as a result of the movement of Na^+ during the generation of an action potential.

Deterministic model A method of identifying the critical features of a motor skill as part of a qualitative analysis. Deterministic models require that the analyst first establish the outcome of the motor skill and then identify the factors that determine the outcome. These factors are placed in a hierarchy, such that each factor is determined by those factors appearing immediately below it either by addition or by a biomechanical principle.

Diathermy The use of high-frequency electromagnetic waves to elicit a thermal response in biologic tissue. Short-wave diathermy techniques typically use a frequency of approximately 27 MHz with a wavelength of 11 m, while microwave diathermy employs shorter wavelengths applied at much higher frequencies. Diathermy can be used as a passive heating method to increase intramuscular temperature as part of a warm-up, although its effectiveness relative to physical performance remains to be demonstrated.

Differential calculus A division of calculus that is used to calculate the rate of change in a variable with respect to another variable to which it has a functional relationship.

Differential learning A form of practice schedule that emphasizes the variability in an athlete's natural movements by deliberately precluding repetitions of the same movements. The increased variability in coordination during the acquisition of skilled movement provides greater information to the learner about his or her capabilities by exploring a greater region of the perceptual-motor workspace.

Differentiation A mathematical technique whereby the rate of change in one variable is expressed with respect to the change in another variable to which it has a functional relationship. Typically in biomechanics, the central difference method is used in the differentiation process.

Dihydropyridine receptors Receptors located on the transverse tubules that mediate the release of Ca^{2+} from the sarcoplasmic reticulum in response to an action potential during the activation of a skeletal muscle. Dihydropyridine receptors interact with ryanodine receptors located on the sarcoplasmic reticulum.

Direct perception   A major tenet of ecological psychology whereby patterns of ambient energy found in the environment (e.g., light, sound) are attended to directly by the performer to provide information that can guide movement.

Discharge doublets   Consecutive action potentials with an interspike interval of less than 10 ms. They are often observed during the periods of high-rate coding at the onset of voluntary contraction, and it is likely that they are also responsible for achieving high rates of force development.

Discrete motor skill   A motor skill that has a specified beginning and ending.

Distance advantage   In the context of a lever system, a mechanical advantage less than 1. This results in the linear distance moved through by the point of application of the external (resistance) force being amplified.

Double-split routine   In the context of a resistance training workout, a program of comprising two workouts per training day, each emphasizing different muscle groups. These routines can increase training frequency.

Downhill sprinting   A form of sprint training in which the athlete sprints down an incline. Downhill sprinting produces greater sprinting speeds than those attained on a horizontal surface due to the gravitational force propelling the athlete forward.

Drop jump   A vertical jump in which the athlete drops from a height prior to landing and then jumps for maximal height. Drops jumps are considered fast stretch–shortening cycle tasks.

Duration   In the context of an exercise stimulus, the length of the work periods. The combination of duration and frequency provide the volume of the exercise stimulus.

Dynamical systems theory   An interdisciplinary framework used to describe and examine different types of systems (i.e., biological, ecological, social) that are in a constant state of flux, changing and evolving over time. Principles derived from dynamical systems theory that have been used to explain the coordination and control of movement during the execution of motor skills include attractor states, coordinative structures, self-organization, stability, control parameters, and order parameters.

Dynamic flexibility   A form of flexibility that is related to the passive resistance to the range of motion available about a joint or group of joints.

Dynamic stretching   Stretching techniques that involve elongating the target muscle group in a controlled manner through the active range of motion before returning to its original length. The elongated position is not held for any substantial time.

Eccentric muscle action   A muscle action where the muscle exerts tension while lengthening.

Eccentric utilization ratio   A measure of the ability of an athlete to utilize the stretch–shortening ratio, calculated as the difference in the height achieved during a countermovement vertical jump compared to that achieved during a static vertical jump.

Ecological psychology   A school of psychology that emphasizes the concept of direct perception, whereby patterns of ambient energy found in the environment are attended to directly by the performer to provide information that can guide movement; this is known as perception–action coupling. Ecological psychology promotes the notion that reciprocity between movements and the information found within the environment is such that the information constrains the observed movements while the movement reveals further information within the environment. The concept of affordances is central to the coupling between the direct perception of environmental information and the subsequent movement.

Effective mass   A variable that determines the rate at which momentum is transferred between bodies involved in a collision. The effective mass reflects the proportion of mass that is arrested immediately during the collision. If a rigid body is involved in the collision, then the effective mass is equal to the mass of the body. In contrast, if the body is nonrigid—such as the human body, which comprises segments that are able to displace relative to one another about joints—then the effective mass can be reduced during the collision. During the absorption phase of a landing task, an athlete is able to flex the joints of the lower body, reducing the effective mass such that the magnitude of the ground reaction force is attenuated, thereby minimizing the risk of injury.

Effective mechanical advantage   The ratio of the external force (e.g., ground reaction force) acting on a joint to the muscular forces at the joint.

Efficiency   The ratio of mechanical work to the energy expenditure during a movement.

Elastin   A microfibrillar protein found in tendon that is responsible for the elasticity of the tissue.

Electromechanical delay   The delay between the activation of a muscle and the detection of the tensile force. Typically, this delay ranges between 25 ms and 100 ms.

Electromyography   A technique for analyzing the motor unit action potentials associated with the activation of skeletal muscles. The amplitude and the frequency of the electromyographic signal provide important information.

Electron transport chain   One part of oxidative phosphorylation, in which the energy generated in the transfer of the electrons from hydrogen ions is conserved as chemical potential energy in the form of ATP. The electrons are transported to the electron transport chain by the high-energy reducing equivalents NADH and $FADH_2$.

Endomysium   A connective tissue sheath that surrounds each muscle fiber within a skeletal muscle.

Endotenon   A connective tissue layer that surrounds bundles of collagen fibers in a tendon. Blood vessels and nerves are contained within the endotenon.

End-plate potential   Depolarization of the membrane of a muscle fiber at the postsynaptic terminals caused by the influx of Na^+ as a result of the action of the neurotransmitter acetylcholine during the activation of a skeletal muscle. An end-plate potential generates a muscle fiber action potential.

Energy, mechanical   The capacity of a body to do mechanical work (symbol E). The SI unit of measurement of mechanical energy is the joule (J). *See also* Gravitational potential energy; Kinetic energy; Strain potential energy.

Energy expenditure   The total amount of energy expended by an athlete.

Enthesis   The junction between a tendon and a bone. The tensile forces at the enthesis have been proposed to be four times greater than those experienced in other regions of a tendon.

Environmental constraints   Constraints to the coordination and control of movements that are associated with the physical properties of the environment in which the athlete is performing as well as societal expectations.

Epimysium   A connective tissue sheath that surrounds groups of fascicles within a skeletal muscle.

Epitenon   A connective tissue layer below the paratenon in tendons. The paratenon and the epitenon serve to reduce friction between the adjacent tissues.

Equations of motion   A series of equations that express the relationships between the kinematic variables of position, velocity, and acceleration.

Equilibrium potential   The resting membrane potential required to maintain the concentrations of ions on either side of the membrane if it were freely permeable to the specific ion. The equilibrium potential occurs when the electrical and chemical forces are equal and there is no movement of the specific ion across the membrane. The equilibrium potential for Na^+ is 71 mV, while that for K^+ is -95 mV.

Event space   A control space used when describing coordination in motor skills where the position of a body segment or joint angle is specified at any given time during the activity. Event space is useful for tasks in which time is considered a constraint. *See also* Angle–angle diagram.

Excitation–contraction coupling   The processes involved in the conversion of an α-motoneuron action potential into the development of muscular tension.

Excitation–transcription coupling   The processes involved in the conversion of an α-motoneuron action potential into the transcription of specific cellular proteins in response to different modes of exercise.

Explicit learning   Learning that occurs when the athlete is consciously aware of the to-be-learned coordination pattern. It results in conscious control of movement that can be easily perturbed.

Explosive muscular strength   An index of muscular strength that is characterized by high rates of force development and can be measured during both dynamic and isometric tasks.

Exponent   A mathematical operation that denotes the repeated multiplication of a base within a specific term.

External attentional focus   A form of attentional focus in which the athlete focuses on variables external to the body and the outcome of the movement. An external attentional focus precludes the constraint imposed on the movement from adopting an internal attentional focus that would possibly interfere with the natural self-organizing properties associated with the motor system.

Extrafusal fiber   *See* Muscle fiber.

Faded feedback   A form of feedback in which the frequency of the provision of information to the learner after the performance of a motor skill is gradually reduced ("faded") during practice.

Fascicle   A bundle of muscle fibers within a skeletal muscle that is contained within a connective tissue sheath known as the perimysium.

Fatigue   A reversible decline in the mechanical output associated with contractile activity that is marked by a progressive reduction in the contractile response of the active muscle. The mechanisms of fatigue can be categorized as those associated with the central nervous system (central fatigue) and those associated directly with the motor units themselves (peripheral fatigue).

Feedback   Information provided to the learner after the performance of a motor skill relating to his or her performance. Typically, the athlete will receive information about the outcome of the movement relative to the goal of the motor skill after each repetition, known as knowledge of results. Other types of feedback can be provided to the performer that the individual would not normally receive simply by completing the movement, such as verbal feedback or observing a video of the performer's movement following the completion of the motor skill, known as knowledge of performance.

Fine motor skill   A motor skill that involves small muscle groups.

First central difference   The finite difference that appears as the numerator in the equation associated with the first central difference method.

First central difference method   A formula taken from finite difference calculus that returns the first derivative of a variable with respect to another variable to which it has a functional relationship.

Flexibility   The range of motion available at a joint or group of joints without inducing an injury to the surrounding structures. *See also* Dynamic flexibility and Static flexibility.

Flight phase   The phase of a jump or a running stride when the athlete is airborne.

Force   An agent that changes, or tends to change, the state of rest or motion of a body (symbol F). The SI unit of measurement of force is the newton (N).

Force advantage   In the context of a lever system, a mechanical advantage greater than 1. It results in the amplification of the muscular force such that a large external load can be overcome through the application of a lesser muscular force.

Force plate   A device that contains transducers to convert mechanical signals (forces) into electrical signals, allowing the magnitude of forces applied to the device to be recorded. The transducers used in commercially available force plates are usually piezoelectric or strain gauges.

Force–velocity relationship   A relationship seen in skeletal muscle that demonstrates the dependence of the tension developed on the velocity of either shortening or lengthening of the muscle.

Free body diagram   A graphical method of determining the effects of external forces acting on a body of interest, in which the forces are represented as arrows with the magnitude of the forces denoted by the length of the arrow and the direction of the forces determined by the orientation of the arrow within a specified reference frame.

Free weights   In the context of resistance training exercises, those exercises that use freely moveable masses to provide the resistance, including barbells, dumbbells, associated benches and racks, medicine balls, throwing implements, body mass, and augmented body mass (e.g., weighted vests, limb weights).

Frequency   In the context of an exercise stimulus, the number of repetitions, sets, training sessions, or other elements. The combination of duration and frequency provides the volume of the exercise stimulus.

Friction   A force induced whenever two bodies in contact move or tend to move relative to each other. The components of the ground reaction force that act along the anteroposterior and mediolateral axes are frictional components.

Frictional force   *See* Friction.

Frontal plane   A plane of motion that divides the body into anterior and posterior halves.

Functional overreaching   Decrements in performance that accompany a short period of increased training volume. The performance decrements occur in the absence of severe psychological disturbances or other negative symptoms. When the training volume is reduced, the decrements in performance associated with functional overreaching dissipate, and the functional capacity of the athlete is enhanced through the adaptation response.

Functional physiological cross-sectional area   The cross-sectional area of a muscle that reflects a section orthogonal to the direction of muscle fibers within the muscle.

Fundamental theorem of calculus   A theorem that relates the two concepts of derivatives and integrals; in practical terms, differentiation and integration are the opposite of one another.

Fusiform   Referring to a skeletal muscle, one that has the fibers (fascicles) arranged parallel along the length of the muscle.

Gait retraining   Training strategies that seek to change the coordination patterns of distance runners in an attempt to either improve performance or reduce the risk of injuries by means of practice and the provision of specific instructions and feedback.

γ-motoneurons   Efferent neurons that innervate the polar regions of the intrafusal fibers. Activation of the γ-motoneurons results in the shortening of the intrafusal fiber at the polar regions and a concomitant stretch of the equatorial region, thereby altering the responsiveness of the fiber to a given rate and magnitude of stretch. The γ-motoneurons therefore modulate the feedback to the central nervous system in response to an imposed stretch of a skeletal muscle.

General motion   The combination of linear and angular motion that describes human movements.

General motor program   A form of memory representation that contains invariant features (e.g., sequencing, relative timing, relative force) that are common to movements within a given class. Generalized motor programs are central to information processing approaches used to explain the coordination and control of movements during the execution of motor skills.

Gibbs free energy   A measure of the energy released in a chemical reaction that can be used, determined by how far a given reaction is from equilibrium. The Gibbs free energy (ΔG) for adenosine-5′-triphosphate hydrolysis is 31 kJ/mol under standard conditions ($\Delta G°$).

Global Positioning System   A U.S.-owned utility that uses 24 satellites orbiting the Earth at a height of approximately 20,200 km to provide accurate positioning and timing information of bodies under analysis.

Glycolysis   The degradation of glucose 6-phosphate to pyruvate through a series of reactions that provide the energy to resynthesize ATP. The fate of pyruvate gives rise to either alactic glycolysis (pyruvate to acetyl-CoA conversion) or lactic glycolysis (pyruvate to lactate conversion). The reactions take place in the cytosol, so glycolysis is one of the metabolic pathways of substrate-level phosphorylation. The rate-limiting enzymes in glycolysis are phosphorylase and phosphofructokinase.

Golgi tendon organ   Groups of Ib afferents and extrafusal fibers enclosed within a capsule located in the musculotendinous junction. Discharge of a Ib afferent in response to an increase in tension developed by a muscle may inhibit the α-motoneurons of the homonymous muscle while exciting those of the antagonistic muscle.

Gravitational force   An attractive force between bodies that possess mass. From Newton's law of universal gravitation, the strength of the gravitational force is proportional to the masses involved and inversely proportional to the square of the distance between the masses.

Gravitational potential energy   The energy that a body possesses due to its position within a gravitational field (symbol E_{GP}). The SI unit of measurement of gravitational potential energy is the joule (J).

Gross motor skill   A motor skill that involves large muscle groups.

Ground reaction force   A force exerted by the ground back onto a body that is in contact with it. It is a consequence of Newton's law of reaction. The ground reaction force has a normal component (perpendicular to the surface) and frictional components (parallel to the surface).

Guided discovery   A general principle in learning that promotes the active engagement of the learner in problem-solving exercises while receiving guidance from a teacher to construct task-relevant knowledge. When applied to the acquisition of motor skills from the constraints-led perspective, this principle promotes the emergence of functional movement task solutions from the confluence of constraints that surround the athlete (organismic, environmental, task constraints) as a result of practice under the guidance offered by a coach. The guidance comes from the manipulation of constraints by the coach during practice that allows the appropriate movement solutions to emerge naturally (self-organization under constraint). Guided discovery has been associated with implicit learning and is in contrast with traditional, repetitive drill-based approaches to the acquisition of motor skills where the to-be-learned movement patterns are prescribed a priori by the coach. These traditional approaches are associated with explicit learning.

High-load speed-strength   A form of speed-strength that is assessed as the peak force generated during movements in which the external load is more than 30% of the athlete's maximal dynamic muscular strength.

Hot water immersion   In the context of a warm-up routine, a passive method of raising intramuscular temperature whereby the athlete is immersed in hot water (~40°C).

Hydrolysis   The chemical process whereby the bonds of a molecule are broken by the addition of water, such as when the high-energy bonds of an ATP molecule are broken to release chemical energy. The product of the hydrolysis of an ATP molecule is adenosine diphosphate, inorganic phosphate, and a hydrogen ion.

Hyperplasia   An increase in the number of fibers within a skeletal muscle. Hyperplasia is unlikely to contribute significantly to the increase in muscle cross-sectional area observed in humans.

Hypertrophy   An increase in the cross-sectional area of the muscle fibers.

Hysteresis   Viscoelastic behavior of a material where there is a difference between the stress–strain curve during loading and unloading cycles of the material.

Impact phase   In the context of landing tasks, the first 100 ms from initial ground contact.

Implicit learning   Learning that occurs without conscious awareness of the to-be-learned coordination pattern. Implicit learning has been shown to be resistant to factors including anxiety, emotions, and changes in environmental constraints that act to perturb the learned movements.

Impulse of force   The product of the magnitude of force and the time over which it acts (symbol J). The SI unit of measurement of impulse is newton-second (Ns).

Impulse–momentum relationship   A mechanical relationship that demonstrates the equality between the impulse of the force applied to a body and the resulting change in momentum of the body.

Indirect calorimetry   A technique that provides an estimate of energy expenditure via the quantities of respiratory gases oxygen and carbon dioxide in the inspired and expired air.

Inertia   The property of a body that resists a change in the state of linear motion. The mass of the body provides a measure of the inertia. For a body in rotation, the mass moment of inertia is the equivalent property and depends on both the amount and the distribution of the mass of the body relative to an axis of rotation.

Information processing approach   An approach to explaining the coordination and control of movements during the execution of motor skills that emphasizes cognitive processes, particularly memory processes, and involves model structures that are analogous to a computer, with the storage and execution of "programs" for specific movement tasks based on sensory information. Central concepts to recent information processing approaches include the generalized motor program and schema.

Informational constraints   Constraints to the coordination and control of movements associated with the provision of specific instructions presented to the athlete prior to the execution of a motor skill and the feedback provided to the athlete upon completion of the motor skill. Informational constraints can be considered a form of task constraints, as they may influence the goal of the task. *See also* Task constraints.

Injury   Damage to biological tissue resulting from either acute trauma or repetitive stresses associated with loading during exercise. An event is classified as an injury if it results in time absent from the sport or activity, affects the level of play, or is diagnosed by a medical professional.

Innervation ratio   The number of muscle fibers within a motor unit.

Instructions   Task-relevant information presented to an athlete prior to executing a motor skill that can alter the athlete's intentions and channel his or her search for an appropriate movement solution. Instructions include verbal information provided by the coach as well as a demonstration provided by a model that is live or videoed. Instructions represent a form of informational constraint.

Insulin/insulin-like growth factor   An intracellular signaling pathway that is involved in muscle fiber hypertrophy.

Integration   A mathematical technique that returns the integral (the area under a curve between specified points). Typically in biomechanics, the trapezoid method of integration is used.

Integrative calculus   A division of calculus that is used to calculate the area under a curve between specified points.

Intensity   In the context of an exercise stimulus, the rate of performing work/expending energy. The intensity of resistance training exercises is provided by the load used and is typically expressed relative to the maximal strength of the athlete.

Internal attentional focus   A form of attentional focus in which the athlete focuses on variables associated with the body and the movement itself. It is proposed that an internal attentional focus may prevent the natural self-organizing tendencies when learning motor skills.

Interneurons   A neuron that modulates the interaction of the neurons involved in afferent–efferent couplings. Interneurons can change the membrane potentials of neurons, thereby changing the excitability of the neuron.

Intrafusal fiber   *See* Muscle spindle.

Isoinertial   In the context of resistance training exercises, any exercise performed against a constant external mass.

Isokinetic   *See* Isokinetic dynamometer.

Isokinetic dynamometer   In the context of resistance training exercises, a device where the resistance, provided by an electronic servo-motor or a hydraulic valve, is manipulated such that the velocity of the movement remains constant over a specific range of the movement.

Isometric muscle action   A muscle action where the muscle exerts tension while maintaining a constant length.

Jump   A ballistic movement that requires the athlete to project himself or herself into a flight phase so as to displace the center of mass vertically or horizontally. Standing jumps are initiated from a starting position where the athlete does not possess any horizontal motion, while running jumps are executed with the athlete possessing horizontal motion at the beginning of the ground contact phase preceding takeoff.

Kinematic variable   A variable that allows the description of the motion of a body without reference to variables that act to change the motion of the body. Kinematic variables include position, velocity, and acceleration.

Kinetic energy   The energy that a body possesses due to motion. The SI unit of measurement of kinetic energy is the joule (J). *See* Transitional kinetic energy.

Kinetic variable   A variable that acts to change the motion of a body, such as forces.

Knowledge of performance   A form of feedback whereby the learner is provided with information regarding the execution of a motor skill that would not otherwise be available to the learner simply by completing the motor skill. Knowledge of performance typically contains information about the movements used when executing a motor skill. *Compare to* Knowledge of results.

Knowledge of results   A form of feedback whereby the learner receives information about the outcome of the movement relative to the goal of the motor skill. *Compare to* Knowledge of performance.

Lactate   A product of the reaction between pyruvate and NADH that is catalyzed by the lactate dehydrogenase enzyme. Lactate formation occurs at times when the demand for ATP is high, such as during the transition from rest to exercise, and the associated oxygen deficit or the exercise intensity is sufficiently high.

Lactate dehydrogenase   The enzyme that catalyzes the formation of lactate from pyruvate. The lactate dehydrogenase reaction is important because it oxidizes NADH, allowing NAD^+ to reenter glycolysis.

Lactate threshold   An exercise intensity that is associated with a substantial increase in blood lactate concentration during an incremental exercise test. Various methods are employed to determine the "substantial increase." Exercising at intensities above that associated with the lactate threshold has been associated with the occurrence of the slow component of VO_2.

Lactic glycolysis   Glycolysis ending with pyruvate being converted to lactate.

Landing   The phase following flight during a jump where the momentum of the center of mass gained at takeoff must be altered. Stationary landing tasks require the motion of the center of mass to be arrested (e.g., a drop–landing), while preparatory landing tasks require another movement to be executed following the absorption phase (e.g., the first landing phase during a drop–jump).

Landing distance   The horizontal distance between the center of mass and the feet upon landing during a horizontal jump.

Lateral sacs   *See* Terminal cisternae.

Law of cosines   A trigonometric equation that relates the length of the sides of a triangle to the cosine of one of the angles.

Law of sines   A trigonometric equation that relates the lengths of the sides of a triangle to the sine of the angles.

Laxity   A lack of stability of a joint, which is influenced by the ligaments and capsular structures that surround the joint rather than the extensibility of the musculotendinous units.

Learning   A relatively permanent improvement in the performance of a motor skill. Learning is assessed through the use of retention and transfer tests. The process of learning involves a search for and stabilization of specific, functional movement task solutions across the perceptual-motor workspace as the performer adapts to a new variety of changing constraints.

Leg stiffness   The resistance of the leg to a deformation. Leg stiffness is determined from the interaction of the stiffness of the hip, knee, and ankle joints during a given task.

Length–tension relationship   A relationship seen in skeletal muscle that demonstrates the dependence of the tension developed on the length of the muscle.

Level of evidence   In the context of evidence-based practice, a method of establishing the strength of the evidence presented in a research article, based largely upon the design of the study. The level of evidence is the first step undertaken by practitioners when critiquing a research article.

Lever system   The arrangement of a muscle and the skeleton. A lever system comprises a rigid beam (bone) that rotates about a fulcrum (anatomic joint) due to the action of forces (muscular forces and those associated with gravity and external loads).

Linear displacement   The change in linear position of a body within a three-dimensional mechanical reference frame. The SI unit of measurement of linear position is the meter (m), and it is represented by the symbol *s*.

Longitudinal axis   An axis of rotation that is perpendicular to the transverse plane.

Low-load speed-strength   A form of speed-strength that is assessed as the peak force generated during movements in which the external load is 30% or less of the athlete's maximal dynamic muscular strength.

Machine weights   In the context of resistance training exercises, plate-loaded and selectorizer devices, electronically braked devices, hydraulic devices, and rubber-band devices that offer resistance in a guided or restricted manner.

Magnetic resonance spectroscopy   A technique that can detect nuclei including carbon (^{13}C), phosphorus (^{31}P), and hydrogen (^{1}H), allowing the direct determination of concentrations of substrates and metabolites in skeletal muscle. Magnetic resonance spectroscopy provides a noninvasive method of assessing the contributions of the energy systems during exercise.

Maintenance of maximal speed phase   In the context of sprint running, the third phase that is characterized by a negative slope of the speed–time curve.

Mass   The quantity of matter contained within a body (symbol m). The SI unit of mass is the kilogram (kg).

Massage   The mechanical manipulation of biological tissue that is applied in a rhythmical manner. Massage techniques such as effleurage can be employed as a passive heating method to increase intramuscular temperature as part of a warm-up, although their effectiveness in terms of improving physical performance remains to be demonstrated.

Maximal dynamic muscular strength   An index of muscular strength determined by the greatest load that can be lifted in a given movement for a single repetition.

Maximal isometric muscular strength   An index of muscular strength determined by the peak force that is measured as an athlete exerts a force against an immovable body.

Mechanical advantage   The ratio of the moment arm of a muscular force to the moment arm of an external force that allows the functional categorization of lever systems.

Mediolateral axis   An axis of rotation that is perpendicular to the sagittal plane.

Mitochondria   The organelles within cells that are responsible for supplying cellular energy.

Mitochondrial biogenesis   The process by which new mitochondria are formed in a cell.

Model template   In the context of the qualitative approach to technique analysis, an "ideal" representation of a technique used in a specific motor skill; this technique is often the one employed by an elite performer.

Moment arm   The perpendicular distance between the line of action of a force and the axis of rotation used to calculate the moment of force.

Moment of force   The rotational effect of a force applied to a body (symbol M). The SI unit of the moment of force is the newton-meter (Nm).

Momentum   The product of mass and velocity that describes the quantity of motion possessed by a body (symbol p). The SI unit of measurement of linear momentum is kilogram-meter per second (kg m/s). The SI unit of measurement of angular momentum is newton-meter per second (kg m^2/s) and is represented by the symbol L.

Monocarboxylate transporters   Specialized proteins that facilitate the transport of monocarboxylates such as lactate across the sarcolemma. There are 14 variants of monocarboxylate transporters (MCTs), and MCT1 and MCT4 have been identified in skeletal muscle. There is some evidence that the MCT1 variant, which is largely expressed in slow, oxidative muscle fibers, facilitates the uptake of lactate from the circulation and other fibers in close proximity.

Motion   A change in the position of a body with respect to time. In a strict mechanical sense, the motion of a body is quantified by momentum. However, given that the mass of the bodies during biomechanical analyses can be assumed to remain constant, velocity can be used to quantify the motion of a body.

Motion analysis system   A device that uses images collected from either video or opto-reflective cameras to provide kinematic data about the movement being analyzed.

Motoneuron   A nerve cell that transmits an action potential during the activation of a skeletal muscle. α-motoneurons are responsible for transmitting actions potentials from the spinal cord to skeletal muscle to activate a skeletal muscle, while γ-motoneurons modulate the feedback to the central nervous system in response to an imposed stretch of a skeletal muscle.

Motor program   A concept central to the information processing approaches to explain the coordination and control of movement. Although the exact definition of a motor program is subject to disagreement, it is generally defined as a form of memory representation that contains a set of movement commands. The concept of the motor program emanated from the notion that the sequencing of movements observed in motor skills was preplanned prior to their execution.

Motor skill   An action or task that requires voluntary movements of the body, head, and/or limbs to achieve its goal. Skilled behavior is reflected in the optimization of the control process during the execution of a motor skill.

Motor unit   A single motoneuron and the muscle fibers that it innervates, forming the functional unit used by the central nervous system during the activation of a skeletal muscle.

Movement   The behavioral characteristics of the body, head, and/or limbs that are component parts of motor skills.

Movement phases   Distinct elements within a motor skill that have a specific function. The reduction of a motor skill into separate phases aids the analyst when observing motor skills.

Muscle biopsies   Invasive procedures in which a small sample of muscle tissue is removed from the participant. Muscle biopsies can provide concentrations of both substrates and metabolites prior to and following exercise and therefore offer an indication of the contribution of each of the energy systems to the provision of energy during the exercise bout.

Muscle fiber   The cell of a skeletal muscle. Muscle fibers contain myofibrils.

Muscle-specific hormone-sensitive lipase   An enzyme that catalyzes the oxidation of triglycerides.

Muscle spindle   A series of intrafusal fibers enclosed in a connective tissue capsule that are innervated by group Ia and II afferent nerve endings, and that discharge action potentials in response to a change in length as part of the stretch reflex.

Myofascial release techniques   Techniques to enhance flexibility that include foam rolling of the target tissue. These techniques are proposed to increase the extensibility of the musculotendinous unit by relieving spasms, breaking adhesions, and increasing blood flow and lymphatic drainage.

Myofibril   A structural element of a muscle fiber that contains the myofilaments.

Myofilament   The contractile proteins of actin, myosin, and titin, which are responsible for the tension developed within a sarcomere.

Myonuclear domain   The sarcoplasmic volume that is controlled by each nucleus. The myonuclear domain limits the increase in fiber size (hypertrophy) by controlling the accretion of protein within the sarcoplasm.

Myosin   One of three contractile proteins (myofilaments) that are responsible for the tension developed within a sarcomere. The other contractile proteins are actin and titin.

Myosin heavy chain   The motor protein of the myosin myofilament that endows the fiber with its main functional characteristics, thereby determining the muscle fiber type.

Myotendinous junction   The connection between muscle fibers and a tendon. The myotendinous junction has been identified as the weakest region of the musculotendinous unit.

Nebulin   The protein that the actin molecules are arranged around in the thin myofilament. The inextensibility of nebulin renders the thin myofilament inelastic.

Needs analysis   An analysis of a specific sport undertaken by a strength and conditioning practitioner, enabling the practitioner to develop an effective training program. The needs analysis should include an assessment of the energy system demands of the sport, the movements used, the common injuries incurred in the sport, and the goals of the athlete and coach.

Neurogenic adaptations   Cellular and molecular responses to an exercise stimulus that lead to changes within the central nervous system, resulting in functional enhancements in specific movement tasks.

Neuromuscular junction   The connection between α-motoneurons and muscle fibers. The neuromuscular junction comprises the presynaptic membrane (terminal region of an α-motoneuron), the synaptic cleft, and the postsynaptic membrane (sarcolemma).

Newton's law of acceleration   The second of Newton's laws of motion, which states that the change in the motion of a body is proportional to and acts in the same direction as the net force acting on the body.

Newton's law of inertia   The first of Newton's laws of motion, which states a body at rest will remain at rest while a body in motion will remain in uniform motion unless acted upon by unbalanced external forces.

Newton's law of reaction   The third of Newton's laws of motion, which states that when one body exerts a force upon another body, the force of the first body is counteracted by a force exerted by the second body back onto the first that is equal in magnitude but opposite in direction.

Nonfunctional overreaching   Decrements in performance that accompany a period of increased training volume without a reduction in the stresses experienced by the athlete. The performance decrements are accompanied by severe psychological disturbances or other negative symptoms. Nonfunctional overreaching is regarded as a precursor to overtraining syndrome.

Normal force   A reaction force that acts perpendicular to the surface.

Normalized tendon length   The ratio of the tendon slack length (threshold length at which a stretched tendon develops force) and the optimal muscle fiber length (length at which active fibers develop maximum force). The normalized tendon length provides an indication of the ability of the musculotendinous unit to store and return strain potential energy.

Notational analysis and time-motion analysis Methods of performance analysis that provide data on physical efforts, movement patterns, and technical actions of the players and relates these data to their relative success.

Nuclear bag fibers A type of intrafusal fiber in which the nuclei are arranged in a central group. Nuclear bag fibers are innervated mainly by group Ia afferents.

Nuclear chain fibers A type of intrafusal fiber in which the nuclei are arranged sequentially along their length. Nuclear chain fibers are innervated by both group Ia and II afferents.

Nuclei The organelles within cells that contain genetic material.

Open motor skill A motor skill that is performed in an unstable and unpredictable environment.

Order parameter A variable that describes the coordination pattern during a motor skill by identifying both the macroscopic aspects of a system and the "collective behavior" of the component subsystems involved. Relative phase is an order parameter.

Organismic constraints Constraints to the coordination and control of movements that are associated with the performer and include the physical properties of the motor system (e.g., height, mass, limb lengths) as well as biomechanical/physiological variables (e.g., heart rate, fatigue, muscle strength, flexibility) and psychological variables (e.g., motivation, attentional focus).

Overtraining syndrome Chronic maladaptations to training that are manifested as performance decrements, disrupted physiological functions (increased resting heart rate and blood pressure, loss of body mass), and behavioral disturbances (decreased appetite, irritability, loss of sleep).

Oxidative phosphorylation Metabolic pathways that provide the energy to resynthesize ATP, taking place exclusively in the mitochondria. The energy is provided by the breakdown of carbohydrates, lipids, or proteins. The citric acid cycle and the electron transport chain are the two parts of oxidative phosphorylation.

Oxygen debt The elevated VO_2 during recovery following the completion of an exercise bout. The elevated VO_2 is associated with the replenishment of myoglobin O_2 stores, PCr resynthesis, and the removal of metabolites (inorganic phosphate, lactate).

Oxygen deficit The apparent lag between the rise in VO_2, which reflects energy provision from oxidative phosphorylation, and the energy demand that is observed during the transition from rest to exercise or during a transition to a higher intensity when exercising (work-to-work transition). A large oxygen deficit results in a depletion of high-energy phosphates and a build-up of metabolites associated with substrate-level phosphorylation. The oxygen deficit is due to the finite time for the oxidative pathway to establish ATP resynthesis at the required rate or a limitation in O_2 supply (blood flow) to the mitochondria.

Parallelogram method A method of vector addition in which the components are placed tail-to-tail and the resultant vector becomes the diagonal across the parallelogram that is formed.

Paratenon A loose connective tissue that surrounds tendon. The paratenon and the epitenon serve to reduce friction between the adjacent tissues.

Part-task practice A form of practice structure in which a motor skill is decomposed into component parts, with some of the components being practiced in isolation before the motor skill is executed in its entirety.

Passive cooling methods Methods of decreasing intramuscular temperature. Examples include the application of ice and cold water immersion.

Passive heating methods Methods of increasing intramuscular temperature as part of a warm-up that do not require the athlete to engage in physical activity. Passive heating methods include immersion in hot water, thermal clothing, massage, and diathermy. They may increase the temperature of the muscle tissue beyond the 1°C that is required for an improved mechanical response, although they will not induce the physiological alterations that accompany active methods that can enhance exercise performance (e.g., post-activation potentiation, accelerated O_2 kinetics).

Patellofemoral pain An injury to the knee characterized by diffuse pain over the anterior knee that is aggravated by any activities that increase the compressive forces at the patellofemoral joint. Patellofemoral pain is the most prevalent complaint reported by runners.

Pennation angle The angle between the direction of the muscle fibers and the line of action of force associated with the muscle.

Perceptual attunement The process of detecting specifying information (task-relevant environmental information that acts to constrain the movements) when learning motor skills.

Perceptual-motor recalibration The process of allowing the athlete to become attuned to affordances following changes in measurable dimensions of the athlete's body (body-scaled affordances) or the perception of an athlete's physical capabilities (action-scaled affordances). This process is likely to be important as the athlete progresses through a training program.

Perceptual-motor workspace   A theoretical construct comprising perceptual information associated with a to-be-learned motor skill, the constraints of the to-be-learned motor skill, and the intrinsic dynamics of the performer. The perceptual-motor workspace represents the context in which an athlete learns a motor skill through experience (practice, game play, free play). The perceptual-motor workspace is represented as a topological landscape in which deep regions represent attractor states.

Performance   The product or outcome of a sequence of movements.

Performance indicators   Action variables that can define some or all aspects of performance of an individual athlete, a team, or an element of a team.

Perimysium   A connective tissue sheath that surrounds each fascicle within a skeletal muscle. The perimysium contributes significantly to passive stiffness of the musculotendinous unit.

Periodization   The planned variation in training methods and means on a cyclic or periodic basis. A periodized training program is divided into hierarchical cycles including macrocycles (the longest training cycles, typically lasting months), mesocycles (the intermediate training cycles, typically lasting weeks), and microcycles (the shortest training cycles, typically lasting days). *See* Blocked periodization; Undulating periodization.

Peripheral fatigue   Mechanisms of fatigue that are associated with the motor units.

Phase portrait   A plot of a body segment/joint angle against the body segment/joint angular velocity. The topological characteristics of phase portraits reveal information about the coordination of the degrees of freedom during the execution of a motor skill in state space. The phase portraits of two body segments/joints can be used to calculate the relative phase between the body segments/joints.

Phenotypic adaptations   Cellular and molecular responses to an exercise stimulus that lead to anatomic, morphologic, and physiologic changes, resulting in functional enhancements in specific movement tasks.

Phosphagen system   Three reactions involved in the resynthesis of ATP (creatine kinase reaction, adenylate kinase reaction, AMP deaminase reaction). These reactions are included in substrate-level phosphorylation.

Phosphofructokinase   A rate-limiting enzyme in glycolysis. Both ADP and inorganic phosphate activate phosphofructokinase.

Phosphorylase   An enzyme that controls the rate of degradation of glycogen to glucose 1-phosphate (glycogenolysis) in glycolysis. Inorganic phosphate is a substrate for phosphorylase while hydrogen ions inhibit phosphorylase.

Pivot mechanism   The rotation of the center of mass about the takeoff leg during the ground contact phase of a running long jump. The pivot mechanism allows the transformation of large horizontal velocity of the center of mass at touchdown into vertical velocity of the center of mass takeoff, increasing the takeoff angle and horizontal distance of the jump.

Plane of motion   An imaginary two-dimensional plane through a body or between orthogonal axes within a reference frame in which motion occurs.

Planned task   A task where the athlete has prior knowledge of the movements that are required to achieve the goal of the task before the athlete has initiated his or her movement (i.e., the direction of the cut during a preparatory landing task). *Contrast with* Unplanned task.

Plyometric exercises   Resistance training exercises that that involve the stretch–shortening cycle during their execution.

Pneumatic/hydraulic resistance training exercises   Use of resistance training devices in which the force applied by the athlete is resisted by the motion of a fluid through an aperture, with the resistance offered being determined by the size of the aperture. These devices remove the constraint of ensuring that the momentum of the load is zero at the end of the movement. This allows for the generation of greater force and power compared to resistance training exercises where momentum is imparted to a mass.

Position   The location of a body within a reference frame. If the location of the system is measured in linear units (SI unit of linear position is the meter [m]) relative to the origin, then the linear displacement of the system can be determined (symbol s). If the location of the system is measured as a plane angle (SI unit of angular position is the radian [rad]), then the angular displacement of the system can be determined (symbol θ).

Position transducer   A device that converts the change in position of a cable attached to the body under investigation into a voltage, allowing the velocity of the body to be measured.

Post-activation potentiation   An acute increase in the mechanical output of a muscle induced by the completion of maximal or near-maximal voluntary muscle actions.

Power   The rate of doing mechanical work (symbol *P*). The SI unit of power is the watt (W).

Power rule   In differential calculus, a method of calculating the derivative of a known function.

Pre-cooling methods   Various methods employed as part of a warm-up to prevent a rise in the body core temperature. An increase in the body core temperature above $39.7 \pm 0.15°C$ has been associated with exhaustion during endurance exercise. Pre-cooling methods include reduction of the ambient temperature, cooling fans, evaporative cooling garments, ice vests, cold drink ingestion, and cold water immersion.

Predictive approach   A method of technique analysis that involves the use of computer-generated mathematical models of the human motor system to identify the most effective techniques.

Pre-exhaustion   In the context of a resistance training workout, routines in which single-joint exercises are performed to exhaustion before multijoint exercises involving similar muscles. Pre-exhaustion routines have been shown to reduce the muscle activation during the multijoint exercise, so they are unlikely to be effective at improving muscular strength.

Preparatory landing tasks   Landing tasks in which the athlete is required to execute another movement following the absorption phase (e.g., the first landing phase during a drop–jump).

Pressure insole   An insole that contains pressure sensors that can be inserted into athletic shoes to record the plantar pressure during locomotory tasks including walking and running.

Primary endings   The terminus of the group Ia afferents in an intrafusal fiber.

Primary messengers   Signals associated with an exercise stimulus that are responsible for activating intracellular signaling pathways that result in the transcription of specific cellular proteins to support the enhanced functional capacity of the systems of the body. Primary messengers associated with skeletal muscle include the mechanical stretch of the sarcolemma, Ca^{2+} flux, redox potential, and phosphorylation potential.

Priming exercise   An exercise bout performed above the lactate threshold as part of a warm-up. Priming exercises increase the primary response of VO_2 kinetics and reduce the amplitude of the VO_2 slow component due to an increase in muscle O_2 availability, increased muscle oxidative enzyme activation, and altered motor unit recruitment patterns during the exercises performed after the priming bout.

Principle of overload   In relation to the general process of adaptation, positive cellular responses are elicited when the stimulus applied exceeds that which the cell typically experiences so long as there is adequate recovery provided between the applications of repeated stimuli.

Principle of specificity   In relation to the general process of adaptation, the influence of the correspondence between the exercise stimulus and the movements being trained (in terms of the mechanical and bioenergetics characteristics) on the functional consequences of adaptation. A high degree of correspondence will elicit a positive transfer of training effect.

Principle of variation   In relation to the general process of adaptation, appropriate manipulation of exercise selection and the intensity and the volume of the exercises within the training program are required for the prolongation of adaptations accrued from long-term training.

Proprioceptive neuromuscular facilitation   Stretching techniques involving the performance of voluntary muscle actions immediately prior to or during an imposed stretch that are proposed to increase the range of motion available at a given joint via an enhancement in neuromuscular relaxation caused by autogenic inhibition and reciprocal inhibition.

Propulsive phase   In the context of a jump, the phase between the first positive vertical motion of the center of mass when the athlete is in contact with the ground until takeoff.

Pyruvate dehydrogenase   The enzyme that catalyzes the conversion of pyruvate to acetyl-coenzyme A. Pyruvate dehydrogenase (PDH) regulates glycolytic flux to the citric acid cycle and determines the rate of glycolysis and lactate formation. PDH is activated in response to high levels of pyruvate and cystolic Ca^{2+} as well as the phosphorylation and redox potentials of the cell.

Q_{10}   A temperature coefficient that represents the thermal dependence of biological and chemical processes. It is calculated as the rate of change in a given variable in response to a $10°C$ temperature change, with a Q_{10} greater than 1.0 indicating a positive thermal dependence for the process under investigation.

Qualitative approach   A method of technique analysis whereby biomechanical principles are applied to guide observations of the athlete and the subjective interpretation and evaluation of the technique.

Quantitative approach   A method of technique analysis that involves the direct measurement of the mechanical aspects of a motor skill that are related to technique.

Radial acceleration   The acceleration experienced by a rotating body that keeps the body moving along the rotational path. The radial acceleration acts inward, toward the axis of rotation, as the result of a centripetal force acting on the body.

Random practice   A form of practice structure in which multiple motor skills are executed in a random order.

Rate coding   The rate at which a motoneuron discharges action potentials.

Rate of force development   An index of the rate at which force rises during a given movement task that is derived from a force–time trace. Various measurements are used to determine the rate of force development, including peak rate of force development, average rate of force development, and rate of force development across finite time periods. Rate of force development provides a measure of explosive strength.

Rate limiter   A constraint that precludes the attainment of a task-relevant coordination pattern until a particular threshold is surpassed.

Ratio scaling   A method of normalizing measures of muscular strength by dividing the measure of strength by the body mass of the athlete. Ratio scaling methods assume that muscular force is directly proportional to body mass and have actually been shown to bias the measure of muscular strength in the favor of the less massive athlete.

Reactive muscular strength   An index of muscular strength that is determined by the ability to tolerate high stretch loads and rapidly transition from eccentric to concentric muscle actions in tasks involving the stretch–shortening cycle.

Reactive strength index   A method of quantifying reactive strength during a drop–jump task as the ratio of jump height to contact time. A high reactive strength index is characterized by the application of a large relative impulse in a short time.

Real-time ultrasonography   A technique in which deep tissue structures can be observed by recording the reflections of ultrasonic waves applied to the tissue. Real-time ultrasonographic techniques have been used to measure the microstructure of musculotendinous units.

Reciprocal inhibition   The reduced excitability of a target muscle due to the activation of the opposing muscle (antagonist) during an imposed stretch of the target muscle, which causes excitation of Ia-inhibitory interneurons.

Reciprocal ponderal index   A ratio of height scaled to body mass (height/body mass$^{2/3}$) that provides a measure of the "shape" of the athlete.

Reference frame   A three-dimensional coordinate system used to describe the location of a body that is the focus of a biomechanical analysis. The three axes, x, y, and z, are described as being orthogonal (90°) to one another.

Relative phase   The difference between the phase angles calculated from the phase portraits plotted for two body segments/joints during the execution of a motor skill. Relative phase represents the topological characteristics of the movement, revealing information about the coordination of the degrees of freedom.

Relative projection height   The difference in the height of the center of mass at takeoff and landing during the execution of a horizontal jump.

Repeated-sprint activities   An activity pattern in which an athlete is required to perform short-duration maximal-speed sprints (10 s or less) and repeat them following a short recovery (60 s or less).

Repetition maximum testing   A method for determining the maximal dynamic strength of an athlete from the load moved during a specific movement. For example, the greatest load that can be lifted in a given movement for a single repetition is the one-repetition maximum (1-RM) for the athlete.

Repolarization   The act of the electrical potential associated with an excitable membrane (i.e., muscle fiber membrane, motoneuron membrane) becoming less negative as a result of the movement of Na^+ during the generation of an action potential.

Representative learning   The generalization of task constraints in practice to the constraints encountered in the specific performance environments of athletes. A congruency between the two would promote perception–action coupling, which is an important element of the ecological approach to the coordination and control of movements.

Resistance training   A method of physical training that involves any exercises that use movements performed against resistances to elicit gains in muscular strength.

Resisted sprint training methods   Training methods whereby the motion of the athlete when sprinting is resisted by means of towing a weighted sled, a parachute, or running uphill.

Respiratory control   An increase in the mitochondrial ATP production for a given concentration of ADP as a result of the increase in the mitochondrial mass of the muscle fiber (mitochondrial biogenesis).

Respiratory exchange ratio   The ratio of CO_2 to O_2 that provides an indication of the substrate being oxidized during exercise.

Resting membrane potential   The membrane potential (difference in electrical charge) of an excitable membrane (i.e., muscle fiber membrane, motoneuron membrane) that is inactive. The resting membrane potential for a muscle fiber is approximately -90 mV.

Resultant vector   The vector returned following the addition of two or more vectors.

Retention test   A method of assessing learning in which a test of the motor skill is administered after a period of time during which the performer has not been practicing the skill. The period of abstinence from practice allows the dissipation of other factors that could influence performance of the motor skill, such that the degree of permanence of performance level can be determined.

Reverse power rule   In integrative calculus, a method of calculating the integral of a known function.

Rotation   Motion of a body characterized by angular displacement.

Rotation–extension strategy   A specific muscle activation pattern that is used during the acceleration phase of sprint running, whereby the forceful extension of the stance leg is delayed until the center of mass is rotated over the stance leg. This strategy requires the reciprocal activation of the biarticular hamstrings and rectus femoris muscles during the stance phase and satisfies the requirements of maximizing the horizontal velocity and minimizing the vertical velocity of the center of mass at takeoff. It represents a task constraint during accelerative sprinting.

Ryanodine receptors   Receptors located on the sarcoplasmic reticulum that mediate the release of Ca^{2+} from the sarcoplasmic reticulum in response to an action potential during the activation of a skeletal muscle. Dihydropyridine receptors located on the transverse tubules interact with ryanodine receptors.

Sagittal plane   A plane of motion that divides the body into left and right halves.

Sarcolemma   The excitable membrane of a muscle fiber.

Sarcomere   The smallest functional unit of a skeletal muscle, which contains the contractile proteins (myofilaments) that are responsible for developing tension during muscle actions.

Sarcopenia   A loss of muscle mass usually associated with aging muscle. Sarcopenia is distinct from disuse atrophy due to the loss of muscle fibers (hypoplasia) that accompanies fiber atrophy, which is believed to be caused by the activation of proteolytic processes and apoptosis within the affected muscle fibers.

Sarcoplasm   The fluid enclosed by the sarcolemma of a muscle fiber, which contains fuel sources and organelles including the mitochondria and the nuclei.

Sarcoplasmic reticulum   The organelle within a muscle fiber that stores calcium ions.

Satellite cell   A myogenic progenitor cell located within the basal lamina of a muscle fiber.

Scalar   A variable used in biomechanical analyses that requires reference only to its magnitude to fully describe its mechanical effects. Examples of scalars include speed, work, and mechanical energy.

Scalar product   The procedure for multiplying vectors that returns a scalar. Also known as the dot product.

Schema   A rule that describes the relationship between the outcomes of the execution of previous motor programs and the parameters of the programs associated with those attempts. A recall schema describes the relationship between the parameters associated with a motor program and the outcome of the movement. A recognition schema describes the relationship between the past sensory consequences of the motor program and the outcome of the motor program. Schemas are central to recent information processing approaches that seek to explain the coordination and control of movements during the execution of motor skills.

Second central difference   The finite difference that appears as the numerator in the equation associated with the second central difference method.

Second central difference method   A formula taken from finite difference calculus that returns the second derivative of a variable with respect to another variable to which it has a functional relationship.

Secondary endings   The termini of the group II afferents in an intrafusal fiber.

Self-organization   A process associated with complex systems characterized by spontaneous pattern generation as a consequence of the interaction of a very large collection of degrees of freedom that may change in response to changing internal and external conditions. When applied to the coordination and control of movements during the execution of motor skills, the process implies that coordination patterns can emerge without any explicit prescription of the pattern.

Sensitivity to strain   Viscoelastic behavior of a material, whereby the material is more deformable under conditions where the rate of strain is low, with its stiffness increasing under high strain rates.

Serial practice   A form of practice structure in which a number of motor skills are executed successively.

Simplification   The process of reducing key performance variables during practice—such as the velocities of objects and other performers, the distances between surfaces and objects, and the forces of objects and other performers—while maintaining the natural performance conditions. The simplification process maintains the important perceptual information that is available to the learner, thereby ensuring reciprocity between the movements and the environment.

Size principle   The specific order of recruitment of motor units during a given muscle action, beginning with the small motor units and progressing to large motor units. Various morphological features of the motoneuron have been used as a marker of size, including the diameter of the neuron cell body, the surface area, the number of dendrites, and the responses of the membrane to stimulation.

Skill   An action or task that has a specific goal to achieve. A motor skill requires voluntary movements of the body, head, and/or limbs to achieve its goal. Skilled behavior is reflected in the optimization of the control process during the execution of a motor skill.

Skill acquisition   An ongoing process involving the search for functional movement task solutions.

Sliding filament theory   The interaction of the crossbridges on the myosin myofilament with the active sites on the actin myofilament during a muscle action. Rotation of the crossbridges pulls the actin myofilaments toward the center of the sarcomere, shortening the sarcomere and developing tension.

Small-sided games   Practices where field-sport athletes participate in games that involve a reduced number of players within a reduced playing area. Small-sided games ensure that the players are exposed to sport-specific information and constitute representative learning. They are more effective at developing agility performance in field-sport athletes compared to change of direction drills, as they promote decision making based on sport-specific information, thereby enhancing perceptual attunement.

Sodium bicarbonate (NaHCO₃)   A salt that can increase the buffering capacity of skeletal muscle. The ingestion of sodium bicarbonate is proposed to increase plasma bicarbonate concentrations, buffering H^+ through the formation of carbonic acid, eventually forming H_2O and CO_2, which is excreted via ventilation (nonmetabolic CO_2).

Sodium citrate   A salt that is proposed to increase the buffering capacity of skeletal muscle when ingested in conjunction with sodium bicarbonate. The combination of the two salts is proposed to reduce the gastrointestinal disturbances that often accompany the ingestion of sodium bicarbonate.

Somatosensory receptors   Receptors located within skeletal muscle that are sensitive to mechanical stimuli, conveying afferent feedback to the central nervous system. Muscle spindles and Golgi tendon organs are somatosensory receptors that can modulate the tension developed by a muscle.

Specific tension   The force capacity of a muscle fiber relative to the cross-sectional area of the fiber. Specific tension reflects the number of myofibrils per unit of cross-sectional area (the myofilament packing density).

Speed strength   An index of muscular strength that is determined by the peak force generated during movements performed against different external loads. Low-load speed-strength is assessed as the peak force generated during movements in which the external load is 30% or less of the athlete's maximal dynamic muscular strength, while high-load speed-strength is assessed as the peak force generated during movements in which the external load is more than 30% of the athlete's maximal dynamic muscular strength.

Split routine   In the context of a resistance training workout, a program of consecutive training days where the focus of each day differs (i.e., day 1 involves lower-body exercises, day 2 involves upper-body exercises), allowing for increased training frequency.

Sprint running   The fastest form of running, which is characterized by an acceleration phase, an attainment of maximal velocity phase, and a maintenance of maximal velocity phase. These phases have different mechanical demands, such that sprint running can be regarded as a multidimensional skill.

Stability   In the context of a coordination pattern, the capacity of a system to quickly return to a coordination pattern after perturbation. The constraints-led approach to the coordination and control of movements proposes that changing the constraints will lead to instabilities in the coordination pattern and the formation of different coordinative structures to satisfy the goal of the task.

Stabilization phase   In the context of landing tasks, the event from 100 ms after initial ground contact to the lowest vertical position of the center of mass.

Stages of learning   A three-stage model of learning that includes the stages of coordination (the learner establishes the coordination pattern), control (the learner gains control of coordinative structures), and skill (the learner optimizes control). Learning is regarded as a discontinuous process, characterized by nonlinear changes in coordination in response to the interacting constraints on the system and the continual search of the perceptual-motor workspace, rather than being a linear progression through the three stages. These stages are useful in guiding the development of practices to enhance learning.

Stance distance   In the context of a running stride or step, the horizontal distance traveled by the center of mass during each stance phase. Stance distance is the sum of touchdown distance (the horizontal distance between the stance foot and the center of mass at touchdown) and takeoff distance (the horizontal distance between the stance foot and the center of mass at takeoff).

Stance phase   In the context of a running stride or step, the event in which a foot is in contact with the ground.

Stance time   In the context of a running stride or step, the duration of the stance phase.

Standing long jump   A jumping task that involves projecting the center of mass horizontally and that is initiated from a starting position in which the athlete does not possess any horizontal motion.

Standing vertical jump   A jumping task that involves projecting the center of mass vertically and that is initiated from a starting position in which the athlete does not possess any horizontal motion.

State space   A control space used when describing coordination in motor skills where the position of a body segment/joint angle and the velocity of body segment/joint angle are specified simultaneously during the activity. State space is useful for tasks in which velocity is considered a constraint. *See also* Phase portrait.

Static equilibrium   The state of a body that is not in motion and is not experiencing any linear or angular accelerations due to the forces and moments of force acting on the body being balanced.

Static flexibility   A form of flexibility related to the extensibility of the musculotendinous unit and the ability of the athlete to tolerate the stretch as the joint is moved toward its maximal range of motion.

Static stretching   Stretching techniques that involve taking a joint to the maximal range of motion, usually determined by the onset of pain, and holding this position for a predetermined time before returning the joint to its resting position. The stretch is then repeated a number of times following a predetermined recovery period.

Static vertical jump   A vertical jump that requires the athlete to begin the propulsive phase from an initial stationary squat position, thereby removing the stretch-shortening cycle.

Stationary landing tasks   Landing tasks that require the athlete to arrest the motion of the center of mass (e.g., a drop–landing).

Step   The event between touchdown of the stance leg and the next contralateral touchdown when running. A step comprises both stance and aerial phases.

Sticking region   A period of decreasing vertical velocity as the barbell ascends during resistance training exercises such as the back squat and bench press; it is evident when performing these lifts with near-maximal loads.

Stiffness   The ratio between the force applied to a body and the deformation caused by the force.

Strain   The ratio of the elongation of the material to its initial length. Strain is expressed as a percentage of the change in length to the original length of the material.

Strain injury   An acute injury of a skeletal muscle caused by the fibers being strained during lengthening of an active muscle when they absorb energy. Strain injuries are characterized by disruption to the structure and functioning of the specific muscle. Hamstring strain injuries are common when sprinting.

Strain potential energy   The energy that a body possesses due to the deformation induced by the work done by a force (symbol E_{SP}). The SI unit of measurement of strain potential energy is the joule (J).

Strength, muscular   The ability of a muscle or a group of muscles to produce a force against an external resistance. Different indices of muscular strength exist, including maximal dynamic strength, maximal isometric strength, explosive strength, speed-strength, and reactive strength.

Stress   The ratio of force applied to a material to the cross-sectional area of the material. The SI unit of stress is the pascal (Pa).

Stress fracture   An injury to a bone defined as a focal structural weakness resulting from repeated application of sub-fracture threshold stresses. Tibial stress fractures are often incurred by distance runners, with the middle and distal thirds of the medial border of the bone being the most common site of injury. Large vertical loading rates and large tibial accelerations have been implicated in the etiology of tibial stress fractures.

Stress relaxation   Viscoelastic behavior of a material characterized by a reduction in the stress experienced by the material over time in response to a constant deformation.

Stretching   The act of moving a joint through a specific range of motion. Stretching techniques include dynamic stretching, static stretching, and proprioceptive neuromuscular facilitation.

Stretch reflex   A spinal reflex that results in an acute increase in the contractile activity of a stretched muscle and a reduction in the output of the antagonistic muscle.

Stretch–shortening cycle   A specific sequence of muscle actions in which a concentric action follows immediately after an eccentric action. Fast stretch–shortening cycle tasks are characterized by short contraction times (less than 250 ms) and low joint displacements (e.g., drop jumps), while slow stretch–shortening cycle tasks are characterized by longer contraction times and greater joint displacements (e.g., countermovement jumps).

Stride   The event between touchdown of the stance leg and the next ipsilateral touchdown when running. A stride comprises both stance and flight phases.

Stride frequency   The inverse of stride time (the sum of stance and flight time) during a running stride.

Stride length   The horizontal distance between ipsilateral stance phases during a running stride.

Substrate-level phosphorylation   The anaerobic metabolic pathways that are available for the resynthesis of ATP following hydrolysis (phosphagen system, glycolysis). These metabolic pathways take place in the cytosol rather than the mitochondria.

Supercompensation   An increase in the functional capacity of an athlete that results in improved performance when training volume is reduced.

Support moment   The sum of the moments of force at the hip, knee, and ankle joints when an athlete is in contact with the supporting surface.

Supramaximal eccentric resistance training exercises   Resistance training exercises that involve eccentric-only movements performed against loads that are greater than those associated with the concentric capabilities of the athlete.

Système Internationale d'Unités (SI units)   The system of standardized units that the scientific community uses when measuring and recording physical quantities.

Takeoff angle   The angle of the velocity vector of the center of mass with respect to the horizontal axis of the reference frame at the point of takeoff when executing a jump.

Takeoff distance   The horizontal distance between the takeoff foot and the center of mass at the point of takeoff during the execution of a horizontal jump or during a running step/stride. During an event such as the long jump, takeoff distance is defined as the horizontal

distance between the takeoff board and the center of mass at the point of takeoff.

Takeoff height   The displacement of the center of mass above that associated with the upright standing posture at the point of takeoff. Takeoff height is caused by the athlete raising onto the toes, raising the arms (if an arm swing is used during the jump), or raising the non-takeoff leg (if performing a unilateral jump) prior to takeoff.

Tangent   A line that touches a curve at only one point.

Target-repetition maximum   In the context of resistance training exercises, the maximum number of repetitions that the athlete can perform with a given submaximal load.

Task agonist   A muscle that is responsible for the motion observed during a given task.

Task antagonist   A muscle that opposes the motion observed during a given task.

Task constraints   Constraints to the coordination and control of movements that are associated with the goal of a given motor task, including the instructions provided to the athlete, any rules specifying the movements used to achieve the goal (e.g., swimming strokes, race walking), and biomechanical constraints (e.g., the rotation–extension strategy in accelerative sprinting).

Technique   A specific sequence or pattern of movements performed during a skill that results in the effective completion of the skill.

Technique analysis   Analytical methods that seek to understand the way in which sports skills are performed so as to provide a basis for improving performance.

Teleoanticipatory model   A model of exercise regulation that proposes that the intensity of exercise is regulated throughout a given bout, and a specific pace (e.g., power output, running speed) is adopted at any given time in anticipation of the end-point of the exercise to ensure that changes in physiological systems that could interfere with performance are limited. Pace is therefore regulated by the athlete in advance of the attainment of catastrophic disturbances in the muscles and other organs, while a certain level of physiological disturbance is tolerated (e.g., decline in energy substrates, increase in metabolic by-products, increased heat storage).

Tendon   A dense band of connective tissue that transmits force from skeletal muscle to bone.

Tendon function   A specific action of a biarticular muscle in which it operates isometrically, acting like a stiff cable, effectively connecting the two joints that it crosses. The tendon function of biarticular muscles allows the energy generated by monoarticular muscles to be transported between joints.

Tension   A pulling force.

Terminal cisternae   Part of a membranous system within skeletal muscle fibers that contain Ca^{2+}. The terminal cisternae are located close to the transverse tubules and release Ca^{2+} in response to an action potential associated with the activation of the muscle.

Thermal clothing   A passive heating method in which the clothing worn by an athlete includes battery-power heating elements that maintain an increase in intramuscular temperature as part of a warm-up.

Thixotropy   A mechanical characteristic of skeletal muscle in which the stiffness of the tissue is reduced when the muscle is moved through a range of motion either by passive or active means.

Time–motion analysis   A method of performance analysis that provides data on the physical efforts, movement patterns, and technical actions of the players, and that relates these data to the players' relative success.

Timing gates   Devices that use photocell technology to record the time taken for a body in motion to cover a given distance, allowing the speed of the body under investigation to be determined.

Titin   One of three contractile proteins (myofilaments) that are responsible for the tension developed within a sarcomere. The other contractile proteins are actin and myosin.

Topological characteristics   In the context of movements, the form and shape of the relative motion of the limbs as expressed in angle–angle diagrams or phase portraits. The topological characteristics of movements reveal the coordination of the degrees of freedom during the execution of motor skills.

Torque treadmill   A treadmill with a servo-motor that acts to minimize the loss of belt speed during each stance phase caused by friction as an athlete runs on it.

Touchdown distance   The horizontal distance between the stance foot and the center of mass at touchdown during a running step.

Transfer of training effect   A training effect characterized by the adaptations accrued through training resulting in increased (positive transfer) or decreased (negative transfer) performance. The transfer of training effect is influenced by the specificity of the training exercises.

Transfer test   A method of assessing learning in which the performance of a motor skill is assessed in a different context than the practice trials or in a novel variation of the practiced skill. A transfer test allows the adaptability of the learned skill to be assessed.

Translation   Motion of a body characterized by linear displacement.

Translational kinetic energy   A form of kinetic energy whereby the body possesses energy due to translational motion (symbol E_{TK}).

Transverse plane   A plane of motion that divides the body into superior and inferior halves.

Transverse tubules   Invaginations of the sarcolemma that transmit the action potential into the interior of the muscle fiber. The terminal cisternae are located close to the transverse tubules and release Ca^{2+} in response to an action potential associated with the activation of the muscle.

Trapezoid rule   A method of integration that allows the calculation of the area under a curve by reducing the area into smaller trapezoids and then summing the trapezoids between specified points.

Tropomyosin   A protein on the actin myofilament that regulates the exposure of the active binding sites on the actin myofilament through its interaction with troponin, thereby regulating the tension developed within a sarcomere.

Troponin   A protein on the actin myofilament that regulates the exposure of the active binding sites on the actin myofilament through its interaction with calcium, thereby regulating the tension developed within a sarcomere.

Undulating periodization   A form of periodization of resistance training in which the intensity and repetitions of the exercise are manipulated during each workout performed within a microcycle.

Unilateral   Any task in which the mechanical output is generated from the limbs acting separately.

Unit vectors   A method used in vector analysis to express the number of units along each of the axes associated with the reference frame that are required to describe the vectors being analyzed. The terms i, j, and k are used to denote unit vectors along the y, z, and x axes, respectively.

Unplanned task   A task in which the athlete is unaware of the specific movement that will be required to successfully achieve the goal of the task, requiring the performer to make a decision as to the most appropriate movement and execute it in response to the presentation of a stimulus. *Contrast with* Planned task.

Unstable surface   In the context of resistance training exercises, the completion of the exercises on an unstable surface (e.g., physioballs, BOSU, wobble-boards).

Uphill sprinting   A form of sprint training in which the athlete sprints up an incline. Uphill sprinting produces lower sprinting speeds than those attained on a horizontal surface due to the gravitational force acting to retard the horizontal motion of the athlete.

Variability   In the context of technique or coordination patterns, the magnitude of the difference between repetitions of the same motor skill expressed with a statistic such as the standard deviation, root mean square error, or coefficient of variation. A consequence of the enormous number of degrees of freedom associated with the motor system, variability is proposed to serve a functional purpose by allowing the performer to adapt to changing task and environmental constraints, preventing injuries in repetitive cyclical movements such as running, and signifying a transition between coordination patterns.

Variable resistance training exercises   Resistance training exercises that provide increased resistance to the athlete's motion during the exercise through either the addition of elastic bands to the load that resist the motion or the addition of chains to the load whereby the mass is increased as the load is lifted due to a greater proportion of chain links being supported by the athlete.

Vector   A variable used in biomechanical analyses that requires reference to both the magnitude and the direction to fully describe its mechanical effect. Examples of vectors include velocity, force, momentum, impulse, and moment of force.

Vector composition   In vector analysis, the process of determining a resultant vector from the addition of two or more vectors.

Vector product   The procedure for multiplying vectors that returns a vector. Also known as the cross product.

Vector resolution   In vector analysis, the process of determining the components of a resultant vector.

Velocity   The rate of change in position of a body; the first derivative of position with respect to time; the time integral of acceleration. The SI unit of measurement of linear velocity is meter per second (m/s) and is represented by the symbol v. The SI unit of measurement of angular velocity is radian per second (rad/s) and is represented by the symbol ω.

Vibration   Oscillation of a body as a result of the application of a mechanical stimulus.

Viscoelasticity   Time-dependent mechanical behavior of a material characterized by sensitivity to strain, stress relaxation, creep, and hysteresis.

Voluntary maximum strength   A measure of maximal muscular strength that requires the athlete to generate maximal force voluntarily as opposed to using electrically evoked measures of maximal force that are measured during absolute maximum strength tests.

VO_2   The volume of O_2 consumed by an athlete. Typically, it is measured at the mouth by means of a gas analysis system, reflecting pulmonary VO_2. Evidence indicates that pulmonary VO_2 can be used to estimate muscle VO_2. VO_2 can be used to calculate energy expenditure via indirect calorimetry.

VO_2 kinetics   The exponential rise in VO_2 measured during rest-to-work or work-to-work transitions where the intensity of the exercise is increased. The primary response of VO_2 kinetics represents the predominant rise in VO_2 during these transitions. A more rapid primary response of VO_2 (accelerated VO_2 kinetics) reduces the oxygen deficit.

VO_2 slow component   The continued rise in VO_2 above that which would be predicted from the power output during an exercise bout. The VO_2 slow component is incurred when exercising above the lactate threshold, reflecting inefficient muscle activity because the energy cost of exercise as measured by VO_2 is increased above that which would be expected for a given power output.

Volume   In the context of an exercise stimulus, the combination of the duration and frequency.

Warm-up   A general term referring to any activities undertaken prior to a physical performance that enhance the physical and mental capacity of the performer and may reduce the risk of injury.

Whole-body vibration   Vertical oscillations applied to an athlete by means of a vibrating platform on which the athlete stands while performing activities that are either dynamic or static in nature. The vibration stimulus is believed to activate the muscle spindles, causing inhibition of the antagonistic muscles (reciprocal inhibition); increase muscle temperature, owing to increased blood flow and muscle perfusion; and/or induce the post-activation potentiation response, which may be responsible for an acute improvement in short-duration events requiring high power outputs.

Work, mechanical   The product of a force applied to a body and the displacement undergone by the body in the same direction as the force acts (symbol W). The SI unit of work is the joule (J).

Work-energy theorem   A mechanical relationship that demonstrates the equality between the work done by a force applied to a body and the resulting change in mechanical energy of the body.

Young's modulus   The slope of the linear region of the stress–strain curve for a given material, which provides a measure of the elasticity of the material.

Z-discs   Discs that are composed of many different proteins and that define the lateral borders of sarcomeres. They are important for the mechanical stability of sarcomeres as well as the signaling processes involved in the transcription of specific cellular proteins in response to different mechanical inputs. The term is derived from the German *zwischenscheibe*, which means "in-between discs."

Index

Page numbers followed by *f* or *t* indicate material in figures or tables.